Deformable Models
in Medical Image Analysis

Deformable Models
in Medical Image Analysis

Ajit Singh
Dmitry Goldgof
Demetri Terzopoulos

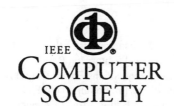

IEEE
COMPUTER
SOCIETY

Los Alamitos, California

Washington • Brussels • Tokyo

Library of Congress Cataloging-in-Publication Data

Deformable models in medical image analysis / [edited by] Ajit Singh, Dmitry Goldgof,
    Demetri Terzopoulos
                p.   cm.
        Includes bibliographical references.
        ISBN 0-8186-8521-2
            1. Diagnostic imaging—Digital techniques.   2. Computer vision.   I. Singh, Ajit, 1963– .
    II. Goldgof, Dmitry B.   III. Terzopoulos, Demetri.
            [DNLM: 1. Image Interpretation, Computer-assisted methods.   2. Diagnosic Imaging.
    3. Models, Anatomic.   4. Models, Biological.   5. Computer Simulation.   WB 141 D315 1998]
    RC78.7.D53D44   1998
    616.07 ' 54 ' 0285—dc21
    DNLM/DLC for Library of Congress   98-23491
                                                                                                  CIP

IEEE Computer Society Press Order Number BP08521
Library of Congress Number 98-23491
ISBN 0-8186-8521-2

Additional copies can be ordered from

IEEE Computer Society Press
Customer Service Center
10662 Los Vaqueros Circle
P.O. Box 3014
Los Alamitos, CA 90720-1314
Tel: (714) 821-8380
Fax: (714) 821-4641
Email:
cs.books@computer.org

IEEE Service Center
445 Hoes Lane
P.O. Box 1331
Piscataway, NJ 08855-1331
Tel: (732) 981-1393
Fax: (732) 981-9667
mis.custserv@computer.org

IEEE Computer Society
Watanabe Building
1-4-2 Minami-Aoyama
Minato-ku, Tokyo 107-0062
JAPAN
Tel: +81-3-3408-3118
Fax: +81-3-3408-3553
tokyo.ofc@computer.org

Publisher: Matt Loeb
Technical Editor: Jon Butler
Developmental/Acquisitions Editor: Cheryl Baltes
Advertising/Promotions: Tom Fink
Production Editor: Lisa O'Conner
Cover Design: Alex Torres

Printed in the United States of America

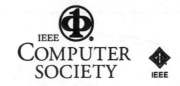

Contents

SECTION II: Segmentation and Reconstruction

SECTION III: Motion Analysis and Tracking

Preface

Deformable models were proposed about ten years ago in the research of Demetri Terzopoulos and his coworkers as physics-based models of nonrigid objects for use in computer vision and computer graphics. Terzopoulos, Andrew Witkin, and Michael Kass developed a technique for reconstructing three-dimensional deformable models of objects from images and for estimating motion by enabling these models to track moving objects in image sequences. A special case of their general physics-based formalism, the two-dimensional deformable contours known as snakes were the first to gain popularity in medical image analysis. Noninvasive medical imaging technologies continue their rapid development while deformable models are becoming increasingly important for medical image analysis, in part because nonrigidity is a fundamental characteristic of soft tissues in the human body and other biological structures.

Deformable models are a powerful, physics-based technique for representing, reconstructing, recognizing, and manipulating nonrigid curves, surfaces, and solids from their images and image sequences. Their basic features are as follows:

- Unlike previous, purely geometric models, deformable models respond to applied simulated forces analogous to the way objects respond to forces in the physical world. The interactive or automatic manipulation of deformable models with forces is therefore very natural and intuitive.

- Image data may be transformed into external forces that act on deformable models. Likewise, shape constraints such as continuity and symmetry act as internal forces. Under the influence of internal and external forces, the models evolve to conform to imaged structures of interest.

- Deformable models are fundamentally dynamic; hence, they unify the analysis of shape and motion. This makes them especially amenable to studying natural objects in motion—beating hearts, moving lips, articulating limbs, and so on.

Considerable research over the last five years has focused on the theoretical and practical aspects of deformable models. Medical image analysis has been both the motivator and the beneficiary of much of this work. Two-dimensional and, more recently, three-dimensional deformable models have been used for segmentation, visualization, tracking, and quantification of organs such as the heart, brain, spine, lungs, liver, blood vessels, and so

forth in images from various modalities such as X-ray, computed tomography (CT), angiography, magnetic resonance (MR), ultrasound, single photon emission computed tomography (SPECT), and positron emission tomography (PET). The flavor of this research spans a wide spectrum from the theoretically inclined to the clinically motivated. Some researchers have concentrated on developing novel deformable modeling techniques and have used medical images primarily to illustrate the capabilities of their algorithms. Others have concentrated on developing full-fledged systems and validating them in a clinical setting.

This book brings together representative pieces of the existing body of research into a single volume. It comprises 32 chapters divided into three parts. While most of the chapters are reprints of published papers, some chapters were prepared especially for this volume to survey the relevant literature and put it into perspective.

Part I is devoted to the theoretical background of deformable models and their general applicability to medical imaging. Part II deals with segmentation and reconstruction. Part III concentrates on motion analysis and tracking. The wide range of medical image analysis problems, representing different imaging modalities, biological structures, and diagnostic issues, that are addressed in these three parts indicate the potentially important role that deformable models can play in medical image analysis. Their usefulness in routine clinical practice, however, can be established only through extensive clinical validation and comparison with the established gold standards in diagnostic radiology. There is a need to juxtapose various techniques based on deformable models, compare their advantages and pitfalls, bring together the best of all approaches, and build clinically oriented systems for validation, and eventual deployment in routine clinical practice. We hope that this book will contribute to fostering such efforts.

This volume would not have been possible without the contributions of many people. We would like to thank the authors of the papers that have been reproduced herein.

Ajit Singh would like to thank his colleagues at Siemens—Ali Banihashemi, Ekkehard Blanz, Indranil Chakravarty, Ming-Yee Chiu, Paul Finn, Thomas Grandke, Alok Gupta, Dietmar Hentschel, Gerhard Laub, and Thomas O'Donnell—for numerous discussions during the period this volume was conceived. He is grateful to Lee Adler and David Wilson at Case Western Reserve University; Mark Haacke at Washington University St. Louis; Michael Modic and Richard White at The Cleveland Clinic; and Todd Parrish and Norbert Wilke at the

University of Minnesota for their collaboration during the days (and nights!) of the "Cardiac Project." Finally he is indebted to his wife, Princy, for her patience.

Demitry Goldgof would like to thank his colleagues and students at the Image Analysis Research Lab at the University of South Florida.

Demetri Terzopoulos would like to thank Ingrid Carlbom and the other members of the former Visualization group at Digital's Cambridge Research Lab, including Richard Szeliski, Keith Waters, Gudrun Klinker, and William Hsu, for providing him the impetus to explore biomedical applications of deformable models and for much fruitful collaboration. He would also like to acknowledge the former collaboration of Andrew Witkin at Carnegie Mellon University, Michael Kass at Apple Computer, Kurt Fleischer at CalTech, and John Platt at Synaptics on the early development of deformable mod-els, as well as more recent collaborations with Tim McInerney, Robert Majka, and David Tonnesen at the University of Toronto, and with Dimitri Metaxas at the University of Pennsylvania, that have resulted in important new results. He would like to thank Kristen Harris of the Harvard Medical School and John Stevens, director of the Eye Research Institute of Canada for their interest in this research. He is grateful for the financial support of the Information Technologies Research Center of Ontario and the Natural Sciences and Engineering Research Council of Canada. Demetri Terzopoulos is a fellow of the Canadian Institute for Advanced Research.

SECTION I
Background

Deformable models in medical image analysis: a survey

Tim McInerney* and Demetri Terzopoulos

Department of Computer Science, University of Toronto, Toronto, ON, Canada M5S 3H5

Abstract
This article surveys deformable models, a promising and vigorously researched computer-assisted medical image analysis technique. Among model-based techniques, deformable models offer a unique and powerful approach to image analysis that combines geometry, physics and approximation theory. They have proven to be effective in segmenting, matching and tracking anatomic structures by exploiting (bottom-up) constraints derived from the image data together with (top-down) *a priori* knowledge about the location, size and shape of these structures. Deformable models are capable of accommodating the significant variability of biological structures over time and across different individuals. Furthermore, they support highly intuitive interaction mechanisms that, when necessary, allow medical scientists and practitioners to bring their expertise to bear on the model-based image interpretation task. This article reviews the rapidly expanding body of work on the development and application of deformable models to problems of fundamental importance in medical image analysis, including segmentation, shape representation, matching and motion tracking.

Keywords: deformable models, matching, motion tracking, segmentation, shape modeling

Received December 4, 1995; revised March 15, 1996; accepted March 18, 1996

1. INTRODUCTION

The rapid development and proliferation of medical imaging technologies is revolutionizing medicine. Medical imaging allows scientists and physicians to glean potentially life-saving information by peering non-invasively into the human body. The role of medical imaging has expanded beyond the simple visualization and inspection of anatomic structures. It has become a tool for surgical planning and simulation, intra-operative navigation, radiotherapy planning, and for tracking the progress of disease. For example, ascertaining the detailed shape and organization of anatomic structures enables a surgeon preoperatively to plan an optimal approach to some target structure. In radiotherapy, medical imaging allows the delivery of a necrotic dose of radiation to a tumor with minimal collateral damage to healthy tissue.

With medical imaging playing an increasingly prominent role in the diagnosis and treatment of disease, the medical image analysis community has become preoccupied with the challenging problem of extracting—with the assistance

*Corresponding author
(e-mail: tim@vis.toronto.edu)

of computers—clinically useful information about anatomic structures imaged through CT, MR, PET, and other modalities (Stytz *et al.*, 1991; Robb, 1994; Ayache, 1995a, b; Bizais *et al.*, 1995). Although modern imaging devices provide exceptional views of internal anatomy, the use of computers to quantify and analyze the embedded structures with accuracy and efficiency is limited. Accurate, repeatable, quantitative data must be efficiently extracted in order to support the spectrum of biomedical investigations and clinical activities from diagnosis, to radiotherapy, to surgery.

Segmenting structures from medical images and reconstructing a compact geometric representation of these structures is difficult due to the sheer size of the datasets and the complexity and variability of the anatomic shapes of interest. Furthermore, the shortcomings typical of sampled data, such as sampling artifacts, spatial aliasing and noise, may cause the boundaries of structures to be indistinct and disconnected. The challenge is to extract boundary elements belonging to the same structure and integrate these elements into a coherent and consistent model of the structure. Traditional low-level image-processing techniques which consider only local information can make incorrect assumptions during this integration process and generate infeasible object boundaries.

As a result, these model-free techniques usually require considerable amounts of expert intervention. Furthermore, the subsequent analysis and interpretation of the segmented objects is hindered by the pixel- or voxel-level structure representations generated by most image-processing operations.

This article surveys deformable models, a promising and vigorously researched model-based approach to computer-assisted medical image analysis. The widely recognized potency of deformable models stems from their ability to segment, match and track images of anatomic structures by exploiting (bottom-up) constraints derived from the image data together with (top-down) *a priori* knowledge about the location, size and shape of these structures. Deformable models are capable of accommodating the often significant variability of biological structures over time and across different individuals. Furthermore, deformable models support highly intuitive interaction mechanisms that allow medical scientists and practitioners to bring their expertise to bear on the model-based image interpretation task when necessary. We will review the basic formulation of deformable models and survey their application to fundamental medical image analysis problems, including segmentation, shape representation, matching and motion tracking.

2. MATHEMATICAL FOUNDATIONS OF DEFORMABLE MODELS

The mathematical foundations of deformable models represent the confluence of geometry, physics and approximation theory. Geometry serves to represent object shape, physics imposes constraints on how the shape may vary over space and time, and optimal approximation theory provides the formal underpinnings of mechanisms for fitting the models to measured data.

Deformable model geometry usually permits broad shape coverage by employing geometric representations that involve many degrees of freedom, such as splines. The model remains manageable, however, because the degrees of freedom are generally not permitted to evolve independently, but are governed by physical principles that bestow intuitively meaningful behavior upon the geometric substrate. The name 'deformable models' stems primarily from the use of elasticity theory at the physical level, generally within a Lagrangian dynamics setting. The physical interpretation views deformable models as elastic bodies which respond naturally to applied forces and constraints. Typically, deformation energy functions defined in terms of the geometric degrees of freedom are associated with the deformable model. The energy grows monotonically as the model deforms away from a specified natural or 'rest shape' and often includes terms that constrain

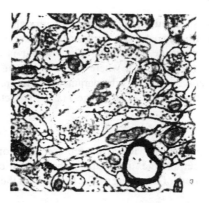

Figure 1. Snake (white) attracted to cell membrane in an EM photomicrograph (Carlbom *et al.*, 1994).

the smoothness or symmetry of the model. In the Lagrangian setting, the deformation energy gives rise to elastic forces internal to the model. Taking a physics-based view of classical optimal approximation, external potential energy functions are defined in terms of the data of interest to which the model is to be fitted. These potential energies give rise to external forces which deform the model such that it fits the data.

Deformable curve, surface and solid models gained popularity after they were proposed for use in computer vision (Terzopoulos *et al.*, 1988) and computer graphics (Terzopoulos and Fleischer, 1988) in the mid-1980s. Terzopoulos introduced the theory of continuous (multidimensional) deformable models in a Lagrangian dynamics setting (Terzopoulos, 1986a), based on deformation energies in the form of (controlled-continuity) generalized splines (Terzopoulos, 1986b). Ancestors of the deformable models now in common use include Fischler and Elshlager's spring-loaded templates (1973) and Widrow's rubber mask technique (1973).

The deformable model that has attracted the most attention to date is popularly known as 'snakes' (Kass *et al.*, 1988). Snakes or 'deformable contour models' represent a special case of the general multidimensional deformable model theory (Terzopoulos, 1986a). We will review their simple formulation in the remainder of this section in order to illustrate with a concrete example the basic mathematical machinery that is present in many deformable models.

Snakes are planar deformable contours that are useful in several image analysis tasks. They are often used to approximate the locations and shapes of object boundaries in images based on the reasonable assumption that boundaries are piecewise continuous or smooth (Figure 1). In its basic form, the mathematical formulation of snakes draws from the theory of optimal approximation involving functionals.

2.1. Energy-minimizing deformable models

Geometrically, a snake is a parametric contour embedded in the image plane $(x, y) \in \Re^2$. The contour is represented as $v(s) = (x(s), y(s))^\top$, where x and y are the coordinate functions and $s \in [0, 1]$ is the parametric domain. The shape of the contour subject to an image $I(x, y)$ is dictated by the functional

$$\mathcal{E}(v) = \mathcal{S}(v) + \mathcal{P}(v). \tag{1}$$

The functional can be viewed as a representation of the energy of the contour and the final shape of the contour corresponds to the minimum of this energy. The first term of the functional,

$$\mathcal{S}(v) = \int_0^1 w_1(s) \left| \frac{\partial v}{\partial s} \right|^2 + w_2(s) \left| \frac{\partial^2 v}{\partial s^2} \right|^2 \, ds, \tag{2}$$

is the internal deformation energy. It characterizes the deformation of a stretchy, flexible contour. Two physical parameter functions dictate the simulated physical characteristics of the contour: $w_1(s)$ controls the 'tension' of the contour while $w_2(s)$ controls its 'rigidity'[a]. The second term in (1) couples the snake to the image. Traditionally,

$$\mathcal{P}(v) = \int_0^1 P(v(s)) \, ds, \tag{3}$$

where $P(x, y)$ denotes a scalar potential function defined on the image plane. To apply snakes to images, external potentials are designed whose local minima coincide with intensity extrema, edges and other image features of interest. For example, the contour will be attracted to intensity edges in an image $I(x, y)$ by choosing a potential $P(x, y) = -c |\nabla[G_\sigma * I(x, y)]|$, where c controls the magnitude of the potential, ∇ is the gradient operator, and $G_\sigma * I$ denotes the image convolved with a (Gaussian) smoothing filter whose characteristic width σ controls the spatial extent of the local minima of P.

In accordance with the calculus of variations, the contour $v(s)$ which minimizes the energy $\mathcal{E}(v)$ must satisfy the Euler–Lagrange equation

$$-\frac{\partial}{\partial s} \left(w_1 \frac{\partial v}{\partial s} \right) + \frac{\partial^2}{\partial s^2} \left(w_2 \frac{\partial^2 v}{\partial s^2} \right) + \nabla P(v(s, t)) = \mathbf{0}. \tag{4}$$

This vector-valued partial differential equation expresses the balance of internal and external forces when the contour rests

[a] The values of the non-negative functions $w_1(s)$ and $w_2(s)$ determine the extent to which the snake can stretch or bend at any point s on the snake. For example, increasing the magnitude of $w_1(s)$ increases the 'tension' and tends to eliminate extraneous loops and ripples by reducing the length of the snake. Increasing $w_2(s)$ increases the bending 'rigidity' of the snake and tends to make the snake smoother and less flexible. Setting the value of one or both of these functions to zero at a point s permits discontinuities in the contour at s.

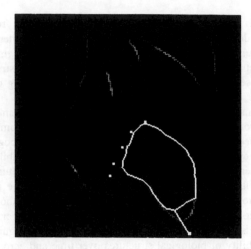

Figure 2. Snake deforming towards high gradients in a processed cardiac image, influenced by 'pin' points and an interactive 'spring' which pulls the contour towards an edge (McInerney and Terzopoulos, 1995a).

at equilibrium. The first two terms represent the internal stretching and bending forces respectively, while the third term represents the external forces that couple the snake to the image data. The usual approach to solving (4) is through the application of numerical algorithms (section 2.3).

2.2. Dynamic deformable models

While it is natural to view energy minimization as a static problem, a potent approach to computing the local minima of a functional such as (1) is to construct a dynamical system that is governed by the functional and allow the system to evolve to equilibrium. The system may be constructed by applying the principles of Lagrangian mechanics. This leads to dynamic deformable models that unify the description of shape and motion, making it possible to quantify not just static shape, but also shape evolution through time. Dynamic models are valuable for medical image analysis, since most anatomical structures are deformable and continually undergo non-rigid motion *in vivo*. Moreover, dynamic models exhibit intuitively meaningful physical behaviors, making their evolution amenable to interactive guidance from a user (Figure 2).

A simple example is a dynamic snake which can be represented by introducing a time-varying contour $v(s, t) = (x(s, t), y(s, t))^\top$ with a mass density $\mu(s)$ and a damping density $\gamma(s)$. The Lagrange equations of motion for a snake with the internal energy given by (2) and external energy given by (3) is

$$\mu \frac{\partial^2 v}{\partial t^2} + \gamma \frac{\partial v}{\partial t} - \frac{\partial}{\partial s} \left(w_1 \frac{\partial v}{\partial s} \right) + \frac{\partial^2}{\partial s^2} \left(w_2 \frac{\partial^2 v}{\partial s^2} \right) = -\nabla P(v(s, t)). \tag{5}$$

The first two terms on the left-hand side of this partial differential equation represent inertial and damping forces. Referring to (4), the remaining terms represent the internal stretching and bending forces, while the right-hand side represents the external forces. Equilibrium is achieved when the internal and external forces balance and the contour comes to rest (i.e. $\partial v/\partial t = \partial^2 v/\partial t^2 = 0$), which yields the equilibrium condition (4).

2.3. Discretization and numerical simulation

In order to compute a minimum energy solution numerically, it is necessary to discretize the energy $\mathcal{E}(v)$. The usual approach is to represent the continuous geometric model v in terms of linear combinations of local-support or global-support basis functions. Finite elements (Zienkiewicz and Taylor, 1989), finite differences (Press et al., 1992) and geometric splines (Farin, 1993) are local representation methods, whereas Fourier bases (Ballard and Brown, 1982) are global representation methods. The continuous model $v(s)$ is represented in discrete form by a vector u of shape parameters associated with the basis functions. The discrete form of energies such as $\mathcal{E}(v)$ for the snake may be written as

$$E(u) = \tfrac{1}{2}u^\top Ku + P(u) \qquad (6)$$

where K is called the *stiffness matrix*, and $P(u)$ is the discrete version of the external potential. The minimum energy solution results from setting the gradient of (6) to 0, which is equivalent to solving the set of algebraic equations

$$Ku = -\nabla P = f \qquad (7)$$

where f is the generalized external force vector.

The discretized version of the Lagrangian dynamics equation (5) may be written as a set of second-order ordinary differential equations for $u(t)$:

$$M\ddot{u} + C\dot{u} + Ku = f, \qquad (8)$$

where M is the mass matrix and C is a damping matrix. The time derivatives in (5) are approximated by finite differences and explicit or implicit numerical time-integration methods are applied to simulate the resulting system of ordinary differential equations in the shape parameters u.

2.4. Probabilistic deformable models

An alternative view of deformable models emerges from casting the model fitting process in a probabilistic framework. This permits the incorporation of prior model and sensor model characteristics in terms of probability distributions. The probabilistic framework also provides a measure of the uncertainty of the estimated shape parameters after the model is fitted to the image data (Szeliski, 1990).

Let u represent the deformable model shape parameters with a prior probability $p(u)$ on the parameters. Let $p(I|u)$ be the imaging (sensor) model—the probability of producing an image I given a model u. Bayes' theorem

$$p(u|I) = \frac{p(I|u)p(u)}{p(I)} \qquad (9)$$

expresses the posterior probability $p(u|I)$ of a model given the image, in terms of the imaging model and the prior probabilities of model and image.

It is easy to convert the internal energy measure (2) of the deformable model into a prior distribution over expected shapes, with lower energy shapes being the more likely. This is achieved using a Boltzmann (or Gibbs) distribution of the form

$$p(u) = \frac{1}{Z_s} \exp(-S(u)), \qquad (10)$$

where $S(u)$ is the discretized version of $S(v)$ in (2) and Z_s is a normalizing constant (called the partition function). This prior model is then combined with a simple sensor model based on linear measurements with Gaussian noise

$$p(I|u) = \frac{1}{Z_I} \exp(-P(u)), \qquad (11)$$

where $P(u)$ is a discrete version of the potential $\mathcal{P}(v)$ in (3), which is a function of the image $I(x, y)$.

Models may be fitted by finding u which locally maximize $p(u|I)$ in (9). This is known as the maximum *a posteriori* solution. With the above construction, it yields the same result as minimizing (1), the energy configuration of the deformable model given the image.

The probabilistic framework can be extended by assuming a time-varying prior model, or system model, in conjunction with the sensor model, resulting in a Kalman filter. The system model describes the expected evolution of the shape parameters u over time. If the equations of motion of the physical snakes model (8) are employed as the system model, the result is a sequential estimation algorithm known as 'Kalman snakes' (Terzopoulos and Szeliski, 1992).

3. MEDICAL IMAGE ANALYSIS WITH DEFORMABLE MODELS

Although originally developed for application to problems in computer vision and computer graphics, the potential of deformable models for use in medical image analysis has been quickly realized. They have been applied to images generated by imaging modalities as varied as X-ray, CT, angiography, MR and ultrasound. Two-dimensional and three-dimensional deformable models have been used to segment, visualize,

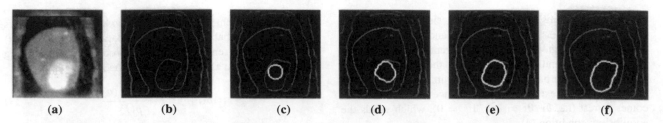

Figure 3. (**a**) Intensity CT image slice of LV. (**b**) Edge detected image. (**c**) Initial snake. (**d**)–(**f**) Snake deforming towards LV boundary, driven by 'inflation' force. (McInerney and Terzopoulos, 1995a).

track and quantify a variety of anatomic structures ranging in scale from the macroscopic to the microscopic. These include the brain, heart, face, cerebral, coronary and retinal arteries, kidney, lungs, stomach, liver, skull, vertebra, objects such as brain tumors, a fetus, and even cellular structures such as neurons and chromosomes. Deformable models have been used to track the non-rigid motion of the heart, the growing tip of a neurite and the motion of erythrocytes. They have been used to locate structures in the brain, and to register images of the retina, vertebra and neuronal tissue.

In the following sections, we review and discuss the application of deformable models to medical image interpretation tasks including segmentation, matching and motion analysis.

3.1. Image segmentation with deformable curves

The segmentation of anatomic structures—the partitioning of the original set of image points into subsets corresponding to the structures—is an essential first stage of most medical image analysis tasks, such as registration, labeling and motion tracking. These tasks require anatomic structures in the original image to be reduced to a compact, analytic representation of their shapes. Performing this segmentation manually is extremely labor-intensive and time-consuming. A primary example is the segmentation of the heart, especially the left ventricle (LV), from cardiac imagery. Segmentation of the left ventricle is a prerequisite for computing diagnostic information such as ejection-fraction ratio, ventricular volume ratio, heart output, and for wall motion analysis which provides information on wall thickening etc. (Singh *et al.*, 1993).

Most clinical segmentation is currently performed using manual slice editing. In this scenario, a skilled operator, using a computer mouse or trackball, manually traces the region of interest on each slice of an image volume. Manual slice editing suffers from several drawbacks. These include the difficulty in achieving reproducible results, operator bias, forcing the operator to view each 2-D slice separately to deduce and measure the shape and volume of 3-D structures, and operator fatigue.

Segmentation using traditional low-level image-processing techniques, such as region growing, edge detection and mathematical morphology operations, also requires consid-

erable amounts of expert interactive guidance. Furthermore, automating these model-free approaches is difficult because of the shape complexity and variability within and across individuals. In general, the underconstrained nature of the segmentation problem limits the efficacy of approaches that consider local information only. Noise and other image artifacts can cause incorrect regions or boundary discontinuities in objects recovered by these methods.

A deformable-model-based segmentation scheme, used in concert with image preprocessing, can overcome many of the limitations of manual slice editing and traditional image-processing techniques. These connected and continuous geometric models consider an object boundary as a whole and can make use of *a priori* knowledge of object shape to constrain the segmentation problem. The inherent continuity and smoothness of the models can compensate for noise, gaps and other irregularities in object boundaries. Furthermore, the parametric representations of the models provide a compact, analytical description of object shape. These properties lead to a robust and elegant technique for linking sparse or noisy local image features into a coherent and consistent model of the object.

Among the first and primary uses of deformable models in medical image analysis was the application of deformable contour models, such as snakes (Kass *et al.*, 1988), to segment structures in 2-D images (Berger, 1990; Cohen, 1991; Ueda and Mase, 1992; Rougon and Prêteux, 1993; Cohen and Cohen, 1993; Leitner and Cinquin, 1993; Carlbom *et al.*, 1994; Gupta *et al.*, 1994; Lobregt and Viergever, 1995; Davatzikos and Prince, 1995). Typically users initialized a deformable model near the object of interest (Figure 3) and allowed it to deform into place. Users could then use the interactive capabilities of these models and manually fine-tune them. Furthermore, once the user is satisfied with the result on an initial image slice, the fitted contour model may then be used as the initial boundary approximation for neighboring slices. These models are then deformed into place and again propagated until all slices have been processed. The resulting sequence of 2-D contours can then be connected to form a continuous 3-D surface model (Lin and Chen, 1989; Chang *et al.*, 1991; Cohen, 1991; Cohen and Cohen, 1993).

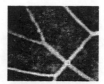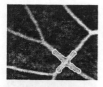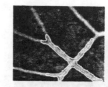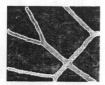

Figure 4. Image sequence of a clipped angiogram of a retina showing an automatically subdividing snake flowing and branching along a vessel (McInerney and Terzopoulos, 1995b).

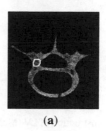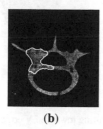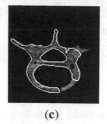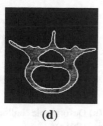

| **(a)** | **(b)** | **(c)** | **(d)** |

Figure 5. Segmentation of a cross sectional image of a human vertebra phantom with a topologically adaptable snake (McInerney and Terzopoulos, 1995b). The snake begins as a single closed curve and becomes three closed curves.

The application of snakes and other similar deformable contour models to extract regions of interest is, however, not without limitations. For example, snakes were designed as interactive models. In non-interactive applications, they must be initialized close to the structure of interest to guarantee good performance. The internal energy constraints of snakes can limit their geometric flexibility and prevent a snake from representing long tube-like shapes or shapes with significant protrusions or bifurcations. Furthermore, the topology of the structure of interest must be known in advance since classical deformable contour models are parametric and are incapable of topological transformations without additional machinery.

Various methods have been proposed to improve and further automate the deformable contour segmentation process. Cohen and Cohen (1993) used an internal 'inflation' force to expand a snakes model past spurious edges towards the real edges of the structure, making the snake less sensitive to initial conditions [inflation forces were also employed in Terzopoulos et al. (1988)]. Amini et al. (1990) used dynamic programming to carry out a more extensive search for global minima. Poon et al. (1994) and Grzeszczuk and Levin (1994) minimized the energy of active contour models using simulated annealing which is known to give global solutions and allows the incorporation of non-differentiable constraints.

Poon et al. (1994) also used a discriminant function to incorporate region-based image features into the image forces of their active contour model. The discriminant function allows the inclusion of additional image features in the segmentation and serves as a constraint for global segmentation consistency (i.e. every image pixel contributes to the discriminant function). The result is a more robust energy functional and a much better tolerance to deviation of the initial guess from the true boundaries. Others researchers (Rougon and Prêteux, 1991; Herlin et al., 1992; Chakraborty et al., 1994; Gauch et al., 1994; Chakraborty and Duncan, 1995; Mangin et al., 1995) have also integrated region-based information into deformable contour models in an attempt to decrease sensitivity to insignificant edges and initial model placement.

Recently, several researchers (Leitner and Cinquin, 1991; Caselles, et al., 1993, 1995; Whitaker, 1994; Malladi et al., 1995; Mc Inerney and Terzopoulos, 1995b; Sapiro et al., 1995) have been developing topology-independent shape modeling schemes that allow a deformable contour or surface model not only to represent long tube-like shapes or shapes with bifurcations (Figure 4), but also dynamically to sense and change its topology (Figure 5).

3.2. Volume image segmentation with deformable surfaces

Segmenting 3-D image volumes slice by slice, either manually or by applying 2-D contour models, is a laborious process and requires a post-processing step to connect the sequence of 2-D contours into a continuous surface. Furthermore, the resulting surface reconstruction can contain inconsistencies or show rings or bands. The use of a true 3-D deformable surface model, on the other hand, can result in a faster, more robust segmentation technique which ensures a globally smooth and coherent surface between image slices. Deformable surface models in 3-D were first used in computer vision (Terzopoulos et al., 1988). Many researchers have since explored the use of deformable surface models for segmenting structures in

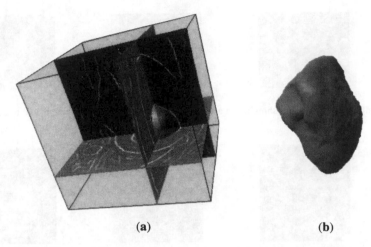

(a)   (b)

Figure 6. (**a**) Deformable 'balloon' model embedded in volume image deforming towards LV edges. (**b**) Reconstruction of LV (McInerney and Terzopoulos, 1995a).

medical image volumes. Miller (1991) constructed a polygonal approximation to a sphere and geometrically deformed this 'balloon' model until the balloon surface conforms to the object surface in 3-D CT data. The segmentation process is formulated as the minimization of a cost function where the desired behavior of the balloon model is determined by a local cost function associated with each model vertex. The cost function is a weighted sum of three terms: a deformation potential that 'expands' the model vertices towards the object boundary, an image term that identifies features such as edges and opposes the balloon expansion, and a term that maintains the topology of the model by constraining each vertex to remain close to the centroid of its neighbors.

Cohen and Cohen (1992b; 1993) and McInerney and Terzopoulos (1995a) used finite-element and physics-based techniques to implement an elastically deformable cylinder and sphere, respectively. The models are used to segment the inner wall of the LV of the heart from MR or CT image volumes (Figure 6). These deformable surfaces are based on a thin-plate under tension surface spline, the higher dimensional generalization of Equation (2), which controls and constrains the stretching and bending of the surface. The models are fitted to data dynamically by integrating Lagrangian equations of motion through time in order to adjust the deformational degrees of freedom. Furthermore, the finite-element method is used to represent the models as a continuous surface in the form of weighted sums of local polynomial basis functions. Unlike Miller's (1991) polygonal model, the finite element method provides an analytic surface representation and the use of high-order polynomials means that fewer elements are required to represent an object accurately. Pentland and Sclaroff (1991) and Nastar and Ayache (1993a) also developed physics-based

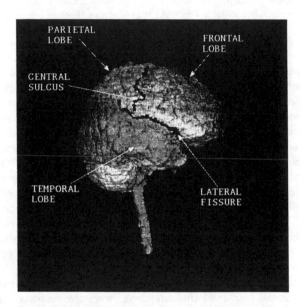

Figure 7. The result of matching a labeled deformable atlas to a morphologically preprocessed MR image of the brain (Sandor and Leahy, 1995).

models but used a reduced modal basis for the finite elements (see section 3.5).

Staib and Duncan (1992b) described a 3-D surface model used for geometric surface matching to 3-D medical image data. The model uses a Fourier parameterization which decomposes the surface into a weighted sum of sinusoidal basis functions. Several different surface types are developed such as tori, open surfaces, closed surfaces and tubes. Surface finding is formulated as an optimization problem using gradient ascent which attracts the surface to strong image gradients in the vicinity of the model. An advantage of the Fourier parameterization is that it allows a wide variety of smooth surfaces to be described with a small number of parameters. That is, a Fourier representation expresses a function in terms of an orthonormal basis and higher indexed basis functions in the sum represent higher spatial variation. Therefore, the series can be truncated and still represent relatively smooth objects accurately.

In a different approach, Szeliski *et al.* (1993) used a dynamic, self-organizing oriented particle system to model surfaces of objects. The oriented particles, which can be visualized as small, flat disks, evolve according to Newtonian mechanics and interact through external and interparticle forces. The external forces attract the particles to the data while interparticle forces attempt to group the particles into a coherent surface. The particles can reconstruct objects with complex shapes and topologies by 'flowing' over the data, extracting and conforming to meaningful surfaces. A triangulation is then performed which connects the particles into a continuous global model that is consistent with the inferred object surface.

Other notable work involving 3-D deformable surface models and medical image applications can be found in Delingette *et al.* (1992), Whitaker (1994), Tek and Kimia (1995), Davatzikos and Bryan (1995) as well as several models described in the following sections.

3.3. Incorporating *a priori* knowledge

In medical images, the general shape, location and orientation of objects is known and this knowledge may be incorporated into the deformable model in the form of initial conditions, data constraints, constraints on the model shape parameters, or into the model fitting procedure. The use of implicit or explicit anatomical knowledge to guide shape recovery is especially important for robust automatic interpretation of medical images. For automatic interpretation, it is essential to have a model that not only describes the size, shape, location and orientation of the target object but that also permits expected variations in these characteristics. Automatic interpretation of medical images can relieve clinicians from the labor-intensive aspects of their work while increasing the accuracy, consistency and reproducibility of the interpretations.

A number of researchers have incorporated knowledge of object shape into deformable models by using deformable shape templates. These models usually use 'hand-crafted' global shape parameters to embody *a priori* knowledge of expected shape and shape variation of the structures and have been used successfully for many applications of automatic image interpretation. The idea of deformable templates can be traced back to the early work on spring-loaded templates by Fischler and Elshlager (1973). An excellent example

in computer vision is the work of Yuille *et al.* (1992) who constructed deformable templates for detecting and describing features of faces, such as the eye. In medical image analysis, Lipson *et al.* (1990) noted that axial cross sectional images of the spine yield approximately elliptical vertebral contours and consequently extracted the contours using a deformable ellipsoidal template.

Deformable models based on superquadrics are another example of deformable shape templates that are gaining in popularity in medical image research. Superquadrics contain a small number of intuitive global shape parameters that can be tailored to the average shape of a target anatomic structure. Furthermore, the global parameters can often be coupled with local shape parameters such as splines resulting in a powerful shape representation scheme. For example, Metaxas and Terzopoulos (1993) employed a dynamic deformable superquadric model (Terzopoulos and Metaxas, 1991) to reconstruct and track human limbs from 3-D biokinetic data. Their models can deform both locally and globally by incorporating the global shape parameters of a superellipsoid with the local degrees of freedom of a membrane spline in a Lagrangian dynamics formulation. The global parameters efficiently capture the gross shape features of the data, while the local deformation parameters reconstruct the fine details of complex shapes. Using Kalman filtering theory, they developed and demonstrated a biokinetic motion tracker based on their deformable superquadric model.

Vemuri and Radisavljevic (1993, 1994) constructed a deformable superquadric model in an orthonormal wavelet basis. This multiresolution basis provides the model with the ability to transform continuously from local to global shape deformations thereby allowing a continuum of shape models to be created and to be represented with relatively few parameters. They applied the model to segment and reconstruct anatomical structures in the human brain from MRI data.

As a final example, Bardinet *et al.* (1995, 1996a, b) fitted a deformable superquadric to segmented 3-D cardiac images and then refined the superquadric fit using a volumetric deformation technique known as free form deformations (FFDs). FFDs are defined by tensor product trivariate splines and can be visualized as a rubber-like box in which the object to be deformed (in this case the superquadric) is embedded. Deformations of the box are automatically transmitted to embedded objects. This volumetric aspect of FFDs allows two superquadric surface models to be simultaneously deformed in order to reconstruct the inner and outer surfaces of the LV of the heart and the volume in between these surfaces. Further examples of deformable superquadrics can be found in Pentland and Horowitz (1991) and Chen *et al.* (1994) (see section 3.5).

Several researchers cast the deformable model fitting process in a probabilistic framework (see section 2.4) and include prior knowledge of object shape by incorporating prior probability distributions on the shape variables to be estimated (Staib and Duncan, 1992a; Worring *et al.*, 1993; Vemuri and Radisavljevic, 1994). For example, Staib and Duncan (1992a) used a deformable contour model on 2-D echocardiograms and MR images to extract the LV of the heart and the corpus callosum of the brain, respectively. This closed contour model is parameterized using an elliptic Fourier decomposition and *a priori* shape information is included as a spatial probability expressed through the likelihood of each model parameter. The model parameter probability distributions are derived from a set of example object boundaries and serve to bias the contour model towards expected or more likely shapes.

Szekely *et al.* (1996) have also developed Fourier parameterized models. Furthermore, they have added elasticity to their models to create 'Fourier snakes' in 2-D and elastically deformable Fourier surface models in 3-D. By using the Fourier parameterization followed by a statistical analysis of a training set, they define mean organ models and their eigen-deformations. An elastic fit of the mean model in the subspace of eigenmodes restricts possible deformations and finds an optimal match between the model surface and boundary candidates.

Cootes *et al.* (1994) and Hill *et al.* (1993) presented a statistically based technique for building deformable shape templates and use these models to segment various organs from 2-D and 3-D medical images. The statistical parameterization provides global shape constraints and allows the model to deform only in ways implied by the training set. The shape models represent objects by sets of landmark points which are placed in the same way on an object boundary in each input image. For example, to extract the LV from echocardiograms, they chose points around the ventricle boundary, the nearby edge of the right ventricle, and the top of the left atrium. The points can be connected to form a deformable contour. By examining the statistics of training sets of hand-labeled medical images, and using principal component analysis, a shape model is derived that describes the average positions and the major modes of variation of the object points. New shapes are generated using the mean shape and a weighted sum of the major modes of variation. Object boundaries are then segmented using this 'point distribution model' by examining a region around each model point to calculate the displacement required to move it towards the boundary. These displacements are then used to update the shape parameter weights.

3.4. Matching

Matching of regions in images can be performed between the representation of a region and a model (labeling) or between the representation of two distinct regions (registration). Reg-

istration of 2-D and 3-D medical images is necessary in order to study the evolution of a pathology in an individual, or to take full advantage of the complementary information coming from multimodality imagery. Recent examples of the use of deformable models to perform medical image registration are found in Bookstein (1989), Moshfeghi (1991), Moshfeghi *et al.* (1994), Gueziec and Ayache (1994), Feldmar and Ayache (1994), Thirion (1994), Hamadeh *et al.* (1995), Lavallée and Szeliski (1995). These techniques primarily consist in constructing highly structured descriptions for matching. This operation is usually carried out by extracting regions of interest with an edge-detection algorithm, followed by the extraction of landmark points or characteristic contours (or curves on extracted boundary surfaces in the case of 3-D data). In 3-D, these curves usually describe differential structures such as ridges, or topological singularities. An elastic matching algorithm can then be applied between corresponding pairs of curves or contours where the 'start' contour is iteratively deformed to the 'goal' contour using forces derived from local pattern matches with the goal contour (Moshfeghi, 1991).

An example of matching where the use of explicit *a priori* knowledge has been embedded into deformable models is the extraction and labeling of anatomic structures in the brain, primarily from MR images. The anatomical knowledge is made explicit in the form of a 3-D brain atlas. The atlas is modeled as a physical object and is given elastic properties. After an initial global alignment, the atlas deforms and matches itself onto corresponding regions in the brain image volume in response to forces derived from image features. The assumption underlying this approach is that at some representational level, normal brains have the same topological structure and differ only in shape details. The idea of modeling the atlas as an elastic object was originated by Broit (1981), who formulated the matching process as a minimization of a cost function. Subsequently, Bajcsy and Kovacic (1989) implemented a multiresolution version of Broit's system where the deformation of the atlas proceeds step-by-step in a coarse-to-fine strategy, increasing the local similarity and global coherence. The elastically deformable atlas technique has since become a very active area of research and is being explored by several researchers (Evans *et al.*, 1991; Bookstein, 1991; Bozma and Duncan, 1992; Gee *et al.*, 1993; Delibasis and Undrill, 1994; McDonald *et al.*, 1994; Christensen *et al.*, 1995; Declerck *et al.*, 1995; Sandor and Leahy, 1995; Snell *et al.*, 1995; Subsol *et al.*, 1995; Davatzikos *et al.*, 1996).

There are several problems with the deformable atlas approach. The technique is sensitive to initial positioning of the atlas—if the initial rigid alignment is off by too much, then the elastic match may perform poorly. The presence of neighboring features may also cause matching problems—the atlas may warp to an incorrect boundary. Finally, without user interaction, the atlas can have difficulty converging to complicated object boundaries. One solution to these problems is to used image preprocessing in conjunction with the deformable atlas. Sandor and Leahy (1995) used this approach automatically to label regions of the cortical surface that appear in 3-D MR images of human brains (Figure 7). They automatically matched a labeled deformable atlas model to preprocessed brain images, where preprocessing consists of 3-D edge detection and morphological operations. These filtering operations automatically extract the brain and sulci (deep grooves in the cortical surface) from an MR image and provide a smoothed representation of the brain surface to which their 3-D B-spline deformable surface model can rapidly converge.

3.5. Motion tracking and analysis

The idea of tracking objects in time-varying images using deformable models was originally proposed in the context of computer vision (Kass *et al.*, 1988; Terzopoulos *et al.*, 1988). Deformable models have been used to track non-rigid microscopic and macroscopic structures in motion, such as blood cells (Leymarie and Levine, 1993) and neurite growth cones (Gwydir *et al.*, 1994) in cine-microscopy, as well as coronary arteries in cine-angiography (Lengyel *et al.*, 1995). However, the primary use of deformable models for tracking in medical image analysis is to measure the dynamic behavior of the human heart, especially the LV. Regional characterization of the heart wall motion is necessary to isolate the severity and extent of diseases such as ischemia. Magnetic resonance and other imaging technologies can now provide time-varying 3-D images of the heart with excellent spatial resolution and reasonable temporal resolutions. Deformable models are well suited for this image analysis task.

In the simplest approach, a 2-D deformable contour model is used to segment the LV boundary in each slice of an initial image volume. These contours are then used as the initial approximation of the LV boundaries in corresponding slices of the image volume at the next time instant and are then deformed to extract the new set of LV boundaries (Ueda and Mase, 1992; Ayache *et al.*, 1992; Herlin and Ayache, 1992; Singh *et al.*, 1993; Geiger *et al.*, 1995). This temporal propagation of the deformable contours dramatically decreases the time taken to segment the LV from a sequence of image volumes over a cardiac cycle. Singh *et al.* (1993) reported a time of 15 min to perform the segmentation, considerably less than the 1.5–2 h that a human expert takes for manual segmentation. McInerney and Terzopoulos (1995a) have applied the temporal propagation approach in 3-D using a 3-D dynamic deformable 'balloon' model to track the LV (Figures 8 and 9).

In a more involved approach, Amini and Duncan (1992) used bending energy and surface curvature to track and analyze LV motion. For each time instant, two sparse subsets of surface points are created by choosing geometrically significant landmark points, one for the endocardial surface and the other for the epicardial surface of the LV. Surface patches surrounding these points are then modeled as thin, flexible plates. Making the assumption that each surface patch deforms only slightly and locally within a small time interval, for each sampled point on the first surface they construct a search area on the LV surface in the image volume at the next time instant. The best matched (i.e. minimum bending energy) point within the search window on the second surface is taken to correspond to the point on the first surface. This matching process yields a set of initial motion vectors for pairs of LV surfaces derived from a 3-D image sequence. A smoothing procedure is then performed using the initial motion vectors to generate a dense motion vector field over the LV surfaces.

Cohen *et al.* (1992a) also employed a bending energy technique in 2-D and attempt to improve on this method by adding a term to the bending energy function that tends to preserve the matching of high curvature points. Goldgof *et al.* (Goldgof *et al.*, 1988; Mishra *et al.*, 1991; Huang and Goldgof, 1993; Kambhamettu and Goldgof, 1994) have also been pursuing surface shape matching ideas primarily based on changes in Gaussian curvature and assume a conformal motion model (i.e. motion which preserves angles between curves on a surface but not distances).

An alternative approach is that of Chen *et al.* (1994), who used a hierarchical motion model of the LV constructed by combining a globally deformable superquadric with a locally deformable surface using spherical harmonic shape modeling primitives. Using this model, they estimated the LV motion from angiographic data and produced a hierarchical decomposition that characterizes the LV motion in a coarse-to-fine fashion.

Pentland and Horowitz (1991) and Nastar and Ayache (1993a, b) were also able to produce a coarse-to-fine characterization of the LV motion. They used dynamic deformable models to track and recover the LV motion and make use of modal analysis, a well-known mechanical engineering technique, to parameterize their models. This parameterization is obtained from the eigenvectors of a finite element formulation of the models. These eigenvectors are often referred to as the 'free vibration' modes and variable detail of LV motion representation results from varying the number of modes used.

The heart is a relatively smooth organ and consequently there are few reliable landmark points. The heart also undergoes complex non-rigid motion that includes a twisting (tangential) component as well as the normal component of motion. The motion recovery methods described above

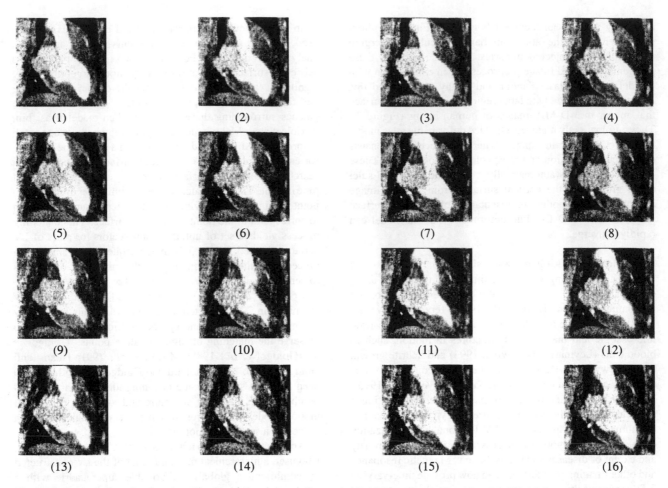

(1)   (2)   (3)   (4)

(5)   (6)   (7)   (8)

(9)   (10)   (11)   (12)

(13)   (14)   (15)   (16)

Figure 8. Sagittal slice of successive CT volumes over one cardiac cycle (1–16) showing motion of canine LV (McInerney and Terzopoulos, 1995a).

are, in general, not able to capture this tangential motion without additional information. Recently, magnetic resonance techniques, based on magnetic tagging (Axel and Dougherty, 1989) have been developed to track material points on the myocardium in a non-invasive way. The temporal correspondence of material points that these techniques provide allow for quantitative measurement of tissue motion and deformation including the twisting component of the LV motion. Several researchers have applied deformable models to image sequences of MR tagged data (Young et al., 1993, 1995; Ducan et al., 1994; Kumar and Goldgof, 1994; Amini et al., 1995; Kraitchman et al., 1995; Park et al., 1996). For example, Amini et al. (1995) and Kumar and Goldgof (1994) used a 2-D deformable grid to localize and track SPAMM (spatial modulation of magnetization) tag points on the LV tissue. Park et al. (1995, 1996) fitted a volumetric physics-based deformable model to MRI-SPAMM data of

the LV. The parameters of the model are functions which can capture regional shape variations of the LV such as bending, twisting and contraction. Based on this model, the authors quantitatively compared normal hearts and hearts with hypertrophic cardiomyopathy.

Another problem with most of the methods described above is that they model the endocardial and epicardial surfaces of the LV separately. In reality the heart is a thick-walled structure. Duncan et al. (1994) and Park et al. (1995, 1996) developed models which consider the volumetric nature of the heart wall. These models use the shape properties of the endocardial and epicardial surfaces and incorporate mid-wall displacement information of tagged MR images. By constructing 3-D finite element models of the LV with nodes in the mid-wall region as well as nodes on the endocardial and epicardial surfaces, more accurate measurements of the LV motion can be obtained. Young and Axel (1992, 1995) and Creswell (1992) have also

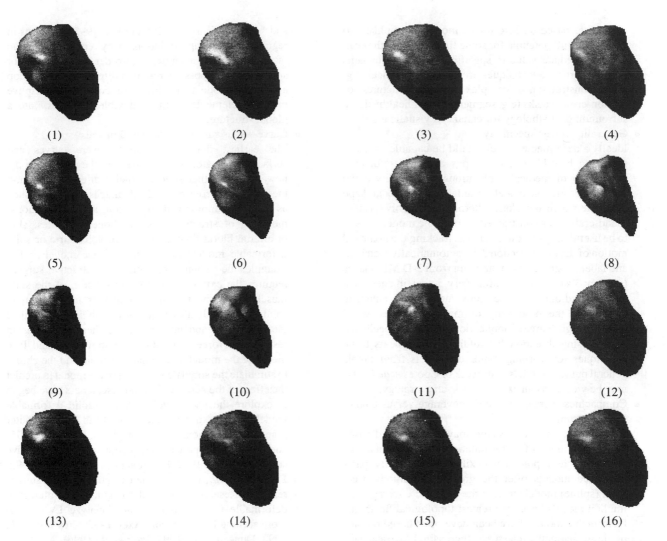

Figure 9. Tracking of the LV motion during one cardiac cycle (1–16) using deformable balloon model (McInerney and Terzopoulos, 1995a).

constructed 3-D finite element models from the boundary representations of the endocardial and epicardial surfaces.

4. DISCUSSION

In the previous sections we have surveyed the considerable and rapidly expanding body of work on deformable models in medical image analysis. The survey has revealed several issues that are relevant to the continued development of the deformable model approach. This section summarizes the key issues and indicates some promising research directions.

- Automation versus control
  Interactive (semiautomatic) algorithms and fully automatic algorithms represent two alternative approaches

to computerized medical image analysis. Certainly automatic interpretation of medical images is a desirable, albeit very difficult, long-term goal, since it can potentially increase the speed, accuracy, consistency and reproducibility of the analysis. However, the interactive or semiautomatic methodology is likely to remain dominant in practice for some time to come, especially in applications where erroneous interpretations are unacceptable. Consequently, the most immediately successful deformable-model-based techniques are likely be those that drastically decrease the labor-intensiveness of medical image processing tasks through partial automation, while still allowing for interactive guidance or editing by the medical expert. Although fully automatic techniques based on deformable models are unlikely to reach their full potential for some time to come, they can be of immediate value in specific application domains where interactive techniques are either impractical (e.g. 3-D reconstruction of complex vascular structures) or for non-critical tasks (e.g. segmentation of healthy tissue surrounding a pathology for enhanced visualization).

- Generality versus specificity

Ideally a deformable model should be capable of representing a broad range of shapes and be useful in a wide array of medical applications. Generality is the basis of deformable model formulations with local shape parameters such as snakes. Alternatively, highly specific, 'hand-crafted' or constrained deformable models appear to be useful in applications such as tracking the non-rigid motion of the heart (section 3.5), automatically matching and labeling structures in the brain from 3-D MR images (section 3.4), or segmenting very noisy images such as echocardiograms. Certainly attempts to automate completely the processing of medical images would require a high degree of application and model specificity. A promising direction for future study appears to be techniques for learning 'tailored' models from simple general purpose models. The work of Cootes *et al.* (1994) may be viewed as an example of such a strategy.

- Compactness versus geometric coverage versus topological flexibility

A geometric model of shape may be evaluated based on the parsimony of its formulation, its representational power and its topological flexibility. Generally, parameterized models offer the greatest parsimony, free-form (spline) models feature the broadest coverage, and implicit models have the greatest topological flexibility. Deformable models have been developed based on each of these geometric classes. Increasingly, researchers are turning to the development of hybrid deformable models that combine complementary features. For objects with a simple, fixed topology and without significant protrusions, parameterized models coupled with local (spline) and/or global deformations schemes appear to provide a good compactness–descriptiveness tradeoff (Terzopoulos and Metaxas, 1991; Pentland and Horowitz, 1991; Vemuri and Radisavljevic, 1994; Chen *et al.*, 1994). On the other hand, the segmentation and modeling of complex, multipart objects such as arterial or bronchial 'tree' structures, or topologically complex structures such as vertebrae, is a difficult task with these types of models. Polygon-based or particle-based deformable modeling schemes seem promising in segmenting and reconstructing such structures. Polygon-based models may be made compacted by removing

and 'retiling' (Turk, 1992; Gourdon, 1995) polygons in regions of low shape variation, or by replacing a region of polygons with a single, high-order finite element or spline patch. A possible research direction is to develop alternative models that blend or combine descriptive primitive elements, such as flexible cylinders, into a global structure.

- Curve versus surface versus solid models

The earliest deformable models were curves and surfaces. Anatomic structures in the human body, however, are either solid or thick-walled. To support the expanding role of medical images into tasks such as surgical planning and simulation, and the functional modeling of structures such as bones, muscles, skin or arterial blood flow, may require volumetric or solid deformable models rather than surface models. For example, the planning of facial reconstructive surgery requires the extraction and reconstruction of the skin, muscles and bones from 3-D images using accurate solid models. It also requires the ability to simulate the movement and interactions of these structures in response to forces, the ability to move, cut and fuse pieces of the model in a realistic fashion, and the ability to stimulate the simulated muscles of the model to predict the effect of the surgery. Several researchers have begun to explore the use of volumetric or solid deformable models of the human face and head for computer graphics applications (Essa *et al.*, 1993; Lee *et al.*, 1995) and for medical applications, particularly reconstructive surgery (Waters, 1992; Pieper *et al.*, 1992; Geiger, 1992; Delingette *et al.*, 1994) and there is much room for further research. Researchers have also begun to use volumetric deformable models to track and analyze LV motion more accurately (Young and Axel, 1992; Creswell *et al.*, 1992; Duncan *et al.*, 1994; Park *et al.*, 1996).

- Accuracy and quantitative power

Ideally it should be possible to measure and control the accuracy of a deformable model. The most common accuracy control mechanisms are the global or local subdivision of model basis functions (Miller *et al.*, 1991), or the repositioning of model points to increase their density in regions of the data exhibiting rapid shape variations (Vasilescu and Terzopoulos, 1992). Other mechanisms that warrant further research are the local control and adaptation of model continuity, parameter evolution (including the rate and scheduling of the evolution), and the automation of all accuracy control mechanisms. The parametric formulation of a deformable model should not only yield an accurate description of the object, but it should also provide quantitative information about the object in an intuitive, convenient form. That is, the model parameters should be useful for operations such as measuring, matching, modification, rendering, and higher-level analysis or geometric reasoning. This 'parameter descriptiveness' criterion may be achieved in a postprocessing step by adapting or optimizing the parameterization to match the data more efficiently or more descriptively. However, it is preferable to incorporate the descriptive parameterization directly into the model formulation. An example of this strategy is the deformable model of Park *et al.* (1995, 1996).

- Robustness
Ideally, a deformable model should be insensitive to initial conditions and noisy data. Deformable models are able to exploit multiple image attributes and high-level or global information to increase the robustness of shape recovery. For example, many snakes models now incorporate region-based image features as well as the traditional edge-based features (section 3.1). Strategies worthy of further research include the incorporation of shape constraints into the deformable model that are derived from low-level image-processing operations such as thinning, medial axis transforms or mathematical morphology. A classical approach to improve the robustness of model fitting is the use of multiscale image preprocessing techniques (Kass *et al.*, 1988; Terzopoulos *et al.*, 1988), perhaps coupled with a multiresolution deformable model (Bajcsy and Kovacic, 1989). A multiresolution technique that merits further research in the context of deformable models is the use of wavelet bases (Strang and Nguyen, 1996) for deformations (Vemuri *et al.*, 1993; Vemuri and Radisavljevic, 1994). A deformable model should be able to easily incorporate added constraints and any other *a priori* anatomic knowledge of object shape and motion. Section 3.3 reviewed several of the most promising techniques to incorporate *a priori* knowledge. For example, for LV motion tracking, a promising research direction is the incorporation of biomechanical properties of the heart and the inclusion of the temporal periodic characteristics of the heart motion. Future directions include modeling schemes that incorporate reasoning and recognition mechanisms using techniques from artificial intelligence such as rule-based systems or neural networks.

5. CONCLUSION

The increasingly important role of medical imaging in the diagnosis and treatment of disease has opened an array of challenging problems centered on the computation of accurate geometric models of anatomic structures from medical images. Deformable models offer an attractive approach to tackling such problems, because these models are able to represent the complex shapes and broad shape variability of anatomical structures. Deformable models overcome many of the limitations of traditional low-level image-processing techniques, by providing compact and analytical representations of object shape, by incorporating anatomic knowledge, and by providing interactive capabilities. The continued development and refinement of these models should remain an important area of research into the foreseeable future.

ACKNOWLEDGEMENTS

We would like to thank Stephanie Sandor and Richard Leahy of the USC Signal and Image Processing Institute for the deformable brain atlas figure, as well as the following individuals for providing citation information that improved the completeness of the bibliography: Amir Amini, Nicholas Ayache, Ingrid Carlbom, Chang Wen Chen, James Duncan, Dmitry Goldgof, Thomas Huang, Stephane Lavallee, Francois Leitner, Gerard Medioni, Dimitri Metaxas, Alex Pentland, Stan Sclaroff, Ajit Singh, Richard Szeliski, Baba Vemuri, Alistair Young and Alan Yuille. T.M. is grateful for the financial support of an NSERC postgraduate scholarship. D.T. is a fellow of the Canadian Institute for Advanced Research. This work was made possible by the financial support of the Information Technologies Research Center of Ontario.

REFERENCES

Amini, A. A. and Duncan, J. S. (1992). Bending and stretching models for LV wall motion analysis from curves and surfaces. *Image and Vision Computing*, 10(6), 418–430.

Amini, A. A., Weymouth, T. E. and Jain, R. C. (1990). Using dynamic programming for solving variational problems in vision. *IEEE Trans. Pattern Anal. Machine Intelligence*, 12(9), 855–867.

Amini, A. A., Curwen, R. W., Klein, A. K., Egglin, T. K., Pollak, J., Lee, F. and Gore, J. C. (1995). Physics based snakes, Kalman snakes, and snake grids for feature localization and tracking in medical images. In (Bizais *et al.*, 1995), pp. 363–364.

Axel, L. and Dougherty, L. (1989). Heart wall motion: Improved method of spatial modulation of magnetization for MR imaging. *Radiology*, 172, 349–350.

Ayache, N. (1995a). Medical computer vision, virtual reality and robotics. *Image and Vision Computing*, 13(4), 295–313.

Ayache, N. (ed.) (1995b). *Proc. First International Conf. on Computer Vision, Virtual Reality and Robotics in Medicine (CVRMed'95), Nice, France, April, 1995.* Lectures Notes in Computer Science, Vol. 905. Berlin, Germany: Springer–Verlag.

Ayache, N., Cohen, I. and Herlin, I. L. (1992). Medical image tracking. Ch. 17 Blake, A. and Yuille, A. (eds), *Active Vision*. Cambridge, MA: MIT Press.

Bajcsy, R. and Kovacic, S. (1989). Multiresolution elastic matching. *Comput. Vision, Graphics Image Process.*, 46, 1–21.

Ballard, D. and Brown, C. (1982). *Computer Vision*. Englewood Cliffs, NJ: Prentice–Hall.

Bardinet, E., Cohen, L. D. and Ayache, N. (1995). Superquadrics and free-form deformations: A global model to fit and track 3D medical data. In (Ayache, 1995b), pp. 319–326.

Bardinet, E., Cohen, L. D. and Ayache, N. (1996a). *Analyzing the deformation of the left ventricle of the heart with a parametric deformable model.* Research report 2797. INRIA, Sophia-Antipolis, France.

Bardinet, E., Cohen, L. D. and Ayache, N. (1996b). A parametric deformable model to fit unstructured 3D data. *Computer Vision and Image Understanding.* In press. Also research report 2617, INRIA, Sophia-Antipolis, France.

Berger, M. O. (1990). Snake growing. In Faugeras, O. (ed.), *Computer Vision – Proc. First European Conf. on Computer Vision (ECCV'90), Antibes, France, April, 1990,* pp. 570–572, Lectures Notes in Computer Science. Springer–Verlag.

Bizais, Y., Barillot, C. and Paola, R. Di (eds) (1995). *Information Processing in Medical Imaging: Proc. 14th Int. Conf. (IPMI'95), Ile de Berder, France, June, 1995.* Computational Imaging and Vision, Vol. 3. Dordrecht, The Netherlands: Kluwer Academic.

Bookstein, F. L. (1989). Principal warps: Thin-plate splines and the decomposition of deformations. *IEEE Trans. Pattern Anal. Machine Intelligence,* 11(6), 567–585.

Bookstein, F. L. (1991). Thin-plate splines and the atlas problem for biomedical images. In Barret, H.H. and Gmitro, A.F. (eds), *Information Processing in Medical Imaging: Proc. 12th Int. Conf. (IPMI'91), Wye, UK, July, 1991,* pp. 326–342, Lectures Notes in Computer Science. Springer–Verlag.

Bozma, I. and Duncan, J. S. (1992). A modular system for image analysis using a game theoretic framework. *Image Vision Comput.,* 10(6), 431–443.

Broit, C. (1981). *Optimal Registration of Deformed Images.* Ph.D. thesis, Computer and Information Science Dept., University of Pennsylvania, Philadelphia, PA.

Carlbom, I., Terzopoulos, D. and Harris, K. (1994). Computer-assisted registration, segmentation, and 3D reconstruction from images of neuronal tissue sections. *IEEE Trans. Med. Imag.,* 13(2), 351–362.

Caselles, V., Catte, F., Coll, T. and Dibos, F. (1993). A geometric model for active contours. *Numerische Mathematik,* 66.

Caselles, V., Kimmel, R. and Sapiro, G. (1995). Geodesic active contours. In *Proc. Fifth International Conf. on Computer Vision (ICCV'95), Cambridge, MA, June, 1995,* pp. 694–699, Los Alamitos, CA: IEEE Computer Society Press.

Chakraborty, A. and Duncan, J. S. (1995). Integration of boundary finding and region-based segmentation using game theory. In (Bizais *et al.,* 1995), pp. 189–200.

Chakraborty, A., Staib, L. H. and Duncan, J. S. (1994). Deformable boundary finding influenced by region homogeneity. In *Proc. Conf. on Computer Vision and Pattern Recognition (CVPR'94), Seattle, WA, June, 1994,* Los Alamitos, CA, pp. 624–627. IEEE Computer Society Press.

Chang, L. W., Chen, H. W. and Ho, J. R. (1991). Reconstruction of 3D medical images: A nonlinear interpolation technique for reconstruction of 3D medical images. *Comput. Vision, Graphics Image Process.,* 53(4), 382–391.

Chen, C. W., Huang, T. S. and Arrott, M. (1994). Modeling, analysis and visualization of left ventricle shape and motion by hierarchical decomposition. *IEEE Trans. Pattern Anal. Machine Intelligence,* 16(April), 342–356.

Christensen, G., Rabbitt, R. D., Miller, M. I., Joshi, S. C., Grenander, U., Coogan, T. A. and van Essen, D. C. (1995). Topological properties of smooth anatomic maps. In (Bizais *et al.,* 1995), pp. 101–112.

Cohen, I., Ayache, N. and Sulger, P. (1992a). Tracking points on deformable objects using curvature information. In Sandini, G. (ed.), *Computer Vision – Proc. Second European Conf. on Computer Vision (ECCV'92), Santa Margherita Ligure, Italy, May, 1992,* pp. 458–466, Lectures Notes in Computer Science. Springer–Verlag.

Cohen, I., Cohen, L. D. and Ayache, N. (1992b). Using deformable surfaces to segment 3D images and infer differential structures. *CVGIP: Image Understanding,* 56(2), 242–263.

Cohen, L. D. (1991). On active contour models and balloons. *CVGIP: Image Understanding,* 53(2), 211–218.

Cohen, L. D. and Cohen, I. (1993). Finite element methods for active contour models and balloons for 2D and 3D images. *IEEE Trans. Pattern Anal. Machine Intelligence,* 15(11), 1131–1147.

Cootes, T., Hill, A., Taylor, C. and Haslam, J. (1994). The use of active shape models for locating structures in medical images. *Image Vision Comput.,* 12(6), 355–366.

Creswell, L. L., Wyers, S. G., Pirolo, J. S., Perman, W. H., Vannier, M. W. and Pasque, M. K. (1992). Mathematical modelling of the heart using magnetic resonance imaging. *IEEE Trans. Med. Imag.,* 11(4), 581–589.

Davatzikos, C. and Bryan, R. N. (1995). Using a deformable surface model to obtain a mathematical representation of the cortex. In *International Symp. on Computer Vision, Coral Gables, FL, November, 1995,* pp. 212–217, Los Alamitos, CA: IEEE Computer Society Press.

Davatzikos, C. A. and Prince, J. L. (1995). An active contour model for mapping the cortex. *IEEE Trans. Med. Imag.,* 14(1), 65–80.

Davatzikos, C. A., Prince, J. L. and Bryan, R. N. (1996). Image registration based on boundary mapping. *IEEE Trans. Med. Imag.,* 15(1), 112–115.

Declerck, J., Subsol, G., Thirion, J. P. and Ayache, N. (1995). Automatic retrieval of anatomic structures in 3D medical images. In (Ayache, 1995b), pp. 153–162.

Delibasis, K. and Undrill, P. E. (1994). Anatomical object recognition using deformable geometric models. *Image Vision Comput.,* 12(7), 423–433.

Delingette, H., Hebert, M. and Ikeuchi, K. (1992). Shape representation and image segmentation using deformable surfaces. *Image Vision Comput.,* 10(3), 132–144.

Delingette, H., Subsol, G., Cotin, S. and Pignon, J. (1994). Virtual reality and craniofacial surgery simulation. In (Robb, 1994), pp. 607–618.

Duncan, J. *et al.* (1994). Towards reliable, noninvasive measurement of myocardial function from 4D images. In *Medical Imaging 1994: Physiology and Function from Multidimensional Medical*

Images, SPIE Proc., Vol. 2168, pp. 149–161, Bellingham, WA: SPIE.

Essa, I., Sclaroff, S. and Pentland, A. P. (1993). Physically-based modeling for graphics and vision. In Martin, R. (ed.), *Directions in Geometric Computing*. Information Geometers, U.K.

Evans, A. C., Dai, W., Collins, L., Neelin, P. and Marrett, S. (1991). Warping of a computerized 3D atlas to match brain image volumes for quantitative neuroanatomical and functional analysis. In *Medical Imaging V: Image Processing*, SPIE Proc., Vol. 1445, pp. 236–246, Bellingham, WA: SPIE.

Farin, G. (1993). *Curves and Surfaces for CAGD*. New York, NY: Academic Press.

Feldmar, J. and Ayache, N. (1994). Locally affine registration of free-form surfaces. In *Proc. Conf. on Computer Vision and Pattern Recognition (CVPR'94), Seattle, WA, June, 1994*, pp. 496–501, Los Alamitos, CA: IEEE Computer Society Press.

Fischler, M. and Elschlager, R. (1973). The representation and matching of pictorial structures. *IEEE Trans. on Computers*, 22(1), 67–92.

Gauch, J. M., Pien, H. H. and Shah, J. (1994). Hybrid boundary-based and region-based deformable models for biomedical image segmentation. In *Mathematical Methods in Medical Imaging III*, SPIE Proc., Vol. 2299, pp. 72–83, San Diego, CA: SPIE.

Gee, J., Reivich, M. and Bajcsy, R. (1993). Elastically deforming 3D atlas to match anatomical brain images. *Journal of Computer Assisted Tomography*, 17(2), 225–236.

Geiger, B. (1992). Three dimensional simulation of delivery for cephalopelvic disproportion. In *First International Workshop on Mechatronics in Medicine and Surgery, Costa del Sol, Spain, October, 1992*, pp. 146–152.

Geiger, D., Gupta, A., Costa, L. A. and Vlontzos, J. (1995). Dynamic programming for detecting, tracking and matching deformable contours. *IEEE Trans. Pattern Anal. Machine Intelligence*, 17(3), 294–302.

Goldgof, D. B., Lee, H. and Huang, T. S. (1988). Motion analysis of nonrigid surfaces. In *Proc. Conf. on Computer Vision and Pattern Recognition (CVPR'88), Ann Arbor, MI, June, 1988*, pp. 375–380, Los Alamitos, CA: IEEE Computer Society Press.

Gourdon, A. (1995). Simplification of irregular surface meshes in 3D medical images. In (Ayache, 1995b), pp. 413–419.

Grzeszczuk, R. P. and Levin, D. N. (1994). Brownian strings: Segmenting images with stochastically deformable contours. In (Robb, 1994), pp. 72–89.

Gueziec, A. and Ayache, N. (1994). Smoothing and matching of 3D space curves. *Int. J. Comput. Vision*, 12(1), 79–104.

Gupta, A., O'Donnell, T. and Singh, A. (1994). Segmentation and tracking of cine cardiac MR and CT images using a 3-D deformable model. In *Proc. IEEE Conf. on Computers in Cardiology, September, 1994*.

Gwydir, S. H., Buettner, H. M. and Dunn, S. M. (1994). Non-rigid motion analysis and feature labelling of the growth cone. In *IEEE Workshop on Biomedical Image Analysis, Seattle, WA, June, 1994*, pp. 80–87, Los Alamitos, CA: IEEE Computer Society Press.

Hamadeh, A., Lavallee, S., Szeliski, R., Cinquin, P. and Peria, O. (1995). Anatomy-based registration for computer-integrated surgery. In (Ayache, 1995b), pp. 212–218.

Herlin, I. L. and Ayache, N. (1992). Features extraction and analysis methods for sequences of ultrasound images. *Image Vision Comput.*, 10(10), 673–682.

Herlin, I. L., Nguyen, C. and Graffigne, C. (1992). A deformable region model using stochastic processes applied to echocardiographic images. In *Proc. Conf. on Computer Vision and Pattern Recognition (CVPR'92), Urbana, IL, June, 1992*, pp. 534–539, Los Alamitos, CA: IEEE Computer Society Press.

Hill, A., Thornham, A. and Taylor, C. J. (1993). Model-based interpretation of 3D medical images. In *Proc. 4th British Machine Vision Conf. (BMVC'93), Surrey, UK, September, 1993*, pp. 339–348, BMVA Press.

Huang, W. C. and Goldgof, D. B. (1993). Adaptive-size meshes for rigid and nonrigid shape analysis and synthesis. *IEEE Trans. Pattern Anal. Machine Intelligence*, 15(3).

Kambhamettu, C. and Goldgof, D. B. (1994). Point correspondence recovery in nonrigid motion. *CVGIP: Image Understanding*, 60(1), 26–43.

Kass, M., Witkin, A. and Terzopoulos, D. (1988). Snakes: Active contour models. *Int. J. Comput. Vision*, 1(4), 321–331.

Kraitchman, D. L., Young, A. A., Chang, C. N. and Axel, L. (1995). Semi-automatic tracking of myocardial motion in MR tagged images. *IEEE Trans. Med. Imag.*, 14(3), 422–432.

Kumar, S. and Goldgof, D. (1994). Automatic tracking of SPAMM grid and the estimation of deformation parameters from cardiac MR images. *IEEE Trans. Med. Imag.*, 13(1), 122–132.

Lavallée, S. and Szeliski, R. (1995). Recovering the position and orientation of free-form objects from image contours using 3D distance maps. *IEEE Trans. Pattern Anal. Machine Intelligence*, 17(4), 378–390.

Lee, Y., Terzopoulos, D. and Waters, K. (1995). Realistic modeling for facial animation. In *Proc. SIGGRAPH'95, Los Angeles, CA, August, 1995, in Computer Graphics Proc., Annual Conf. Series 1995*, pp. 55–62, New York, NY: ACM SIGGRAPH.

Leitner, F. and Cinquin, P. (1991). Complex topology 3D objects segmentation. In *Model-Based Vision Development and Tools*, SPIE Proc., Vol. 1609, pp. 16–26, Bellingham, WA: SPIE.

Leitner, F. and Cinquin, P. (1993). From splines and snakes to Snakes Splines. In Laugier, C. (ed.), *Geometric Reasoning: From Perception to Action*, Lectures Notes in Computer Science, Vol. 708, pp. 264–281, Springer–Verlag.

Lengyel, J., Greenberg, D. P. and Popp, R. (1995). Time-dependent three-dimensional intravascular ultrasound. In *Proc. SIGGRAPH'95, Los Angeles, CA, August, 1995, in Computer Graphics Proc., Annual Conf. Series 1995*, pp. 457–464, New York, NY: ACM SIGGRAPH.

Leymarie, F. and Levine, M. (1993). Tracking deformable objects in the plane using an active contour model. *IEEE Trans. Pattern Anal. Machine Intelligence*, 15(6), 635–646.

Lin, W. C. and Chen, S. Y. (1989). A new surface interpolation technique for reconstructing 3D objects from serial cross-sections. *Comput. Vision, Graphics Image Process.*, 48(Oct.), 124–143.

Lipson, P., Yuille, A. L., O'Keefe, D., Cavanaugh, J., Taaffe, J. and Rosenthal, D. (1990). Deformable templates for feature extraction from medical images. In Faugeras, O. (ed.), *Computer Vision – Proc. First European Conf. on Computer Vision (ECCV'90), Antibes, France, April, 1990*, pp. 477–484, Lectures Notes in Computer Science. Springer–Verlag.

Lobregt, S. and Viergever, M. A. (1995). A discrete dynamic contour model. *IEEE Trans. Med. Imag.*, 14(1), 12–24.

Malladi, R., Sethian, J. and Vemuri, B. C. (1995). Shape modeling with front propagation: A level set approach. *IEEE Trans. Pattern Anal. Machine Intelligence*, 17(2), 158–175.

Mangin, J. F., Tupin, F., Frouin, V., Bloch, I., Rougetet, R., Regis, J. and Lopez-Krahe, J. (1995). Deformable topological models for segmentation of 3D medical images. In (Bizais *et al.*, 1995), pp. 153–164.

McDonald, D., Avis, D. and Evans, A. (1994). Multiple surface identification and matching in magnetic resonance images. In (Robb, 1994), pp. 160–169.

McInerney, T. and Terzopoulos, D. (1995a). A dynamic finite element surface model for segmentation and tracking in multidimensional medical images with application to cardiac 4D image analysis. *Computerized Medical Imaging and Graphics*, 19(1), 69–83.

McInerney, T. and Terzopoulos, D. (1995b). Topologically adaptable snakes. In *Proc. Fifth International Conf. on Computer Vision (ICCV'95), Cambridge, MA, June, 1995*, pp. 840–845, Los Alamitos, CA: IEEE Computer Society Press.

Metaxas, D. and Terzopoulos, D. (1993). Shape and nonrigid motion estimation through physics-based synthesis. *IEEE Trans. Pattern Anal. Machine Intelligence*, 15(6), 580–591.

Miller, J. V., Breen, D. E., Lorensen, W. E., O'Bara, R. M. and Wozny, M. J. (1991). Geometrically deformed models: A method for extracting closed geometric models from volume data. In *Computer Graphics (Proc. SIGGRAPH'91 Conf., Las Vegas, NV, July, 1991)*, Vol. 25(4), pp. 217–226.

Mishra, S. K., Goldgof, D. B. and Huang, T. S. (1991). Non-rigid motion analysis and epicardial deformation estimation from angiography data. In *Proc. Conf. on Computer Vision and Pattern Recognition (CVPR'91), Maui, HI, June, 1991*, pp. 331–336, Los Alamitos, CA: IEEE Computer Society Press.

Moshfeghi, M. (1991). Elastic matching of multimodality medical images. *CVGIP: Graphical Models and Image Processing*, 53, 271–282.

Moshfeghi, M., Ranganath, S. and Nawyn, K. (1994). Three-dimensional elastic matching of volumes. *IEEE Trans. on Image Processing*, 3, 128–138.

Nastar, C. and Ayache, N. (1993a). Fast segmentation, tracking, and analysis of deformable objects. In *Proc. Fourth International Conf. on Computer Vision (ICCV'93), Berlin, Germany, May, 1993*, pp. 275–279, Los Alamitos, CA: IEEE Computer Society Press.

Nastar, C. and Ayache, N. (1993b). Non-rigid motion analysis in medical images: A physically based approach. In Colchester, A.C.F. and Hawkes, D.J. (eds), *Information Processing in Medical Imaging: Proc. 13th Int. Conf. (IPMI'93), Flagstaff, AZ, June, 1993*, pp. 17–32, Lectures Notes in Computer Science. Springer–Verlag.

Park, J., Metaxas, D. and Axel, L. (1995). Volumetric deformable models with parameter functions: A new approach to the 3D motion analysis of the LV from MRI–SPAMM. In *Proc. Fifth International Conf. on Computer Vision (ICCV'95), Cambridge, MA, June, 1995*, pp. 700–705, Los Alamitos, CA: IEEE Computer Society Press.

Park, J., Metaxas, D. and Axel, L. (1996). Analysis of left ventricular wall motion based on volumetric deformable models and MRI-SPAMM. *Medical Image Analysis*, 1(1), 53–72.

Pentland, A. and Horowitz, B. (1991). Recovery of nonrigid motion and structure. *IEEE Trans. Pattern Anal. Machine Intelligence*, 13(7), 730–742.

Pentland, A. and Sclaroff, S. (1991). Closed-form solutions for physically based shape modelling and recognition. *IEEE Trans. Pattern Anal. Machine Intelligence*, 13(7), 715–729.

Pieper, S., Rosen, J. and Zeltzer, D. (1992). Interactive graphics for plastic surgery: A task-level analysis and implementation. In *Proc. ACM 1992 Symposium on Interactive 3D Graphics*, pp. 127–134.

Poon, C. S., Braun, M., Fahrig, R., Ginige, A. and Dorrell, A. (1994). Segmentation of medical images using an active contour model incorporating region-based images features. In (Robb, 1994), pp. 90–97.

Press, W. H., Teukolsky, S. A., Vetterling, W. T. and Flannery, B. P. (1992). *Numerical Recipes in C*. Cambridge University Press.

Robb, R. A. (ed.) (1994). *Proc. Third Conf. on Visualization in Biomedical Computing (VBC'94), Rochester, MN, October, 1994*. SPIE Proc., Vol. 2359, Bellingham, WA: SPIE.

Rougon, N. and Prêteux, F. (1991). Deformable markers: Mathematical morphology for active contour models control. In *Image Algebra and Morphological Image Processing II* SPIE Proc., Vol. 1568, pp. 78–89, Bellingham, WA: SPIE.

Rougon, N. and Prêteux, F. (1993). Directional adaptive deformable models for segmentation with application to 2D and 3D medical images. In *Medical Imaging 93: Image Processing*, SPIE Proc., Vol. 1898, pp. 193–207, Bellingham, WA: SPIE.

Sandor, S. and Leahy, R. (1995). Towards automatic labelling of the cerebral cortex using a deformable atlas model. In (Bizais *et al.*, 1995), pp. 127–138.

Sapiro, G., Kimmel, R. and Caselles, V. (1995). Object detection and measurements in medical images via geodesic deformable contours. In *Vision Geometry IV*, SPIE Proc., Vol. 2573, pp. 366–378, Bellingham, WA: SPIE.

Singh, A., von Kurowski, L. and Chiu, M. Y. (1993). Cardiac MR image segmentation using deformable models. In *Biomedical Image Processing and Biomedical Visualization*, SPIE Proc., Vol. 1905, pp. 8–28, Bellingham, WA: SPIE.

Snell, J. W., Merickel, M. B., Ortega, J. M., Goble, J. C., Brookeman, J. R. and Kassell, N. F. (1995). Model-based boundary estimation of complex objects using hierarchical active surface templates. *Pattern Recog.*, 28(10), 1599–1609.

Staib, L. H. and Duncan, J. S. (1992a). Boundary finding with parametrically deformable models. *IEEE Trans. Pattern Anal. Machine Intelligence*, 14(11), 1061–1075.

Staib, L. H. and Duncan, J. S. (1992b). Deformable Fourier models for surface finding in 3D images. In Robb, R. A. (ed.), *Proc. Second Conf. on Visualization in Biomedical Computing (VBC'92), Chapel Hill, NC, October, 1992*, SPIE Proc., Vol. 1808, pp. 90–104, Bellingham, WA: SPIE.

Strang, G. and Nguyen, T. (1996). *Wavelets and Filter Banks*. Wellesley, MA: Wellesley-Cambridge Press.

Stytz, M., Frieder, G. and Frieder, O. (1991) Three-dimensional medical imaging: Algorithms and computer systems. *ACM Computing Surveys*, 23, 421–499.

Subsol, G., Thirion, J.Ph. and Ayache, N. (1995). A general scheme for automatically building 3D morphometric anatomical atlases: Application to a skull atlas. In *Proc. Second International Symp. on Medical Robotics and Computer Assisted Surgery (MRCAS'95), Baltimore, MD, November, 1995*, pp. 226–233.

Székely, G., Kelemen, A., Brechbuhler, Ch. and Gerig, G. (1996). Segmentation of 2-D and 3-D objects from MRI volume data using constrained elastic deformations of flexible Fourier surface models. *Medical Image Analysis*, 1(1), 19–34.

Szeliski, R. (1990). Bayesian modeling of uncertainty in low-level vision. *Int. J. Comput. Vision*, 5, 271–301.

Szeliski, R., Tonnesen, D. and Terzopoulos, D. (1993). Modeling surfaces of arbitrary topology with dynamic particles. In *Proc. Conf. on Computer Vision and Pattern Recognition (CVPR'93), New York, NY, June, 1993*, pp. 82–87, Los Alamitos, CA: IEEE Computer Society Press.

Tek, H. and Kimia, B. (1995). Shock-based reaction-diffusion bubbles for image segmentation. In (Ayache, 1995b), pp. 434–438.

Terzopoulos, D. (1986a). *On Matching Deformable Models to Images*. Tech. rept. 60. Schlumberger Palo Alto Research. Reprinted in *Topical Meeting on Machine Vision*, Technical Digest Series, Vol. 12, (Optical Society of America, Washington, DC) 1987, 160–167.

Terzopoulos, D. (1986b). Regularization of inverse visual problems involving discontinuities. *IEEE Trans. Pattern Anal. Machine Intelligence*, 8(4), 413–424.

Terzopoulos, D. and Fleischer, K. (1988). Deformable models. *The Visual Computer*, 4(6), 306–331.

Terzopoulos, D. and Metaxas, D. (1991). Dynamic 3D models with local and global deformations: Deformable superquadrics. *IEEE Trans. Pattern Anal. Machine Intelligence*, 13(7), 703–714.

Terzopoulos, D. and Szeliski, R. (1992). Tracking with Kalman snakes. In Blake, A. and Yuille, A. (eds), *Active Vision*, pp. 3–20, Cambridge, MA: MIT Press.

Terzopoulos, D., Witkin, A. and Kass, M. (1988). Constraints on deformable models: Recovering 3D shape and nonrigid motion. *Artif. Intelligence*, 36(1), 91–123.

Thirion, J. P. (1994). Extremal points: Definition and application to 3D image registration. In *Proc. Conf. on Computer Vision and Pattern Recognition (CVPR'94), Seattle, WA, June, 1994*, pp. 587–592, Los Alamitos, CA: IEEE Computer Society Press.

Turk, G. (1992). Re-tiling polygonal surfaces. In *Computer Graphics (Proc. SIGGRAPH'92 Conf., Chicago, IL, July, 1992)*, Vol. 26(2), pp. 55–64, ACM SIGGRAPH.

Ueda, N. and Mase, K. (1992). Tracking moving contours using energy-minimizing elastic contour models. In Sandini, G. (ed.), *Computer Vision – Proc. Second European Conf. on Computer Vision (ECCV'92), Santa Margherita Ligure, Italy, May, 1992*, pp. 453–457, Lectures Notes in Computer Science. Springer–Verlag.

Vasilescu, M. and Terzopoulos, D. (1992). Adaptive meshes and shells: Irregular triangulation, discontinuities and hierarchical subdivision. In *Proc. Conf. on Computer Vision and Pattern Recognition (CVPR'92), Urbana, IL, June, 1992*, pp. 829–832, Los Alamitos, CA: IEEE Computer Society Press.

Vemuri, B. C. and Radisavljevic, A. (1994). Multiresolution stochastic hybrid shape models with fractal priors. *ACM Trans. on Graphics*, 13(2), 177–207.

Vemuri, B. C., Radisavljevic, A. and Leonard, C. (1993). Multiresolution 3D stochastic shape models for image segmentation. In Colchester, A. C. F. and Hawkes, D. J. (eds), *Information Processing in Medical Imaging: Proc. 13th Int. Conf. (IPMI'93), Flagstaff, AZ, June, 1993*, pp. 62–76, Lectures Notes in Computer Science. Springer–Verlag.

Waters, K. (1992). A physical model of facial tissue and muscle articulation derived from computer tomography data. In Robb, R. A. (ed.), *Proc. Second Conf. on Visualization in Biomedical Computing (VBC'92), Chapel Hill, NC, October, 1992*, SPIE Proc., Vol. 1808, pp. 574–583, Bellingham, WA: SPIE.

Whitaker, R. (1994). Volumetric deformable models. In (Robb, 1994).

Widrow, B. (1973). The rubber mask technique, part I. *Pattern Recognition*, 5(3), 175–211.

Worring, M., Smeulders, A. W. M., Staib, L. H. and Duncan, J. S. (1993). Parameterized feasible boundaries in gradient vector fields. In Colchester, A. C. F. and Hawkes, D. J. (eds), *Information Processing in Medical Imaging: Proc. 13th Int. Conf. (IPMI'93), Flagstaff, AZ, June, 1993*, pp. 48–61, Lectures Notes in Computer Science. Springer–Verlag.

Young, A. and Axel, L. (1992). Non-rigid wall motion using MR tagging. In *Proc. Conf. on Computer Vision and Pattern Recognition (CVPR'92), Urbana, IL, June, 1992*, pp. 399–404, Los Alamitos, CA: IEEE Computer Society Press.

Young, A. A., Axel, L., Dougherty, L., Bogen, D. K. and Parenteau, C. S. (1993). Validation of tagging with MR imaging to estimate material deformation. *Radiology*, 188, 101–108.

Young, A. A., Kraitchman, D. L., Dougherty, L. and Axel, L. (1995). Tracking and finite element analysis of stripe deformation in magnetic resonance tagging. *IEEE Trans. Med. Imag.*, 14(3), 413–421.

Yuille, A. L., Hallinan, P. W. and Cohen, D. S. (1992). Feature extraction from faces using deformable templates. *Int. J. Comput. Vision*, 8, 99–111.

Zienkiewicz, O. C. and Taylor, R. L. (1989). *The Finite Element Method*. New York, NY: McGraw–Hill.

Biomedical Imaging Modalities: An Overview

Raj Acharya, Richard Wasserman, Jeffrey Stevens, and Carlos Hinojosa
Biomedical Imaging Group (BMIG)
Department of Electrical and Computer Engineering
201 Bell Hall
State University of New York at Buffalo
Buffalo, NY 14260

1. Introduction

The introduction of advanced imaging technologies has improved significantly the quality of medical care available to patients. Noninvasive imaging modalities allow a physician to make increasingly accurate diagnoses and render precise and measured modes of treatment. Current uses of imaging technologies include laboratory medicine, surgery, radiation therapy, nuclear medicine, and diagnostic radiology. Common medical imaging methodologies may be divided grossly into two general groupings: (1) techniques that seek to image internal anatomical structures and (2) methods that present mappings of physiological function.

Rapid technological advances have made the acquisition of three- and four-dimensional representations of human and animal internal structures commonplace. A multitude of imaging modalities are available currently.

X-ray computed tomography (CT) is a popular modality that is used routinely in clinical practice. CT generates a 3D image set that is representative of a patient's anatomy. CT scanners produce a set of 2D, axial cross-section images that may be stacked to form a 3D data set. The mathematics of CT image reconstruction is also employed in many imaging modalities. The problem associated with CT reconstruction was solved by radon in 1917. The availability of high-speed computers and relatively inexpensive memories allow modern scanners to utilize sophisticated reconstruction algorithms. The majority of current X-ray CT scanners collect 3D images, at the rate of one 2D slice at a time. Specialized scanners are also available that collect an entire 3D volume within a very short time span.

Magnetic resonance imaging (MRI) is similar to CT imaging in that it generates 3D data sets corresponding to a patient's anatomy. However, MRI differs fundamentally from CT in the manner in which images are acquired. CT scanners employ X-ray radiation to generate the data needed to reconstruct internal structures. Alternatively, MRI utilizes radio frequency (RF) waves and magnetic fields to obtain 3D images and is based on the principle of nuclear magnetic resonance (NMR). MRI scanners utilize nonionizing beams and provide unparalleled soft tissue contrast in a noninvasive manner.

Emission computed tomography techniques obtain 3D representations of the location of 3D injected pharmaceuticals. The injected pharmaceuticals are labeled with gamma-ray-emitting radionuclides. The emitted gamma rays are measured at sites external to a patient. Such measured data may be utilized to reconstruct a 3D mapping of internal emission density. A 3D image is generated by reconstructing a measured set of 2D projection images acquired at various angles around the patient. Emission tomography differs from MRI and CT in that it provides physiological function information, such as perfusion and metabolism, as opposed to strictly anatomical information.

Another methodology that gathers functional information is biomagnetic source imaging. This technology allows for the external measurement of the low-level magnetic fields generated by neuron activity. Biomagnetic source imaging allows a clinician to gather data concerning brain function that has previously proved elusive [1].

Ultrasound-based imaging techniques comprise a set of methodologies capable of acquiring both quantitative and qualitative diagnostic information. Many ultrasound-based methods are attractive due to their ability to obtain real-time imagery, employing compact and mobile equipment, at a significantly lower cost than is incurred with other medical imaging modalities. The real-time nature of ultrasound makes it possible for physicians to observe the motion of structures inside a patient's body. This ability has resulted in the widespread use of ultrasound technology in the fields of pediatrics and cardiology. Equipment that employs doppler echo techniques can extract quantitative velocity information such as the rate of blood flow in a vessel of interest. Additionally, the introduction of ultrasound signals into a patient, at the levels currently employed, has been determined to be safe [2]. The lack of negative effects from exposure, portability of equipment, relatively low cost, and quantitative acquisition modes distinguish ultrasound techniques as an important class of medical imaging technology.

This chapter provides an overview of most of the popular imaging modalities currently in clinical use. The foregoing discussion limits the use of advanced mathematical concepts, instead employing intuitive descriptions of each medical modality. It is hoped that a general understanding of the modality from which an image is derived will help researchers in the subsequent analysis of the image data.

The sections to follow include discussions of X-ray computed tomography (section 2), magnetic resonance imaging (section 3), emission-computed tomography (section 4), biomagnetic source imaging (section 5), digital subtraction angiography (section 6), and ultrasound imaging techniques (section 7).

2. X-Ray Computed Tomography

X-ray computed tomography (CT) or computed axial tomography (CAT) is a medical imaging modality capable of noninvasively acquiring a 3D representation of a patient's internal anatomical structure. This 3D representation may be visualized from an arbitrary viewpoint, providing vital information for anatomical mapping, tumor localization, stereotactic surgery planning, and many other diagnostic applications [3].

Physicians have long utilized X-ray-based imaging systems for noninvasive medical diagnostics. In the case of the conventional radiograph, a patient is placed in front of an X-ray source that transmits radiation through the subject's body. Each X-ray incident on the patient is attenuated by the tissues it passes through along its linear flight path. Differing tissue types in the body exhibit differing densities with respect to X-ray radiation. Each tissue type may therefore be assigned a value μ (z, y, z) which denotes the tissue density at Cartesian coordinate (x, y, z). The line integral of these tissue densities,

$$S = \int \mu(x,y,z)\,dl$$

is proportional to the attenuation experienced by an X ray passing along the given path. A 2D projection image or "shadow" of these X rays is imaged by measuring the X-ray energy leaving the patient's body in some 2D region of interest. Conventional radiography is a limited diagnostic modality, in the sense that it produces a 2D projection of a 3D object. Consequently, a large amount of information concerning internal anatomical structure is unavailable to the radiologist.

X-ray CT is a modality that is based upon the same physical principles that form the basis of conventional radiography. Differing tissue types possess different linear attenuation coefficients. This fact is utilized in conjunction with X-ray shadows from multiple viewpoints in order to reconstruct a representation of internal anatomical structure.

The data resultant from a typical CT scan consists of a series of 2D axial slices of a patient, which may be stacked to form a 3D representation (see Figure 1a and 1b). Each 2D slice is a matrix of voxel elements containing the calculated tissue density at each point within the imaged region. Though CT scans typically acquire slice data along the axial plane, it is possible to obtain planar views from other orientations. A mathematical shuffling of the information contained in the array of stacked slices allows a viewer to examine the patient from any viewpoint. However, such manipulation of the image viewpoint results in a degradation of image quality and detail.

In a common CT configuration, an X-ray source is located on one side of the patient's body and an array of X-ray detectors is located on the other side. The X-ray source and detectors are connected in a fixed, collinear arrangement forming a gantry, as illustrated in Figure 2. The X-ray detectors consist of an array of sensors that produce electrical data proportional to the amount of incident X-ray information. This information is stored in the memory of a data acquisition computer unit until it is needed for analysis. The gantry may be rotated around the patient about an origin centered in the axial plane. Improvements in fourth-generation CT devices make use of differing geometrical configurations of sources and detectors, but employ similar physical techniques of image generation.

The imaging problem in conventional radiography is essentially a single step. A patient is placed between a fixed X-ray source and a X-ray detector, the X-ray source is enabled, and the resultant X-ray projections are captured in some useful manner. Conversely, the CT imaging problem can be divided into two distinct parts, slice data acquisition and slice reconstruction.

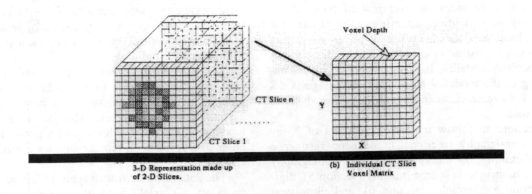

Figure 1: Data representation of reconstructed CT data.

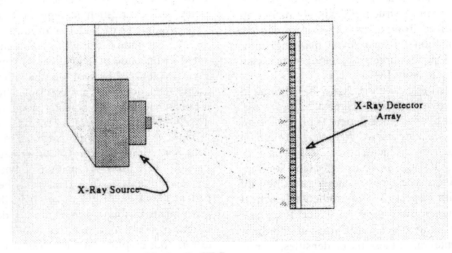

Figure 2. CT Scanner gantry.

The slice data acquisition sequence is initiated by activating a thin X-ray beam that spreads out and enters the patient along the edge of a desired image slice (see Figure 3). As the X-ray energy passes through the patient's body, it will penetrate differentially through various tissue types. The total attenuation along a ray's path is related to a line integral of tissue densities taken along that path. As each ray exits the patient, it strikes an element in the sensor array resulting in a measure of linear tissue density along the ray's path. The set of readings taken from the sensor array is then stored in computer memory. A single array measurement set for a fixed angular displacement of the gantry contains severely limited information. Therefore the gantry must be rotated around the patient, allowing for the acquisition of tissue line density measurements at multiple angular orientations about the center of the axial plane. If the gantry is rotated a full 180 degrees around the patient and a sufficient number of density measurements are taken, then an appropriate algorithm will reconstruct a 2D view of the slice imaged.

A patient undergoing a CT scan is placed typically on a movable couch around which is located the rotating gantry. The data for each CT slice is measured one slice at a time employing the methodology described above. After acquisition of the information for a slice is completed, the couch automatically moves the patient into the correct position to image the next slice. This process is repeated until data has been collected for the entirety of the volume of interest.

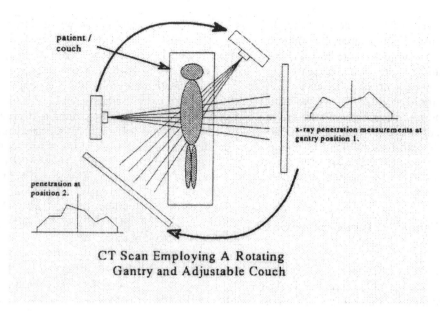

Figure 3. CT scanner methodology.

At the completion of the data acquisition phase of image formation, the CT computer holds information on the line integrals of tissue densities along multiple paths. This information can be combined to reconstruct the internal tissue densities within each slice of the CT scan. The most commonly utilized reconstruction technique is the *filtered back projection* algorithm.

Filtered back-projection is the process by which the 1D projections measured at multiple angles are reconstructed into the final slice matrix. Each slice is reconstructed individually and the resulting slices are stacked to form the final 3D CT representation. The scan and rotate data acquisition sequence, which a CT machine employs for each slice, results in the data set [4]

$$g \equiv g(n,\theta) = \int_L \mu(x,y,z)dl$$

where n is an integer denoting a sensor element in the X-ray detector array and θ is the angular position of the gantry.

The reconstruction is performed by first filtering the 1D projections $g(n,\theta)$ appropriately. This filtering produces the data set

$$\hat{g}(n,\theta) = g(n,\theta) \otimes h(n)$$

where $\otimes$ denotes convolution and $h(n)$ is an appropriate high pass filter.

The contents of the $\hat{g}(n,\theta)$ data set are then "back-projected" onto the slice data matrix. Back projection is performed by the operation:

$$f(x,y) = \int_0^\pi \hat{g}(x\cos\theta + y\sin\theta, \theta)d\theta$$

where $f(x, y)$ is the reconstructed slice data set. After this back-projection process is completed, the slice matrix will contain voxel data corresponding to a slice of the patient's body. A stacking of the reconstructed slice matrices results in a 3D CT volume representation. This three dimensional data set may then be manipulated to provide visualizations of the anatomical data from viewpoints other than the axial plane, provided that slices were acquired without a significant gap between them.

The product of the filtered back-projection algorithm is an array of 2D matrices containing reconstructed voxel data points. In many imaging applications, image elements possess no depth and are termed pixels or picture elements. In the case of CT, each of the imaged slices has a certain thickness that must be taken into account. Therefore, each matrix element in the reconstructed slice actually represents a tissue density within some volume element or voxel. Each element in the reconstructed slice matrix is assigned a CT number. This CT number is a measure of the density (with respect to water) of the tissues located within an individual voxel. The voxel number is calculated for each pixel by the CT reconstruction algorithm. Prior to image display, the CT numbers are quantized to correspond to allowable gray-scale values for the display system in use.

2.1 Dynamic Spatial Reconstructor (DSR)

A dynamic spatial reconstructor (DSR) is an x-ray CT scanner capable of providing dynamic synchronous vol-

23

ume 3D CT images, every 1/60 second [5]. The DSR has 14 source-detector pairs. Each source generates a cone beam that penetrates the subject to create a 2D image at the detector. The gantry rotates 1.5 degrees every 1/60 second, resulting in 14 new projections every 1/60 second. Reconstruction employing these 14 views results in a 3D volume corresponding to the highest temporal resolution. Several such reconstructions, each corresponding to adjacent time intervals, can be combined to obtain a desired spatial resolution. Special reconstruction algorithms have been designed to exploit the temporal nature of the DSR scanner [6].

2.2 Cardiovascular Computed Tomography (CVCT and Cine CT)

CT imaging, as discussed in section 2, is a versatile modality with which to acquire 3D imagery of a patient. However, due to mechanical limitations, CT is best employed when the anatomical area to be imaged has characteristically little motion. Consequently, the head region is an excellent candidate for CT imaging studies. Nonstatic anatomical areas, such as the cardiac region, cannot be examined adequately using typical CT technology. The cardiovascular computed tomography scanner (CVCT) was developed to overcome the aforementioned difficulties that CT encountered when imaging the dynamic cardiac region. The more recent Cine CT or Imatron Cine CT scanners have offered advanced versions of the earlier CVCT units.

CT scanners typically rely upon the mechanical motion of either the radiation source, detector, or both. Popular geometries for mechanical scanning include: translate-rotate, rotate-rotate, and rotate-stationary geometries [7]. The basic imaging processes inherent to CT image acquisition are discussed in section 2. Due to physical constraints, the gantry can be rotated around the patient at a maximum rate of approximately once every second. Due to the relatively slow motion of the gantry with respect to the dynamic system being imaged, accurate visual data cannot be acquired. In order to image a nonstatic system, the CT apparatus must be able to acquire imagery significantly faster than the system's rate of change. If image acquisition is rapid enough, a single reconstructed image can be viewed as having occurred at a single instant of time. Consequently, a series of such high-speed images would present a visual record of a system's motion. Due to the data acquisition techniques employed in CT, rapid image formation requires that the gantry rotate at high speeds. In the case of cardiac imagery, the acquisition time required for each complete image is on the order of milliseconds. Due to the mechanical nature of the CT gantry such rotation speeds are not feasible.

The rate of CT image acquisition can be increased significantly by replacing the mechanical gantry system

with an electrostatic scanning apparatus. As alluded to previously, the angular sampling rate [4] must be increased in order to achieve clinically useful motion imagery of the heart. Electrostatic scanning techniques are capable of generating angular sampling rates at least an order of magnitude higher than those possible via mechanical systems. The common television employs a form of electronic scanning. An electron beam is scanned over the television surface in order to produce the desired picture. The beam is rapidly swept across the entire viewing area of the screen. As long as the beam is swept at a high enough rate, each pixel on the television's monitor appears to be illuminated simultaneously. Such a common example illustrates the high-speed capabilities of electrostatic scanning methods.

The cardiovascular computed tomography scanner (CVCT), developed between 1978 and 1982, utilizes electronic scanning. It is capable of providing multiple 1 cm. slices through the heart at scan rates of 50 ms. The scanner consists of an electron beam source, deflection coils, stationary target rings, detector rings, and a data acquisition system [7]. Electron beams are generated at the head of the scanner. These beams pass through deflection coils, which direct them toward one of four target rings. The target rings are located below the patient under the region of interest.

Each target ring corresponds to two adjacent slices in the subject. The target rings redirect the incident electron beams upward through the patient. This radiation passes through the patient as in the case of CT. The radiation exiting the body is collected by detector rings on the anterior side of the patient. The angular projection information collected can be varied electronically in such a system. Deflection coil characteristics may be altered electronically. Such changes in the coils' characteristics modify the angle at which projection data is obtained. This angular measurement position may be varied rapidly, resulting in the collection of data at a significantly higher rate than is possible in mechanical systems. CVCT scanners employ the discussed methodology to capture cardiac imagery at a high enough rate to allow for motion analysis of a heart under study.

3. Magnetic Resonance Imaging

Magnetic resonance imaging (MR or MRI) represents a major innovation in medical imaging technology. MR imaging can provide detailed images of the human body with unparalleled soft tissue contrast in a noninvasive manner. The phenomenon of nuclear magnetic resonance (NMR) is relatively new to the field of diagnostic medicine. The technique itself has existed for over 45 years in the field of physical chemistry. NMR was first discovered in 1946 by Bloch and Purcell, two researchers working independently at Stanford and Harvard, respectively. Both were awarded the Nobel Prize in 1952 for their work.

3.1 Magnetic Resonance

Resonance, in the physical sense, is defined as the absorption of energy from a source at a specific frequency, often called the *natural* or *resonant* frequency. In the case of MRI or NMR the source is RF energy, and the object resonating is the nuclei of atoms, while in an external magnetic field. Nuclei are promoted to a higher energy state via the absorption of the RF energy. The higher energy or *excited* state cannot be indefinitely maintained. Consequently the nuclei release energy in order to return to their lower energy or *ground* state. RF energy is released by the nuclei when the ground state is returned to. This emitted RF energy can be referred to as the MR signal. The characteristics of the MR signal are dependent upon the specific molecular environment of the emitting nucleus. Diverse types of information can be collected concerning a molecular environment from the MR signal. Figure 4 is a simplified version of NMR. The bar below each side represents the energy in the system.

3.2 Nuclei Properties in External Magnetic Fields

MR imaging cannot be applied to all nuclei. Nuclei must be either rotating, and therefore possessing angular momentum (spin), or must possess an odd number of protons or neutrons. Only nuclei with these characteristics can be made to resonate. Since nuclei possess electrical charge, their spinning produces a magnetic moment $\vec{\mu}$, aligned on the axis of the spin. $\vec{\mu}$ is a vector quantity indicating the strength and direction of the magnetic field surrounding the nucleus. Hence, a spinning nuclei is a dipole (having two poles), and may be thought of as a microscopic bar magnet (Figure 5).

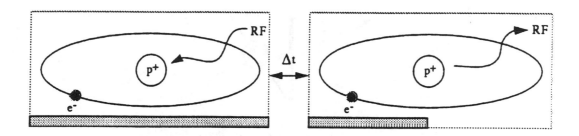

Figure 4. Simplified view of nuclear magnetic resonance.

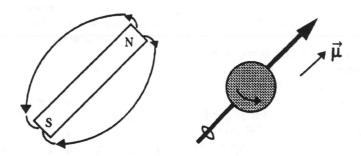

Figure 5. Magnetic nuclei act like microscopic bar magnets.

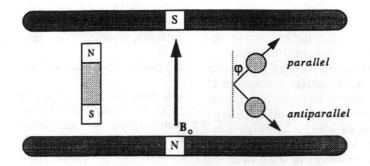

Figure 6. Nuclei alignment in external magnetic fields.

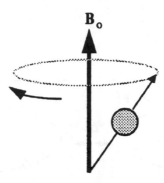

Figure 7. Nuclei precession in external magnetic fields.

In the presence of an external static magnetic field, spins[1] will align with the external field, similar to the manner in which a bar magnet would align in the same field. Quantum physics dictates that a proton has only two allowable quantum states as its spin quantum number, $I = 1/2$. These two states are the parallel (spin up) and anti-parallel (spin down) states, pertaining to low and high energy states respectively. Additionally, these states are slightly askew with respect to the external field direction (Figure 6).

A nucleus containing a single proton is the principal isotope of hydrogen. Hydrogen, ^1H is the element of preference in MRI since ^1H has a high natural abundance and has a high sensitivity to its MR signal.

Hydrogen is the most common element found in biological tissue, concentrated in tissue water. 99 percent of all hydrogen isotopes encountered are ^1H (that is, one proton and no neutrons).

A nucleus' sensitivity to its MR signal is expressed in terms of its gyromagnetic ratio, γ. The gyromagnetic ratio

represents a nucleus' resonance frequency in a 1-Tesla[2] external field. γ is a nuclear constant for every isotope. Sensitivity increases proportionally with signal frequency. Hydrogen has the largest gyromagnetic ratio and therefore has the largest MR signal sensitivity.

When subjected to an external magnetic field, henceforth denoted by B_0, protons align with the field and simultaneously experience a torque due to B_0. As a result, they process about the B_0 axis at a rate given by the *Larmour* relationship.

$$f_{Larmour} = \gamma B_0 \qquad (1)$$

where B_0 is measured in Tesla (T) and γ has units of megahertz per Tesla (MHz/T). For example, the resonance frequency of the hydrogen nucleus ($\gamma = 42.58MHz/T$) with an external field strength of 1 Tesla ($B_0 = 1T$) is 42.58 MHz. An illustration of precession is presented in Figure 7.

The effects of an external magnetic field, B_0, upon a single hydrogen nucleus have been discussed. These re-

---

[1] The terms spin and dipole will be used interchangeably throughout the section, as both are identical for our discussion.

[2] A Tesla is a unit of measurement for magnetic fields.

sults can be extended to a group of protons, analogous to a small volume of tissue.

Within any external magnetic field, there will always be a small net excess of spins within a given volume aligned in the parallel (lower energy) state as opposed to the antiparallel (higher energy) state. This excess parallel state population is represented by the net magnetization vector, $\vec{M}$. $\vec{M}$ increases in direct proportion to external field strength, B_0, as shown in Figure 8.

The net magnetization vector ($\vec{M}$) is ultimately responsible for the emitted MR signal. The need for powerful magnets in MR imaging is apparent from Figure 8. If $\vec{M}$ is maximized then so is the resultant MR signal. The subatomic MRI description is no longer needed for the purposes of this chapter. All that need be understood is that a net magnetization vector exists, $\vec{M}$, representing the aggregate magnetic state of our tissue volume.

At this time, we introduce a coordinate system for further discussions. The patient is placed inside a gantry, which houses the hardware necessary to create the magnetic fields required for MR imaging. The static magnetic field, $\vec{B}_0$, is taken to be in the z direction, from caudal to cranial. The xy plane, referring to axial or transverse slices through the patient, is defined as x from left to right, and y posterior to anterior.

M can be oriented in any direction, unlike $\vec{\mu}$, which has only two orientations (parallel and antiparallel) [8].

3.3 MR Imaging Process

Prior to imaging, $\vec{M}$ is in its equilibrium position, aligned along the z axis of the gantry. There is no detectable MR signal before the imaging sequence begins. The MR receiver coils are oriented such that only the component of $\vec{M}$ in the transverse (xy) plane induces a measurable signal. Components of $\vec{M}$ in the transverse direction are referred to as transverse magnetization, and the components along the z axis as longitudinal magnetization. During the imaging process RF pulses modify $\vec{M}$. This interaction results in the emission of RF energy, which is then detected in the receiver coils. As mentioned previously, this emitted RF energy is referred to as the MR signal.

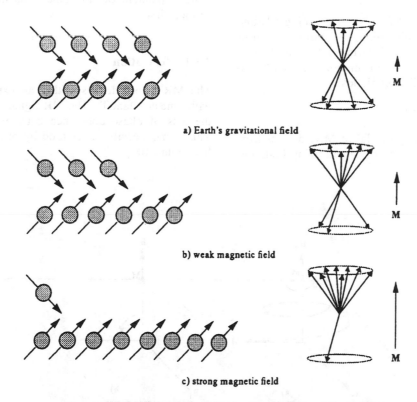

a) Earth's gravitational field

b) weak magnetic field

c) strong magnetic field

Figure 8. Nuclei states in varying external magnetic fields.

Transverse magnetization is created by an RF field, denoted B_1, applied in the transverse plane. If the RF field is oscillating at the *Larmour* frequency, $\vec{M}$ will mutate from its equilibrium alignment along the z axis. There are two methods for visualizing this transition, stationary and rotating frames of reference (Figure 9). A stationary frame of reference views the transitions from outside the system. A complex spiraling motion is viewed due to spins mutated from their equilibrium position while simultaneously precessing. In the case of a rotating frame of reference, the system observation point is situated above the system and rotates at the *Larmour* frequency. Such a reference eliminates the precessional component of the spin's motion. Consequently, the rotation of the $\vec{M}$ vector from equilibrium can be simply viewed. A rotating frame of reference will be assumed throughout the rest of this discussion.

The flip angle denotes the displacement over which $\vec{M}$ is rotated from equilibrium after the application of an RF signal. Figure 9 illustrates a 90° flip angle. Increasing the RF pulse's power will cause a consequent increase in the resultant flip angle. Flip angle can be determined by the relationship

$$\theta = \gamma B_1 t \tag{2}$$

where t is the time duration of the RF pulse. Any flip angle is attainable.

Varied combinations of RF pulses and timing relationships constitute an MR pulse sequence. Pulse sequences can be employed to extract differing information from tissues. Section 3.4 discusses information that can be extracted from tissue via MRI techniques.

3.4 Tissue Characterization

The impressive diagnostic potential of MRI derives from its ability to provide a means of characterizing both normal and pathological tissues. Hydrogen is present in nearly all tissues, therefore it can be assumed that MRI data can be collected from nearly all tissues. Images of tissue hydrogen concentration, $\rho[H]$, can be obtained by MRI techniques. However, variations in hydrogen concentration between tissues are quite small typically, yielding only moderate contrast images. Consequently, hydrogen concentration images are of limited clinical interest.

The most clinically useful information lies almost entirely in the behavior of regional hydrogen, rather than its regional concentration. The molecular environment influences the behavior of nuclei, which in turn influences the characteristics of the MR signal. In the case of MR imaging, the hydrogen nuclei within a tissue volume are observed and characteristics about its magnetic environment are inferred.

Several tissue-related factors influence the emitted MR signal. The most important of these are the relaxation times. For brevity, only the relaxation time factors will be discussed. The interested reader may refer to [8, 9] for discussions of other MR-signal-influencing factors.

Relaxation refers to the process by which the spins respond to the disrupting effects of both their environment and external RF pulses. There are two types of relaxation, T_1 and T_2 relaxation. MR signal strength is more dependent on T_2, hence this method will be described first.

3.5 T_2 Relaxation

The MR signal decays within an exponential envelope with time constant T_2. The MR signal's decay is related to the loss of phase coherence between precessing spins. This is most easily understood by means of an example. See Figure 10.

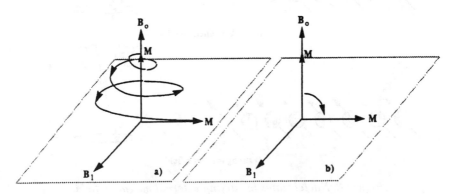

Figure 9. Frames of reference in MR imaging. a) Stationary frame. b) Rotating frame.

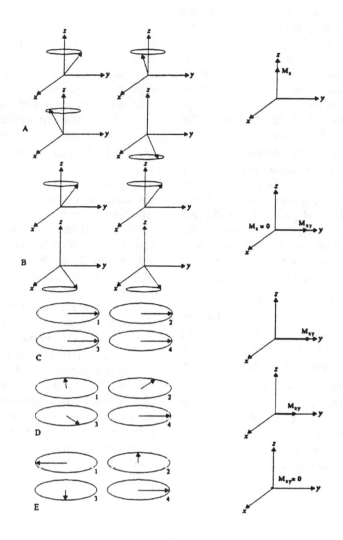

Figure 10. T2 relaxation: a) System prior to pulse sequence. b) After 90° RF pulse. c) Transverse magnetization. d) Dephasing proceeds to reduce transverse magnetization. e) Spins are completely dephased, and transverse magnetization disappears.

Figure 10a presents a finite volume of tissue containing 4 nuclei at equilibrium. Three of the nuclei's spins are in the parallel state and one is in the antiparallel state. All of the illustrated nuclei are processing at random phase angles with respect to a point in the transverse plane. Hence their transverse components cancel and $M_{xy} = 0$. The slight excess of spins in the parallel state creates a net magnetization component in the z direction, M_{xy}. Figure 10b illustrates the nuclei of 10a after an RF pulse at the *Larmour* frequency is applied such that one of the nuclei absorbs energy resonantly and is excited into the antiparallel state. In addition to promoting nuclei 3 to the antiparallel state, the RF pulse also creates phase coherence between the spins [10, 9]. In this case, $\vec{\mu}_i$ for $i = 1, ..., 4$ all project onto the same spot in the transverse plane.

Consequently, the vector sum of the transverse components produces a large net transverse magnetization, $M_{xy} \neq 0$. Projections onto the z axis will therefore cancel, and $M_z = 0$. M_{xy} is responsible for the resultant MR signal. Initially, M_{xy} is large, and for the instantly applied pulse is equal to M_z at equilibrium. This represents an RF pulse with a 90° flip angle. Figure 10c is equivalent to 10b except that arrows now correspond to individual nuclei projections onto the transverse plane, that is, $\vec{\mu}_{xy,i}$ for $i = 1$,

..., 4. Figure 10d illustrates local magnetic field inhomogeneities creating differing effective magnetic environments about each nuclei. As a result, nuclei precess at slightly different rates, given by Equation 1. As demonstrated by Equation 1, nuclei in stronger fields precess faster; those in weaker fields, more slowly. As a result, the vector sum of transverse components is no longer a maximum. A smaller M_{xy} will then result in a weaker MR signal. As time progresses, the MR signal disappears due to dephasing processes. This is illustrated in Figure 10e. After a sufficiently long time, transverse components of the spins return to completely random phases. Consequently, there is no detected signal.

Figure 11 illustrates a typical MR signal known as the free induction decay (FID). The decay envelope corresponding to T_2^* effects is much sharper than that of T_2.

Two types of local field inhomogeneities are caused by dephasing. Dephasing effects resulting from microscopic intrinsic field variations only are termed T_2. T_2 is a measure of how long it takes for M_{xy} to decrease, dependent upon intrinsic microscopic magnetic inhomogeneities only. It is a characteristic parameter of tissue. Dephasing due to both microscopic field variations as well as external static field (B_0) inhomogeneities is referred to as T_2^*. T_2^* is significantly shorter than T_2, as static field inhomogeneities are many orders of magnitude greater than microscopic field variations. Figure 11 illustrates the decay envelopes for both types of decay. The FID is shown within the T_2^* envelope in Figure 11. Information concerning T_2^* largely represents characteristics of the scanner's external static field. Methods exist to remove the effects of external field inhomogeneities [8, 10, 9]. The decay envelopes are exponential in nature, with 63 percent of the signal decaying after one T_2 interval and 84 percent after two T_2 intervals, and so forth.

3.6 T_1 Relaxation

RF stimulation at the *Larmour* frequency causes nuclei to resonantly absorb energy. In order for the system to return to equilibrium, energy must be released, that is, some spins must return to their parallel orientation. This energy is released into the molecular environment.

T_1 is also an exponential time constant. It represents the rate at which M_z returns to its equilibrium value. This concept is most easily understood in terms of $\vec{M}$ (Figure 12).

Figure 12a illustrates a system at rest, that is, the longitudinal component is at a maximum. Figure 12b presents the system of 12a after being disturbed by a 90° RF pulse. Immediately following the pulse, the net magnetization in the z direction is zero, that is, $M_z = 0$ (see section 3.5). Figure 12(c) illustrates the longitudinal component, M_z, after a very short period of time relative to T_1. As time progresses, more energy is released, and M_z begins to grow toward the equilibrium value (12d,e). After a sufficient time interval, the system has returned to its initial state (illustrated in Figure 12f).

T_2 and T_1 relaxation occur simultaneously, and are largely independent. After a time interval of approximately 5 T_2, the system's phase coherence has been completely lost. This dephasing occurs much more rapidly than the release of energy to the surroundings [8, 11]. Combining Figures 10 and 12 illustrates the relaxation processes occurring simultaneously, with Figure 10 occurring between b and c in Figure 12.

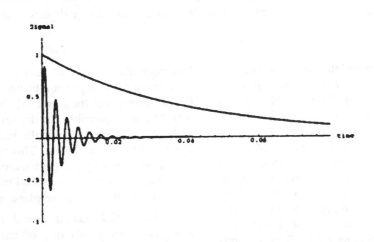

Figure 11. T_2 and T_2^* decay envelopes, FID shown within T_2^* envelope.

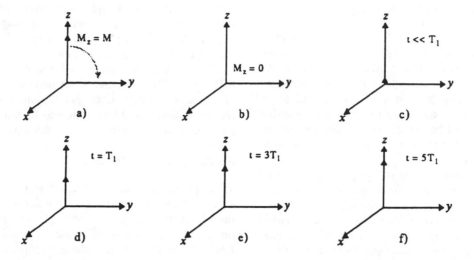

Figure 12. T_1 relaxation: a) System a equilibrium. b) After RF 90° RF pulse. c) Longitudinal component after a short duration of time. d, e, f) Successively longer times.

Through proper RF stimulation, in the form of pulse sequences, it is possible to acquire information regarding either of the two discussed tissue characteristics [8, 10]. MR images created from sequences emphasizing T_1 information are known as T_1-weighted images. Images emphasizing T_2 are analogously referred to as T_2 weighted. Within every pulse sequence, there is a specific time interval during which MR data is acquired. We shall refer to this time period as *TE*. Via proper selection of *TE*, it is possible to obtain good contrast between various tissue types, whether normal or pathological. T_1 and T_2 tissue contrast concepts are illustrated in Figure 13.

It has been found that pathology often exhibits T_1 and T_2 values differing from surrounding healthy tissue.

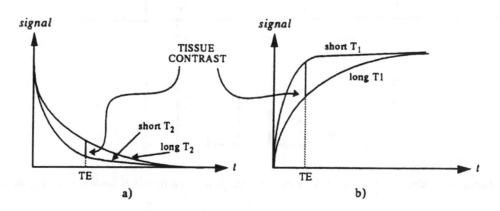

Figure 13. a) T_2 and b) T_1 tissue contrast.

3.7 Spatial Localization in MR Imaging

This section begins a discussion of methods with which to generate clinically useful image data by utilizing the theoretical results of the past sections. Ideally, we would like to somehow divide tissue into tiny volume elements, referred to as voxels. Voxels must have a finite volume in order to contain enough nuclei to produce a measurable signal. Voxels need not be cubic, and are often elongated rectangles. The use of cubic voxel will be assumed, without loss of generality.

Spatial localization of these voxels is achieved through the use of magnetic field gradients. Magnetic gradients are weak nonuniform magnetic fields, at maximum a few percent as powerful as the static magnetic field B_0. Gradients are superimposed over the static field to create a spatially varying magnetic field in the tissue (Figure 14).

The effective magnetic field experienced by a proton after superposition of a gradient is $B_0 + G_x x$. At each location along the direction of the gradient, there is a unique magnetic field. Therefore, by Equation 1, there will also be a unique *Larmour* frequency for each position along the direction of the gradient, given by

$$f_{Larmor} = \gamma B_0 + \gamma G x \cdot x) \tag{3}$$

where the term on the right is the *Larmour* frequency adjustment due to the presence of the magnetic gradient. The gradient technique results in spatial location being encoded into the frequency of the MR signal.

There are several methods for spatially localizing the MR signal. The methods to be reviewed fall into either 2D (planar) strategies, or 3D (volume) strategies. The planar strategies will be considered first, as the 3D strategies are simple extensions of 2D techniques.

3.8 Planar Data Collection

When planar techniques are employed, the first step is to select a plane through the tissue under investigation (Figure 15). A plane is selected by applying a gradient in the z direction to a volume of tissue in a uniform magnetic field, B_0. Each location along z experiences a unique magnetic field, and consequently a unique *Larmour* frequency (Equation 3). Each point along z defines an x-y plane in our coordinate system. All nuclei in this plane experience the same magnetic field and will resonate at the same frequency. If a 90° RF pulse is applied, corresponding to the *Larmour* frequency at z_p, the entire plane $z = z_p$ will acquire a nonzero transverse magnetization, M_{xy}. (Figure 10). Any MR signal subsequently received will be from protons in the selected plane only. This process is known as plane or slice section.

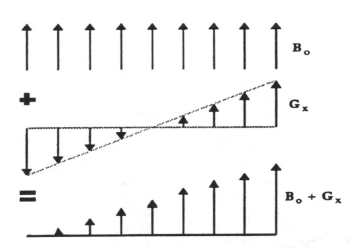

Figure 14. Magnetic field gradients add to the static external field, resulting in a spatially varying magnetic field.

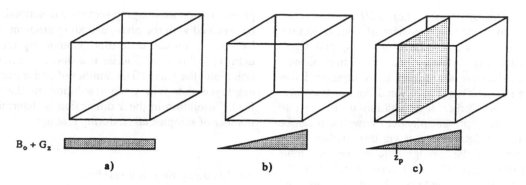

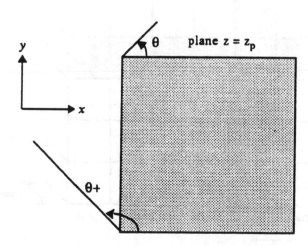

Figure 15. Slice selection utilizing a z gradient.

All protons in the selected plane $z = z_p$ will process at $f_{Larmour} = \gamma B_0 + \gamma (G_{zp} \cdot z_p)$ The slice selection gradient is then removed. Protons return to processing at the rate given by Equation 1. The only volumes (planes have a finite width) with nonzero transverse component are those in the plane $z = z_p$.

3.8.1 Polar data collection
Polar data collection is the simplest of collection strategies, and provides the closest analogy to transmission tomography. A slice is first selected via gradient techniques as described in section 3.8. At signal measurement time, *TE*, additional gradients are applied in both the x and y directions, G_x and G_y. This subjects all protons at an angle $\phi = \arctan G_y/G_x$ to the same magnetic field, that is, there is a gradient along the $\phi + \pi/2$ direction. The simultaneous application of G_y and G_x divide the selected plane into lines. (Figure 16)

The information received from the slice is composed of several frequencies. Each frequency represents the combined signals of protons along a line through the plane. The information may be arranged such that data is acquired on equally spaced intervals along the direction $\phi + \pi/2$. This method results in a projection of the tissue in the selected plane being measured. Projections are collected for $0 \le \phi < \pi$, allowing the use of computed tomography reconstruction algorithms, such as convolution/filtered back-projection for image reconstruction.

Figure 16. Collecting projections via polar data collection.

3.8.2 2D Fourier transform collection, 2DFT

The polar collection strategy consists of slice selection, followed by simultaneous application of G_x and G_y to reduce dimensionality from a plane to a line. Consequently, backprojection is required to reorganize information into an image. Two-dimensional Fourier transform imaging allows the further segmentation of a line into pixels (image pixels represent physical vowels). It can be shown [12] that the data collected via this method is the Fourier Transform of the tomographic image. A simple application of the inverse Fourier transform results in the desired image. Back-projection algorithms are not required.

The method works as follows. A slice of tissue is first selected. A gradient is then applied in the y direction. Spins in different effective magnetic fields along the direction of the gradient process at different frequencies as given by Equation 3 with x replaced by y. Spins along the y direction begin to dephase due to the gradient's nonlinearity. After a brief interval of time, Δt, G_y is removed. The spins return to the resonant frequency determined by the external field, as described by Equation 1. However, the spins are still linearly out of phase, from the brief application of G_y. Spatial location along the y axis is encoded within the phase of the spins. At signal readout time, TE, the G_x gradient is applied to spatially encode location along the x direction into the frequency content of the MR signal. Each point in the plane has a unique phase-frequency pair, which can be written as: (frequency, phase) = $(f(x), \theta(y))$ (Figure 17).

Unfortunately, one such phase encoding is insufficient to fully encode spatial location into the MR signal's phase. The entire imaging sequence described above must be repeated with the phase encoding gradient incremented by a small amount each time. Combining these multiple data sets allows the Fourier transform to determine position along the y axis. The number of phase encoding steps employed determines the resolution in the y direction [11]. Resolution in the x dimension is determined by the number of samples taken during readout.

3.8.3 Imaging time and resolution

The time required for the above imaging processes have similar forms:

$$\text{Imaging Time} = TR * N * NEX \qquad (4)$$

where TR = time to repetition; the time it takes for the plane to return to equilibrium such that it may be excited again. N is equal to the number of phase encoding steps for 2DFT imaging, and the number of angular views for polar collection. NEX is equal to the number of excitations; the number of times the entire imaging process will be repeated (used for signal averaging to improve signal-to-noise ratio). For TR = 1.5 sec., N = 120, and NEX = 2, the time required to collect the data necessary to image one plane is 384 sec. For 20 slices, each 1.0 *mm.* thick, the scan would require over 2 hours. It is easy to see how imaging time could begin to be a practical problem. Fortunately, there exists fast imaging techniques as well as multislice methods to minimize the scan time and optimize patient throughput [8, 13].

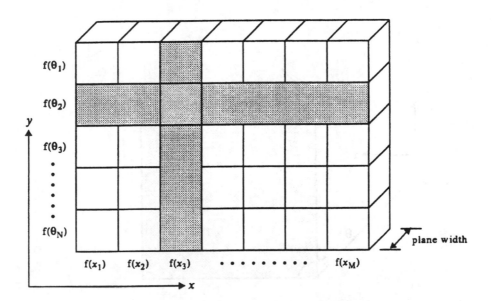

Figure 17. Locations in space have a unique pair of frequency and phase values.

34

3.9 3DFT and Spherical Imaging

3DFT imaging is a simple extension of 2DFT imaging. The only difference is that there is no slice selection. Information for an entire volume is obtained by phase encoding in two directions (x and y), and frequency encoding in the x direction.

Spherical imaging involves simultaneous application of G_x, G_y, and G_z. These gradients are adjusted such that samples are obtained in full azimuthal and polar increments.

3.10 Recent Advances in Magnetic Resonance Imaging

Recent advances in high-speed imaging allow cross-sectional images to be obtained in extremely short periods of time. This opens a new horizon for the use of MRI. The clinical potential of observing motion in both normal and pathological tissue is devastating.

Let us assume that it is possible to generate MR images rapidly enough to observe motion in a single plane. For many processes, this is currently possible. It is often desirable to study the motion of tissue between consecutive time frames. Image processing techniques could be employed to identify tissue contours, and the motion of these contours tracked. However, even if the contours could be properly found, and the correspondence problem solved, any motion seen would simply be that of the inner and outer surfaces of the tissue. Nothing would be known about the motion of tissue between the surfaces. Identifiable and trackable landmarks are needed within the tissue, just as the contours are for the outside of the tissue. Several pre-imaging pulse sequences have been suggested to create such landmarks. These pulse sequences are applied prior to the imaging sequence, and alter the magnetic properties of tissue in such a way as to create landmarks. Since magnetization is a property of tissue, when the tissue moves, the magnetization moves with it. Three of these sequences are described below. These methods are collectively referred to as tagged MRI.

3.10.1 Selective tagging

Selective tagging, introduced by Zerhouni, et al. [14], involves perturbing the magnetization of protons in specified lines, such that these regions exhibit no MR signal. Dark bands are consequently produced in the image. Typically these lines are oriented in a polar fashion (Figure 18). Selective tagging is useful for observing motion most easily seen in polar coordinates, such as the twisting motion of the heart.

3.10.2 Spatial modulation of magnetization

Spatial modulation of magnetization (SPAMM), introduced by Axel and Dougherty [15], makes use of many principles common to 2DFT imaging. This method creates a series of evenly spaced stripes in any direction. For two orthogonal directions, a gridlike pattern is produced (Figure 19).

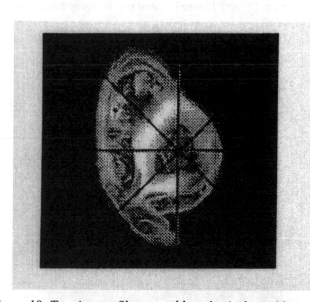

Figure 18: Tagging profile created by selectively exciting planes.

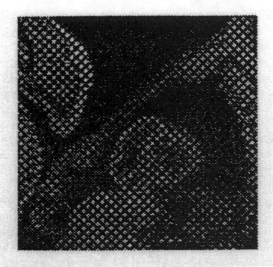

Figure 19. Tagging profile created by spatial modulation of magnetization. Reproduced with permission [12].

The intersection of grid lines creates trackable markers in the tissue. Motion parameters may then be estimated based upon motion of these noninvasive markers.

3.10.3 Striped tagging

Striped tagging (STAG), introduced by Bolster, McVeigh, and Zerhouni [16], is a hybrid of the above two techniques. A series of evenly spaced beads are produced along any line. The motion of these beads may then be followed (Figure 20).

The choice of tagging sequence employed is largely application dependent. Tagging in Figure 18 and Figure 20 were introduced artificially for illustration purposes. Actual tags are not as distinct as shown here.

3.11 Summary

Magnetic resonance imaging offers an abundance of diagnostic information. An inherent physical advantage MRI has over CT, PET, SPECT, and other imaging modalities is that images may be collected physically from any plane through the volume. The other modalities are limited to transaxial or close to transaxial images. There is a wealth of literature regarding MRI principles, imaging, and pre-imaging techniques [11, 8, 9, 17, 10].

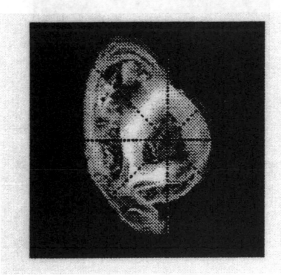

Figure 20. Profile created by striped tagging.

4. Emission Computed Tomography

Emission computed tomography (ECT) has been widely employed in biomedical research and clinical medicine during the past two decades. ECT differs fundamentally from many other medical imaging modalities in that it produces a mapping of physiological functions as opposed to imaging anatomical structure. In the case of transmission mode modalities, such as X-ray CT discussed in section 2, a source of radiation is external to the patient and is perfectly localized before the process of reconstruction. The basic purpose in transmission tomography is the mapping of the absorption coefficient distribution. Internal structural views can then be reconstructed utilizing the absorption distribution.

In the case of positron emission tomography (PET) and single-photon emission (SPECT) (which constitute the two different modalities of ECT), the radiation source utilized is a radioisotope compound that has been introduced into a patient's body. The radioactive compound is metabolically distributed into various organs and tissues and no a priori information concerning the radiation's location is known. The main goal of ECT is the determination of the isotope compound distribution within a patient's body. Measurements are taken of radiation leaving the patient's body using a specially designed detector system. The detector readings are employed as input to a reconstruction algorithm to produce the internal isotope compound distribution.

4.1 Single-photon emission computed tomography

SPECT imaging techniques employ radioisotopes that decay emitting a single gamma photon. This represents the fundamental difference between PET and SPECT. PET systems employ isotopes in which a couple of photons are produced in each individual annihilation. There are a rich variety of isotopes that decay, emitting a single photon and which consequently can be utilized in SPECT. Some of the most commonly employed isotopes are Tc-99m, I-125, and I-131. These isotopes present the advantages of being produced at relatively low cost and of having long half-lives. The long half-lives of these isotopes permits their production in a laboratory external to the hospital.

When the nucleus of a radioisotope disintegrates, a gamma photon is emitted with a random direction that is uniformly distributed in the sphere surrounding the nucleus. If the photon is unimpeded by a collision with electrons or other particle within the body, its trajectory will be a straight line or "ray."

In order for a photon detector external to the patient to discriminate the direction that a ray is incident from, a physical collimation is required. Typically, lead collimator plates are placed prior to the detector's crystal in such a manner that the photons incident from all but a single direction are blocked by the plates. This guarantees that only photons incident from the desired direction will strike the photon detector.

When a gamma photon collides with matter in a patient's body, photoelectric absorption and Compton scattering effects occur. These two types of interactions can be summarized as:

- *photoelectric absorption*: The photon hits an atom and its energy is essentially transferred to the atom or to an electron. The particular gamma photon involved in this collision will consequently not be detected by the detector system.

- *Compton scattering*: The photon strikes one of the electrons surrounding an atom and the gamma ray is deflected from its original path. The photon continues in a new direction with reduced energy. This particular photon may be detected by the camera, however information on its original path will be lost.

Most modern detector systems consist of stacked, circular detector arrays. These detector arrays are often referred to as X-ray cameras. Each detector crystal produces an electrical pulse when it is struck by a gamma photon. The electrical pulses are counted by support hardware and provide a measure of the number of photons incident on each detector in the array during the interval of measurement. The sensor arrays are constructed so that the photon detection process takes place in one plane or slice at a time. Therefore only the gamma rays that lie in this plane will have a chance to be registered or detected.

Considering the collimation process, interaction effects, and measurements being limited to a single slice, one can note that only a small percentage of the original number of the emitted photons will be registered by the detector apparatus. A typical percentage is 5 percent or less. The number of emitted photons cannot be increased limitlessly since this would represent an increase in the gamma ray energy that the patient is exposed to. It seems that these constraints are implicit in SPECT and efficient reconstruction algorithm design must take optimal advantage of the measurement counts of the detector arrays.

In order to avoid further information loss, the registration efficiency of the detector crystals must be close to 100 percent. The most commonly employed detector for SPECT applications is a thallium-activated sodium iodide single crystal due to the relatively high atomic weight of iodine and consequently good gamma-ray absorption properties. Crystal thickness selection must take into account the trade-off between spatial resolution and sensitivity; thick crystals absorb more gamma rays but exhibit poor resolution while thin crystals have good resolution and poor sensitivity. Typically, the crystal thickness lies between 0.375 to 0.5 inches. When a gamma-ray photon enters the crystal, a fast electron is formed due to either photoelectric effects or Compton scattering with the crystal's iodide ions. When this electron decelerates due to interactions with the crystal, a scintillation is produced. This radiation of visible light is sensed by a photomultiplier tube and is converted to an electrical pulse.

Scattering and attenuation of gamma photons within a patient's body produce inaccuracies in the estimation of radioisotope distribution. After a Compton interaction with an electron, gamma photons lose a portion of their original energy and proceed along an altered trajectory. If such an altered photon is detected by the camera, the apparent position of the photon's original emission point will be the location of the Compton interaction. This incorrect determination of the photon's point of initial production results in an inaccurate estimation of the radioisotope distribution. If attenuation effects were ignored, the resultant underestimation of the radioactivity concentration would make most clinical analysis impossible. A large number of the scattered photons can be eliminated from the registered photons by employing the fact that radioisotopes generally emits one or two groups of photons of well-defined energy. Therefore the electronics of the detector system can be designed in such a way that only the photons inside an energy acceptance window are registered. However this window cannot be infinitesimally small in practice, and we still have a good deal of the scattering problem. One simple approximation to improve the distribution estimation is to assume that the transaxial contour of the patient is an ellipse and consists of a single tissue type with a uniform attenuation. A more accurate method is to employ additional attenuation measurements using an external gamma source. A simplified attenuation map of the transaxial section can be used as additional information in the attenuation correction reconstruction algorithm.

The resolution of an image refers to the degree of discrimination that is possible between two small, closely placed objects. When an image reconstruction of a single point of radioisotope concentration is performed, a bell-shape plot is obtained that approximates a Gaussian curve. Typically, the spatial resolution is defined as the width of this curve at half its maximum height (full width at half maximum, or FWHM). A typical transaxial resolution in SPECT ranges from 10 to 20 *mm.*, which is significantly poorer than the fine resolution achieved in transmission tomography (1–2 *mm.*). Resolution in the axial direction specifies the slice thickness and is determined by the collimation properties of the detectors; typically the axial resolution ranges from 10 to 20 *mm.*

4.2 Positron Emission Tomography

The distinguishing physical feature of the radionuclides used in positron emission tomography (PET) is that they decay via the emission of positrons. When this emission occurs inside a patient's body, the positron travels a short distance, approximately 1 *mm.*, before its motion is slowed enough to find a nearby electron and interact with it. A positron is the antiparticle of an electron and is almost identical to it except that positrons possess a negative charge. When a positron and an electron interact, their masses are converted into two photons traveling in opposite directions along a nearly collinear path. This physical process occurs for every matter-antimatter particle pair interaction and it is known as a pair annihilation. Each of the annihilation photons possesses a high energy (511 keV). This energy is equal to one-half of the energy corresponding to the particle's mass.

Annihilation radiation produces high-energy photon rays with opposite collinear trajectories. This permits a unique opportunity to detect the direction of travel of these photons without the use of a physical collimator. This is performed by placing two positron sensitive detectors on opposite sides of the patient. The simplest PET scanner consists of a circular array of gamma-detector-equipped-electronics that can determine instances of gamma rays being simultaneously incident at two detectors. When two photons strike the two members of an opposing pair of detectors in the sensor ring, the system records a "coincident event." A coincident registration usually implies that the annihilation occurred somewhere along the line defined by the two detectors. These coincidence registrations constitute the raw data upon which the reconstruction of a tomographic slice is based. The PET camera has electronic circuits that can distinguish coincidences from every possible pair of detectors. The set of detector bins aligned on a particular angle define a set of projection lines of the object or a "view."

In order to achieve good spatial resolution, the distance between the projection lines should be rather small. The distance should be no greater than the distance between the closest two points of concentration we wish to distinguish in the reconstructed image. This can be accomplished through the design of cameras with small detectors and placing such cameras with the tightest possible packing arrangement. However, the detectors cannot practically be made arbitrarily small, and a large number of detectors substantially increases the camera's cost. In practice, a typical transaxial resolution in PET is approximately 4 to 6 *mm.* FWHM.

In order to increase spatial resolution many PET scanners have a system of "wobbling" motion. This wobbling consists of a small circular motion (1 *cm.* or less) of the ring detector in such a manner that the detectors cover the missing gaps. Of course, this additional information must be treated in the reconstruction algorithm employed for such a scanner.

The attenuation and scattering of gamma photons within the body make PET a difficult imaging task. In some typical chest PET scans, for example, approximately 15 percent of the annihilation photon pairs "headed" to a particular bin detector are registered; the rest of the photons are attenuated. If no correction approach is implemented, attenuation of photons would lead to an underestimation of the radioisotope concentration. Fortunately, attenuation correction techniques can be applied. One approach consists of introducing an attenuation correction factor in the estimation of the radionuclide concentration. This correction factor is the ratio of the measurement of a detector bin when a positron-emitting source point is placed on one side of the PET scan area and a measurement taken with and without a patient in the PET scanner. A complete attenuation correction is then possible, disposing of the correction factor for all detector pairs.

The problem of scattering is more difficult to treat. If a deflected photon continues traveling in the plane of the ring detector after the scattering, this photon may still hit a detector and generate a false coincidence. An energy window approach similar to that employed for SPECT can be implemented for PET scanning. However, this represents only a partial solution due to the finite accuracy in energy measurement by the scintillation crystals employed in PET. New approaches to scatter correction are currently undergoing active research.

Another factor that complicates PET is the presence of "accidental coincidences." The detection system registers a coincidence event when both detectors of a bin are triggered within some resolving time τ, which is typically measured in nsec. Usually these photons are produced by the same annihilation event. However, it is possible that the system can be "tricked" by photons produced in unrelated annihilations. The rate of accidental coincidences per second N is given by

$$N = 2 \times \tau \times S_1 \times S_2$$

where S_1 and S_2 are the counting rates of each of the detectors. The problem of accidental coincidence rapidly increases with the radionuclide concentration. The rate of counts measured by the detectors is proportional to the concentration value. The influence of accidental coincidence can be reduced by subtracting the computed number of random coincidences using the equation above.

4.3 PET Reconstruction Algorithms

Estimation of the positron-emitter compound distribution $f(x, y, z, t)$ is realized through computational algorithms. These algorithms are provided the number of counts M_i associated with the projection lines L_i. If the period Δt in which the data was collected is short enough and if we proceed to reconstruct one transaxial slice at the time, the problem reduces to the determination of the two dimensional function $f(x, y)$. The basic problem can be stated as follows:

Estimate the function $f(x, y)$ from the system of equations

$$c_i = \int_{Li} f(x, y) ds \quad 1 \leq i \leq I$$

where L_i is the i-th line of the I projection lines (detector bin lines in the PET case); $c_i = M_i / V_i$ depends on the attenuation line integral V_i, which can be calculated either from a hypothetical attenuation coefficient or from an experimental measurement.

Reconstruction algorithms can be divided into back-projection methods, Fourier methods, and iterative methods. The first two methods (transform methods) are the most commonly employed due to relative ease of implementation and low computational cost. The images obtained by transform methods are good enough for a great variety of applications. On the other hand, iterative methods provide greater flexibility in the introduction of attenuation correction information to the algorithm and statistical treatment of the data.

A simple reconstruction scheme is the back-projection process. This method consists of reconstructing each transaxial slice image by a method similar to that described in section 2 for CT machines. The filter employed in this filtered back projection is typically a multiplicative combination in Fourier space of a ramp and another filter, such as the Hamming, Butterworth, or Shepp-Logan filter [18].

Iterative reconstruction methods include the algebraic reconstruction technique (ART), the simultaneous iterative reconstruction technique (SIRT), and the least-squared iterative technique. The first two methods involve the alteration of the estimate of the transaxial image around a circle by adding or subtracting from each point to what is called for. The least-squared iterative technique is based on the minimization of the squared error, which is defined as the square of the difference between the measured and calculated projection. The minimization process is performed by calculating the partial derivatives of the squared error with respect to variables of interest and setting this derivative equal to zero [19].

Shepp and Vardi have presented a reconstruction methodology based on statistical methods [20]. Their method is based on the expectation maximization of the emission distribution. Shepp and Vardi take into account the Poisson statistics of radioactive decay. Convergency to a global maximum is guaranteed by the Shepp-Vardi algorithm. However, approaching this maximum value can be exceedingly slow in some cases.

5. Biomagnetic Source Imaging with Squids

Biomagnetic source imaging is a relatively new medical imaging modality that produces representations of the minute magnetic fields created by neuronal activity within the body [1]. As in the case of ECT, images produced via biomagnetic source imaging provide mappings of functional rather than anatomical information. An important goal of this technology is the ability to localize neuron activity in response to specifically applied sensory stimuli [21].

Biomagnetic source imaging is made possible by a solid-state sensor known as a Superconducting Quantum Interference Device (Squid). Squid sensors can be employed to measure the magnetic fields produced in the brain by neural currents. Given a set of external magnetic measurements, it is desirable to generate a visual mapping of the current densities, in three dimensions, that gave rise to the external magnetic field [21]. It is hoped that Squid technology and biomagnetic source imaging will be of significant assistance to researchers investigating epilepsy, Alzheimer's disease, Parkinson's disease, and schizophrenia [1].

6. Digital Subtraction Angiography

A common problem with the radiograph discussed in section 2 is the poor contrast between anatomical structures. This low-contrast resolution limits the utility of such radiographs severely. However, through the use of digital acquisition systems it is possible to greatly increase the utility of 2D projection radiographs for certain, specific applications. Digital subtraction angiography (DSA) is a modality that exploits the digital acquisition of radiographs to produce high-contrast images of blood vessels.

A common problem with radiograph technology is the fact that many internal tissues are superimposed on each other. The projection nature of the radiograph yields a final image in which it is difficult to delineate individual structures. Wherein a specific structure is analyzed, it would be advantageous to acquire a radiograph which displayed only that structure without any subsequent loss of resolution. This result could be achieved in a digital image if the values of all pixels without information on that structure were set to zero and all pixels corresponding to the structure of interest were allowed to maintain their natural values. While such a result could be obtained using image processing techniques, such as segmentation, the resulting loss in resolution would degrade severely an already poor contrast image. However if two images were taken of a subject, in which the contrast of the anatomical structure of interest changed significantly from one image to the next, excellent results could be achieved. The subtraction of two digital images results in a difference image. This difference image retains only the information that has changed from one image to the other. The digital subtraction of radiographs is the concept underlying DSA [22]. This concept is illustrated with a one-dimensional signal in Figure 21.

The basis for a DSA device consists of an x-ray system very similar to that used for a conventional radiograph. The main difference occurs in the technique used to acquire the radiograph. Conventional radiography utilizes typically a film, which after processing will contain an image proportional to the amount of x-ray energy leaving the patient's body. Subtraction angiography has been practiced employing film technology [23]. However such techniques possess disadvantages, such as the long time interval that takes place between subsequent radiographs. Patient movement during the entire radiograph acquisition sequence creates significant problems for the subtraction process since the methodology is premised on registration between the subtracted images.

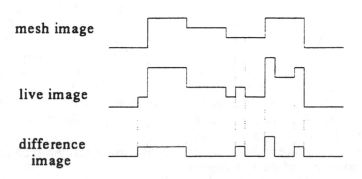

Figure 21. Illustration of DSA signal subtraction concept.

In the case of DSA, the film acquisition apparatus is replaced by a system that can rapidly acquire a high-resolution image of x-ray radiation incident on it. After proper patient positioning, an initial radiograph is taken of a patient. This initial radiograph is called commonly the mask image and contains the base information that will be subtracted from the second image. The mask radiograph is acquired and stored in a computer. A contrast medium is then injected into the patient. This contrast medium is designed to elicit a significant change in the contrast of blood in the vessels of interest. A second radiograph is then taken of the patient with the contrast agent in place. This second image is again acquired and stored in a computer's memory. This image is referred to as the live image in that it contains vessel information that was not present in the mask image. The digital results of these radiographs can now be subtracted and their difference amplified. After subtraction, all information that was in both the mask and live images has been eliminated. The resulting image is now a high-contrast image of the patient's blood vessels in a region of interest. Clinical applications of DSA differ in some ways from the simplistic description above. However such techniques utilized for the improvement of image quality do not affect the underlying methodology described herein.

In the past, prior to the use of digital technology, the above discussed two-image subtraction angiograph encompassed the limits of technology. However, DSA allows for a variety of subtraction techniques including mask or temporal mode subtraction, time difference subtraction, and energy subtraction [23]. All of the subtraction techniques employ the basic methodology discussed previously. Specific DSA subtraction methods differ in the techniques used to select the mask and live images.

The mask or temporal mode subtraction technique seeks to provide a physician with a temporal view of a contrast media through the patient's vessels of interest. When digital acquisition techniques are employed, radiographs can be collected typically as a sequence of images occurring at a fixed time interval (Δt) apart. This method can be utilized to acquire a series of mask radiographs prior to the introduction of the contrast media. One of these mask images is selected as the general mask image $v_g(x,y)$. After the contrast agent is introduced, a series of live digital radiographs $v_i(x,y)$ will be acquired, where i denotes the number of the radiograph in the acquisition sequence. In the subtraction of $v_g(x,y)$ from $v_i(x,y)$ for all values of i, the progress of the contrast media may be viewed temporally. This methodology is limited mainly by patient motion though some correction can be employed via computer-based registration techniques.

A technique referred to as time interval difference subtraction (TID) has been utilized to reduce effects caused by patient motion during the imaging process.

When employing TID, a subtraction is performed continuously between subsequent live images by $v_i - v_{i-1}$. While this method reduces significantly the effects associated with patient motion, it produces images of very poor contrast quality. This poor quality is associated with the closeness of the mask and live images in time. This temporal proximity results in the full contrast that could be generated by the contrast agent not being realized. Due to the summarized drawbacks, the TID technique is not utilized extensively in clinical settings.

Another method that seeks to address the artifacts that can be caused by patient motion and misregistration are energy subtraction methods. Energy subtraction approaches may be subdivided into two subclasses, K-edge subtraction and photoelectric/Compton decomposition.

K-edge subtraction techniques are based upon the x-ray energy absorption properties of the iodine contrast agent that is employed typically in DSA applications. Such contrast agents exhibit excellent energy absorption above the binding energy in the K shell, and little absorption below this K shell [23]. If a radiograph is taken of the patient utilizing x-rays of an energy below this K line, then the contrast agent will not be visible. This image can then be employed as the mask agent for DSA. The patient is then imaged utilizing x-rays above the K line of iodine. This second image will include a high-contrast image of the iodine, which can then be employed as the live image. Digital subtraction can now be performed. Problems associated with this technique involve difficulties in producing proper intensity levels of such monochromatic X-ray photon beams.

A method known as photoelectric/Compton decomposition operates on a principle similar to that of K-edge subtraction. The iodine contrast agent employed commonly for DSA responds differentially to different X-ray photon energy ranges. This knowledge is employed to acquire a mask image and a live image via the utilization of carefully chosen differential energy levels for the X-ray source. Photoelectric/Compton decomposition virtually eliminates effects based on patient motion [23] since the mask and live image are generated only milliseconds apart. The photoelectric decomposition technique requires X-ray generators that can switch rapidly between the required kVp levels.

The major practical difference between the two energy-subtraction-based techniques discussed is the requirements they place on the employed X-ray generator. K-edge subtraction requires difficult-to-produce, monochromatic X-ray beams while the photoelectric subtraction approach employs beams of differing energies. While the decomposition approach utilizes easier-to-produce X-ray beams, it has the disadvantage of a reduction in output signal to noise ratio for low kVp X rays. This drawback is due to the significant attenuation of the low-energy beams by thicker structures in the patient.

7. Ultrasound Imaging

Ultrasound-based imaging techniques comprise a set of methodologies capable of acquiring both quantitative and qualitative diagnostic information. Many ultrasound based methods are attractive due to their ability to obtain real-time imagery employing compact and mobile equipment at a significantly lower cost than is incurred with other medical imaging modalities. The real time nature of ultrasound makes it possible for physicians to observe the motion of structures inside a patient's body. This ability has resulted in the widespread use of ultrasound technology in the fields of pediatrics and cardiology. Equipment that employs Doppler echo techniques can extract quantitative velocity information such as the rate of blood flow in a vessel of interest. Additionally, the introduction of ultrasound signals into a patient at the levels currently employed has been determined to be very safe [2]. The lack of negative exposure effects, portability, relatively low cost, and quantitative acquisition modes makes ultrasound techniques an important class of medical imaging methods.

Ultrasound is classified as sound waves possessing a high temporal frequency. Typical medical instruments for diagnostic ultrasound employ waveforms that oscillate in the range of 1-10 MHz [2]. Such waves can be produced using a single ultrasound transducer or an array of transducers. Ultrasound transducers are capable of producing ultrasound signals when they are excited electrically. Inversely, these transducers produce an electric signal when excited by incident ultrasound rays. Consequently, the same set of ultrasound transducers are typically used for both ultrasound transmission and detection in medical applications.

The sound waves transmitted by the ultrasound transducers are introduced into the patient's body in the area of diagnostic interest. As the waves pass through the body, they travel through differing tissue types with correspondingly differing acoustic properties. At the boundary between two tissue types, a partial reflection of the ultrasound signal will take place. Some portion of the sound waves will be reflected back towards the source transmitter while the remaining portion of the incident ultrasound will continue propagating onward. This process is not idealized in living tissue and results in complex scattering interactions that are out of the scope of this chapter. Reflected waveforms are measured with respect to their time of original transmission by employing the source transducer apparatus as mentioned above. It should be intuitively clear that only waveforms reflected along the incident path will be detectable by the original transducer.

It has been previously mentioned that ultrasound source/detector configurations can consist of a single transducer or an array of transducers. Array-transducer arrangements are often employed in modern medical ultrasound units. These array configurations provide a larger receptor aperture and subsequently improved image reconstruction.

In order to understand the manner in which ultrasound machines acquire images, it is best to first investigate a simple, idealized scenario. One such case might be a task that entails imaging a one-dimensional scene consisting of a single, ideal reflector using a single transmitter located at the origin. If an ultrasound pulse is transmitted at time t_1 and a return pulse is detected at time t_2, then the distance to the target from the transmitter may be calculated as

$$x = \frac{t_2 - t_1}{c}$$

where c is the speed of sound in the instant medium. Extending this approach to medical applications, one can view the body as a series of point sources located at the junctions of tissues with differing characteristic acoustic impedances. Ultrasound units designed to image internal structures for applications such as echographic and pediatric settings are designed to measure the time of reception of ultrasound signals with respect to their time of transmission in real time. This results in the real-time measurement of the distance from the transducer to internal anatomical surfaces, resulting in real-time imagery of these structures.

Information from returned echoes or reflections with respect to time can be presented to the physician in several ways [2]. Two commonly employed techniques are time-amplified and brightness-mode displays. Time-amplified or *A-mode* displays present the amplitudes of the returned ultrasound signals with respect to their time of return as a series of one-dimensional spikes of varying height. Brightness or *B mode* displays present the same data on a single line. The brightness of each point on this line indicates the signal amplitude detected at that time or depth. If an array of detectors is employed with the proper mechanisms, then it is possible to generate a series of B-mode scan lines. The combination of these scan lines results in a 2D fan like view. This 2D view can be generated in real time allowing for the detection and viewing of moving internal structures such as a beating heart. Another mode of image presentation commonly referred to is time motion or *M mode*. M mode employs a display of B-mode lines with respect to a time axis acquired by moving the source/transmitter wand across the area of interest [24].

Quantitative information can be extracted from echo reflections through an understanding and utilization of the Doppler effect. In short, when a signal with frequency f_0 and propagating at speed v_c is reflected from a target moving at a speed v_t, then the frequency of the echoed signal received at the ultrasound detector is shifted by a factor described by the Doppler principle. The frequency of the transmitted wave is shifted by a factor of

$$fd = \frac{2v_c f_0}{v_t}$$

where f_d is the approximate, detected Doppler frequency shift and $f_r = f_d + f_0$, where f_r is the actual frequency received at the detector.

An area in which Doppler techniques are commonly employed is Doppler echocardiography. Doppler echocardiography allows the measurement of the velocity and direction of blood flow at a fixed distance from the ultrasound transducer within a patient's body. The Doppler-shifted frequencies to be measured are produced by the reflection of injected ultrasound waves from flowing red blood cells in the vessels of interest. When utilizing the method of pulsed Doppler echocardiography, short bursts of ultrasound are introduced into the patient. Pulsed-echo techniques keep the target distance fixed and retrieve velocity measurements for targets located at that distance. Since the desired distance of measurement is fixed, the expected echo time is also fixed. Echoes not received in a neighborhood of this expected echo time are not processed by the imaging instrumentation. This technique is often referred to as range gating [2]. An alternative Doppler technique is continuous wave Doppler. When this method is employed, ultrasound is continuously injected into the patient. Such an approach is advantageous in that it allows for very accurate, high-velocity measurements. Unfortunately, when continuous Doppler is employed, the depth at which the velocity is being measured cannot be determined due to the fact that no range gating takes place. For either of the Doppler principle-based techniques, the echoed signal's frequency components are measured to determine the Doppler frequency shift using the fast Fourier transform (FFT).

8. Conclusion

Advancing technology is steadily increasing the radiologist's ability to learn accurate and precise information about a patient in a noninvasive manner. Current medical imaging modalities are capable of acquiring data on internal anatomical structures, as well as mappings of physiological function. Advanced software reconstruction algorithms and analytic techniques seek to maximize the information derived from current medical modalities while driving the development of even more advanced technologies.

An overview has been provided of some of the more popular medical imaging modalities currently in clinical use. It is hoped that a general understanding of the modality from which an image is derived will help researchers in the subsequent analysis of the image data.

References

[1] "Biomagnetic Source Imaging with Squids: A New Method for Functional Brain Diagnosis," *Cryogenic News,* Vol. 30, Aug. 1990, p. 740.

[2] E.A. Geiser and L.H. Oliver, "Echocardiography: Physics and instrumentation," in *Cardiac Imaging and Image Processing*, S.M. Collins and D.J. Skorton, eds., McGraw Hill, New York, N.Y., 1986, pp. 3–23.

[3] P. Sprawls, "The Principles of Computed Tomography, Image Formation and Quality," in *Essentials of Body Computed Tomography*, R.K. Gedgaudas-McClees and W.E. Torres, eds., W.B. Saunders Company, Philadelphia, Penn., 1990, pp. 1–9.

[4] A.K. Jain. *Fundamentals of Digital Image Processing*. Prentice Hall, N.J., 1989.

[5] R.A. Robb et al., "High Speed 3d X-ray CT: The Dynamic Spatial Reconstructor," *Proc. IEEE*, Vol. 71, No. 3, Mar. 1983, pp. 308–319.

[6] R.S. Acharya et al., "High Speed 3d Imaging of the Beating Heart Using Temporal Estimation, *Computer Vision Graphics and Image Processing*, Sept. 1987, pp. 259–270.

[7] D.P. Boyd and D.W. Farmer, "Cardiac Computed Tomography," in *Cardiac Imaging and Image Processing,* S.M. Collins and D.J. Skorton, eds., McGraw Hill, New York, N.Y., 1986, pp. 57–87.

[8] R.R. Edelman, M.D. and J.R. Hesselink, M.D., *Clinical Magnetic Resonance Imaging*. W.B. Saunders Co., Toronto, Canada, 1990.

[9] D.D. Stark and W.G. Bradly, Jr., *Magnetic Resonance Imaging*, Mosby Year Book, Toronto, Canada, 2nd ed., 1992.

[10] D. Kean and M. Smith, *Magnetic Resonance Imaging*, Williams and Wilkins, Baltimore, Md., 1986.

[11] D.W. Chakeres and P. Schmalbrock, *Fundamentals of Magnetic Resonance Imaging*. Williams and Wilkins, Baltimore, Md., 1992.

[12] K.F. King and P.R. Moran, "A Unified Description of NMR Imaging, Data Collection Strategies and Reconstruction," *Medical Physics*, Vol. 11, No. 1, Jan/Feb 1984.

[13] S. Riederer, "Recent Advances in Magnetic Resonance Imaging, *Proc. IEEE*, Vol. 76, No. 9, Sept. 1988.

[14] E.A. Zerhouni, MD et al., "Human Heart: Tagging with MR Imaging—A Method for Noninvasive Assessment of Myocardial Motion," *Radiology*, Vol. 169, 1988, pp. 59–63.

[15] L. Axel Ph.D., M.D. and L. Dougherty, "MR Imaging of Motion with Spatial Modulation of Magnetization," *Radiology*, Vol. 171, 1989, pp. 841–845.

[16] B.D Bolster, E.R. McVeigh, Ph.D., and E.A. Zerhouni, MD, "Myocardial Tagging in Polar Coordinates with Use of Striped Tags," *Radiology*, Vol. 177, 1990, pp. 769–772.

[17] W.H. Oldendorf and W. Oldendorf Jr., *Basics of Magnetic Resonance Imaging*, Martinus Nijhoff, Boston, Mass., 1988.

[18] G.T. Herman, *Image Reconstruction from Projections: Implementation and Applications,* Academic Press, New York, N.Y., 1980.

[19] Budinger and Gullberg, "Three-Dimensional Reconstruction in Nuclear Medicine Emission Imaging, *IEEE Trans. Nuclear Science*, Vol. 21, 1974, pp. 2–20.

[20] L.A. Shepp and Y. Vardi, "Maximum Likelihood Reconstruction for Emission Tomography," *IEEE Trans. Medical Imaging*, Vol. MI1, No. 2, Oct. 1982, pp. 113–121.

[21] J.C. Mosher, P.S. Lewis, and R.M. Leahy, "Multiple Dipole Modeling and Localization from Spatio-Temporal MEG Data," *IEEE Trans. Biomedical Engineering*, Vol. 39, No. 6, June 1992, pp. 541–559.

[22] R.A. Kruger and S.J. Riederer, *Basic Concepts of Digital Subtraction Angiography,* G.K. Hall Medical Publishers, Boston, Mass., 1984.

[23] T. Villafana, "Basic Physics and Instrumentation for Digital Subtraction Angiography, in *Digital Subtraction Imaging in Infants and Children*, E.N. Faerber, ed., Futura Publishing Company, Inc., Mount Kisco, N.Y., 1989, pp. 1–36.

[24] H. Feigenbaum, *Echocardiography*, 5th ed., Lea and Febiger, Philadelphia, Penn., 1994.

Snakes: Active Contour Models

MICHAEL KASS, ANDREW WITKIN, and DEMETRI TERZOPOULOS
Schlumberger Palo Alto Research, 3340 Hillview Ave., Palo Alto, CA 94304

Abstract

A snake is an energy-minimizing spline guided by external constraint forces and influenced by image forces that pull it toward features such as lines and edges. Snakes are active contour models: they lock onto nearby edges, localizing them accurately. Scale-space continuation can be used to enlarge the capture region surrounding a feature. Snakes provide a unified account of a number of visual problems, including detection of edges, lines, and subjective contours; motion tracking; and stereo matching. We have used snakes successfully for interactive interpretation, in which user-imposed constraint forces guide the snake near features of interest.

1 Introduction

In recent computational vision research, low-level tasks such as edge or line detection, stereo matching, and motion tracking have been widely regarded as autonomous bottom-up processes. Marr and Nishihara [11], in a strong statement of this view, say that up to the 2.5D sketch, no "higher-level" information is yet brought to bear: the computations proceed by utilizing only what is available in the image itself. This rigidly sequential approach propagates mistakes made at a low level without opportunity for correction. It therefore imposes stringent demands on the reliability of low-level mechanisms. As a weaker but more attainable goal for low-level processing, we argue that it ought to provide sets of alternative organizations among which higher-level processes may choose, rather than shackling them prematurely with a unique answer.

In this paper we investigate the use of energy minimization as a framework within which to realize this goal. We seek to design energy functions whose local minima comprise the set of alternative solutions available to higher-level processes. The choice among these alternatives could require some type of search or high-level reasoning. In the absence of a well-developed high-level mechanism, however, we use an interactive approach to explore the alternative organizations. By adding suitable energy terms to the minimization, it is possible for a user to push the model out of a local minimum toward the desired solution. The result is an active model that falls into the desired solution when placed near it.

Energy minimizing models have a rich history in vision going back at least to Sperling's stereo model [16]. Such models have typically been regarded as autonomous, but we have developed interactive techniques for guiding them. Interacting with such models allows us to explore the energy landscape very easily and develop effective energy functions that have few local minima and little dependence on starting points. We hope thereby to make the job of high-level interpretation manageable yet not constrained unnecessarily by irreversible low-level decisions.

The problem domain we address is that of finding salient image contours—edges, lines, and subjective contours—as well as tracking those contours during motion and matching them in stereopsis. Our variational approach to finding image contours differs from the traditional approach of detecting edges and then linking them. In our model, issues such as the connectivity of the contours and the presence of corners affect the energy functional and hence the detailed structure of the locally optimal contour. These issues can, in principle, be resolved by very high-

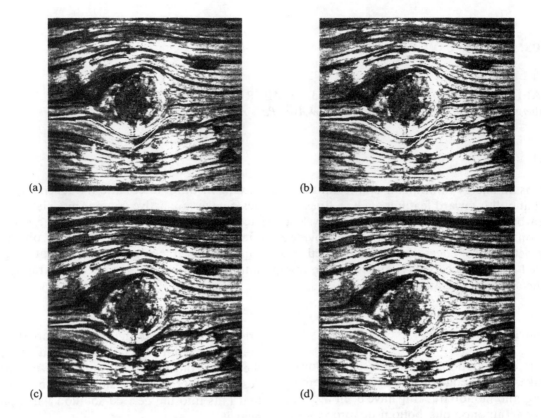

Fig. 1. Lower-left: Original wood photograph from Brodatz. Others: Three different local minima for the active contour model.

level computations. Perhaps more importantly, high-level mechanisms can interact with the contour model by pushing it toward an appropriate local minimum. Optimization and relaxation have been used previously in edge and line detection, [3,5,13,24,25], but without the interactive guiding used here.

In many image interpretation tasks, the correct interpretation of low-level events can require high-level knowledge. Consider, for example, the three perceptual organizations of two dark lines in figure 1. The three different organizations correspond to three different local minima in our line-contour model. It is important to notice that the shapes of the lines are materially different in the three examples, not just because of a different linking of line segments. The segments themselves are changed by the perceptual organization.

Without detailed knowledge about the object in view, it is difficult to justify a choice among the three interpretations. Knowing that wood is a layered structure, or perhaps inferring its layered structure from elsewhere in the picture could help to rule out interpretation (b). Beyond that, the 'correct' interpretation could be very task dependent. In many domains, such as analyzing seismic data, the choice of interpretation can depend on expert knowledge. Different seismic interpreters can derive significantly different perceptual organizations from the same seismic sections depending on their knowledge and training. Because a single 'correct' interpretation cannot always be defined, we suggest low-level mechanisms which seek appropriate local minima instead of searching for global minima.

Unlike most other techniques for finding salient contours, our model is *active*. It is always minimizing its energy functional and therefore exhibits dynamic behavior. Because of the way the contours slither while minimizing their energy, we call them snakes. Changes in high-level interpretation can exert forces on a snake as it continues its minimization. Even in the absence of such forces, snakes exhibit hysteresis when exposed to moving stimuli.

Snakes do not try to solve the entire problem of finding salient image contours. They rely on other mechanisms to place them somewhere near the desired contour. However, even in cases where no satisfactory automatic starting mechanism exists, snakes can still be used for semi-automatic image interpretation. If an expert user pushes a snake close to an intended contour, its energy minimization will carry it the rest of the way. The minimization provides a 'power assist' for a person pointing to a contour feature.

Snakes are an example of a more general technique of matching a deformable model to an image by means of energy minimization. In spirit and motivation, this idea shares much with the rubber templates of Widrow [23]. From any starting point, the snake deforms itself into conformity with the nearest salient contour. We have applied the same basic techniques to the problem of 3D object reconstruction from silhouettes by using energy minimizing surfaces with preferred symmetries [17]. We expect this general approach will find a wide range of applicability in vision.

In section 2 we present a basic mathematical description of snakes along with their Euler equations. Then in section 3 we give details of the energy terms that can make a snake attracted to different types of important static, monocular features such as lines, edges, and subjective contours. Section 4 addresses the applicability of snake models to stereo correspondence and motion tracking. Finally, section 5 discusses further refinements and directions of our current work.

2 Basic Snake Behavior

Our basic snake model is a *controlled continuity* [18] spline under the influence of image forces and external constraint forces. The internal spline forces serve to impose a piecewise smoothness constraint. The image forces push the snake toward salient image features like lines, edges, and subjective contours. The external constraint forces are responsible for putting the snake near the desired local minimum. These forces can, for example, come from a user interface, automatic attentional mechanisms, or high-level interpretations.

Representing the position of a snake parametrically by $\mathbf{v}(s) = (x(s), y(s))$, we can write its energy functional as

$$E^*_{\text{snake}} = \int_0^1 E_{\text{snake}}(\mathbf{v}(s)) \, ds$$

$$= \int_0^1 E_{\text{int}}(\mathbf{v}(s)) + E_{\text{image}}(\mathbf{v}(s))$$

$$+ E_{\text{con}}(\mathbf{v}(s)) \, ds \qquad (1)$$

where E_{int} represent the internal energy of the spline due to bending, E_{image} gives rise to the image forces, and E_{con} gives rise to the external constraint forces. In this section, we develop E_{int} and give examples of E_{con} for interactive interpretation. E_{image} is developed in section 3.

2.1 Internal Energy

The internal spline energy can be written

$$E_{\text{int}} = (\alpha(s)|\mathbf{v}_s(s)|^2 + \beta(s)|\mathbf{v}_{ss}(s)|^2)/2 \qquad (2)$$

The spline energy is composed of a first-order term controlled by $\alpha(s)$ and a second-order term controlled by $\beta(s)$. The first-order term makes the snake act like a membrane and the second-order term makes it act like a thin plate. Adjusting the weights $\alpha(s)$ and $\beta(s)$ controls the relative importance of the membrane and thin-plate terms. Setting $\beta(s)$ to zero at a point allows the snake to become second-order discontinuous and develop a corner. The controlled continuity spline is a generalization of a Tikonov stabilizer [19] and can formally be regarded as *regularizing* [14,15] the problem.

Details of our minimization procedure are given in the appendix. The procedure is an $O(n)$ iterative technique using sparse matrix methods. Each iteration effectively takes implicit Euler steps with respect to the internal energy and explicit Euler steps with respect to the image and external constraint energy. The numeric considerations are relatively important. In a fully explicit Euler method, it takes $O(n^2)$ iterations each of $O(n)$ time for an impulse to travel down the length of a snake. The resulting snakes are flaccid. In order to erect more rigid snakes, it is vital to use a more stable method that can accommodate the large internal forces. Our semi-implicit method allows forces to travel the entire length of a snake in a single $O(n)$ iteration.

2.2 Snake Pit

In order to experiment with different energy functions for low-level visual tasks, we have developed a user-interface for snakes on a Symbolics Lisp Machine. The interface allows a user to select starting points and exert forces on snakes interactively as they minimize their energy. In addition to its value as a research tool, the user-interface has proven very useful for semiautomatic image interpretation. In order to specify a particular image feature, the user has

only to push a snake near the feature. Once close enough, the energy minimization will pull the snake in the rest of the way. Accurate tracking of contour features can be specified in this way with little more effort than pointing. The snake energy minimization provides a 'power assist' for image interpretation.

Our interface allows the user to connect a spring to any point on a snake. The other end of the spring can be anchored at a fixed position, connected to another point on a snake, or dragged around using the mouse. Creating a spring between x_1 and x_2 simply adds $-k(x_1 - x_2)^2$ to the external constraint energy E_{con}.

In addition to springs, the user interface provides a $1/r^2$ repulsion force controllable by the mouse. The $1/r$ energy functional is clipped near $r = 0$ to prevent numerical instability, so the resulting potential is depicted by a volcano icon. The volcano is very useful for pushing a snake out of one local minimum and into another.

Figure 2 shows the snake-pit interface being

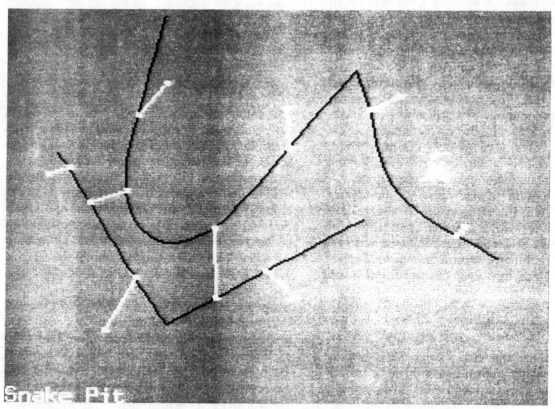

Fig. 2. The Snake Pit user-interface. Snakes are shown in black, springs and the volcano are in white.

used. The two dark lines are different snakes which the user has connected with two springs shown in white. The other springs attach points on the snakes to fixed positions on the screen. In the upper right, the volcano can be seen bending a nearby snake. Each of the snakes has a sharp corner which has been specified by the user.

3 Image Forces

In order to make snakes useful for early vision we need energy functionals that attract them to salient features in images. In this section, we present three different energy functionals which attract a snake to lines, edges, and terminations. The total image energy can be expressed as a weighted combination of the three energy functionals

$$E_{\text{image}} = w_{\text{line}}E_{\text{line}} + w_{\text{edge}}E_{\text{edge}} + w_{\text{term}}E_{\text{term}}$$

$$(3)$$

By adjusting the weights, a wide range of snake behavior can be created.

3.1 Line Functional

The simplest useful image functional is the image intensity itself. If we set

$$E_{\text{line}} = I(x, y) \qquad (4)$$

then depending on the sign of w_{line}, the snake will be attracted either to light lines or dark lines. Subject to its other constraints, the snake will try to align itself with the lightest or darkest nearby contour. This energy functional was used with the snakes shown in figure 1. By pushing with the

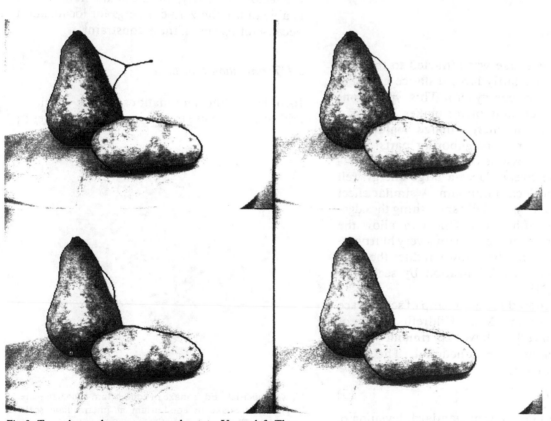

Fig. 3. Two edge snakes on a pear and potato. Upper-left: The user has pulled one of the snakes away from the edge of the pear. Others: After the user lets go, the snake snaps back to the edge of the pear.

volcano, a user can rapidly move a snake from one of these positions to another. The coarse control necessary to do so suggests that symbolic attentional mechanisms might be able to guide a snake effectively.

3.2 Edge Functional

Finding edges in an image can also be done with a very simple energy functional. If we set $E_{edge} = -|\nabla I(x,y)|^2$, then the snake is attracted to contours with large image gradients. An example of the use of this functional is shown in figure 3. In the upper left, a user has placed two snakes on the edges of the pear and potato. He has then pulled part of the snake off the pear with a spring. The remaining pictures show what happens when he lets go. The snake snaps back rapidly to the boundary of the pear.

3.3 Scale Space

In figure 3, the snake was attracted to the pear boundary from a fairly large distance away because of the spline energy term. This type of convergence is rather common for snakes. If part of a snake finds a low-energy image feature, the spline term will pull neighboring parts of the snake toward a possible continuation of the feature. This effectively places a large energy well around a good local minimum. A similar effect can be achieved by spatially smoothing the edge- or line-energy functional. One can allow the snake to come to equilibrium on a very blurry energy functional and then slowly reduce the blurring. The result is minimization by scale-continuation [20,21].

In order to show the relationship of scale-space continuation to the Marr–Hildreth theory of edge-detection [10], we have experimented with a slightly different edge functional. The edge-energy functional is

$$E_{line} = -(G_\sigma * \nabla^2 I)^2 \tag{5}$$

where G_σ is a Gaussian of standard deviation σ. Minima of this functional lie on zero-crossings of $G_\sigma * \nabla^2 I$ which define edges in the Marr–

Hildreth theory. Adding this energy term to a snake means that the snake is attracted to zero-crossings, but still constrained by its own smoothness. Figure 4 shows scale-space continuation applied to this energy functional. The upper left shows the snake in equilibrium at a very coarse scale. Since the edge-energy function is very blurred, the snake does a poor job of localizing the edge, but is attracted to this local minimum from very far away. Slowly reducing the blurring leads the snake to the position shown in the upper right and finally to the position shown in the lower left. For reference, the zero-crossings of $G_\sigma * \nabla^2 I$ corresponding to the energy function of the snake in the lower left are shown superimposed on the same snake in the lower right. Note that the snake jumps from one piece of a zero-crossing contour to another. At this scale, the shapes of the zero-crossings are dominated by the small-scale texture rather than the region boundary, but the snake nevertheless is able to use the zero-crossings for localization because of its smoothness constraint.

3.4 Termination Functional

In order to find terminations of line segments and corners, we use the curvature of level lines in

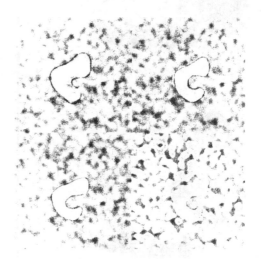

Fig. 4. Upper-left: Edge snake in equilibrium at coarse scale. Upper-right: Snake in equilibrium at intermediate scale. Lower-left: Final snake equilibrium after scale-space continuation. Lower-right: Zero-crossings overlayed on final snake position.

a slightly smoothed image. Let $C(x, y) = G_\sigma(x, y) * I(x, y)$ be a slightly smoothed version of the image. Let $\theta = \tan^{-1}(C_y/C_x)$ be the gradient angle and let $\mathbf{n} = (\cos\theta, \sin\theta)$ and $\mathbf{n}_\perp = (-\sin\theta, \cos\theta)$ be unit vectors along and perpendicular to the gradient direction. Then the curvature of the level contours in $C(x, y)$ can be written

$$E_{\text{term}} = \frac{\partial\theta}{\partial\mathbf{n}_\perp} \tag{6}$$

$$= \frac{\partial^2 C/\partial\mathbf{n}_\perp^2}{\partial C/\partial\mathbf{n}} \tag{7}$$

$$= \frac{C_{yy}C_x^2 - 2C_{xy}C_xC_y + C_{xx}C_y^2}{(C_x^2 + C_y^2)^{3/2}} \tag{8}$$

By combining E_{edge} and E_{term}, we can create a snake that is attracted to edges or terminations. Figure 5 shows an example of such a snake exposed to a standard subjective contour illusion [7]. The shape of the snake contour between the edges and lines in the illusion is entirely determined by the spline smoothness term. The variational problem solved by the snake is very closely related to a variational formulation proposed by Brady et al. [2] for the interpolation of subjective contours. Ullman's [22] proposal of interpolating

using piecewise circular arcs would probably also produce a very similar interpolation. An appealing aspect of the snake model is that the same snake that finds subjective contours can very effectively find more traditional edges in natural imagery. It may, moreover, provide some insight into why the ability to see subjective contours is important.

A further unusual aspect of the snake model that bears on the psychophysics of subjective contours is hystheresis. Since snakes are constantly minimizing their energy, they can exhibit hysteresis when shown moving stimuli. Figure 6 shows a snake tracking a moving subjective contour. As the horizontal line segment on the right moves over, the snake bends more and more until the internal spline forces overpower the image forces. Then the snake falls off the line and reverts to a smoother shape. Bringing the line segment close enough to the snake makes the snake reattach. While it is difficult to show the hysteresis in a still picture, the reader can easily verify the corresponding hysteresis in human vision by recreating the moving stimulus. This type of hysteresis is uncharacteristic of purely bottom-up processes and global optimizations.

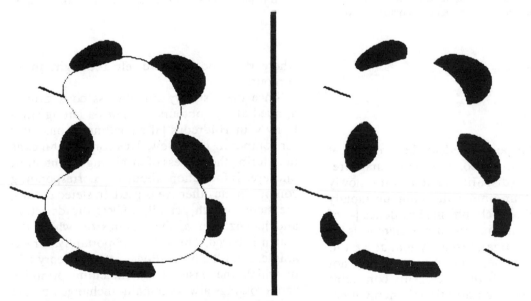

Fig. 5. Right: Standard subjective contour illusion. Left: Edge/termination snake in equilibrium on the subjective contour.

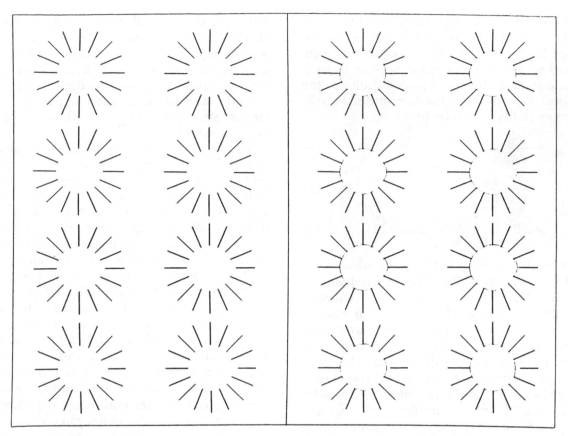

Fig. 6. Above left: Dynamic subjective contour illusion. Sequence is left to right, top to bottom. Above Right: Snake attracted to edges and terminations. As the moving horizontal line slides to the right, the snake bends until it falls off the line. Bringing the line close enough makes the snake reattach.

4 Stereo and Motion

4.1 Stereo

Snakes can also be applied to the problem of stereo matching. In stereo, if two contours correspond, then the disparity should vary slowly along the contour unless the contour rapidly recedes in depth. Psychophysical evidence [4] of a disparity gradient limit in human stereopsis indicates that the human visual system at least to some degree assumes that disparities do not change too rapidly with space. This constraint can be expressed in an additional energy functional for a stereo snake:

$$E_{\text{stereo}} = (\mathbf{v}_s^L(s) - \mathbf{v}_s^R(s))^2 \tag{9}$$

where $\mathbf{v}^L(s)$ and $\mathbf{v}^R(s)$ are left and right snake contours.

Since the disparity smoothness constraint is applied along contours, it shares a strong similarity with Hildreth's [8] smoothness constraint for computing optic flow. This constraint means that during the process of localizing a contour in one eye, information about the corresponding contour in the other eye is used. In stereo snakes, the stereo match actually affects the detection and localization of the features on which the match is based. This differs importantly, for example, from the Marr–Poggio stereo theory [12] in which the basic stereo matching primitive zero-crossings always remain unchanged by the matching process.

Figure 7 shows an example of a 3D surface reconstructed from disparities measured along a

52

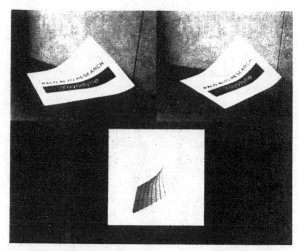

Fig. 7. Bottom: Stereogram of a bent piece of paper. Below: Surface reconstruction from the outline of the paper matched using stereo snakes. The surface model is rendered from a very different viewpoint than the original to emphasize that it is a full 3D model, rather than a 2.5D model.

single stereo snake on the outline of a piece of paper. The surface is rendered from a very different viewpoint than the original to emphasize that a 3D model of the piece of paper has been computed rather than merely a 2.5D model.

4.2 Motion

Once a snake finds a salient visual feature, it 'locks on.' If the feature then begins to move slowly, the snake will simply track the same local minimum. Movement that is too rapid can cause a snake to flip into a different local minimum, but for ordinary speeds and video-rate sampling, snakes do a good job of tracking motion. Figure 8 shows eight selected frames out of a two-second video sequence. Edge-attracted snakes were initialized by hand on the speaker's lips in the first frame. After that, the snakes tracked the lip movements automatically.

The motion tracking was done in this case without any interframe constraints. Introducing such constraints will doubtless make the tracking

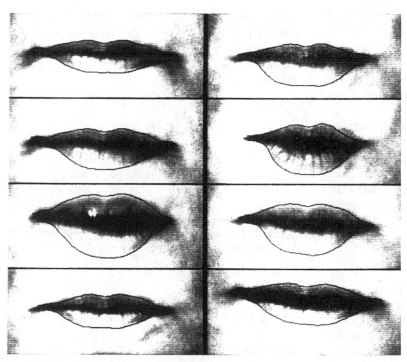

Fig. 8. Selected frames from a 2-second video sequence showing snakes used for motion tracking. After being initialized to the speaker's lips in the first frame, the snakes automatically track the lip movements with high accuracy.

more robust. A simple way to do so is to give the snake mass. Then the snake will predict its next position based on its previous velocity.

5 Conclusion

Snakes have proven useful for interactive specification of image contours. We have begun to use them as a basis for interactively matching 3D models to images. As we develop better energy functionals the 'power assist' of snakes becomes increasingly effective. Scale-space continuation can greatly enlarge the capture region around features of interest.

The snake model provides a unified treatment to a collection of visual problems that have been treated differently in the past. Edges, lines, and subjective contours can all be found by essentially the same mechanisms. Tracking these features through motion and matching them in stereo is easily handled in the same framework.

Snakes, perhaps, embody Marr's notion of 'least commitment' [9] more than his bottom-up 2.5D sketch. The snake provides a number of widely separated local minima to further levels of processing. Instead of committing irrevocably to a single interpretation, snakes can change their interpretation based on additional evidence from higher levels of processing. They can, for example, adjust monocular edge-finding based on binocular matches.

We believe that the ability to have all levels of visual processing influence the lowest-level visual interpretations will turn out to be very important. Local energy-minimizing systems like snakes offer an attractive method for doing this. The energy minimization leaves a much simpler problem for higher level processing.

Acknowledgments

Kurt Fleischer helped greatly with the snake pit user-interface and created the all-important volcano icon. John Platt helped us develop snake theory and guided us around the infinite abyss of numerical methods. Snake-lips Atkinson provided the visual motion stimulus.

Appendix: Numerical Methods

Let $E_{ext} = E_{image} + E_{con}$. When $\alpha(s) = \alpha$, and $\beta(s) = \beta$ are constants, minimizing the energy functional of equation (1) gives rise to the following two independent Euler equations:

$$\alpha x_{ss} + \beta x_{ssss} + \frac{\partial E_{ext}}{\partial x} = 0 \qquad (10)$$

$$\alpha y_{ss} + \beta y_{ssss} + \frac{\partial E_{ext}}{\partial y} = 0 \qquad (11)$$

When $\alpha(s)$ and $\beta(s)$ are not constant, it is simpler to go directly to a discrete formulation of the energy functional in equation (2). Then we can write

$$E^*_{snake} = \sum_{i=1}^{n} E_{int}(i) + E_{ext}(i) \qquad (12)$$

Approximating the derivatives with finite differences and converting to vector notation with $\mathbf{v}_i = (x_i, y_i) = (x(ih), y(ih))$, we expand $E_{int}(i)$

$$E_{int}(i) = \alpha_i |\mathbf{v}_i - \mathbf{v}_{i-1}|^2 / 2h^2$$
$$+ \beta_i |\mathbf{v}_{i-1} - 2\mathbf{v}_i + \mathbf{v}_{i+1}|^2 / 2h^4 \qquad (13)$$

where we define $\mathbf{v}(0) = \mathbf{v}(n)$. Let $f_x(i) = \partial E_{ext}/\partial x_i$ and $f_y(i) = \partial E_{ext}/\partial y_i$ where the derivatives are approximated by a finite difference if they cannot be computed analytically. Now the corresponding Euler equations are

$$\alpha_i(\mathbf{v}_i - \mathbf{v}_{i-1}) - \alpha_{i+1}(\mathbf{v}_{i+1} - \mathbf{v}_i)$$
$$+ \beta_{i-1}[\mathbf{v}_{i-2} - 2\mathbf{v}_{i-1} + \mathbf{v}_i]$$
$$- 2\beta_i[\mathbf{v}_{i-1} - 2\mathbf{v}_i + \mathbf{v}_{i+1}]$$
$$+ \beta_{i+1}[\mathbf{v}_i - 2\mathbf{v}_{i+1} + \mathbf{v}_{i+2}]$$
$$+ (f_x(i), f_y(i)) = 0 \qquad (14)$$

The above Euler equations can be written in matrix form as

$$\mathbf{Ax} + \mathbf{f}_x(\mathbf{x}, \mathbf{y}) = 0 \qquad (15)$$

$$\mathbf{Ay} + \mathbf{f}_y(\mathbf{x}, \mathbf{y}) = 0 \qquad (16)$$

where $\mathbf{A}$ is a pentadiagonal banded matrix.

To solve equations (15) and (16), we set the right-hand sides of the equations equal to the product of a step size and the negative time derivatives of the left-hand sides. Taking into account derivatives of the external forces we use requires changing **A** at each iteration, so we achieve faster iteration by simply assuming that $\mathbf{f}_x$ and $\mathbf{f}_y$ are constant during a time step. This yields an explicit Euler method with respect to the external forces. The internal forces, however, are completely specified by the banded matrix, so we can evaluate the time derivative at time t rather than time $t - 1$ and therefore arrive at an implicit Euler step for the internal forces. The resulting equations are

$$\mathbf{A}\mathbf{x}_t + \mathbf{f}_x(\mathbf{x}_{t-1}, \mathbf{y}_{t-1}) = -\gamma(\mathbf{x}_t - \mathbf{x}_{t-1}) \qquad (17)$$

$$\mathbf{A}\mathbf{y}_t + \mathbf{f}_y(\mathbf{x}_{t-1}, \mathbf{y}_{t-1}) = -\gamma(\mathbf{y}_t - \mathbf{y}_{t-1}) \qquad (18)$$

where γ is a step size. At equilibrium, the time derivative vanishes and we end up with a solution of equations (15) and (16).

Equations (17) and (18) can be solved by matrix inversion:

$$\mathbf{x}_t = (\mathbf{A} + \gamma\mathbf{I})^{-1}(\mathbf{x}_{t-1} - \mathbf{f}_x(x_{t-1}, y_{t-1})) \qquad (19)$$

$$\mathbf{y}_t = (\mathbf{A} + \gamma\mathbf{I})^{-1}(\mathbf{y}_{t-1} - \mathbf{f}_y(x_{t-1}, y_{t-1})) \qquad (20)$$

The matrix $\mathbf{A} + \gamma\mathbf{I}$ is a pentadiagonal banded matrix, so its inverse can be calculated by *LU* decompositions in $O(n)$ time [6,1]. Hence equations (19) and (20) provide a rapid solution to equations (15) and (16). The method is implicit with respect to the internal forces, so it can solve very rigid snakes with large step sizes. If the external forces become large, however, the explicit Euler steps of the external forces will require much smaller step sizes.

References

1. A. Benson, and D.J. Evans, ACM TRANS. MATHEMATICAL SOFTWARE, vol. 3, pp. 96–103, 1977.
2. M. Brady, W.E.L. Grimson, and D. Langridge, "Shape encoding and subjective contours," PROC. AM. ASSOC. ARTIF. INTEL., Stanford University, 1980.
3. D.J. Burr, "Elastic matching of line drawings," IEEE TRANS. PAMI-8, p. 708, 1986.
4. P. Burt, and B. Julesz, "A disparity gradient limit for binocular fusion," SCIENCE, vol. 208, pp. 615–617, 1980.
5. M.A. Fischler, and R.A. Elschlager, "The representation and matching of pictorial structure," IEEE TRANS. ON COMPUTERS, vol. C-22, pp. 67–92, 1973.
6. I. Gladwell, and R. Wait (eds.), A SURVEY OF NUMERICAL METHODS FOR PARTIAL DIFFEREN-TIAL EQUATIONS. Clarendon: Oxford, 1979.
7. Kanisza, "Subjective contours," SCIENTIFIC AMERICAN, vol. 234, pp. 48–52, 1976.
8. E. Hildreth, "The computation of the velocity field," PROC. ROY. SOC. (LONDON), vol. B221, pp. 189–220.
9. D. Marr, VISION. Freeman: San Francisco, 1982.
10. D. Marr and E. Hildreth, "A theory of edge detection," PROC. ROY. SOC. (LONDON), vol. B207, pp. 187–217, 1980.
11. D. Marr and H.K. Nishihara, "Visual information processing: Artificial Intelligence and the sensorium of sight," TECHNOLOGY REVIEW, vol. 81(1), October 1978.
12. D. Marr and T. Poggio, "A computational theory of human stereo vision," PROC. ROY. SOC. (LONDON), vol. B204, pp. 301–328, 1979.
13. A. Martelli, "An application of heuristic search methods to edge and contour detection," CACM, vol. 19, p. 73, 1976.
14. T. Poggio and V. Toree, "Ill-posed problems and regularization analysis in early vision," PROC. AARPA Image Understanding Workshop, New Orleans, L.A., Baumann (ed.), pp. 257–263, 1984.
15. T. Poggio, V. Toree, and C. Koch, "Computational vision and regularization theory," NATURE, vol. 317(6035), pp. 314–319, 1985.
16. G. Sperling, "Binocular vision: a physical and a neural theory," AM. J. PSYCHOLOGY, vol. 83, pp. 461–534, 1970.
17. D. Terzopoulos, A. Witkin, and M. Kass, "Symmetry-seeking models for 3D object reconstruction," INT. J. COMPUTER VISION, vol. 3, 1987.
18. D. Terzopoulos, "Regularization of inverse visual problems involving discontinuities," IEEE TRANS. PAMI-8, p. 413, 1986.
19. A.N. Tikhonov, "Regularization of incorrectly posed problems," SOV. MATH. DOKL., vol. 4, pp. 1624–1627, 1963.
20. A. Witkin, "Scale space filtering," PROC. EIGHTH INT. JOINT CONF. ARTIF. INTEL., Karlsruhe, pp. 1019–1021, 1983.
21. A. Witkin, D. Terzopoulos, and M. Kass, "Signal matching through scale space," PROC. AM. ASSOC. ARTIF. INTEL., Philadelphia, pp. 714–719, 1986.
22. S. Ullman, "Filling the gaps: The shape of subjective contours and a model for their generation," BIOLOGICAL CYBERNETICS, vol. 25, 1976.
23. B. Widrow, "The rubber mask technique, parts I and II," PATTERN RECOGNITION, vol. 5, pp. 175–211, 1973.
24. S. Zucker, R. Hummel, and A. Rosenfeld, "An application of relaxation labeling to line and curve enhancement," IEEE TRANS. ON COMPUTERS, vol. C-26, p. 394, 1977.
25. S. Zucker, "Computational and psychophysical experiments in grouping: Early orientation selection." In HUMAN AND MACHINE VISION, Jacob Beck, et al. (eds.), Academic Press: New York, pp. 545–567, 1983.

NOTE
On Active Contour Models and Balloons

Laurent D. Cohen

INRIA, Domaine de Voluceau, Rocquencourt, B.P. 105, 78153 Le Chesnay Cedex, France*

Received November 8, 1989; accepted June 26, 1990

The use of energy-minimizing curves, known as "snakes," to extract features of interest in images has been introduced by Kass, Witkin & Terzopoulos (*Int. J. Comput. Vision* 1, 1987, 321–331). We present a model of deformation which solves some of the problems encountered with the original method. The external forces that push the curve to the edges are modified to give more stable results. The original snake, when it is not close enough to contours, is not attracted by them and straightens to a line. Our model makes the curve behave like a balloon which is inflated by an additional force. The initial curve need no longer be close to the solution to converge. The curve passes over weak edges and is stopped only if the edge is strong. We give examples of extracting a ventricle in medical images. We have also made a first step toward 3D object reconstruction, by tracking the extracted contour on a series of successive cross sections. © 1991 Academic Press, Inc.

I. INTRODUCTION

We introduce a new model for active contours, which significantly improves the detection quality of closed edges. Our model was used to segment automatically noisy ultrasound and magnetic resonance images of the beating heart, in both 2 and 3 dimensions. We present the features of this new model, with a number of various significant experimental results, and we discuss future research.

The use of deformable contour models to extract features of interest in images was introduced by Kass and co-workers [1, 2]. These models are known as "snakes" or energy-minimizing curves.

We are looking for mathematical descriptions of the shapes of objects appearing in images. We assume that the objects we are looking for are smooth. We thus define an elastic deformable model as in [1]. The model is placed on the image and is subject to the action of "external forces" which move and deform it from its initial position to best fit it to the desired features in the image.

We are interested in extracting good edges. Usually in edge detection, after the gradient of the image is com-

puted, the maxima are extracted and then edges are linked together. Here we do it another way; we start with a continuous curve model and we try to localize it on the maxima of the gradient. We draw a simple curve close to the intended contours and let the action of the image forces push the curve the rest of the way. The final position corresponds to the equilibrium reached at the minimum of the model's energy.

The external forces are derived from the image data or imposed as constraints. Internal forces define the physical properties of the model.

If this original idea is due to [1, 3, 4], our model presents the following interesting new features which can solve some of the problems encountered with the original snake method:

- The external image forces applied on the curve to push it to the high gradient regions are modified to give more stable results.
- The original "snake" model, when it is not submitted to any external forces, finds its equilibrium at a point or a line according to the internal parameters and boundary conditions. Also, a snake which is not close enough to contours is not attracted by them. We define a new active contour model by adding an inflation force which makes the curve behave well in these cases. The curve behaves like a balloon which is inflated. When it passes by edges, it is stopped if the edge is strong, or passes through if the edge is too weak with respect to the inflation force. This avoids the curve's being "trapped" by spurious isolated edge points, and makes the result much more insensitive to the initial conditions.
- We take into account *edge points* previously extracted by a local edge detector. This allows to combine the quality of a good *local* edge detector, e.g. a Canny–Deriche edge extractor [5–7], with a *global* active model.

After the main ideas of "snakes" are reviewed in the next section, the following section describes the new aspects of our method. We illustrate our technique by showing the results of feature extraction in medical images. Finally, we give the first 3D reconstruction results obtained by propagating the segmentation in a series of successive slices.

* The author is now at CEREMADE, U.R.A. CNRS 749, Université Paris IX–Dauphine, Place du Marechal de Lattre de Tassigny 75775 Paris Cedex 16, France.

"On Active Contour Models and Balloons" by L.D. Cohen from *CVGIP: Image Understanding,* Vol. 53, No. 2, Mar. 1991, pp. 211–218. Copyright © 1991 Academic Press, Inc. Reprinted with permission.

2. ENERGY MINIMIZING CURVES

2.1. *Active Contour Model*

Snakes are a special case of deformable models as presented in [2].

The deformable contour model is a mapping:

$$\Omega = [0, 1] \rightarrow \Re^2$$

$$s \mapsto v(s) = (x(s), y(s)).$$

We define a deformable model as a space of admissible deformations Ad and a functional E to minimize. This functional represents the energy of the model and has the form

$$E: \quad Ad \rightarrow \Re$$

$$v \mapsto E(v) = \int_\Omega w_1|v'(s)|^2 + w_2|v''(s)|^2 + P(v(s))ds,$$

where the primes denote differentiation and where P is the potential associated to the external forces. It is computed as a function of the image data according to the desired goal. So if we want the snake to be attracted by edge points, the potential should depend on the gradient of the image. In the following, the space of admissible deformations Ad is restricted by the boundary conditions $v(0)$, $v'(0)$, $v(1)$, and $v'(1)$ given. We can also use periodic curves or other types of boundary conditions.

The mechanical properties of the model are controlled by the functions w_j. Their choice determines the elasticity and rigidity of the model.

If v is a local minimum for E, it satisfies the associated Euler–Lagrange equation:

$$\begin{cases} -(w_1v')' + (w_2v'')'' + \nabla P(v) = 0 \\ v(0), \, v'(0), \, v(1), \text{ and } v'(1) \text{ being given.} \end{cases} \quad (1)$$

In this formulation each term appears as a force applied to the curve. A solution can be seen either as realizing the equilibrium of the forces in the equation or as reaching the minimum of the energy.

Thus the curve is under control of two forces:

● The internal forces (the first two terms) which impose the regularity of the curve. w_1 and w_2 impose the elasticity and rigidity of the curve.
● The image force (the potential term) pushes the curve to the significant lines which correspond to the desired attributes. It is defined by a potential of the shape $\int_0^1 P(v(s))ds$ where

$$P(v) = -|\nabla I(v)|^2.$$

I denotes the image. The curve is then attracted by the local minima of the potential, which means the local maxima of the gradient, that is edges (see [8] for a more complete relation between minimizing the energy and locating contours).

● other external forces can be added to impose constraints defined by the user.

2.2. *Numerical Solution*

We discretize the equation by finite differences.

If $F(v) = (F_1(v), F_2(v)) = -\nabla P(v) + \ldots$ is the sum of image and external forces, the equation

$$-(w_1v')' + (w_2v'')'' = F(v)$$

becomes after finite differences in space (step h)

$$\frac{1}{h}(a_i(v_i - v_{i-1}) - a_{i+1}(v_{i+1} - v_i))$$

$$+ \frac{b_{i-1}}{h^2}(v_{i-2} - 2v_{i-1} + v_i)$$

$$- 2\frac{b_i}{h^2}(v_{i-1} - 2v_i + v_{i+1})$$

$$+ \frac{b_{i+1}}{h^2}(v_{i+2} - 2v_{i+1} + v_i)$$

$$-(F_1(v_i), F_2(v_i)) = 0$$

where we defined $v_i = v(ih)$; $a_i = w_1(ih)/h$; $b_i = w_2(ih)/h^2$.

This can be written in the matrix form

$$AV = F,$$

where A is pentadiagonal and V and F denote the vectors of positions v_i and forces at these points $F(v_i)$.

Since the energy is not convex, there are many local minima of E. But we are interested in finding a good contour in a given area. We suppose in fact we have a rough estimate of the curve. We impose the condition to be "close" to this initial data by solving the associated evolution equation

$$\begin{cases} \dfrac{\partial v}{\partial t} - (w_1v')' + (w_2v'')'' = F(v) \\ v(0, s) = v_0(s) \\ v(t, 0) = v_0(0) \quad v(t, 1) = v_0(1) \\ v'(t, 0) = v_0'(0) \quad v'(t, 1) = v_0'(1) \end{cases} \quad (2)$$

We find a solution of the static problem when the previous solution $v(t)$ stabilizes. Then the term $\partial v/\partial t$ tends to 0 and we achieve a solution of the static problem.

The evolution problem becomes after finite differences in time (step τ) and space (step h):

$$(I_d + \tau A)v^t = (v^{t-1} + \tau F(v^{t-1})) \quad (3)$$

where I_d denotes the identity matrix.

Thus, we obtain a linear system and we have to solve a pentadiagonal banded symmetric positive system. We compute the solution using a LU decomposition of $(I_d + \tau A)$. The decomposition need be computed only once if the w_i remain constant through time. We stop iterating when the difference between iterations is small enough.

3. IMPROVING THE MODEL

Solving the formulation described in the previous section leads to two difficulties for which we give solutions in this section. In both cases we give a new definition of the forces, focusing on the evolution equation formulation even though the forces no longer derive from a potential.

3.1. *Instability due to Image Forces*

Let us examine the effect of the image force $F = -\nabla P$ as defined in the previous section.

The direction of F implies steepest descent in P, which is natural since we want to get a minimum of P. Equilibrium is achieved at points where P is a minimum in the direction normal to the curve.

However, even though the initial guess can be close to an edge, instabilities can occur due to the discretization of the evolution problem. We see from Eq. (3) that the position at time t, v^t, is obtained after moving v^{t-1} along vector $\tau F(v^{t-1})$ and then solving the system, which can be seen as smoothing the curve. This leads to the following remarks:

Time Discretization. If $\tau F(v^{t-1})$ is too large the point v^{t-1} can be moved too far across the desired minimum and never come back (see Fig. 1). So the curve can pass through the edge and then make large oscillations without reaching equilibrium, or stabilize to a different minimum. This problem was avoided by the authors of [1] by manual tuning of the time step.

If we choose τ small enough such that the move $\tau F(v^{t-1})$ is never too large, for example never larger than a pixel size, then the previous problem is avoided.

However, only very few high gradient points will attract the curve and small F will not affect much the curve (see Fig. 5) since they are too small compared with the internal forces. So instead of acting on the time step, we modify the force by normalizing it, taking $F = -k \nabla P / \|\nabla P\|$, where τk is on the order of the pixel size. So the steps cannot be too large, and since the magnitude for F

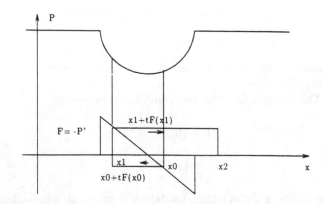

FIG. 1. Instability due to time discretization. Starting from $x0$, $tF(x0)$ is too large and we go away from the good minimum to $x2$ which is also an equilibrium.

is about one pixel, when a point of the curve is close to an edge point, it is attracted to the edge and stabilizes there if there is no conflict with the smoothing process. Thus, smaller and larger image gradients have the same influence on the curve. This is not a difficulty since, in either case, the points on the curve find their equilibrium at local minima of the potential, along edge points.

Space Discretization. The force F is known only on a discrete grid corresponding to the image, and therefore, there can be a zero-crossing without any zero in the grid. This means that in the best case a point always oscillates between the pixels neighboring the minimum (see Fig. 2). This problem is simply solved by bilinear interpolation of F at noninteger positions. Thus we have a continuous definition of F and equilibrium points correspond to the zeros of F.

Accounting for Previous Local Edge Detection. We want to account for a previous local edge detection, obtained for instance with a Canny–Deriche edge detector

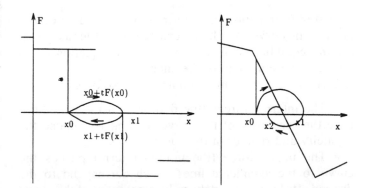

FIG. 2. Instability due to space discretization. On the left, with the discrete force there is no equilibrium point. There is an oscillation between the points $x0$ and $x1$. On the right, after continuous interpolation of F, there is convergence after a few iterations.

[5–7]. We would like the curve to be attracted by these detected edges. To do this, we define the attraction forces by simulating a potential defined by convolving the binary edge image with a Gaussian impulse response. This can be used either as the only image forces or together with an intensity-gradient image to enforce the detected edges. This is useful when the detected edges are broken into small segments which are not linked together. Using energy-minimizing curves in this case is a way to close contours. For example if we use a high threshold in order to keep only the points that are very likely to be real contours, the curve both closes and smooths the contour.

Remark that even though the equation changed, the curve is still pushed to minimize the potential and the energy.

We give below examples of results applying this method, first to a drawn line and then to medical images. In Fig. 3, we see how the corners are slightly smoothed due to the regularization effect. The corner on the left seems to be better, but it is due to the discretization needed to superimpose the curve on the image; the right angle is more precise in the horizontal–vertical corner than in the rotated one.

In Fig. 4, the top image is taken from a time sequence of ultrasound images during a cardiac cycle and the problem is to detect and follow the deformation of the mitral valve in the heart. As mentioned above, we used the Canny detector [5] as implemented recursively by Deriche [6] to compute the image gradient.

The other image is a slice from a 3D NMR image in the heart area. We want to extract the left ventricle. We use here the 3D edge detector [7] obtained by generalization of the 2D Canny–Deriche filter.

We give in comparison examples of what happens when we do not normalize the image force (Fig. 5). If the time step is too large, the force $\tau F(v^{t-1})$ is too large and beginning from the result in Fig. 4, we get instabilities. These are such that points that are slightly on one side of

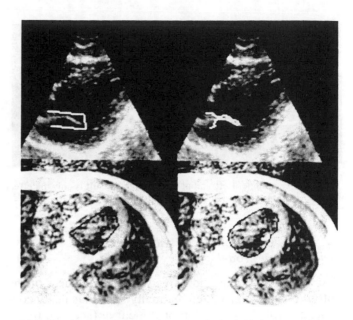

FIG. 4. Above: ultrasound image. Left: initial curve; right: the valve is detected. Below: NMR image of the heart. Left: initial curve; right: the ventricle is detected.

a contour are moved far away on the other side. On the contrary, when the time step is too small, we see that, taking the same initial curve as in Fig. 4, in the left region of the curve, the image forces are too small and smoothing occurs only.

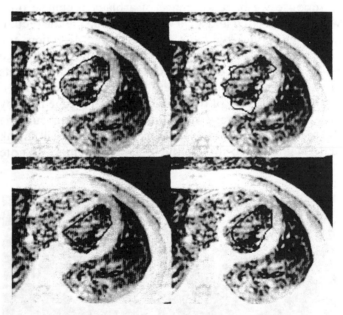

FIG. 5. Instabilities. Above: time step too large. Left: initial curve; right: result after one iteration. Below: time step too small. Left: initial curve; right: result. In the left part of the curve the regularization forces were dominant.

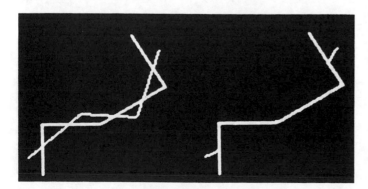

FIG. 3. Left: initial curve; right: result.

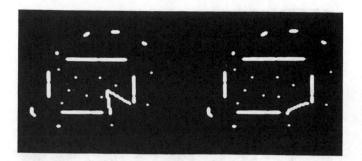

FIG. 6. Rectangle. Left: initial curve; Right: result is only the effect of regularization since no edges are close enough.

3.2. *Localization of the Initial Guess.*
The Balloon Model

To make the snake find its way, an initial guess of the contour has to be provided manually. This has many consequences for the evolution of the curve (see Fig. 6).

- If the curve is not close enough to an edge, it is not attracted by it.
- If the curve is not submitted by any forces, it shrinks on itself.

The finite difference formulation of the problem makes the curve behave like a set of masses linked by zero length strings. This means that if there is no image force ($F = 0$), the curve shrinks on itself and vanishes to a point or straightens to a line depending on the boundary conditions. This happens if the initial curve or part of it is placed in a constant area.

Suppose we have an image of a black rectangle on a white background and a curve is placed inside the rectangle. Even though we have a perfect edge detection, the curve vanishes. If a point is close enough to an edge point, it is attracted by it and neighboring curve points also stick to the edge. If there are enough such points, eventually the rest of the curve follows the edge little by little. On the contrary, if the initial curve is surrounding the rectangle, even if it is far from the edges, it will shrink and, as it does so, stick to the rectangle. Let us also note

that, often, due to noise, some isolated points are gradient maxima and can stop the curve when it passes by (see Fig. 7).

All these remarks suggest we add another force which makes the contour have a more dynamic behavior. We now consider our curve as a "balloon" (in 2D) that we inflate. From an initial oriented curve we add to the previous forces a pressure force pushing outside as if we introduced air inside. The force F now becomes

$$F = k_1 \mathbf{n}(s) - k \frac{\nabla P}{\|\nabla P\|}$$

where $\mathbf{n}(s)$ is the normal unitary vector to the curve at point $v(s)$ and k_1 is the amplitude of this force. If we change the sign of k_1 or the orientation of the curve, it will have an effect of deflation instead of inflation. k_1 and k are chosen such that they are of the same order, which is smaller than a pixel size, and k is slightly larger than k_1 so an edge point can stop the inflation force. The curve then expands and it is attracted and stopped by edges as before. But since there is a pressure force, if the edge is too weak the curve can pass through this edge if it is a singularity with regard to the rest of the curve being inflated. This means that it tends to create a tangent discontinuity at this point. The smoothing effect with the help of the inflation force then removes the discontinuity and the curve passes through the edge. (See bottom left of Fig. 11).

In the gradient image of the rectangle above, we have removed some edges and added some spurious ones to illustrate those remarks. Starting from the same small curve as in the previous examples, we obtain the whole rectangle (see Fig. 8). When the curve passes by a noise point in the rectangle image, it sticks to the point. But since the curve is expanding, the noise point becomes a singular point of the curve and it is removed by the regularization effect after a few iterations. When the balloon reaches an equilibrium, the points which stick to edges are slightly outside of the real contour since the edge force has to be in equilibrium with the inflation and regu-

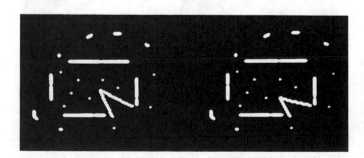

FIG. 7. Rectangle. Left: initial curve; right: result is stopped at one edge point.

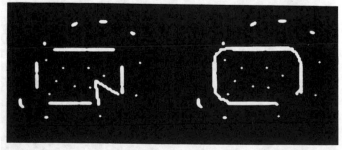

FIG. 8. Rectangle. Left: initial curve; right: result after the balloon, is inflated.

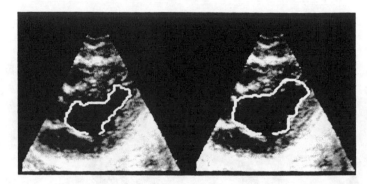

FIG. 9. Ultrasound image. Left: initial cavity; right: result.

larization forces. We can then reduce the inflation force to localize the position of the curve.

3.3. *Optimizing Elasticity and Rigidity Coefficients*

The coefficients of elasticity and rigidity have great importance for the behavior of the curve along time iterations. If w_1 and w_2 are around unity, the internal energy has a major influence and the image forces have small effect. In this case the curve is only regularized.

A correct choice for parameters is guided by numerical analysis considerations. We wish that the coefficients of the rigidity matrix all have the same order of magnitude. We obtain good results when the parameters are of the order of h^2 for w_1 and h^4 for w_2, where h is the space discretization step.

When we have an initial curve detected which is known to lie inside the object, our balloon technique is particularly efficient. For example, we are looking for the boundary of a cavity in an ultrasound image of the heart (see Fig. 9). An approximation of the cavity is given by thresholding the image at a low value after applying mathematical morphology operations. We know that this approximation lies inside the real cavity. By taking the approximated boundary as the initial value for v, we expand the balloon and it comes to stick more precisely to the cavity boundary.

In Fig. 10 we give another application of balloons to the same problem as in Fig. 4, but we now take a curve which is not close to the ventricle, either in shape or in position. After a few steps of evolution of the balloon, we obtain almost the same final result as before, but it takes more iterations. In fact the final curve in Fig. 10 is slightly external to the ventricle. As we noted above, if we now cancel the expansion force, we obtain the same result as in Fig. 4.

We show in Fig. 11 the same steps as in Fig. 10, but superimposed on the potential image. We can see in the two middle steps how a point of the curve is stuck to an edge and creates a singularity there. This is removed after a few iterations by the cumulative effect of the pressure force and smoothing.

The directions of our research after contour extraction is surface extraction in 3D images.

A first step is to follow the contour from one slice to

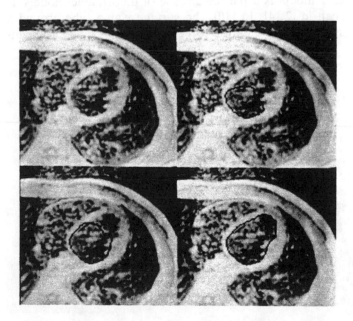

FIG. 10. NMR image. Evolution of the balloon curve to detect the left ventricle.

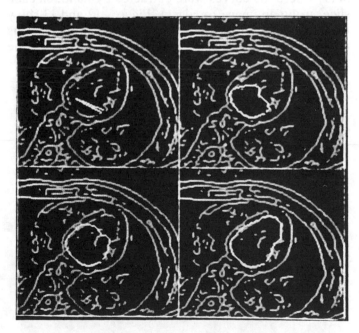

FIG. 11. NMR image. Evolution of the balloon curve to detect the left ventricle superimposed on the potential image.

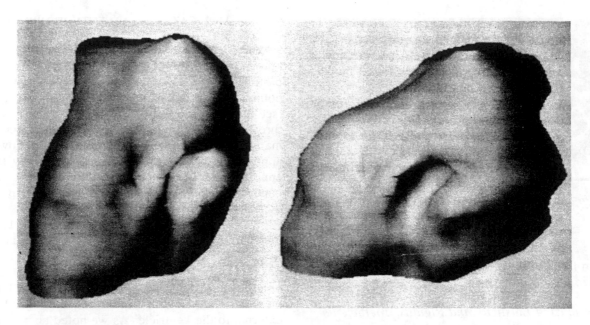

FIG. 12. Two views of the reconstructed inside cavity of the left ventricle.

the other. With our method, we experimented with the reconstruction of a 3D surface by initializing a balloon model in an intermediate cross section, and by propagating the result to neighboring cross-sections, initializing the curve in a cross-section with the result obtained in the previously processed connected section (as was done for motion tracking in [1]). We made a first approach to 3D reconstruction by extracting the contour slice by slice (as in [9] where the curves were extracted by hand, on each slice, using an image of edges). Figures 12 and 13 show the reconstruction of the left and right ventricles. This reconstruction is almost automatic. Indeed, when the

contour undergoes a big change from one slice to the next, the initial curve in that slice may have to be redefined in order to obtain a good contour, a problem which can be avoided by adding interpolated slices when necessary.

The next step is to follow the deformation in time of this surface. This can be done either slice by slice or globally by generalizing to a 3D surface model as in [10], or to a 3D balloon. This is possible since the active contour model is a particular case of deformable models as seen in [2, 4]. In [10], the surface was a tube around a spine and an inflation force was used to control expan-

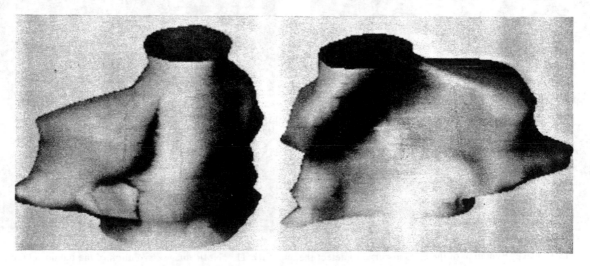

FIG. 13. Two views of the reconstructed inside cavity of the right ventricle.

sion and contraction of the tube around the spine. The two ends of the tube were cinched shut using contraction force and inflation was used to counteract smoothing. So the use of an inflation force in our "balloon" model is significantly different from that in [10].

We can add internal forces to control the deformation so as to follow the desired contours. This is possible if we have a physical model of the desired object (for example, to follow the deformation of a ventricle during a cycle), or to make the curve expand or collapse from the initial data using some knowledge of the deformation.

Another application of our research is the elastic matching of extracted features to an atlas, which is related to the work in [11]. This was also studied in [12] with simple geometric shapes as templates which are deformed to match the image.

5. CONCLUSION

We presented a model of deformation which can solve some of the problems encountered with the "snake" model of [1]. We modified the definition of external forces deriving from the gradient of the image to obtain more stable results. We also introduced a pressure force which makes the curve model behave like a balloon. This enables us to give an initial guess of the curve which is far from the desired solution. We showed promising results of our model on MR (magnetic resonance) and ultrasound images to extract features like the contour of a heart ventricle on 2D slices. Using a series of such contours in successive cross sections, we made a 3D reconstruction of the inside surface of the ventricles. This method has been tested for several applications in medical image analysis. Our main goal is to generalize this method to obtain surface boundaries in 3D images.

6. ACKNOWLEDGMENTS

The author thanks the reviewer for useful comments on this paper and also Nicholas Ayache and Isaac Cohen for their constant help during this work.

REFERENCES

1. Michael Kass, Andrew Witkin, and Demetri Terzopoulos, Snakes: Active contour models, *Int. J. Comput. Vision* **1**, 1987, 321–331.
2. Demetri Terzopoulos, On matching deformable models to images, in *Topical Meeting on Machine Vision*, pp. 160–167, *Technical Digest Series*, Vol. 12, Optical Society of America, 1987.
3. Andrew Blake and Andrew Zisserman, *Visual Reconstruction*, MIT Press, Cambridge, MA, 1987.
4. Demetri Terzopoulos, The computation of visible-surface representations, *IEEE Trans. Pattern Anal. Machine Intelligence* **PAMI-10**(4), 1988, 417–438.
5. John Canny, A computational approach to edge detection, *IEEE Trans. Pattern Anal. Machine Intelligence* **PAMI-8**(6), 1986, 679–698.
6. Rachid Deriche, Using Canny's criteria to derive a recursively implemented optimal edge detector, *Int. J. Comput. Vision*, 1987, 167–187.
7. O. Monga and R. Deriche, 3d edge detection using recursive filtering application to scanner images, in *Proceedings of Computer Vision and Vision and Pattern Recognition, San Diego, June 1989*.
8. Pascal Fua and Yvan G. Leclerc, Model driven edge detection, in *DARPA Image Understanding Workshop, 1988*.
9. N. Ayache, J. D. Boissonnat, E. Brunet, L. Cohen, J. P. Chièze, B. Geiger, O. Monga, J. M. Rocchisani, and P. Sander, Building highly structured volume representations in 3d medical images, in *Computer Aided Radiology*, Berlin, 1989.
10. Demetri Terzopoulos, Andrew Witkin, and Michael Kass, Constraints on deformable models: Recovering 3d shape and nonrigid motion, *AI J.* **36**, 1988, 91–123.
11. Ruzena Bajcsy and Stane Kovacic, Multiresolution elastic matching, *Comput. Vision Graphics Image Process.* **46**, 1989, 1–21.
12. A. L. Yuille, D. S. Cohen, and P. W. Hallinan, Feature extraction from faces using deformable templates, in *Proceedings of Computer Vision and Pattern Recognition, San Diego, June 1989*.

Correspondence

Dynamic Programming for Detecting, Tracking, and Matching Deformable Contours

Davi Geiger, Alok Gupta, Luiz A. Costa, and John Vlontzos

Abstract—The problem of segmenting an image into separate regions and tracking them over time is one of the most significant problems in vision. Terzopoulos et al have proposed an approach to detect the contour regions of complex shapes, assuming a user selected initial contour not very far from the desired solution.

We propose to further explore the information provided by the user's selected points and apply an optimal method to detect contours which allows a segmentation of the image. The method is based on dynamic programming (DP), and applies to a wide variety of shapes. It is exact and not iterative. We also consider a multiscale approach capable of speeding up the algorithm by a factor of 20, although at the expense of losing the guaranteed optimality characteristic.

The problem of tracking and matching these contours is addressed. For tracking, the final contour obtained at one frame is sampled and used as initial points for the next frame. Then, the same DP process is applied. For matching, a novel strategy is proposed where the solution is a smooth displacement field in which unmatched regions are allowed while cross vectors are not. The algorithm is again based on DP and the optimal solution is guaranteed.

We have demonstrated the algorithms on natural objects in a large spectrum of applications, including interactive segmentation and automatic tracking of the regions of interest in medical images.

Index Terms—Dynamic programming, deformable contours, snakes, contour segmentation, tracking, matching, optimal solutions.

I. Introduction

The problem of segmenting an image into separate regions is one of the most significant problems of vision. If a sequence of images is provided, one may need to track these regions through time. A way to represent these regions is by their enclosing contours. Many natural objects cannot be described by simple geometric shapes (e.g., circle, ellipse) but need to be represented with complex contours. To model these complex shape contours, Terzopoulos, Witkin, and Kass [13], [21] have introduced the idea of snakes, also known as deformable contours. Some interesting extensions include [6], [16], [17], [24]. In particular this approach as applied to medical images, the main domain of applications considered in this paper, was first considered in [2], [7], [11]. The formulation of the cost functions has been influenced by their work.

Minimizing an energy function is a typical way to detect deformable shapes. A limitation of this approach has been that the algorithms are slow, iterative, and not guaranteed to find the global minimum. Moreover, we argue that some of the user input information has not been utilized by previous methods.

Manscript received June 30, 1993; revised August 14, 1994.

D. Geiger is with Courant Institute, NYU, 251 Mercer St., New York, NY 10012; e-mail geiger@cs.nyu.edu.

A. Gupta and J. Vlontzos are with Siemens Corporate Research, Inc., 755 College Rd. East, Princeton, NJ 08540; e-mail alok@scr.siemens.com.

L.A. Costa is with LSI-USP, Av. Prof. Luciano Gualberto, 158, Sao Paulo, SP, Brazil.

IEEECS Log Number P95030.

A. Detection

To detect these contours, we have devised a non-iterative method which is guaranteed to find the global minimum. We first consider a list of uncertainty for each point selected by the user wherein the point is allowed to move. Then, a search window is created from two consecutive lists. We argue that, in this way, the information provided by the user is properly utilized. We then apply a dynamic programming (DP) algorithm [5] to obtain the optimal contour passing through these lists of uncertainty. Moreover, the deformable model is a consequence of having to consider all possible deformations and all possible contours. We are allowing the selected points to move as well, but we stress that the method is not iterative. Note that the guaranteed optimality is with respect to the selected window.

The drawback of DP algorithms is that they require large memory and are slow. Therefore, we consider a multiscale approach capable of speeding up the algorithm by a factor of 20, although at the expense of losing the guaranteed optimality characteristic. Other heuristics to speed up the algorithm are also considered.

B. Tracking

Once the contours have been detected in one image, we consider tracking consecutive frames (through time) or different slices (through space). The contour obtained in the previous frame is sampled at high curvature points (typically 3% of the points are kept) and applied as the initial points for the next frame. The method is applied again. A multiscale strategy can be used to speed up the algorithm.

C. Matching

Finally, we consider the problem of matching these contours and present a novel strategy. We suggest four requirements for matching: 1) the uniqueness of the match is relaxed such that elements of one contour need not have a match in the other contour (occluded elements), 2) the size of each unmatched region should be small, 3) no cross displacements are allowed (each match gives a displacement vector), and 4) the displacements field should be smooth. The algorithm is again based on DP and the optimal solution is guaranteed.

D. Applications

The domain of applications includes different medical modalities. Doctors would like to automatically, or semi-automatically, detect arteries or the time evolution of the left and right ventricle of the heart (to diagnose abnormalities of the heart). The image modalities considered are Magnetic Resonance Images (MRI), Digitally Subtracted Angiograms (DSA), and Computer Tomography (CT). In particular, the algorithm with the tracking technique has been extensively tested on MRI cardiac data and is now being transferred to clinical use by doctors.

The matching strategy can also help the interpolation of a sequence of images. By identifying the correspondence between an artery undergoing some motion, we can create an intermediate image where the artery displacement can be taken into account.

We have also applied our technique to the problems of detecting human features, such as the head boundaries or the hand contour. Other applications include the detection of man-made objects under different illuminations.

Reprinted from *IEEE Trans. Pattern Analysis and Machine Intelligence*, Vol. 17, No. 3, Mar. 1995, pp. 294–402.

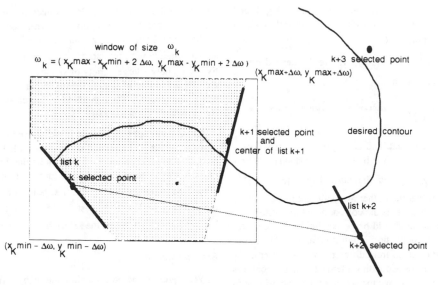

Fig. 1. Four selected points, from k to $k + 3$, three lists of uncertainty, from $list_k$ to $list_{k+2}$, and a window for DP search, $\omega = \left(\omega_k^x, \omega_k^y \right)$. The desired contour is also shown. The search space is denoted by the shaded region. Note that $list_{k+1}$ is perpendicular to the straight line connecting k to $k + 2$ and analogously for $list_{k+2}$.

E. Previous dynamic programming work

Contour detection: Our contour detection algorithm differs from previously proposed methods based on DP in the following ways: Amini et al [1] applied an iterative algorithm where at each step DP was applied to improve the current contour result a "little", by just allowing small changes of the contour's shape. Other approaches, like that of Pope et al [18], have assumed one variable contour (e.g., the radial r coordinate in the (r, θ) space), thus a much more restrictive class of contours.

Our proposed dp has similar characteristics as the original work of Montanari [14], followed by Wu and Maitre [23], Ballard and Brown [3], Mortensen et al [15], Sashua and Ullman [20], and Barzohar and Cooper [4]. However, none of them have considered the problem of utilizing the selected user interface by introducing lists of uncertainty and their corresponding search windows. The lists of uncertainty eliminate the constraint that the path must pass thorough the start-end points. Moreover, the size of the contours is not fixed. This flexibility requires special adaptation of the DP algorithm.

Furthermore, none of the previous methods, other than Wu and Maitre, have considered multiscale techniques to speed up their algorithms. Wu and Maitre have used multiscale by adding one extra constraint (the size of the contour becomes dependent upon the "median size" of the contour). This constraint fixes the size of the contours. Alternatively, we allow larger deformations in our multiscale strategy.

Contour tracking: A previous method of tracking contour using DP has been proposed by Ueda and Mase [22]. They impose a cost for the deformation of the contour to make contour detection robust. However, their assumption is not always valid, especially for contours undergoing deformations. Unlike them, we tailor our tracking scheme to contours that are only deforming but not moving (translating) much. In particular, this assumption is valid for the spatial and temporal propagation of the left ventricle slices from MRI data.

Contour moatching: A matching strategy has been proposed by Hospital et al [12] for recognition of a sequence of linear segments. They proposed an N-stage DP algorithm

which differs from ours since their cost function is tailored to a different application. For our cost function a one-stage DP algorithm can be derived. Gregor and Thomason [10] have applied DP to DNA sequence matching, but their algorithm does not incorporate the constraints outlined in the previous section and is a rather simple algorithm, unsuitable for our application. Our approach is closely related to dynamic time warping [19] as applied to speech processing, although we consider the displacements to be a vector field (not a scalar distance) and introduce the smoothness of the displacement field as a measure. Wu and Maitre [23] have also proposed a matching algorithm to register the contours of SPOT and SAR images. However, their matching is based on very simple criteria (similarity measure) and, thus, does not have the extensions presented here.

II. DETECTING DEFORMABLE CONTOURS

To solve the problem of detecting complex shapes via user selected points, an energy formulation was first suggested by [13], [21] which has since been used by many authors. Typically, the shape with minimal energy "correctly" represents the segmented region. Thus, the problem of segmentation involves minimizing the energy of the deformable shape, starting with an initial approximate shape (polygonal approximation), usually derived from the user interface or some higher level operator. In our applications the image "forces" (used to attract the contour) are usually given by the magnitude of the intensity gradient of the image or, in some applications, by the intensity itself.

A. The search constraints provided by the user

The user first selects a few points, say S selected points. In the past a simple polygonal approximation of the contour has been used. We argue that more information exists and can be used. Our main argument is that, as illustrated in Fig. 1, given three consecutive points, say k, $k + 1$, and $k + 2$, the contour point at $k + 1$ should be able to move roughly perpendicular to the straight line connecting k and $k + 2$. One way to formulate it is by considering the probability of a user selecting a set of S points, $\{\vec{X}_k = (x_k, y_k), k = 0, ..., S-1\}$, given that the set of points $\{\vec{X}_{c_k} = (x_{c_k}, y_{c_k})\}$ are the desired points belonging to the "actual" contour as:

$$P\left(\{\vec{X}_k\}|\{\vec{X}_{c_k}\}\right) = C\prod_{k=0}^{S-1} e^{-[(\vec{X}_{c_k} - \vec{X}_k)(\vec{X}_{k-1} - \vec{X}_{k+1})]/|(\vec{X}_{k-1} - \vec{X}_{k+1})|},$$

where C is a normalization constant, and appropriate boundary conditions are set at $k = 0$ and $k = S - 1$. We have used the standard definitions, $\vec{X}_k . \vec{X}_{k-1} = x_{k-1}x_k + y_{k-1}y_k$ and the norm $|X_k| = \left(x_k^2 + y_k^2\right)^{1/2}$. This probability emphasizes that the farther away a point in the contour is from the selected point, the larger is the cost, and that the vector connecting it to the k selected point should be perpendicular to the vector $(x_{k+1} - x_{k-1}, y_{k+1} - y_{k-1})$. This assumption is intuitive and could be supported by the following experiment: from different images collect many user selected points and the corresponding elements on the contours and analyze the covariance matrix. We expect that the errors will be in the direction that we have described. Although we have not done this experiment in a formal way, we have observed such occurrence. Within a Bayesian approach, this probability can be combined with the energy function to provide the posterior probability.

We simplify the above formulation by considering a maximum distance, say M, to the selected point (beyond which the probability becomes zero), and also by just considering pixel elements perpendicular to the line connecting $k - 1$ and $k + 1$. This small set of pixels ($2M + 1$ elements) constitute a list of uncertainty, say $list_k^M$. This list is centered at the selected pixel k and is perpendicular to the straight line connecting the points $k - 1$ and $k + 1$.

Secondly, we can formulate a probability distribution that $\vec{X} = (x, y)$ belongs to the contour given that $\vec{X}_{c_k} = (x_{c_k}, y_{c_k})$ is the element of the contour belonging to the uncertainty list. This gives $P(X|\vec{X}_{c_k})$. More precisely, given two selected points, say k and $k + 1$, and their uncertainty lists, say $list_k^M$ and $list_{k+1}^M$, a search window ω_k is created within which the contour must lie. A few different criteria for choosing an appropriate window are necessary for the variety of applications we have considered. These windows are equivalent to setting the probability distribution to be constant through the window and zero outside. The additional constraint is that one point in the contour must lie on the uncertainty list.

We have considered the following method for most of the applications. The window is created from the extrema points of the two lists, $list_k^M$ and $list_{k+1}^M$, allowing an extra offset $\Delta\omega$. More precisely, from $list_k^M$ and $list_{k+1}^M$ we select the x and y coordinates (independently) with minimum and maximum values, say $x_k^{min}, y_k^{min}, x_k^{max}, y_k^{max}$. The index k refers to the window ω_k in the sense that x_k^{min} can belong to either $list_k^M$ or $list_{k+1}^M$. Then the window $\omega = (\omega_k^x, \omega_k^y)$ has sizes $(x_k^{max} - x_k^{min} + 2\Delta\omega, y_k^{max} - y_k^{min} + 2\Delta\omega)$ as shown in Fig. 1. Note that the choice of the coordinates $x_k^{min}, y_k^{min}, x_k^{max}, y_k^{max}$ for one window must not be carried to the next window, even though one of the lists is in common.

To further reduce the search window, we just consider the portion of the rectangle that is in between the lines passing through the two lists. In this way we avoid "contour repetition" when going from one

window to the next (which also reduces the search space). We have used this restriction when applying the method to images of the heart.

Another criteria is to augment the search window by considering a square window with the larger size between ω_k^x and ω_k^y. The objective is to allow a large variety of shapes when the two selected points are aligned in one of the directions; otherwise, thin rectangular windows would result. Thus, creation of search windows can be tailored for each application domain.

Closed and open contours: If the desired contour is open, the extrema points must be treated differently. A list of size M is still created, but now generated by a perpendicular line created by just the initial (or end) point and the next (previous) point. If the contour is closed the initial list (list of the first point, or $list_0^M$) is created using the second ($k = 1$) and the last ($k = S - 1$) selected points, while the last list ($list_{S-1}^M$) considers the selected points $k = S - 2$ and $k = 0$.

B. Cost function

We represent the deformable contour by a field $c(x, y)$ that is 1 if the contour occupies the location (x, y) in the image plane and 0 otherwise. When an image plane of size N is discretized, say in a square lattice with $i, j = 0, 1, ..., N - 1$, then we use the representation $c_{ij} = c(x(j), y(i))$, where (i, j) are the indices along the $-y$ and x coordinates. $c_{ij} = 1$ represents the presence of the field c at pixel (i, j). When $c_{ij} = 0$, the contour is not present at the pixel. Another representation for the contour is a parametric one, $c(x(s), y(s))$ or just c_s, where s is a parameter that, when varied from 0 to L, causes c_s to cover the entire contour.

We first consider the sequence of the S selected points to be $\{(i_k, j_k)\}$, indexed by k, such that $k = 0, 1, ..., S - 1$. Given the input, we define the cost (energy) for detecting the deformable contours. This cost is a sum of costs between two consecutive points, say k and $k + 1$, and is given by

$$E(C) = \sum_{k=0}^{S-1} \sum_{(i,j) = (i_k, j_k)}^{(i_k + \omega_k^x, j_k + \omega_k^y)} c_{ij}\left\{\frac{1}{l_{ij}^2 + \rho} + \mu\gamma_{ij}(C)\right\}, \quad (1)$$

where l_{ij} takes values between 0 and 1, giving a measure of the magnitude of the intensity gradient, $\|\nabla_{ij}I\|$. $\gamma_{ij}(c)$ represents the curvature of the contour at pixel (i, j). The parameter $\rho \ll 1$ works as threshold for the cost of passing through pixels with no intensity gradients, in the sense that the cost does not become too large for $l_{ij} \approx 0$. μ controls smoothness of the desired contour. Throughout all the experiments we have set $\rho = 0.01$ and $\mu = 1$. The window $\omega_k = (\omega_k^x, \omega_k^y)$ is created between two consecutive selected points, defining a region where the contour can be present. The energy terms ensure that the contour localizes where there are large intensity differences (edges) and that it is smooth. Minimizing the total cost causes the optimal path to be as short as possible (analogous to a stretching energy). The smoothness criterion asserts that the path should be smooth and no abrupt changes are allowed, i.e., the path curvature should be small (analogous to a bending energy). We define curvature to simply be "the change" of the image gradient:

$$\gamma_{ij}(C) = \left|\phi_{ij}I - \phi_{i_p, j_p}I\right| \text{ where } \phi_{ij}I = arctan\left(\frac{\nabla_y I}{\nabla_x I}\right). \quad (2)$$

This definition assumes the curvature of the contours to coincide with the appropriate changes of intensity. It does not require isointensity

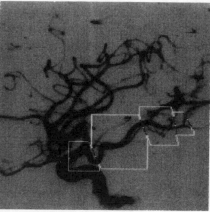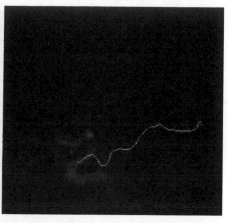

Fig. 2. Centerline detection in digitally subtracted angiograms (DSA). The input points are shown on the left image, the search space on the energy image in the center, and recovered centerline on the right.

contours as in Cohen et al [7], but is closely related to their formulation. The null space of $\gamma_{ij}(c)$ includes other intensity variations. More generally, we can consider three points: the current pixel being tested (i, j), its possible predecessor (i_p, j_p) and *its* predecessor (i_{p-1}, j_{p-1}). In this case the problem can still be solved but at the expense of a larger search, i.e., search on neighbors and next neighbors (e.g., see [1]). We have found that our assumptions were acceptable to the domain of applications we have considered. Thus, the energy (1) can be re-written as

$$E(C) = \sum_{k=0}^{S-1} \sum_{(i,j)=(i_s,j_s)}^{(i_s+\omega_k^x, j_s+\omega_k^y)} c_{ij} \left\{ \frac{1}{l_{ij}^2 + \rho} + \mu \left| \phi_{ij} I - \phi_{i_p,j_p} I \right| \right\}.$$

Given a set of C_k contour points, $\{(i_c, j_c); c = 0, 1, ..., C_k - 1\}$, for each window ω_k the total energy (cost) can also be written as:

$$E(C) = \sum_{k=0}^{S-1} E_k(C_k) \sum_{k=0}^{S-1} \sum_{c=0}^{C_k - 1, (i_c, j_c) \in \omega_k} H_{i_c, j_c}, \tag{3}$$

where $H_{i_c, j_c} = \frac{1}{l_{i_c, j_c}^2 + \rho} + \mu \left| \phi_{i_c, j_c} I - \phi_{i_c^p, j_c^p} I \right|$, (i_c^p, j_c^p) are the predecessors to (i_c, j_c). Note that C_k also has to be estimated and the constraint is that the initial and last points, (i_0, j_0) and $\left(i_{C_k-1}, j_{C_k-1}\right)$, belong to the list of uncertainty.

C. Connectivity: hard constraint

The above energy formulation does not guarantee that the contour is a *connected* chain. This requirement is met by just considering connected paths between two selected points so that, given a pixel element of the contour, we guarantee that a neighbor pixel must also belong to the contour. It can be easily imposed with the DP technique described next.

D. Dynamic Programming

Let us consider the problem of finding the optimal path passing near the selected pixels (i_k, j_k) and (i_{k+1}, j_{k+1}). Two lists of size M, perpendicular to the straight line connecting the points are created, $list_k^M$ and $list_{k+1}^M$. Then a search window is produced including all of the list elements (see Section II.A and Fig. 1).

Why DP: The main property explored by dp is that

$$\begin{aligned} min_C E(C) &= min_{C-C_0} min_{C_0} E(C) \\ &= min_{C-C_0} \left\{ E(C) - E_0(C_0) + min_{C_0} E_0(C_0) \right\} \\ min_{C_k} E_k(C_k) &= min_{C_k-c_0} min_{c_0} E(C_k) \\ &= min_{C_k-c_0} \left\{ \left(E_k(C_k) - H_{i_0, j_0} \right) + min_{c_0} \left[H_{i_0, j_0} \right] \right\} \end{aligned} \tag{4}$$

where all C_k contours are considered among the ones inside the window ω_k and are restricted to start and end at the uncertainty lists. This restriction is easily implemented by setting the initial costs high if the initial element does not belong to the list. The same applies for the end point. Note that this formula is valid for any size C_k of contour. We have to additionally check that the total cost remains unchanged once a contour has reached an end list point before C_k steps. Thus, the full search can be accomplished by taking decisions orderly and locally. Since the interaction of each contour element is with just the previous one we can use a one-stage dynamic programming.

For every pixel (i, j) the eight connected neighborhood defines the set $P_{(i,j)}$ of possible predecessors. Let us consider $minC_k$ to be the longest straight line between elements of $list_k^M$ and $list_{k+1}^M$. The number of steps we consider in our DP, for each window ω_k, is four times this minimum size, i.e., the largest possible contour we consider is $4minC_k$. One could allow larger contours to exist without compromising the algorithm or its complexity (the maximum contour size in each window has size less than $\omega_k^x \cdot \omega_k^y$) but, in our experiments, it was not necessary. After $4minC_k$ steps, every element of $list_{k+1}^M$ has a cost "vector" associated with it, where each element of the vector refers to the corresponding predecessors. This cost vector will be the starting vector for the next window computations. More precisely, for the next window $(k+1)$, an infinite cost is assigned everywhere except for the elements of the $list_{k+1}^M$.

Complexity: The computational complexity of the DP algorithm is $O\left(C\sum_{k=0}^{S-1} min C_k \cdot \omega_k^x \cdot \omega_k^y\right)$. C is less than 100 since, for every chosen element, eight possible neighbors have been considered. The depth of the algorithm is the maximum length, namely $4minC_k$.

Detection of open contour: Results: We show the results of this algorithm (Fig. 2) applied to detecting the centerline of an artery in a Digitally Subtracted Angiogram image (DSA). Only five approximate points were given. The densitometric profile of the DSA projection of the blood lumen has maximum intensity near the center of the artery.

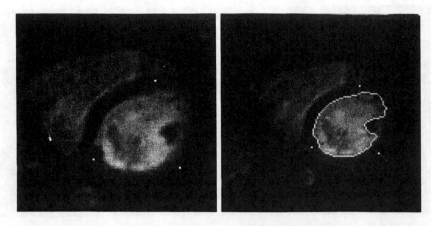

Fig. 3. Cardiac MR image: The inner wall of the left ventricle is detected using the "two-loop" method. Three points were selected (displayed on the left image). The initial fixed point, for the first loop, is on the white list, and the fixed point of the second loop belongs to the contour (it has moved along the uncertainty list from its original position, shown in white).

The modified DP cost function, obtained by replacing l_{ij} in (1) with I_{ij} (the normalized intensity at i, j) gives the desired contour. Centerline detection is a crucial step in 3D reconstruction of vessel tree from multiple projections.

E. Closed contours

We have described a DP algorithm suitable for open contours. If the contours are constrained to be closed, (i.e., the first and the last point are the same) we can apply the same algorithm in the following way. The initial and end lists are considered to be made of one (and the same) point only, given by any element of the initial list, $list_0^M$. This element is kept fixed by the DP, while other points are free to move about in their lists. The DP algorithm will return the best contour under this constraint. By running the algorithm for each choice of initial (and end) point among $list_0^M$, choosing the best run will give the optimal result. Thus, in the case of a closed contour, the same algorithm runs M times.

Note that more information regarding closed contours can be incorporated in the algorithm. The two sides of the uncertainty lists can be assigned to be the "inner list" and the "outer list" for a closed contour. This allows better control over the search space by restricting the inner and outer search space as desired by the user. For example, an inflating balloon will not have an inner search list, or a shrinking contour can have a smaller outer list than the inner list.

Speeding up the algorithm: We propose (and present results for) a fast "two-loop" method that takes just two runs instead of the M runs of the DP algorithm. In the first run of the DP algorithm the first point (the same as the last point) is kept fixed while all other points are allowed to move in their uncertainty lists. For the second run, the contour is reordered so as to start and terminate from the second point, which is now fixed in its new estimated position. This allows all the points to move in only two iterations (see Fig. 3). The final contour is not guaranteed to be optimal, but the experiments gave very close to the optimal solution.

Detection of closed contours: We demonstrate the result of detecting a closed contour corresponding to the inner wall of the left ventricle on a cardiac magnetic resonance (MR) image (see Fig. 3). Three points were specified, and the two-loop method was used. Fig. 4 shows results with a different input on the same image. Only a center point and the approximate radius were given by the user. Six points were sampled on the circle to obtain the initial approximation to the contour. The two-loop method (shown in Fig. 4(b)) increases the speed by an order of magnitude and, in our experiments, gave us the same result as optimal DP. We discuss the multiscale analysis to further speed up DP in the next section.

F. Multiscale Analysis

To reduce the computational complexity of the detecting contours we investigated the use of a pyramid strategy. We have chosen a pyramid structure [8] since it preserves the discontinuity map.

Solving at the coarsest scale: Once we have the discontinuity map at a desired coarse scale, the selected points are carried up through the scaled image and we run the DP algorithm at the coarsest scale. Because of the complexity of the algorithm ($O\left(\sum_{k=0}^{S-1} min\, C_k \cdot \omega_k^x \cdot \omega_k^y\right)$), we can obtain speedup factors of $(2^3)^l$ on computational time, where l is the number of scale levels. This is because, at each scale level reduction, the maximum length, $4minC_k$, and the window size, ω_k, are reduced by a factor of 2. Thus, for three scale levels ($l = 3$), the complexity of the algorithm diminishes by $\left(2^3\right)^3 = 512$.

Coarse-to-fine strategy: Once we have computed the contour at the coarsest scale we have to compute it at the next finer scale and so on until it reaches the original scale. At each new scale each contour element can be mapped to a 2×2 window. We assume that each element contour maps to the pixel with the largest gradient value among the four possible ones. The problem is then to find the best connected contour passing through (or near) two consecutive "chosen" pixels. A simple technique of interpolation can accomplish this task. We can also apply DP to find this contour. For each selected pixel, an uncertainty list of size three (including the selected pixel) is considered as prescribed by the algorithm, i.e., by passing a perpendicular line to the line between the neighbor selected pixels. Thus, between two consecutive points, a small window of uncertainty is considered and the algorithm is applied. Note that this contour must be smaller than 36 pixels and $4minC_k = 10$ is reasonable. Then, the complexity of the algorithm at each scale l is approximately $100 \times 10 \times 6^2 \times N_{l+1}$, where N_l is the size of the contour at scale l. Since there are l scales, and the size of the contour is approximately doubled for each finer level, the algorithm spends $72\,000 \times l \times N_l$ more time to obtain the final result.

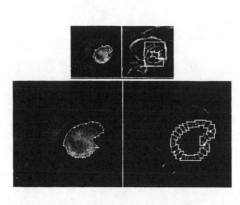

(a) Two-loop DP with multiscale

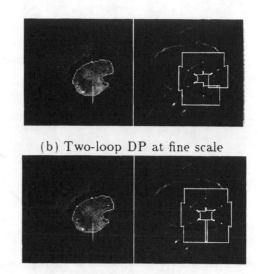

(b) Two-loop DP at fine scale

(c) Optimal DP at fine scale

Fig. 4. (a) Multiscale (two scales) recovery of a closed contour using DP. The result obtained at the coarsest scale is carried to the fine scale, where small search windows are used by DP. The results are compared with those obtained using the two-loop DP algorithm (b), and using the optimal DP (c). The images on the right show the six starting points and the search windows on the edge image.

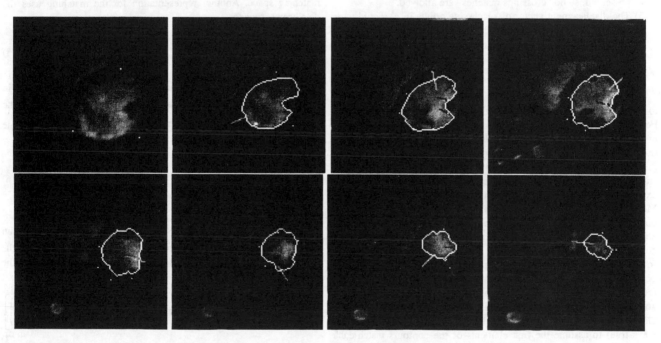

Fig. 5. Spatial tracking of contours for the left ventricle of the heart in MR images using the two-loop method.

In practice, for a closed contour shown in Fig. 4(c), a seven minute algorithm takes 36 seconds. Moreover, in this case (closed contour) the "two loop" approach further reduces it to 8.0 seconds (see Fig. 4(a)).

Multiscale results: Results for the multiscale approach are shown in Fig. 4 for the heart image. The resulting contour is quite close to that obtained by optimal DP and the two-loop DP without the multiscale analysis. The speed up obtained is six times the fine scale two-loop DP and 50 times the fine scale optimal DP.

The criteria for deciding the coarse scale to start the whole process depends on the structure being detected, the image modality, and the application domain. In case of cardiac MR images, the proximity of the inner and outer walls of the left ventricle limits l to 2. The contours for the head silhouette were detected at $l = 3$.

ust deal with unmatched features. We would also like to develop a matching strategy that can easily absorb other constraints, possibly coming from a higher level estimate. One may sometimes have the matching information for some of the points of the contour and may use this information to help to match the full contour.

1) *Uniqueness constraint*: Every element of c^1 (the smaller contour) has one match in the other contour.

69

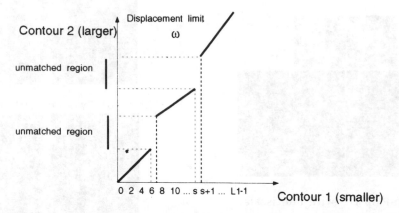

Fig. 6. The matching space and a possible solution to the matching problem. Note that only vertical jumps are allowed since every element of c^1 has a match. $\omega = L^2 - L^1$ is the displacement limit and so no matches are allowed out of the limit. Also, due to the monotonicity constraint, no matches will occur below the diagonal line. The path is monotonic so as to guarantee the ordering (no crosses).

2) *Monotonicity constraint*: The ordering of the contour must be preserved, so no "crossings matches" are allowed,

3) The displacement vector of successive points in c^1 should vary smoothly and the match should be translational invariant (could be extended to rotation invariance).

4) The size of unmatched regions in c^2 (the larger contour) should be as small as possible.

The *uniqueness constraint* can be relaxed to allow elements of c^1 to be left unmatched, requiring a slight modification of the algorithm. For the problems we have considered, the *uniqueness constraint* holds. The *monotonicity constraint* is a natural one since most of the transformations will preserve the order of the contour elements. The third constraint is aimed at dealing with contours that deform smoothly. This is the case for the applications we have considered, expanding balloons or time evolution of heart wall chambers. Moreover, translational invariance is necessary so that, by translating one contour, the results are the same (plus the translation). We could also consider rotation invariance. In this case the formulation becomes more difficult (but possible). We discuss this at the end. The fourth constraint applies to the expansion of a balloon, when it could be easier to leave a large portion of the expanded contour unmatched (see Fig. 7). It can also be applied to the heart wall chamber problem and to many other problems. Finally, when the contours are not closed (e.g., artery of angiography data) it is natural (though not always true) to assume the first elements of the contours match each other, i.e., c_0^1 matches c_0^2. Our model can easily incorporate this constraint.

A. The Cost Function

We propose an energy function minimization scheme to match the contours. One possible representation for the matching of contour elements c_s^1 and c_k^2 is given by the matching unit $M_{s,k}$ such that $M_{s,k} = 1$ if there is a match and $M_{s,k} = 0$ otherwise. A matching space is then the natural place to visualize the possible solutions. The matching space is a two dimensional space with the x-axis taking the elements of the smaller contour, c^1, and the y-axis taking the elements from the larger contour, c^2. Each element of the space takes the value of the matching unit M, 1 if there is a match and 0 otherwise. We

show in Fig. 6 a possible solution to the matching problem in the matching space. Another representation for the matching uses the displacement vector,

$$\vec{D}_s(M_{s,k}) = \sum_{k=0}^{L^2-1} M_{s,k}\left(x_k^2 - x_s^1, y_k^2 - y_s^1\right), \tag{5}$$

where each element s in contour c^1 and each matched element k in contour c^2 defines a displacement $\vec{D}_s = \left(x_k^2 - x_s^1, y_k^2 - y_s^1\right)$. When the matched element k is unknown the above equation defines $\vec{D}_s$. Due to the *uniqueness constraint*, we have

$$\sum_{k=0}^{L^2-1} M_{s,k} = 1 \quad \forall s. \tag{6}$$

The *uniqueness constraint* can be relaxed to allow for unmatched elements on c^1 by rewriting it as $\sum_{k=0}^{L^2-1} M_{s,k}\ 0,1 \quad \forall s$. We suggest an energy function, depending upon the displacement vector and the matching units, $M_{s,k}$, (the displacement vector depends on the matching units), of the form

$$E(M) = \sum_{s=1}^{L^1-1}\left[\mu\left\|\vec{D}_s(M) - \vec{D}_{s-1}(M)\right\| + \eta\left(\sum_{k,k^p=0}^{L^2-1} M_{s,k}M_{s-1,k^p}\left(k - k^p\right)^2\right)\right]. \tag{7}$$

The first term enforces the smoothness of the displacement field (dependent upon the matching field). Moreover, it is translational invariant ($\vec{D}_s' = \vec{D}_s + \vec{T} \Rightarrow \left\|\vec{D}_s' - \vec{D}_{s-1}'\right\| = \left\|\vec{D}_s - \vec{D}_{s-1}\right\|$), thus satisfying requirement three. The second term penalizes larger jumps more, satisfying requirement four. μ and η are parameters to be estimated. Notice that for $\mu = 0$ we obtain the "normalization length" method, i.e., becomes equivalent to parameterize curves 1 and 2 with $\rho_1 \in [0, 1]$ and $\rho_2 \in [0, 1]$, respectively, and to match the elements with the same ρ_1 and ρ_2. The limit in which $\eta = 0$ where we obtain large regions of unmatched points is shown in Fig. 7(c).

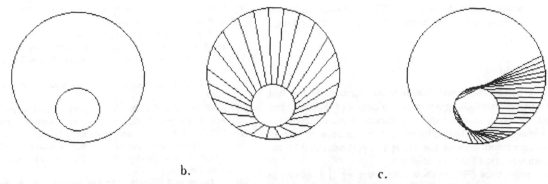

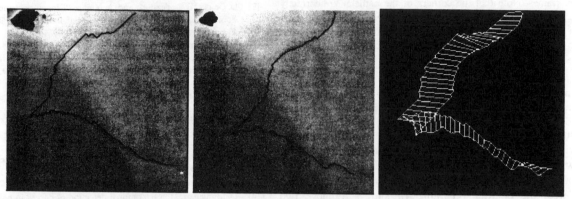

Fig. 7. Matching two eccentric circles: (a) edge map of two circles. (b) matching pixels of two active contours connected with lines. $\mu = 1$ and $\lambda = 0.1$. Every fifth match is displayed for clarity. (c) for $\lambda = 0$ no penalty for large jumps is imposed and the result is of less interest.

Fig. 8. Matching two open contours (catheters) corresponding to a fluoroscopic sequence. On the right we display the displacement vectors.

Possible extensions: We could have included a term for similarity based on the grey level of the image, e.g.,

$$\sum_{s=1}^{L^1-1} \sum_{k=0}^{L^2} M_{s,k} |T_s - T_k|,$$

where $|T_s - T_k|$ is a measurement of the similarity between the image at pixel s in one frame and at pixel k in the other frame. The algorithm we have devised would not be much altered but, for the applications we have considered, this was not necessary, i.e., we assumed $|T_s - T_k|$ to be the same for every pixel pair of the contours. Moreover, one could consider an energy function that is rotation invariant. In this case one could re-represent the contour by its tangent angles, then, by imposing a translation invariance on these elements, we would achieve rotation invariance (and translation invariance, since tangent angles are already invariant under translation). We plan to further explore this idea.

Displacement limit: We note that a displacement limit exists. Given two contours, c^1 and c^2, with sizes L^1 and L^2, such that $L^2 > L^1$, the maximum possible jump (or equivalently maximum possible size of an unmatched region of c^2) is $L^2 - L^1$. This is because of *uniqueness*, where every element of c^1 has to have a match:

$$M_{s,k} = 1 \Rightarrow k - s \leq L^2 - L^1. \tag{8}$$

B. DP for Matching Active Contours

Our objective is to find a path in the matching space such that just L^1 points from the contour c^2 matches all the L^1 points from the contour $c^1 (c_0^1, c_1^1, ..., c_{L^1-1}^1)$.

Hard constraints: We apply the *uniqueness constraint* by just considering the best match for each element of c^1. We use the *monotonicity constraint* to restrict the space of possible solutions. If c_s^1 matches c_k^2, i.e., if $M_{s,k} = 1$, than the previous candidates for c_{s-1}^1 are restricted to $c_{k^p}^2$ such that $k^p < k$.

Why DP: Let us assume K to be a set of $k_0, k_1, ..., k_{L^1-1}$ so that k_i is the index of the contour c_2 that matches the element $c_{s_i}^1$. We can write:

$$K = \left\{ k_i \middle| M_{s_i,k_i} = 1, i = 0, ..., N \right\}, \tag{9}$$

where $N = L^1 - 1$ and the constraints $k_i \geq s_i$ and $k_i < k_{i+1}$.

Then our goal is to find K^* that minimize the energy function $E(M)$, since M will depend only on K. Let us define H_i as:

$$H_i = \mu D(k_i, k_{i-1}) + \eta (k_i - k_{i-1})^2, \; i = 1, ..., N \tag{10}$$

where $D(k_i, k_{i-1}) = \left\| \vec{D}_{s_i} - \vec{D}_{s_{i-1}} \right\|$ and H_0 we can define as $H_0 = \eta (k_0)^2$. Then, the main proper of (7) is:

$$\min_K E(K) = \min_{K-\{k_N\}} \min_{\{k_N\}} E(K) = \min_{K-\{k_N\}} \left\{ (E(K) - H_N) + \min_{k_N} [H_N] \right\}. \tag{11}$$

If we apply the above property, until k_0 we can find the minimum of $E(K)$.

The search goes from left to right, column by column, from the bottom to the top. Our strategy is an adaptation of the one suggested in [9] for stereo matching with occlusions. The kth element of the resulting array *match*, is an index of a contour element in c^2 matching a contour element c_s^1.

C. Matching results

In Figs. 7 and 8 we present matching experiments. In the first (Fig. 7) we show the matching between two circles of different sizes and centers. One may consider this experiment as the matching between two images of an inflating balloon. It can be seen that the algorithm produces uniform matches along the perimeter despite the large difference in size of the two contours.

The next experiment (Fig. 8) shows the matching of a catheter in fluoroscopy data (the catheter has already been identified). This matching can help interpolate the displacement of the catheter in between frames. Note that the corners of the catheter are correctly matched to each other. It should be noted that, because of the restricted search space, the DP matching algorithm is very fast, matching two contours of 500 points in a few milliseconds.

V. Conclusions

We have proposed methods to detect, track, and match deformable contours. When detecting the contours our contribution has been to

1) suggest ways to further explore the information provided by the user selected points by creating lists and windows of uncertainty,
2) build an energy and apply a one-stage DP to optimally detect the contour (guaranteed), and 3) propose two speed up procedures, one using a non-linear multiscale technique to obtain factors of 20 and the other, for closed contours, using a "two-loop" technique.

In particular, the algorithm with the tracking technique has been extensively tested on MRI cardiac data and is now being transferred to be used by doctors for clinical analysis. The use of the algorithm for other medical domains is now being tested, e.g., segmentation of very thin blood vessels in arterial tree in angiography.

For tracking we have simply selected 3% of the contour points as initial information for the next frame. Then the same algorithm was applied to detect the contours. Other methods for tracking, such as using Kalman filtering, can be incorporated into the algorithm but further experimentation and elaborations would be necessary.

For matching contours we have proposed a novel cost function and two constraints. The cost function enforces the smoothness of the match and small jumps of unmatched elements. The first constraint guarantees *uniqueness*; each contour element of the smallest contour has just one match. Thus some elements of the larger contour are left unmatched. The second constraint, *monotonicity*, is an ordering type of constraint and it guarantees that no cross displacement vectors are allowed. One of the features of our matching strategy is that it is easy to absorb more information (higher level information). If one knows that some features match each other one can use it to reduce the space of possible solutions and to speed up the algorithm.

References

[1] A. Amini, T. Weymouth, and R. Jain, "Using dynamic programming for solving variational problems in vision," *IEEE Trans. Pattern Analysis and Machine Intelligence*, vol. 12, no. 9, pp. 855–867, 1990.

[2] N. Ayache, I. Cohen, and I. Herlin, "Medical image tracking," *Active Vision*, A. Blake and A. Yuille, eds., chap. 20, MIT Press, Cambridge, Mass., 1992.

[3] D.H. Ballard and C.M. Brown, *Computer Vision*, Prentice Hall, Englewood Cliffs, N.J., 1982.

[4] M. Barzohar and D.B. Cooper, "Automatic finding of main roads in aerial images by using geometric-stochastic models and estimation," *Proc. IEEE Conf. Computer Vision and Pattern Recognition*, pp. 459–464, 1993.

[5] R. E. Bellman, *Applied Dynamic Programming*, Princeton Univ. Press, 1962.

[6] A. Blake and R. Cipollo, "The dynamic analysis of apparent contours," *First ECCV*, pp. 73–82, Springer-Verlag, Antibes, France, Apr. 1990.

[7] I. Cohen, L.D. Cohen, and N. Ayache, "Using deformable surfaces to segment 3D images and infer differential structures," *Computer Vision, Graphics, and Image Processing*, vol. 56, no. 2, pp. 242–263, Sept. 1992.

[8] D. Geiger and J. Kogler, "Scaling images and image features via the renormalization group," *Proc. IEEE Conf. Computer Vision and Pattern Recognition*, 1993.

[9] D. Geiger, B. Ladendorf, and A. Yuille, "Binocular stereo with occlusion," *Computer Vision-ECCV92*, G. Sandini, ed., vol. 588, pp. 423–433, Springer-Verlag, Santa Margherita, Italy, 1992.

[10] J. Gregor and M.G. Thomason, "Dynamic programming alignment of sequences representing cyclic patterns," *IEEE Trans. Pattern Analysis and Machine Intelligence*, vol. 15, no. 2, pp. 129–135, 1993.

[11] A. Gueziec and N. Ayache, "Smoothing and matching of 3D-space curves," *Second ECCV*, Springer-Verlag, Santa Margherita, Italy, May 1992.

[12] M. Hospital, H. Yamada, T. Kasvand, and S. Umeyama, "3D curve based matching method using dynamic programming," *Proc. Int'l Conf. Computer Vision*, pp. 728–732, 1987.

[13] M. Kass, A. Witkin, and D. Terzopoulos, "Snakes: Active contour models," *Proc. Int'l Conf. Computer Vision*, pp. 259–268, London, England, June 1987.

[14] U. Montanari, "On the optimal detection of curves in noisy pictures," *Comm. ACM*, pp. 335–345, 1971.

[15] E. Mortensen, B. Morse, W. Barrett, and J. Udupa, "Adaptive boundary detection using *live-wire* two dimensional dynamic programming," *Computers and Cardiology*, pp. 635–638, 1992.

[16] A. P. Pentland and B. Horowitz, "Recovery of nonrigid motion and structure," *IEEE Trans. Pattern Analysis and Machine Intelligence*, vol. 13, no. 7, July 1991.

[17] A.P. Pentland and J.R. Williams, "Good vibrations: Modal dynamics for graphics and animation," *Proc. ACM SIGGRAPH*, pp. 215–222, 1989.

[18] D. Pope, D. Parker, P. Clayton, and D. Gustafson, "Left ventricular border recognition using a dynamic search algorithm," *Radiology*, vol. 155, no. 2, pp. 513–517, 1985.

[19] H. Sakoe and S. Chiba, "Dynamic programming algorithm optimization for spoken word recognition," *IEEE Trans. Acoustics, Speech, Signal Processing*, vol. 26, no. 1, pp. 43–49, May 1978.

[20] A. Shashua and S. Ullman, "Structural saliency: The detection of globally salient structures using a locally connected network," *Proc. Int'l Conf. Computer Vision*, pp. 321–327, 1988.

[21] D. Terzopoulos, A. Witkin, and M. Kass, "Symmetry-seeking models for 3D object reconstruction," *Proc. Int'l Conf. Computer Vision*, pp. 269–276, London, England, June 1987.

[22] N. Ueda and K. Mase, "Tracking moving contours using energy-minimizing elastic contour models," *Computer Vision-ECCV92*, G. Sandini, ed., vol. 588, pp. 453–457, Springer-Verlag, Santa Margherita, Italy, 1992.

[23] Y. Wu and H. Maitre, "Registration of a spot image and a SAR image using multiresolution representation of a coastline," *Proc. Int'l Conf. Pattern Recognition*, pp. 913–917, 1990.

[24] A. Yuille and P. Hallinan, "Deformable templates," *Active Vision*, A. Blake and A. Yuille, ed., MIT Press, Cambridge, Mass, 1992.

Constraints on Deformable Models: Recovering 3D Shape and Nonrigid Motion*

Demetri Terzopoulos, Andrew Witkin and Michael Kass

Schlumberger Palo Alto Research, 3340 Hillview Avenue, Palo Alto, CA 94304, U.S.A.

Recommended by AAAI-87 Program Committee

ABSTRACT

Inferring the 3D structures of nonrigidly moving objects from images is a difficult yet basic problem in computational vision. Our approach makes use of dynamic, elastically deformable object models that offer the geometric flexibility to satisfy a diversity of real-world visual constraints. We specialize these models to include intrinsic forces inducing a preference for axisymmetry. Image-based constraints are applied as extrinsic forces that mold the symmetry-seeking model into shapes consistent with image data. We describe an extrinsic force that applies constraints derived from profiles of monocularly viewed objects. We generalize this constraint force to incorporate profile information from multiple views and use it to exploit binocular image data. For time-varying images, the force becomes dynamic and the model is able to infer not only depth, but nonrigid motion as well. We demonstrate the recovery of 3D shape and nonrigid motion from natural imagery.

1. Introduction

A primary goal of early vision is to recover the shapes and motions of 3D objects from their images. To achieve this goal, we must synthesize visual models that satisfy a bewildering variety of constraints. Some constraints derive from the sensory information content of images. Others reflect background knowledge about image formation and about the shapes and behaviors of real-world objects. Exploiting diverse constraints in combination has proven to be a challenge. We need models which not only integrate constraints, but which escape the confines of conventional representations that impose simplify-

---

* This paper was the most outstanding paper in the subfield "Perception-Vision" at the AAAI-87 Conference.

ing assumptions about shape and motion. Computational vision calls for general-purpose models having the capability to accurately represent the free-form shapes and nonrigid motions of natural objects—objects with which the human visual system copes routinely. Clearly, we need new models that can accommodate deformation, nonconvexity, nonplanarity, inexact symmetry, and a gamut of localized irregularities.

We propose a physically based modeling framework for shape and motion reconstruction of free-form flexible objects from their images. In this framework, objects are modeled as elastically deformable bodies subject to continuum mechanical laws. Constraints are expressed as forces applied to these bodies. The applied forces deform the elastic models and propel them through potentially complicated motions such that they satisfy the available constraints over time. We develop algorithms for inferring from natural images the structures and motions of flexible objects moving nonrigidly in three dimensions. The algorithms compute detailed 3D object models directly from image intensity data without making use of intermediate optic-flow fields or 2.5D surface representations.

To reconstruct models directly from natural images that possibly involve significant occlusions, we must exploit several powerful constraints in unison. Our physical models focus the constraints in a natural way—by summing together the associated forces. There are two types of forces: Intrinsic forces encode constraints internal to our deformable models. Extrinsic forces couple the models to the external image data and provide an avenue for user interaction.

1.1. Intrinsic constraints

The intrinsic constraints reflect generically valid assumptions about natural objects. Our deformable models apply a basic constraint that is characteristic of physical bodies: surface coherence. The constraint is inherent in the elastic forces prescribed by the physics of deformable continua—these forces elicit piecewise continuous deformations.

A second generic constraint built into our models is symmetric regularity, an attribute of many natural and synthetic objects. Rather than imposing strict symmetries through explicit parameterization, we design more liberal *symmetry-seeking* intrinsic forces. These forces constrain the deformations of the model in order to give it a preference for certain desired symmetries. Representing symmetry as constrained deformation rather than through geometric parameterization frees the model from the shackles of particular parametric shape families such as, say, the quadrics—spheres, cylinders, ellipsoids, etc.

Our work to date considers the reconstruction of the 3D shape and nonrigid motion of objects possessing approximate axial symmetry. Our axisymmetry-seeking model of shape is essentially a deformable tube surrounding and coupled to a deformable spine. The coupling results from intrinsic forces that imbue the combined model with a preference for axisymmetry. In this regard, our model is close in spirit to the generalized cylinder representation first recommended in 1971 by Binford as a convenient description of 3D surfaces for the purposes of vision [1].

Generalized cylinders often are overly restrictive in that they can represent with accuracy only perfectly axisymmetric shapes. Since some amount of asymmetry is evident in many synthetic and most natural shapes, generalized cylinders can result in a loss of crucial information about objects. By contrast, the symmetry-seeking model accommodates deviations from symmetry by deforming. Only as the intrinsic forces are strengthened does the symmetry-seeking model tend to impose the strict symmetries of a generalized cylinder. As the intrinsic forces are weakened, however, the model will be able to faithfully represent increasingly asymmetric shapes, although axisymmetric shapes have greater stability and hence are preferred.

1.2. Extrinsic constraints

The extrinsic constraints reflect, in part, observations about the environment that can be extracted from sensory data. Although, in principle, we can exploit within our framework a variety of image-based cues, including shading and texture, the present paper makes exclusive use of information about profiles (the profile of an object, also known as its occluding contour, refers to the curve which outlines the image region covered by the projection of the object). The human visual system has a remarkable ability to infer the 3D shapes of objects from their 2D profiles in images. To demonstrate this ability, David Marr was fond of showing Picasso's "Rites of Spring," which consists entirely of silhouettes (Fig. 1).

Silhouette information in confluence with the a priori constraints intrinsic to symmetry-seeking deformable models proves sufficient to recover 3D shapes. For example, Fig. 2 illustrates the reconstruction of Picasso's "Rites" directly from the silhouettes in Fig. 1 using 43 instances of the symmetry-seeking model. The symmetry-seeking models are embedded in a force field which encodes the profile information. The ambient forces mold the deformable models to make their 3D shapes consistent with the observed 2D profiles of objects or their subparts. Perfect axisymmetries are generally absent from the reconstructed shapes, as dictated by the artistic silhouettes.

Another possible source of extrinsic constraints is a human operator. We augment the ambient force field with forces controlled by computer pointing devices, thereby providing opportunity for a user to willfully guide the reconstruction process. We can create symmetry-seeking models and pull or push them through space while we monitor their shapes and motions as wire-frame projections on the image plane(s). As we bring models near imaged objects of interest, we observe them reconstructing the detailed shapes of these objects.

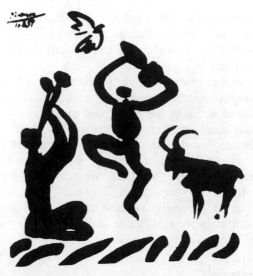

Fig. 1. "'Rites of Spring' by Pablo Picasso. We immediately interpret such silhouettes in terms of particular three-dimensional surfaces—this despite the paucity of information in the image itself. In order to do this, we plainly must invoke certain a priori assumptions and constraints about the nature of the shapes." (D. Marr [2, p. 213]).

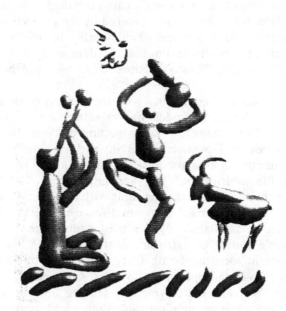

Fig. 2. 3D rendition of Picasso's "Rites." This 3D reconstruction employs 43 instances of the symmetry-seeking model. The instances were reconstructed semi-automatically from the silhouettes in Fig. 1 (see text).

On a sufficiently powerful computer, deformable models offer an interactive modeling medium of practical interest in its own right. Nonetheless, our long-range goal in the context of machine vision is to replace the user with fully automatic top-down control processes, possibly linked to knowledge bases.

1.3. The reconstruction method

In this paper, we first review the special case of shape recovery from a static monocular view [3], then we generalize our approach to shape and motion recovery from input data consisting of a temporal sequence of binocular image pairs.

Figure 3 illustrates the reconstruction of a crook-necked squash from its monocular image using a symmetry-seeking model. The user initializes the

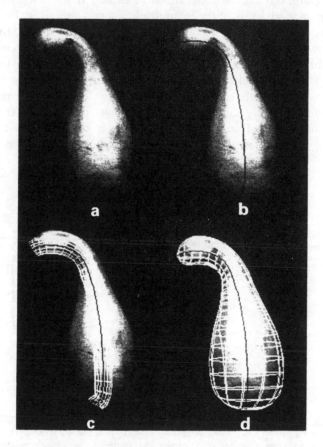

Fig. 3. Reconstruction of a 3D symmetry-seeking model. (a) Squash image. (b) User-initialized spine shown in black. (c) Initial tube. (d) Reconstructed model displayed as a wire frame projected into the image.

model by specifying the projection of the spine in the image plane near the medial axis of the object. In the monocular case the model is subject to extrinsic forces expressed as the gradient of an image potential function. The potential is a measure of the local contrast in the image after an appropriate smoothing transformation. Hence, the high contrast contour in the image (by assumption, the profile of the object) attracts the occluding boundary of the model (the occluding boundary of a 3D solid refers to the locus of points along which lines of sight graze its surface). The shape of model achieves a fixed point in the ambient force field. At equilibrium, the model's occluding boundary, relative to the viewpoint associated with the image is consistent with the shape of the object profile in the image. The model's intrinsic continuity and symmetry forces specify 3D shape over the remainder of its surface. Figure 4 sketches the monocular reconstruction scenario.

The image potential can be generalized to exploit more complete geometric information provided by profiles in multiple images acquired from different viewpoints around an object. For the particular case of stereo, the potential incorporates two images from slightly different vantage points. Deprojection of its gradient through a binocular camera model creates a stereo force field in space. Points on the model's occluding boundaries with respect to both the left and right eye are sensitive to the stereo force field. The forces position boundary points laterally and in depth such that their binocular projections coincide as much as possible with object profiles in both images. By attending

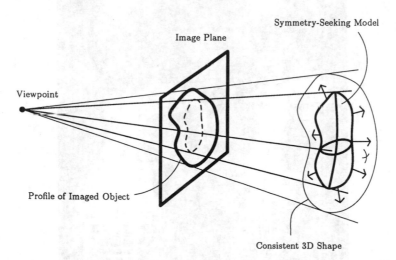

Fig. 4. Monocular reconstruction scenario. The arrows depict extrinsic forces in space which act on the symmetry-seeking model's occluding boundary as seen from the viewpoint. The forces deform the 3D model so as to make its image plane projection (dotted curve) more consistent with the 2D profile of the imaged object. The model comes to equilibrium as soon as its 3D shape achieves maximal consistency with the image data.

to the occluding boundary associated with each image individually, our method overcomes the difficulties that boundaries of smooth objects are known to present to conventional stereo matching techniques.

When the objects under consideration move, the ambient force field becomes dynamic. It carries the model through nonrigid motions, continually molding its shape to maintain maximal consistency with the evolving image data. The evolution of the model is computed by numerically integrating the partial differential equations of motion for the deformable body as it reacts to the dynamic force field.

The remainder of this paper is organized as follows: Section 2 discusses our approach relative to other work in vision and modeling. Section 3 describes the geometry and dynamics of the deformable symmetry-seeking model. Section 4 describes the image forces; first the monocular force, then the more general motion–stereo force. Section 5 briefly overviews the implementation of the model reconstruction algorithm. Section 6 presents results. Section 7 concludes the paper with a discussion.

2. Background

2.1. Constraint-based modeling

The work in this paper develops further a constraint-based modeling paradigm which has been successful on a variety of problems in computer graphics and animation as well as in computer vision: Terzopoulos et al. [4] apply physical constraints to deformable curve, surface, and solid models to construct and animate computer graphics objects made of simulated rubber, cloth, and other flexible materials. Witkin et al. [5] apply geometric constraints to parameterized shape primitives such as cylinders or spheres to automatically dimension, assemble, and animate objects constructed from such parts. Barzel and Barr [6] assemble articulated objects with dynamic constraints and simulate these objects with accurate Newtonian dynamics.

Witkin et al. [7] subject a deformable sheet in image coordinates to constraint forces derived from area correlation to perform stereo reconstruction in the style of the 2.5D sketch (Fig. 5(c)). Terzopoulos et al. [3] use symmetry-seeking models in a limited way to perform object reconstruction from static monocular profiles (Fig. 5(d)). Kass et al. [8] apply image-based constraints to deformable planar curves, dubbed "snakes," to interactively locate and track edges and other image features (Fig. 6). Platt [9] extends a deformable space curve model into a space-time surface, and uses it to recover rigid motion.

2.2. Comparison to conventional models

The elastically deformable models developed in this paper have evolved from variational models for visual surface reconstruction [10]. A number of features

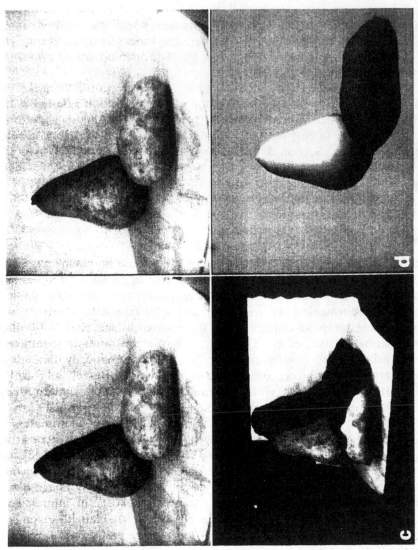

Fig. 5. Reconstructions of a still life scene. (a)–(b) Stereo images. (c) 2.5D reconstruction of stereo pair using a deformable sheet disparity model (from [7]). Left image is mapped on the reconstructed surface which is rendered from an oblique viewpoint to show depth discontinuities as gaps in surface. (d) 3D reconstruction of objects in left image using a symmetry-seeking deformable model (from [3]).

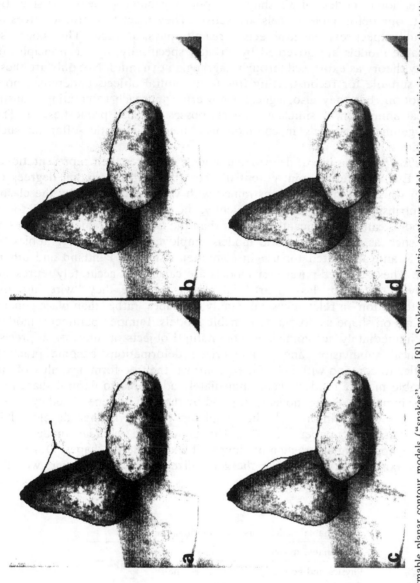

Fig. 6. Deformable planar contour models ("snakes"—see [8]). Snakes are elastic contour models subject to extrinsic forces that attract them towards image features such as lines and edges. After allowing two snakes to capture the outline of the pear and the potato, the user pulls one of the snakes away from the edge of the pear using an interactive spring force. When the user releases the snake, it is pulled back to the edge of the pear.

distinguish our modeling approach from the norm in computational vision. The comparison is summarized by Table 1.

Conventional models of 3D shape are purely geometric, hence passive. By contrast, our deformable models are active. They react to extrinsic forces as one would expect real elastic objects to react to physical forces. This is because deformable models are governed by physics; specifically, by the principles of elasticity theory as expressed through Lagrangian dynamics. Not only are these models suitable for reconstructing free-form natural objects undergoing non-rigid motion, but they also suggest a powerful approach to creating realistic graphical animation of simulated objects possessing such properties [4]. The purely geometric models in common use, being kinematic, offer no such possibilities.

The *distributed* nature of deformable models enhances their representational power. Every material point potentially contributes three spatial degrees of freedom which are mutually constrained with variable tightness by the elastic forces intrinsic to the model. Consequently, the geometric coverage of deformable models can be significantly broader than the *lumped*-parameter families of shapes such as the superquadric models employed in computer graphics by Barr [11] and advocated for use in computer vision by Pentland and others [12, 13]. These lumped-parameter models are capable of accurately representing only a restricted class of artificial objects because they "wire into the parameterization" a relatively small family of shapes, rather than place generic constraints on shape as do our deformable models. Lumped-parameter models cannot immediately accommodate most natural objects of interest, so precise hierarchical subdivision and parameterized deformations become practical necessities to contend with [14, 15]. By contrast, the free-form flexibility of our deformable models renders them immediately adaptable to natural shapes.

Our symmetry-seeking model is inspired by the idea of generalized cylinders first proposed by Binford [1], then implemented and further developed in several subsequent papers [16–22]. The generalized cylinder model is an intuitively appealing abstraction of elongated, axisymmetric shapes. Our model captures axisymmetry much like the generalized cylinder; however, we take

Table 1
Deformable models versus conventional models

Deformable models	Conventional models
Physics and geometry	Only geometry
Active	Passive
Dynamic	Kinematic
Distributed	Lumped parameter
Broad coverage	Narrow coverage
Controlled constraints	Strict constraints

seriously the fact that many objects of interest are only approximately symmetric.

A major difference between our deformable model and generalized cylinders is that, while generalized cylinders *impose* symmetry constraints on objects they represent—inevitably with some loss of detailed shape information—the forces intrinsic to our model express *preference* for certain symmetries, but the model is not limited to strictly symmetric shapes. As the intrinsic forces are strengthened, the symmetry-seeking model will tend to impose the strict symmetries of a generalized cylinder. Conversely, by weakening the intrinsic forces, the model acquires the capacity to represent irregular objects with significant fine structure (assuming, of course, that sufficient constraint is maintained so that the reconstruction problem remains well-conditioned for the image data under consideration). Shape representations capable of applying constraint in this controllable manner are desirable for reconstruction and recognition; an early example is the spring–template shape model proposed by Fischler and Elschlager [23].

2.3. Recovery of nonrigid motion

Among the contributions of the present paper is a technique for recovering from image data the structure and motion of nonrigid objects in space. The significantly simpler case of recovering rigid motion has a long history and continues to attract much attention in computational vision. The literature is replete with analyses of the minimal sets of pointwise motion data sufficient to solve the structure-from-motion problem uniquely, subject to a rigidity assumption (see the survey [24]). However, a rigid-body assumption can be sensitive to noise, and it is clearly inappropriate when dealing with flexible objects.

In recent years, a desire to relax rigidity assumptions has begun to motivate new investigations into using motion information to invert the optical projection equations. Initial computational analyses treat restricted types of nonrigid motion—such as articulated bodies [25, 26]—while subsequent work recognizes the need for further generalization. Webb and Aggarwal [27] shed the global rigid-body assumption in favor of assuming local rigidity of planar patches. Under orthogonal projection, this implies a measurable affine distortion in the image plane. They are able to recover surface orientations from intensity and motion information. Chen [28] discusses the representation of nonrigid objects from the perspective of linear elasticity theory and generalizes the method of Webb and Aggarwal to handle perspective projection while presupposing a weaker assumption: that object surfaces deform isometrically (only bending occurs, so that distances along the surface are preserved). Koenderink and van Doorn [29] pursue a similar surface isometry assumption and they present an algorithm for recovering local aspects of shape from two views of a seven-point polygonal model. Ullman [30] considers the problem of recovering the structure of arbitrarily deforming "objects" consisting of a set of points in space from the projected positions of these points at several successive time instants. His algorithm incrementally adjusts the 3D positions of points in a model to best account for the projected positions, while maximizing the model's rigidity across successive frames, as measured by the weighted sum of squared deviations of 3D distances between all pairs of points (global interaction).

Our approach goes beyond the above methods in significant ways, while retaining some of their best features. Our methods apply successfully to raw image sequences of extended natural objects undergoing nonrigid motion, not just to pointwise synthetic data. Our models accommodate arbitrary deformations, including bending, stretching, and shearing components. In principle, they also permit piecewise continuous deformations with explicit treatment of discontinuities (although the present paper does not pursue discontinuities). The underlying formulation is based on elasticity theory, and the elastic deformation forces are computable by local interaction in the discretized elastic body.

2.4. Multimodal integration and multiple views

The continuum mechanical equations of motion that govern our models provide a conceptually simple mechanism for integrating multiple visual modalities and information from multiple views. Each information source makes a contribution to the net force field acting on the model (cf. [31]).

Techniques have been developed for constructing volumetric descriptions of objects by intersecting projective cones associated with profiles in images taken from multiple viewpoints [32, 33]. Active sensors have been incorporated as well [34]. Although it makes use of profiles in multiple images, the volume intersection approach is fundamentally different from ours.

We demonstrate multimodal and multiview integration by combining stereo with motion in order to recover the evolving shape in proper depth robustly. Several researchers have investigated motion–stereo fusion as a means of facilitating the recovery of 3D velocity information from images [35–39]. Typically, they treat the case of observers moving through static environments.

Our approach is intended to handle flexible objects moving independently. It extracts 2D shape information directly from profiles and is able to estimate depth over each object's surface from profiles in stereo image pairs. Our current algorithms to do not involve explicit stereo or motion correspondence matching computations; each model simply tracks its associated object via the evolving force field to produce a 3-space velocity field over the entire surface of the object (including hidden surfaces) in proper depth.

3. The Symmetry-Seeking Model

Before we review the formulation of the symmetry-seeking model proposed in [3], here is an informal description. Consider a deformable sheet made of elastic material (a membrane–thin-plate hybrid). Roll this sheet to form a tube. Next, pass a deformable spine made of similar material down the length of the tube. At regularly spaced points along the spine, couple it to the tube with radially projecting forces so as to maintain the spine in approximate axial position within the tube. Include additional forces that coerce the tube into a quasi-symmetric shape around the spine. Finally, provide extra control over the shape by introducing expansion/compression forces radiating from the spine. The rigidities of the spine and the tube are independently controllable, and their natural rest metrics and curvatures can either be prescribed or modified dynamically. If the circumferential metric of the tube is set to zero, for instance, the tube will tend to contract around the spine, unless the other forces prevail. The model will shorten or lengthen as the longitudinal metrics of the tube and spine are modified. In short, a variety of interesting behavior (including viscoelasticity and fracture) can be obtained by adjusting the control variables designed into the model.

We represent the spine and tube as geometric mappings from material coordinate domains into Euclidean 3-space $\mathbb{R}^3$. We express the mappings as vectors whose component functions denote time-varying components of position in space. The spine is a deformable space curve defined by mapping a univariate material coordinate domain $s \in [0, 1]$ into $\mathbb{R}^3$: $v(s, t) = (X(s, t), Y(s, t), Z(s, t))$. The tube is made from a deformable space sheet defined by mapping a bivariate material coordinate domain $(x, y) \in [0, 1]^2$ into $\mathbb{R}^3$: $v(x, y, t) = (X(x, y, t), Y(x, y, t), Z(x, y, t))$.

A functional $\mathscr{E}(v)$ characterizes the deformable material by associating a nonnegative strain energy with any admissible mapping. In our deformable models, $\mathscr{E}$ is an instance of the controlled-continuity spline functions defined in [40].

The continuum mechanical equation

$$\mu \frac{\partial^2 v}{\partial t^2} + \gamma \frac{\partial v}{\partial t} + \frac{\delta \mathscr{E}(v)}{\delta v} = f(v) \tag{1}$$

governs the nonrigid motion of a body in response to a net extrinsic force $f(v)$, where μ is the mass density function of the deformable body and γ is the viscosity function of the ambient medium [41]. The third term on the left-hand side of the equation is the variational derivative of the strain energy functional $\mathscr{E}$ [42]; it expresses the elastic force internal to the body.

The deformation energy associated with the spine mapping $v(s, t)$ is given by

$$\mathscr{E}^S(\boldsymbol{v}) = \int_0^1 w_1 \left| \frac{\partial \boldsymbol{v}}{\partial s} \right|^2 + w_2 \left| \frac{\partial^2 \boldsymbol{v}}{\partial s^2} \right|^2 \, \mathrm{d}s \,, \qquad (2)$$

where vertical bars denote Euclidean vector norms. Here, $w_1(s, t)$ determines the local tension along the spine, while $w_2(s, t)$ determines its local rigidity.

The deformation energy associated with the sheet mapping $\boldsymbol{v}(x, y, t)$ is given by the functional

$$\mathscr{E}^T(\boldsymbol{v}) = \int_0^1 \int_0^1 w_{10} \left| \frac{\partial \boldsymbol{v}}{\partial x} \right|^2 + w_{01} \left| \frac{\partial \boldsymbol{v}}{\partial y} \right|^2$$

$$+ w_{20} \left| \frac{\partial^2 \boldsymbol{v}}{\partial x^2} \right|^2 + 2 w_{11} \left| \frac{\partial^2 \boldsymbol{v}}{\partial x \partial y} \right|^2 + w_{02} \left| \frac{\partial^2 \boldsymbol{v}}{\partial y^2} \right|^2 \, \mathrm{d}x \, \mathrm{d}y \,. \qquad (3)$$

The weighting functions $w_{10}(x, y, t)$ and $w_{01}(x, y, t)$ locally control the tension of the sheet along each material coordinate curve, while $w_{20}(x, y, t)$, $w_{11}(x, y, t)$, and $w_{02}(x, y, t)$ locally control its rigidities.

Aside from boundary terms, the variational derivatives of $\mathscr{E}^S$ and $\mathscr{E}^T$ expressing the elastic forces are given as follows:

$$\frac{\delta \mathscr{E}^S}{\delta \boldsymbol{v}} = \frac{\partial^2}{\partial s^2} \left(w_2 \frac{\partial^2 \boldsymbol{v}}{\partial s^2} \right) - \frac{\partial}{\partial s} \left(w_1 \frac{\partial \boldsymbol{v}}{\partial s} \right), \qquad (4)$$

$$\frac{\delta \mathscr{E}^T}{\delta \boldsymbol{v}} = \frac{\partial^2}{\partial x^2} \left(w_{20} \frac{\partial^2 \boldsymbol{v}}{\partial x^2} \right) + 2 \frac{\partial^2}{\partial x \partial y} \left(w_{11} \frac{\partial^2 \boldsymbol{v}}{\partial x \partial y} \right) + \frac{\partial^2}{\partial y^2} \left(w_{02} \frac{\partial^2 \boldsymbol{v}}{\partial y^2} \right)$$

$$- \frac{\partial}{\partial x} \left(w_{10} \frac{\partial \boldsymbol{v}}{\partial x} \right) - \frac{\partial}{\partial y} \left(w_{01} \frac{\partial \boldsymbol{v}}{\partial y} \right). \qquad (5)$$

The weighting functions in the above expressions control the elastic properties. When necessary, we can regulate the natural shapes of the deformable bodies—i.e., their equilibrium shapes exclusive of external forces—through suitably defined control functions. For instance we can encourage the spine to maintain a nonzero natural arc length $L_1(s)$, by defining

$$w_1 = K_1 \left(\left| \frac{\partial \boldsymbol{v}}{\partial s} \right| - L_1 \right),$$

where K_1 is a tension factor. Similarly we can define

$$w_{10} = K_{10} \left(\left| \frac{\partial \boldsymbol{v}}{\partial x} \right| - L_{10} \right), \qquad w_{01} = K_{01} \left(\left| \frac{\partial \boldsymbol{v}}{\partial y} \right| - L_{01} \right)$$

to encourage natural lengths $L_{10}(x, y)$ and $L_{01}(x, y)$ for the sheet along the x

and y material coordinate directions respectively. Analogous expressions for w_2 will encourage a natural nonzero curvature for the spine, while for w_{20}, w_{11}, and w_{02} they will encourage natural curvatures for the sheet.

To allow discontinuities to occur in the spine at any material point s_0, we set $w_1(s_0, t) = w_2(s_0, t) = 0$ which permits a position discontinuity, or $w_2(s_0, t) = 0$ which permits a tangent discontinuity. The obvious extensions hold with regard to the five control functions associated with the sheet. See [40] for further details regarding discontinuities.

The tube is formed by prescribing boundary conditions on two opposite edges of the sheet that "seam" these edges together. We seam the edge $x = 0$ to the edge $x = 1$, letting y span the length of the tube. The required periodic boundary conditions are

$$v(0, y, t) = v(1, y, t), \qquad \frac{\partial v}{\partial x}\bigg|_{(0,y,t)} = \frac{\partial v}{\partial x}\bigg|_{(1,y,t)}. \qquad (6)$$

To couple the two components, we first identify $y \equiv s$, bringing into correspondence the spine coordinate with the coordinate along the length of the tube (see Fig. 7). We then distinguish the mapping function of the spine $v^S(s, t)$ from that of the tube $v^T(x, s, t)$ with superscripts S and T.

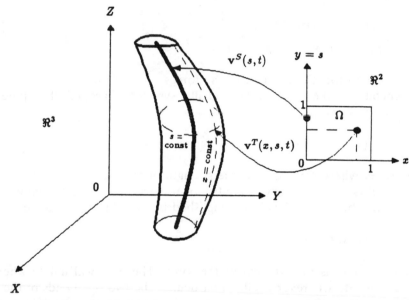

Fig. 7. Geometric representation of the symmetry-seeking model. For fixed time t, the spine and tube components of the model map material coordinates $y = s$ and (x, s), respectively, into positions in $\mathbb{R}^3$.

87

We define

$$\bar{v}^{\mathrm{T}}(s) = \frac{1}{l} \int_0^1 v^{\mathrm{T}} \left| \frac{\partial v^{\mathrm{T}}}{\partial x} \right| \mathrm{d}x$$

to be the centroid of the coordinate curve ($s = \text{constant}$) circling the tube, whose length is given by

$$l(s) = \int_0^1 \left| \frac{\partial v^{\mathrm{T}}}{\partial x} \right| \mathrm{d}x .$$

We also define the tube's radial vector function with respect to the spine as $r(x, s) = v^{\mathrm{T}} - v^{\mathrm{S}}$, the unit radial vector function $\hat{r}(x, s) = r/|r|$, and

$$\bar{r}(s) = \frac{1}{l} \int_0^1 |r| \left| \frac{\partial v^{\mathrm{T}}}{\partial x} \right| \mathrm{d}x$$

as the mean radius of the coordinate curve $s = \text{constant}$.

The spine is coerced into an axial position within the tube by introducing the following forces on the spine and tube respectively:

$$\begin{aligned} f_a^{\mathrm{S}}(s, t) &= a(\bar{v}^{\mathrm{T}} - v^{\mathrm{S}}) , \\ f_a^{\mathrm{T}}(x, s, t) &= -(a/l)(\bar{v}^{\mathrm{T}} - v^{\mathrm{S}}) , \end{aligned} \tag{7}$$

where $a(s)$ controls the strength of the forces.

To encourage the tube to be radially symmetric around the spine, we introduce the force

$$f_b^{\mathrm{T}}(x, s, t) = b(\bar{r} - |r|)\hat{r} \tag{8}$$

on the tube, where $b(s)$ controls the strength of the force.

Finally, it is useful to provide control over expansion and contraction of the tube around the spine. This is accomplished by introducing the force

$$f_c^{\mathrm{T}}(x, s, t) = c\hat{r} , \tag{9}$$

where $c(s)$ controls the strength of the force. The tube will inflate wherever $c > 0$ and deflate wherever $c < 0$. In particular, the two open ends of the tube can be cinched shut by assigning large negative values to $c(0)$ and $c(1)$, thereby creating a sausage-like surface. This force is also useful for counteracting a tendency of the tube to contract around the spine due to the quadratic curvature approximations appearing in $\mathcal{E}$. Use of the true curvature tensor in $\mathcal{E}$ will alleviate the contraction problem directly, but at the expense of non-linearities that are computationally expensive and badly behaved numerically.

Summing the above coupling forces into the equations of motion (1) associated with the spine and tube, we obtain the following dynamic system describing the motion of the symmetry-seeking model:

$$\mu\,\frac{\partial^2 \boldsymbol{v}^S}{\partial t^2} + \gamma\,\frac{\partial \boldsymbol{v}^S}{\partial t} + \frac{\delta \mathcal{E}^S}{\delta \boldsymbol{v}^S} = \frac{\delta P^S}{\delta \boldsymbol{v}^S} + \boldsymbol{f}_a^S\,,$$

$$\mu\,\frac{\partial^2 \boldsymbol{v}^T}{\partial t^2} + \gamma\,\frac{\partial \boldsymbol{v}^T}{\partial t} + \frac{\delta \mathcal{E}^T}{\delta \boldsymbol{v}^T} = \frac{\delta P^T}{\delta \boldsymbol{v}^T} + \boldsymbol{f}_a^T + \boldsymbol{f}_b^T + \boldsymbol{f}_c^T\,.$$

(10)

The elasticity terms on the left-hand side of these coupled equations are given by (4) and (5) (with $y \equiv s$ in the latter).

$P^S(\boldsymbol{v}^S)$ and $P^T(\boldsymbol{v}^T)$ are generalized potential functions associated with the spine and tube respectively. Their variational derivatives express the extrinsic forces that act on these bodies.

4. Extrinsic Force Fields

This section explains how we transform one or more input images into generalized potential functions suitable for reconstruction. The resulting force field brings instances of the symmetry-seeking model into maximal consistency with the images, and it maintains the consistency over time in the dynamic case.

More specifically, profiles in the images exert an attraction over the model such that the deformable tube, as projected into the image planes through a suitable camera model, accounts as much as possible for the observed profiles. In this paper, the spine of the model experiences no image-based forces ($P^S = 0$), although we project it into the image plane along with the tube for display purposes.

To simplify the potential functions, we consider objects with subdued texture which are imaged in front of a contrasting background. Hence, we can expect that the stronger image intensity gradients are associated with object profiles. The force fields that we propose yield interesting results, their simplicity notwithstanding.

4.1. Monocular potential

We first define a generalized potential function P^T to couple the tube to a static, monocular image. Given the image of an object, the ambient force field resulting from this potential deforms the symmetry-seeking model to make its shape consistent with the object's profile in the image. The occluding boundary of the deformable tube with respect to the viewpoint is made sensitive to this force field which attracts it towards significant intensity gradients in the image.

Let $I(\xi, \eta)$ be the image intensity function. We define the potential

$$P^{T}(\boldsymbol{v}^{T}) = \beta |\nabla(G_{\sigma} * I(\Pi[\boldsymbol{v}^{T}]))| , \tag{11}$$

which imparts on the tube boundary an affinity for large image intensity changes. The operations symbolized by the expression are as follows: The operator Π denotes an imaging projection. $\Pi[\boldsymbol{v}^{T}]$ expresses the projection of the tube $\boldsymbol{v}^{T}(x, s) = (X^{T}(x, s), Y^{T}(x, s), Z^{T}(x, s))$ from 3-space into the image plane (ξ, η). The expression $G_{\sigma} * I$ denotes the image convolved with a (Gaussian) smoothing filter whose characteristic width is σ. The operator ∇ denotes the gradient of the smoothed image, and the vertical bars signify the magnitude of this gradient.

The weighting function $\beta(x, s)$ is nonzero only for material points (x, s) near occluding boundaries of the tube which are not obscured behind other objects. We activate points near occluding boundaries by defining

$$\beta(x, s) = \begin{cases} 1, & \text{if } |\boldsymbol{i} \cdot \boldsymbol{n}| < \tau , \\ 0, & \text{otherwise} , \end{cases} \tag{12}$$

where τ is a small threshold (nominally 0.05),

$$\boldsymbol{n}(x, s) = \left(\frac{\partial \boldsymbol{v}^{T}}{\partial x} \times \frac{\partial \boldsymbol{v}^{T}}{\partial s} \right) \bigg/ \left| \frac{\partial \boldsymbol{v}^{T}}{\partial x} \times \frac{\partial \boldsymbol{v}^{T}}{\partial s} \right|$$

is the unit normal over the surface of the tube, and $\boldsymbol{i}(x, s)$ is a unit vector from the imaging focal point to any point (x, s) on the tube.

While a perspective projection is generally appropriate for Π, we have obtained satisfactory results in the examples considered below using orthographic projection $\Pi : (\xi, \eta) = (X, Y)$. Everywhere over the tube in this case, $\boldsymbol{i}$ is the unit normal to the image plane, and the resulting force field acts on the tube in a direction parallel to the image plane.

Figure 8 illustrates the effect of the image operations for progressively larger values of σ (we used similar operations in [8]). The ambient force field adjusts the 3D shape of the model's occluding boundary in space so as to maximize the magnitude of the image gradient (darkness) along the projected model profile in the image. By using potential functions at several scales, we can trade off localization accuracy against long-range attraction. As is evident from the figure, broad wells surround the local minima of the image potential at the coarser scales. Such wells attract the model from a considerable distance, but the associated minima are blurred and localize the profiles in the image data rather poorly. Continuous scale space [43] provides a good medium for obtaining both long-range attraction and good localization. We can apply a

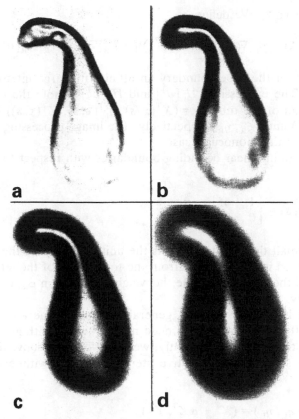

Fig. 8. Creating an image potential function. Result of applying image operations (see text) to the squash image of Fig. 3. (a)–(d) σ increases progressively. Darkness indicates magnitude of local gradient of the Gaussian blurred image. Each processed image has been rescaled to span the available intensity range.

continuation method in the image potential scale space, parameterized by σ, which allows the model to equilibrate at a coarse scale, then continuously reduces the smoothing σ to track an equilibrium trajectory from coarse to fine scale [7].

4.2. Binocular potential

The next refinement is to match the deformable model to an object's profiles in a binocular image pair. The symmetry-seeking model is free to undergo motion in 3-space while deforming such that its stereoscopic projection through the binocular camera model best accounts for the observed profiles in both images.

Let $I_L(\xi_L, \eta_L)$ represent the left and $I_R(\xi_R, \eta_R)$ the right image intensity function. The binocular potential function P^T is a straightforward extension of the monocular case. We define

$$P^{\mathrm{T}}(v^{\mathrm{T}}) = \beta_{\mathrm{L}}|\nabla(G_{\sigma} * I_{\mathrm{L}}(\Pi_{\mathrm{L}}[v^{\mathrm{T}}]))| + \beta_{\mathrm{R}}|\nabla(G_{\sigma} * I_{\mathrm{R}}(\Pi_{\mathrm{R}}[v^{\mathrm{T}}]))|, \qquad (13)$$

which imparts on the tube boundary an affinity for large intensity changes in both images. The expressions $\Pi_{\mathrm{L}}[v^{\mathrm{T}}]$ and $\Pi_{\mathrm{R}}[v^{\mathrm{T}}]$ denote the two-component stereoprojection of the tube $v^{\mathrm{T}} = (X^{\mathrm{T}}(x, s), Y^{\mathrm{T}}(x, s), Z^{\mathrm{T}}(x, s))$ into the image planes $(\xi_{\mathrm{L}}, \eta_{\mathrm{L}})$ and $(\xi_{\mathrm{R}}, \eta_{\mathrm{R}})$ respectively. The image-processing operations are the same as for the monocular case.

We activate points near occluding boundaries with respect to the left image by defining

$$\beta_{\mathrm{L}}(x, s) = \begin{cases} 1, & \text{if } |i_{\mathrm{L}} \cdot n| < \tau, \\ 0, & \text{otherwise}, \end{cases} \qquad (14)$$

where τ is a small threshold, $n(x, s)$ is the unit normal over the surface of the tube, and $i_{\mathrm{L}}(x, s)$ is a unit vector from the focal point of the left image to any point (x, s) on the tube. We define the weighting function $\beta_{\mathrm{R}}(x, s)$ for the right image similarly.

Although it is possible to use a general binocular camera model (see, e.g., [44, Section 10.6]), its parameters need not be known with great accuracy for our approach to work. Consequently, we have found it convenient to employ the following simplified perspective stereoprojection with eye vergence at infinity:

$$\begin{aligned} \Pi_{\mathrm{L}} : (\xi_{\mathrm{L}}, \eta_{\mathrm{L}}) &= (X^{\mathrm{T}} + \alpha Z^{\mathrm{T}}, Y^{\mathrm{T}}), \\ \Pi_{\mathrm{R}} : (\xi_{\mathrm{R}}, \eta_{\mathrm{R}}) &= (X^{\mathrm{T}} - \alpha Z^{\mathrm{T}}, Y^{\mathrm{T}}), \end{aligned} \qquad (15)$$

where α is a constant. In this case, i_{L} and i_{R} become unit normals to the left and right image planes respectively.

4.3. Dynamic potential

When the images are time-varying the ambient force field becomes dynamic. It carries the model through motions, continually molding its shape to maintain maximal consistency with the evolving image data. Our method for allowing the symmetry-seeking model to track an object undergoing nonrigid motion is as follows. The first frame of the image sequence is presented to the model as if it were a static scene. The model achieves the best possible reconstruction using this initial data. The projected boundary points equilibrate at a fixed point in the ambient force field and the model locks on to the consistent state.

Whereas the equilibrium persists indefinitely in the static case, in the dynamic case we immediately present the model with the next frame of the image sequence. Now the ambient force field is perturbed because of the motions of objects in the scene. The model actively seeks a new consistent state by moving towards the nearest fixed point. If the motion of the object is sufficiently slow and continuous, the model will track the dynamic equilibrium point, thus updating its state in accordance with the new image information available to it. By repeating this procedure with each successive incoming frame, the symmetry-seeking model integrates the incoming information over time.

One possible variant to our standard nonrigid tracking procedure is a two-step rigid-deformable technique. With each incoming frame, we first restrict the model to rigid motion in order to obtain a suboptimal result quickly. Only then do we allow it to deform in order to account for the residual nonrigid motion. This method accelerates the numerical solution when objects under analysis move nearly rigidly.

5. Numerical Solution

The continuous differential equations of motion (10) for the symmetry-seeking model pose a nonlinear initial boundary value problem. To obtain a numerical solution, we first perform a semi-discretization in the material coordinates of the model. We then integrate the resulting coupled system of second-order ordinary differential equations through time using standard techniques. In the static field case, we integrate until the viscous damping (γ-term) dissipates all kinetic energy, thus bringing the model to static equilibrium. In the dynamic field case, we integrate through time, computing the motion of the model in reaction to the evolving force field. Numerically, this amounts to solving a sequence of dynamic equilibrium problems, each solution providing initial conditions to the subsequent problem.

Semi-discretization in material coordinates is carried out using standard finite difference approximations on regular grids of nodes [45]. We approximate the three components of the elastic force $\delta \mathscr{E}^S/\delta v^S$ by discretizing the partial derivatives in (4) on a linear N_s point grid. We use a rectangular $N_x \times N_s$ grid to similarly discretize the partial derivatives in the components of $\delta \mathscr{E}^T/\delta v^T$ in (5). The extrinsic force components $\delta P^T(v^T)/\delta v^T$ are computed numerically in the image domains (ξ, η) using bilinear interpolation between centrally differenced pixel values.

Finally, we approximate the time derivatives in (10) at discrete times using finite differences over regular intervals. We have successfully employed both an explicit Euler time integration scheme and an analogue to successive overrelaxation (SOR) to "solve" the dynamic equilibrium problems in sequence, each a large sparse system of algebraic equations. These iterative solution methods require only local operations, and the former is a parallel scheme. Explicit solvers are relatively inexpensive per time step (linear in the number of nodes), but they quickly become unstable as the intrinsic or extrinsic forces are increased, thus necessitating tiny time steps. As expected, we observe stability over larger time steps when using an implicit Euler time integration scheme in conjunction with matrix factorization methods [45]. The drawback of these robust, direct solution methods is that they become expensive for finely discretized models (cubic in the number of nodes).

A good compromise is to use a hybrid technique that combines some of the benefits of direct and iterative schemes. We have had success with an operator splitting approach used in alternating direction implicit (ADI) methods [45, 46]. This efficient procedure exploits the fact that we are dealing with a rectangular grid of nodes. Each time step of the procedure involves a sweep in the x direction solving N_x independent systems of algebraic equations in N_s unknowns, followed by a sweep in the s direction solving N_s independent systems in N_x unknowns. Our strategic linearizations of the elastic forces permit us to apply the method independently to each of the three tube position components (X^T, Y^T, Z^T). The spine gives rise to an additional system of equations in N_s unknowns for each of its position components (X^S, Y^S, Z^S).

As a consequence of the controlled-continuity deformation model, each of the unidimensional systems of equations has a pentadiagonal matrix of coefficients, and it is efficiently solvable (linear time in the number of unknowns) using direct solution methods. We employ a normalized Cholesky decomposition step followed by a forward–reverse resolution step. See [47] for a derivation of the pentadiagonal matrix and for a discussion of the direct method and [8] for its application to image contour models.

Resolution, a relatively inexpensive step, must be performed at every iteration as the applied forces change. Matrix decomposition is somewhat more expensive, but it is required only when the material properties of the model are altered (e.g., to increase rigidity or to introduce discontinuities). Currently, we perform only an initial decomposition because we have not yet experimented with the variation of material properties during solution.

We find that for larger grid sizes and increasingly rigid material the alternating direction approach evolves solutions faster than the SOR type method that we employed in [3]. This is attributable to the fact that the direct solution of each unidimensional system obtained through operator splitting "immediately" distributes to all nodes along two perpendicular parametric grid lines the effects of forces acting on their common node.

6. Results

Figure 9 shows selected frames from an animation sequence showing the reconstruction of a single symmetry-seeking model from a monocular image. Given an image of the squash (Fig. 3), the user initializes the spine's projection in the image plane somewhere near the medial axis of the squash. The tube

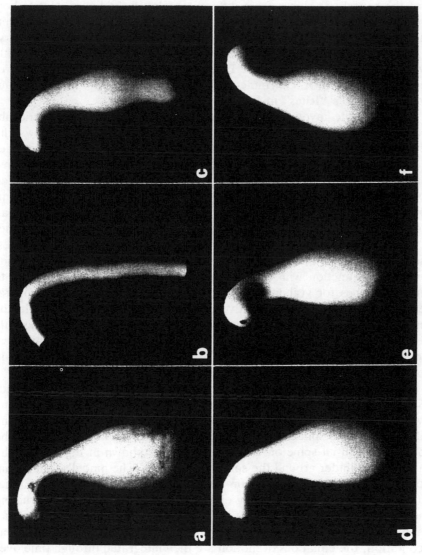

Fig. 9. Reconstruction of a squash. (a) Squash image. Selected frames from an animation sequence are shown: (b) Initial state of the 3D model. (c) Intermediate shape during reconstruction. (d) Final reconstructed model. (e)–(f) Model rotating rigidly in space. The 3D model is rendered as a shaded shell.

begins as a generalized cylinder with uniformly circular cross-section. It inflates due to the action of the internal expansion forces. As the tube approaches a profile, the force field due to the significant intensity edge attracts it strongly. It equilibrates over the profile to reconstruct the nonconvex, quasi-symmetric 3D shape of the squash, as shown from different angles in the figure. Notice how the model begins as a generalized cylinder yet recovers the inexact axisymmetry of the squash in the course of reconstruction. By virtue of the symmetry-seeking constraints intrinsic to the model, hidden surface portions are smoothly extrapolated from portions in view. Essentially the same reconstruction procedure applies to each of 43 symmetry-seeking model instances in the reconstruction of Picasso's "Rites" in Fig. 2.

The next example involves the reconstruction of two quasi-symmetric objects, a pear and a potato, from a single image. Figure 10(a) shows the grey-level image of the still life scene. Notice that the potato partially occludes the pear in the image. Figure 10(b) shows the initial model configurations, manually specified by the user. Figures 10(c) and (d), show the reconstructed 3D models from two points of view. To handle the partial occlusions (incomplete boundaries), we nullify the weighting function $\beta(x, s)$ over portions of an occluded model's surface which are obscured from the viewpoint by another model. Appropriately, the obscured parts of the model feel no image forces, because they are invisible in the image. We use a standard 3D ray-casting technique in conjunction with the projection operation Π in (11) in order to test surface patches for visibility using a depth buffer. The ray-casting operation requires knowledge of the relative depth ordering of the objects. In the monocular case, this information is not available directly, so the user presently specifies the relative depth ordering (although it may be possible to obtain local depth ordering information automatically, through analysis of occlusion cues in the image [48]).

The most direct way of obtaining true depth information is through stereo. The reconstruction method was applied to a stereo–motion sequence consisting of 40 video fields portraying the 3D motion of a human finger. The imaging apparatus was a beam-splitting stereo adaptor mounted on a CCD camera. The user specifies an initial spine on the first stereo pair shown in Fig. 11(a). The initial tube is a cylinder around the spine (Fig. 11(b)). The model's differential equations (using $\mu = 0$) are solved on a $N_x \times N_s = 25 \times 25$ grid for the initial frame (requiring about 40 alternating direction iterations), thus reconstructing the shape of the object in proper depth. Figures 11(c)–(e) show the reconstructed shape rendered from several viewpoints. Using this equilibrium shape as initial condition, the equations of motion are then integrated through time over the remaining frames of the stereo sequence (using 20 alternating direction iterations per frame). This produces a dynamic 3D reconstruction of the finger's shape and motion. Figure 12 shows six representative frames of the sequence along with the corresponding reconstructed shapes in motion.

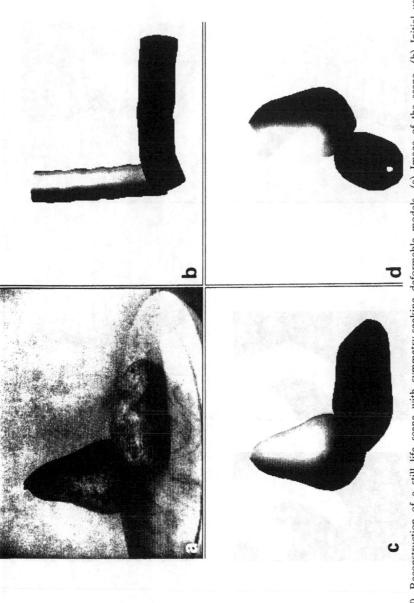

Fig. 10. Reconstruction of a still life scene with symmetry-seeking deformable models. (a) Image of the scene. (b) Initial user-specified configurations of the 3D models. Two rendered views of the reconstructed still life: (c) Frontal view of the 3D models; (d) side view.

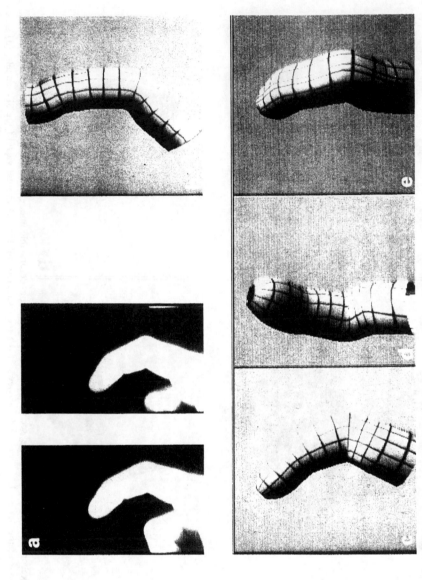

Fig. 11. Initial 3D reconstruction of a finger. (a) Finger stereo pair for first time instant. (b) User-initialized cylinder. (c)–(e) Initial reconstructed shape from three viewpoints. Every other grid line has been drawn on the surface.

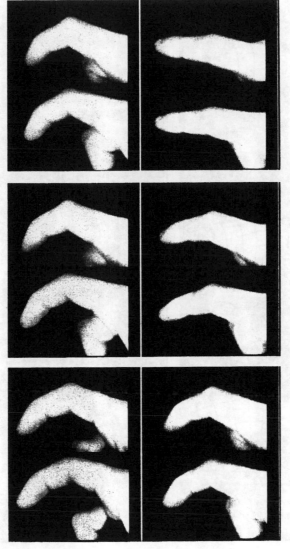

Fig. 12(a). Six frames of the stereo sequence.

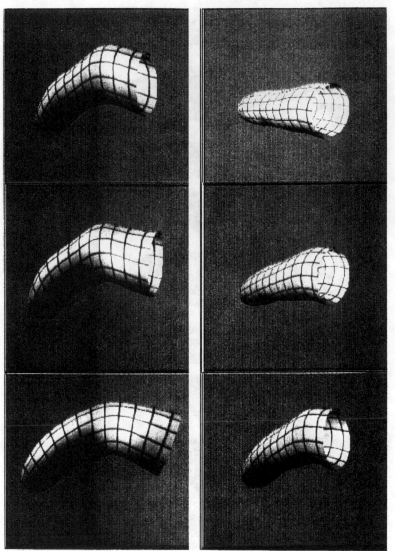

Fig. 12(b). Evolving shape and motion of the model.

7. Discussion

Referring back to Fig. 5, we can compare the 3D model reconstruction with a 2.5D visible-surface reconstruction of the still life scene. The 2.5D reconstruction of the stereo images shown is generated by a stereo algorithm that we developed in [7]. The algorithm generates depth discontinuities along the occluding boundaries of the objects. Profiles of smooth objects and the occluding boundaries which generate them are known to present difficulties to conventional stereo matching techniques. This is mainly because profiles observed in the left and right image map to different occluding boundaries on smooth objects. Our method for reconstructing models directly from images overcomes this problem. The use of a full 3D model in tandem with separate left and right projection operators simplifies the association of each image profile with the suitable occluding contour on the model.

In our experience, the user need not initialize the spine (or tube) of the model with any great accuracy. Typically, the user draws rough medial axes running more or less the length of the objects of interest in the image. Figure 13(a) shows a typical set of initial spines. With the tubes starting out as cylinders extruded along these spines, the reconstruction process makes the necessary adjustments to both the spine and tube (Fig. 13(c)). Figure 13(b) shows the projections of the final spines. Compared to the initial axes, the final axes are improved; they are smoother and have suitable lengths. It appears possible, therefore, to instantiate reasonable spines automatically using medial axis transform [49] or smoothed local symmetry [50] algorithms, and perhaps our reconstruction method, where applicable, could improve the axes generated by such algorithms.

In the restricted case of computing 3D models of objects from a single monocular image, we tacitly assume that a suitable viewpoint has been chosen such that all significant object features are visible, and that the axis of the object is not severely inclined away from the image plane. However, in the more general case where we make use of stereo information, we experience little difficulty in tracking the shape and motion of an object even if its axis tilts away from the image plane significantly.

A shortcoming of our current algorithms stems from the fact that profile information alone, even moving stereo profiles, provide incomplete information about objects. When image data is not utilized over substantial portions of the object's surface, the symmetry-seeking model may yield a reconstructed shape more symmetric than the actual one. Also, it is difficult to detect rotations around the object's axis exclusively from moving profile information. Region-based measures over the surface would be helpful in this regard.

Despite the limitations of our current implementation, a crucial advantage of our approach is the ease of integrating additional constraints into the solution. For instance, we can straightforwardly generalize the binocular potential

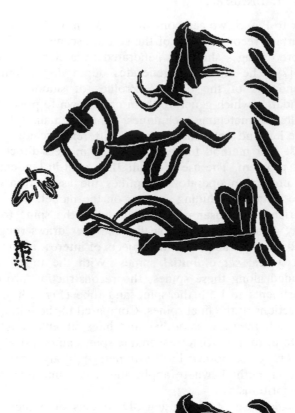

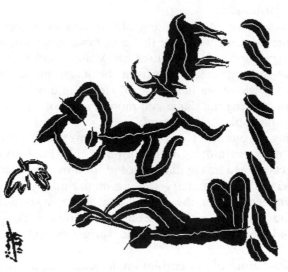

Fig. 13. Spines for the symmetry-seeking models. (a) Projections of the initial spines drawn by the user. (b) Projections of the final spines.

102

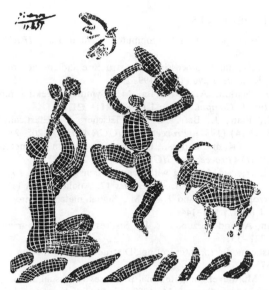

Fig. 13(c). Full resolution wire-frame grids of the reconstructed models.

function (13) as a sum over any number of views taken from known viewpoints around the object (cf. [33]). A focus of our current work is the formulation and implementation of extrinsic constraints that exploit shading and texture information over the entire visible surface, as well as stereo–motion constraints based on local area correlation which promise to effectively supplement our current edge-based information. By applying more sophisticated image-processing methods, we expect to obtain extrinsic forces that can deal with textured objects and more general imaging conditions. We also look forward to incorporating more sophisticated analytic camera models into the generalized potential functionals and to automatically solve for the camera parameters as an integral part of the reconstruction procedure.

We are investigating the use of scale space continuation methods [7] to partially automate the initialization of models. For the time being, however, our algorithms remain interactive, and it is up to the user to supply reasonable initial conditions. Nonetheless, our approach suggests force constraint mechanisms for automatically bringing higher-level knowledge to bear on the reconstruction process. The development of such mechanisms is an interesting topic for future research.

ACKNOWLEDGMENT

We thank the following people: Kurt Fleischer assisted us in rendering models. Keith Nishihara digitized the Picasso. John Platt contributed to the development of our ideas. Marty Tenenbaum provided suggestive interpretations of some of the figures.

REFERENCES

1. Binford, T.O., Visual perception by computer, Invited Talk, *IEEE Systems and Control Conference*, Miami, FL (1971).
2. Marr, D., Visual information processing: The structure and creation of visual representations, *Proc. Roy. Soc. London B* **290** (1980) 199–218.
3. Terzopoulos, D., Witkin, A. and Kass, M., Symmetry-seeking models and 3D object reconstruction, *Int. J. Comput. Vision* **1** (1987) 211–221.
4. Terzopoulos, D., Platt, J., Barr, A. and Fleischer, K., Elastically deformable models, *Comput. Graph.* **21** (4) (1987) (*Proceedings SIGGRAPH-87*) 205–214.
5. Witkin, A., Fleischer, K. and Barr, A., Energy constraints on parameterized models, *Comput. Graph.* **21** (4) (1987) (*Proceedings SIGGRAPH-87*) 225–232.
6. Barzel, R. and Barr, A., Modeling with dynamic constraints, in: *Topics in Physically-Based Modeling, ACM SIGGRAPH '87 Course Notes* **17**, Anaheim, CA (1987).
7. Witkin, A., Terzopoulos, D. and Kass, M., Signal matching through scale space, *Int. J. Comput. Vision* **1** (1987) 133–144.
8. Kass, M., Witkin, A. and Terzopoulos, D., Snakes: Active contour models, *Int. J. Comput. Vision* **1** (1987) 321–331.
9. Platt, J., An elastic model for interpreting 3D structure from motion of a curve, Unpublished Manuscript (1987).
10. Terzopoulos, D., Multilevel computational processes for visual surface reconstruction, *Comput. Vision Graph. Image Process.* **24** (1983) 52–96.
11. Barr, A., Superquadrics and angle-preserving transformations, *IEEE Comput. Graph. Appl.* **18** (1981) 21–30.
12. Pentland, A.P., Parts: Structured descriptions of shape, in: *Proceedings AAAI-86*, Philadelphia, PA (1986) 695–701.
13. Bajcsy, R. and Solina, F., Three dimensional object representation revisited, in: *Proceedings First International Conference on Computer Vision*, London, England (1987) 231–240.
14. Barr, A.H., Global and local deformations of solid primitives, *Comput. Graph.* **18** (3) (1984) (*Proceedings SIGGRAPH-84*) 21–29.
15. Pentland, A.P., Recognition by parts, in: *Proceedings First International Conference on Computer Vision*, London, England (1987) 612–620.
16. Agin, G.A. and Binford, T.O., Computer description of curved objects, *IEEE Trans. Comput.* **25** (1976) 439–449.
17. Hollerbach, J.M., Hierarchical shape description of objects by selection and modification of prototypes, AI-TR-346, MIT AI Lab., Cambridge, MA (1975).
18. Nevatia, R. and Binford, T.O., Description and recognition of curved objects, *Artificial Intelligence* **8** (1977) 77–98.
19. Marr, D., Analysis of occluding contour, *Proc. Roy. Soc. London B* **197** (1977) 441–475.
20. Marr, D. and Nishihara, H.K., Representation and recognition of the spatial organization of three-dimensional shapes, *Proc. Roy. Soc. London B* **200** (1978) 269–294.
21. Brooks, R.A., Symbolic reasoning among 3-D models and 2-D images, *Artificial Intelligence* **17** (1981) 285–348.
22. Shafer, S.A., *Shadows and Silhouettes in Computer Vision* (Kluwer Academic, Boston, MA, 1985).
23. Fischler, M.A. and Elschlager, R.A., The representation and matching of pictorial structures, *IEEE Trans. Comput.* **22** (1973) 67–92.
24. Ullman, S., Recent computational studies in the interpretation of structure from motion, in: J. Beck, B. Hope and A. Rosenfeld (Eds.), *Human and Machine Vision* (Academic Press, New York, 1983) 459–480.
25. Webb, J.A. and Aggarwal, J.K., Visually interpreting the motions of objects in space, *Computer* **14** (1981) 40–46.
26. Hoffman, D.D. and Flinchbaugh, B.E., The interpretation of biological motion, *Biol. Cybern.* **42** (1982) 195–204.

27. Webb, J.A. and Aggarwal, J.K., Shape and correspondence, *Comput. Vision Graph. Image Process.* **21** (1983) 145–160.

28. Chen, S., Structure-from-motion without the rigidity assumption, in: *Proceedings IEEE 3rd Workshop on Computer Vision: Representation and Control*, Bellaire, MI (1985) 105–112.

29. Koenderink, J.J. and van Doorn, A.J., Depth and shape from differential perspective in the presence of bending deformations, *J. Opt. Soc. Am. A* **3** (1986) 242–249.

30. Ullman, S., Maximizing rigidity: The incremental recovery of 3-D structure from rigid and nonrigid motion, *Perception* **13** (1984) 255–274.

31. Terzopoulos, D., Integrating visual information from multiple sources, in: A.P. Pentland (Ed.), *From Pixels to Predicates: Recent Advances in Computational and Robotic Vision* (Ablex, Norwood, NJ, 1986) 111–142.

32. Baumgart, B.G., Geometric modeling for computer vision, AI Memo 249, Stanford Artificial Intelligence Laboratory, Stanford, CA (1974).

33. Martin, W.N. and Aggarwal, J.K., Volumetric description of objects from multiple views, *IEEE Trans. Pattern Anal. Mach. Intell.* **5** (1983) 150–158.

34. Wang, Y.F. and Aggarwal, J.K., On modelling 3-D objects using multiple sensory data, in: *Proceedings IEEE Conf. Robotics and Automation*, Raleigh, NC (1987) 1098–1103.

35. Nevatia, R., Depth measurement from motion stereo, *Comput. Vision Graph. Image Process.* **9** (1976) 203–214.

36. Regan, D. and Beverley, K.I., Binocular and monocular stimuli for motion in depth: Changing disparity and changing size feed the same motion in depth stage, *Vision Res.* **19** (1979) 1331–1342.

37. Ballard, D.H. and Kimball, O.A., Rigid body motion from depth and optical flow, *Comput. Vision Graph. Image Process.* **22** (1983) 95–115.

38. Richards, W., Structure from stereo and motion, *J. Opt. Soc. Am. A* **2** (1985) 343–349.

39. Waxman, A.M. and Sinha, S.S., Dynamic stereo: Passive ranging to moving objects from relative image flows, *IEEE Trans. Pattern Anal. Mach. Intell.* **8** (1986) 406–412.

40. Terzopoulos, D., Regularization of inverse visual problems involving discontinuities, *IEEE Trans. Pattern Anal. Mach. Intell.* **8** (1986) 413–424.

41. Hunter, S.C., *Mechanics of Continuous Media* (Ellis Horwood, Chichester, England, 2nd ed., 1983).

42. Courant, R. and Hilbert, D., *Methods of Mathematical Physics I* (Interscience, London, 1953).

43. Witkin, A., Scale space filtering, in: *Proceedings IJCAI-83*, Karlsruhe, F.R.G. (1983) 1019–1021.

44. Duda, R.O. and Hart, P.E., *Pattern Classification and Scene Analysis* (Wiley, New York, 1973).

45. Lapidus, L. and Pinder, G.F., *Numerical Solution of Partial Differential Equations in Science and Engineering* (Wiley, New York, 1982).

46. Press, W.H., Flannery, B.P., Teukolsky, S.A. and Vetterling, W.T., *Numerical Recipes: The Art of Scientific Computing* (Cambridge University Press, Cambridge, England, 1986).

47. Terzopoulos, D., Matching deformable models to images: Direct and iterative solutions, in: *Topical Meeting on Machine Vision*, *Technical Digest Series* **12** (Optical Society of America, Washington, DC, 1987) 160–167.

48. Rosenberg, D., Levine, M.D. and Zucker, S.W., Computing relative depth from occlusion cues, in: *Proceedings Fourth International Joint Conference on Pattern Recognition*, Tokyo, Japan (1978).

49. Blum, H.A., A transformation for extracting new descriptions of shape, in: *Proceedings Symposium on Models for Perception of Speech and Visual Form*, Boston, MA (1964) 362–380.

50. Brady, J.M. and Asada, H., Smoothed local symmetries and their implementation, *Int. J. Rob. Res.* **3** (1984) 33–61.

Received December 1987

Dynamic 3D Models with Local and Global Deformations: Deformable Superquadrics

Demetri Terzopoulos, *Member, IEEE,* and Dimitri Metaxas

Abstract—This paper presents a physically based approach to fitting complex 3-D shapes using a new class of dynamic models that can deform both locally and globally. We formulate deformable superquadrics which incorporate the global shape parameters of a conventional superellipsoid with the local degrees of freedom of a spline. The local/global representational power of a deformable superquadric simultaneously satisfies the conflicting requirements of shape reconstruction and shape recognition. The model's (six) global deformational degrees of freedom capture gross shape features from visual data and provide salient part descriptors for efficient indexing into a database of stored models. The local deformation parameters reconstruct the details of complex shapes that the global abstraction misses. The equations of motion which govern the behavior of deformable superquadrics make them responsive to externally applied forces. We fit models to visual data by transforming the data into forces and simulating the equations of motion through time to adjust the translational, rotational, and deformational degrees of freedom of the models. We present model fitting experiments involving 2D monocular image data and 3D range data.

Index Terms— Computer vision, physically based modeling, object representation, deformable models, local and global deformations, superquadrics, splines, simulated forces, 3D model fitting, finite element analysis.

I. INTRODUCTION

THE RECONSTRUCTION of shape and the recognition of objects have preoccupied computational vision researchers for several decades. Despite the large body of work on 3D modeling, most models of shape lack the descriptive power to bridge the gap between reconstruction and recognition. The difficulty is one of conflicting requirements.

General-purpose shape reconstruction in low-level visual processing requires models with broad geometric coverage. Reconstruction models must extract meaningful information from noisy sensor data while making the weakest possible assumptions about observed shapes. Generalized spline models that can deform locally subject to generic continuity constraints appear to be well suited to shape reconstruction. By contrast, object recognition is a higher level process that necessitates drastic information reduction and shape abstraction in order to support efficient matching in object databases of manageable size. Volumetric primitives such as spheres, cylinders, and prisms seem appropriate for object recognition since they can decompose composite shapes into natural parts that are compactly expressible using a small set of parameters.

In this paper, we propose an approach to shape modeling that simultaneously satisfies the requirements of reconstruction and recognition and promises a fluent transition between these two aspects of vision. We develop a new family of modeling primitives that have the following features.

Free-Form and Parameterized Geometry: Geometric design makes extensive use of both the free-form and parameterized modeling paradigms. The canonical primitives of these complementary approaches are, respectively, splines with local shape variables and volumetric forms with global shape parameters. One of the goals of our work is to develop a class of hybrid models whose underlying geometric structure intimately combines free-form and parameterized representations. In particular, the present paper combines membrane splines with parameterized superquadric ellipsoids to create a new family of models we dub *deformable superquadrics.*

Local and Global Deformations: Much of the expressive power of modeling primitives stems from their ability to deform into desired shapes. Spline models are free-form because their local shape control variables provide many local degrees of freedom. Consequently, splines have the flexibility to assume diverse shapes, i.e., they have broad geometric coverage. The allowable shapes of parameterized models, on the other hand, are relatively tightly constrained according to a few global parameters such as lengths, radii, and aspect ratios. Our modeling method interprets such parameters as a set of global deformational degrees of freedom. Moreover, we augment our models with the local deformational capabilities of splines. In particular, deformable superquadrics are able to deform both globally like superquadric ellipsoids and locally like membrane splines.

Physics and Dynamics: Concepts from analytic, differential, and computational geometry have fueled much of the shape representation research in vision. Recently, however, some vision researchers have begun to realize that geometry, while adequate for describing the shapes of static objects, is often insufficient when it comes to analyzing the motions and interactions of complex objects. Following our prior work, we remedy the situation by turning to computational physics. In addition to geometry, the formulation of our models includes simulated forces, masses, strain energies, and other physical quantities. Physically based models are fundamentally dynamic, and the behavior of deformable superquadrics is governed by the laws of rigid and nonrigid dynamics expressed through a set of Lagrangian equations of motion.

Manuscript received August 30, 1990; revised November 29, 1990. This work was supported by the Natural Sciences and Engineering Council of Canada and a University of Toronto Open Fellowship.

The authors are with the Department of Computer Science, University of Toronto, Toronto, Canada M5S 1A4.

IEEE Log Number 9100894.

Forces and Interaction: The numerical simulation of the equations of motion determines the evolution of the degrees of freedom of our models under the action of simulated forces and constraints. Forces provide a general and highly intuitive means for coupling the degrees of freedom of a model to various data sets, such as intensity and range data. In response to forces originating at datapoints, the models position and orient themselves properly in space and deform away from their rest shapes to conform to the dataset. In applications where user control over models is desirable, physically based control offers much more than the option of manually adjusting geometric parameters. The machinery supporting dynamics provides a facile interface to the models through the use of force interaction tools. Hence, another objective of our approach to modeling is to support interactive dynamics through the use of efficient numerical simulation methods.

Detail and Abstraction: The local and global deformation parameters along with rigid transformations comprise the degrees of freedom of our dynamic models. The equations of motion permit external forces to position and orient deformable superquadrics freely in space and shape them through the global degrees of freedom—a translation vector, a quaternion (rotation), a scale, three radial aspects, and two squareness parameters—but the forces can also deform the models like splines via the local degrees of freedom. The local degrees of freedom of deformable superquadrics allow the reconstruction of fine scale structure and the natural irregularities of real world data, whereas the global degrees of freedom capture the salient features of shape that are innate to natural parts and appropriate for matching against object prototypes. Our models are therefore suitable for use in both visual reconstruction and recognition tasks.

As an illustration of some of the above ideas, Fig. 1 shows a snapshot of an interactive 3D world inhabited by deformable superquadrics. Through mouse control, the user can initialize models, change their global deformation parameters, apply forces to them, and move the viewpoint. The figure illustrates four deformable superquadrics with different settings for the global deformation parameters. The model at the left is being pulled by a stretchy spring (displayed as a line) activated and dragged by the mouse (arrow). The spring force causes local and global deformations in the model.

A. Overview

Section II provides a background for our work in the context of related research. Section III formulates a general set of dynamic equations governing the motion of deformable superquadrics under the action of externally applied forces. Section IV describes a simplified version of these equations that are suitable for vision applications along with their numerical simulation. Section V discusses techniques for converting visual data into forces that can be applied to deformable superquadrics in data fitting scenarios. Section VI presents experimental results demonstrating the fitting of models to 2D monocular image data and 3D range data. Section VII draws conclusions from our work.

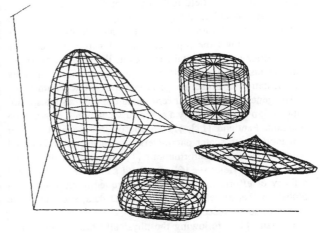

Fig. 1. Interactions with deformable superquadrics.

II. Background

After more than a decade of research, the notion of early visual reconstruction as a data fitting problem using generalized spline models is now in a highly evolved state of development, most evidently so in the context of the surface reconstruction problem [4], [18], [20]. Generalized spline techniques underly the notion of regularization and its application to a variety of reconstruction problems in early vision [14], [19]. The many degrees of freedom and local deformation properties of generalized splines allow them to conform to low-level visual data with ease.

On another front, much effort has gone into the search for suitable models for the purposes of object recognition. Biederman [3] reports the results of psychophysical experiments, suggesting that the recovery of arrangements of two or three major primitive components or parts results in fast recognition of objects, even when the objects are observed from different viewpoints, are occluded, or are unfamiliar. Parameterized part models capture the structure of the world by describing meaningful chunks of data in terms of a few parameters. Such models are beneficial for object representation since dealing with a manageable number of parameters simplifies the problem of indexing into a database of stored models and verifying match hypotheses.

Throughout the 1970's, the research of Binford and his coworkers on generalized cylinders focused on the problem of recovering parameterized models of objects and led to vision systems such as ACRONYM, which use reasoning to recover parameterized parts [5]. Marr and Nishihara [10] were among the first to propose a hierarchical representation of objects in terms of parts. Their work uses generalized cylinders to describe each part, thereby limiting the scope of the representation to objects adequately describable as collections of generalized cylinders.

Motivated by the generalized cylinder idea and the need to go beyond geometry to exploit computational physics in the modeling process, Terzopoulos *et al.* [22] propose a deformable cylinder constructed from generalized splines.

They develop force field techniques for fitting their model to monocular, binocular, and dynamic image data. The distributed nature of this deformable model enhances its descriptive power and allows the representation of natural objects with asymmetries and fine detail. However, the generalized spline components of the model do not explicitly provide an abstract representation of object shape in terms of a few parameters.

The generalized cylinder representation requires the specification of an axis, generally a space curve, and the cross-section function. Pentland [11], [12] proposes the use of a simpler part model with scalar parameters: the superquadric ellipsoid with parameterized deformations [1] (the superquadrics were discovered by Hein; see [6]). Pentland's proposal has spawned a flurry of efforts to reconstruct superquadric ellipsoids with global geometric deformations from 3D data, and these have met with some success [7], [8], [17].

Pentland [13], following the physically based approach of [22], proposes an alternative method for fitting deformable part models based on superquadric ellipsoids. Inspired by modal analysis (a technique for analyzing the vibrations of linear mechanical systems under periodic forcing conditions [2]), he applies polynomial deformation "modes" to superquadrics. Pentland's modeling primitives are not fully dynamic in that the underlying superquadric parameters do not respond to forces and are not fitted to data through force interactions. The deformation modes may make the method efficient for the recovery of smooth, symmetrically deformed parts. On the down side, global deformation modes lack an obvious physical meaning, and they make it difficult to deal with nonlinearities and boundary conditions. Moreover, the representation of complex shapes requires many modes, rendering Pentland's scheme no more efficient than a nodal finite element solution [2].

The present paper develops a new family of primitives with fully dynamic global and local deformations. Our formulation is similar to that of Terzopoulos and Witkin [21] with regard to the dynamics of free rigid-body motions and local deformations, but it includes additional global deformational degrees of freedom that may be inherited from any parameterized family of geometric primitives (in this paper, superquadrics). Our treatment of global deformation dynamics shares similar features with Witkin and Welch's [23] formulation of linearly deformable primitives, but we must deal with the nonlinear deformations of superquadrics. Our treatment of local deformation dynamics is general in that it permits the use of local or global support basis functions (it reduces to modal analysis [2] if we choose a sinusoidal eigenfunction basis). In this paper, we employ local finite element basis functions since they provide greater shape flexibility and are better suited to the purpose of local deformations, i.e., the representation of local detail.

III. FORMULATION OF DEFORMABLE SUPERQUADRICS

In this section, we provide a general formulation of deformable superquadrics. To arrive at the equations of motion that govern these models, we extend some results from [16] and [21].

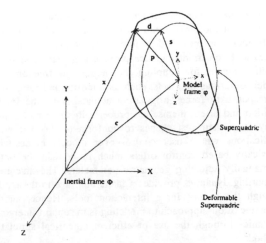

Fig. 2. Geometry of deformable superquadric.

A. Geometry

Geometrically, the models developed in this paper are closed surfaces in space whose intrinsic (material) coordinates are $u = (u, v)$, defined on a domain Ω. The positions of points on the model relative to an inertial frame of reference Φ in space are given by a vector-valued, time-varying function of u:

$$x(u, t) = (x_1(u, t), x_2(u, t), x_3(u, t))^T \qquad (1)$$

where T is the transpose operator. We set up a noninertial, model-centered reference frame ϕ and express these positions as

$$x = c + Rp \qquad (2)$$

where $c(t)$ is the origin of ϕ at the center of the model, and the orientation of ϕ is given by the rotation matrix $R(t)$. Thus, $p(u, t)$ denotes the canonical positions of points on the model relative to the model frame. We further express p as the sum of a reference shape $s(u, t)$ and a displacement function $d(u, t)$:

$$p = s + d. \qquad (3)$$

Fig. 2 illustrates the model geometry.

The ensuing formulation can be carried out for any reference shape given as a parameterized function of u. For concreteness, however, we consider the case of superquadric ellipsoids [1], which yield the reference shape

$$s = a \begin{pmatrix} a_1 C_u^{\epsilon_1} C_v^{\epsilon_2} \\ a_2 C_u^{\epsilon_1} S_v^{\epsilon_2} \\ a_3 S_u^{\epsilon_1} \end{pmatrix} \qquad (4)$$

where $-\pi/2 \leq u \leq \pi/2$ and $-\pi \leq v < \pi$, and where $S_w^\epsilon = \text{sgn}(\sin w)|\sin w|^\epsilon$ and $C_w^\epsilon = \text{sgn}(\cos w)|\cos w|^\epsilon$, respectively. Here, $a \geq 0$ is a scale parameter, $0 \leq a_1, a_2, a_3 \leq 1$ are aspect ratio parameters, and $\epsilon_1, \epsilon_2 \geq 0$ are "squareness" parameters. We collect the superquadric parameters into the parameter vector

$$q_s = (a, a_1, a_2, a_3, \epsilon_1, \epsilon_2)^T. \qquad (5)$$

In general, we can express the displacement d as a linear combination of basis functions $b_i(u)$

$$d = \sum_i \text{diag}(b_i)q_i \qquad (6)$$

where $\text{diag}(b_i)$ is a diagonal matrix formed from the basis functions and where q_i depend only on time and are known as degrees of freedom or generalized coordinates. The basis functions must be admissible, i.e., they must satisfy the kinematic boundary conditions of the model. We will give specific basis functions shortly; however, if we approximate the displacement field using a finite number of basis functions and collect the generalized coordinates into a vector of degrees of freedom $q_d = (\cdots, q_i, \cdots)^T$, we can write

$$d = Sq_d \qquad (7)$$

where S is the shape matrix whose entries are the basis functions.

B. Kinematics

The velocity of points on the model is given by

$$\begin{aligned} \dot{x} &= \dot{c} + \dot{R}p + R\dot{p} \\ &= \dot{c} + B\dot{\theta} + R\dot{s} + RS\dot{q}_d \end{aligned} \qquad (8)$$

where $\theta = (\cdots, \theta_i, \cdots)^T$ is the vector of rotational coordinates of the model, and $B = [\cdots \partial(Rp)/\partial\theta_i \cdots]$. Furthermore

$$\dot{s} = \left[\frac{\partial s}{\partial q_s}\right]\dot{q}_s = J\dot{q}_s \qquad (9)$$

where J is the Jacobian of the superquadric ellipsoid function (see (10) at the bottom of the page). We can therefore write

$$\dot{x} = [I\, B\, RJ\, RS]\dot{q} = L\dot{q} \qquad (11)$$

where $q = (q_c^T, q_\theta^T, q_s^T, q_d^T)^T$, with $q_c = c$ and $q_\theta = \theta$.

C. Dynamics

When fitting the model to visual data, our goal is to recover q, which is the vector of degrees of freedom of the model. The components q_c and q_θ are the global rigid motion coordinates, q_s are the global deformation coordinates, and q_d are the local deformation coordinates of the model. Our approach carries out the coordinate fitting procedure in a physically based way. We make our model dynamic in q by introducing mass, damping, and a deformation strain energy. This allows us, through the apparatus of Lagrangian dynamics, to arrive at a set of equations of motion governing the behavior of our model under the action of externally applied forces.

The derivation in Appendix A shows that the equations of motion take the form

$$M\ddot{q} + C\dot{q} + Kq = g_q + f_q \qquad (12)$$

where M, C, and K are the mass, damping, and stiffness matrices, respectively, where g_q are inertial (centrifugal and Coriolis) forces arising from the dynamic coupling between the local and global degrees of freedom, and where $f_q(u, t)$ are the generalized external forces associated with the degrees of freedom of the model. The appendix provides formulas for the above matrices and vectors.

D. Elasticity

The stiffness matrix K given by (30) determines the elastic properties of the model. We derive K from a deformation energy.

For the applications in this paper, we want the global deformation parameters q_s that stem from the superquadric to freely account for as much of the data as possible. Consequently, we impose no deformation energy on q_s, i.e., we set $K_{ss} = K_{sd} = 0$ in (30). The local deformation parameters q_d, however, must be constrained to yield a small and continuous deformation function.

We impose on q_d a special case of the generalized spline deformation energy proposed in [21], which is a membrane energy given in continuous form by

$$\mathcal{E}(d) = \int w_1\left(\left(\frac{\partial d}{\partial u}\right)^2 + \left(\frac{\partial d}{\partial v}\right)^2\right) + w_0 d^2 du \qquad (13)$$

where the function $w_0(u)$ controls the local magnitude, and $w_1(u)$ controls the local variation of the deformation. In our implementation, we reduce these functions to scalar stiffness parameters w_0 and w_1.

IV. SIMPLIFIED NUMERICAL SIMULATION

Equations (12) along with the expressions in Appendix A give the general equations of motion for a dynamic model with local and global deformations. A full implementation and simulation of the general equations would be appropriate for physically based animation where realistic motion is important [21]. However, in computer vision and geometric design applications involving the fitting of models to data, models governed by simplified equations of motion suffice, as the experiments in Section VI will demonstrate.

We can simplify the equations while preserving useful dynamics by setting the mass density $\mu(u)$ (see (24)) to zero to obtain

$$C\dot{q} + Kq = f_q. \qquad (14)$$

$$J = \begin{pmatrix} a_1 C_u^{\epsilon_1} C_v^{\epsilon_2} & aC_u^{\epsilon_1} C_v^{\epsilon_2} & 0 & 0 & aa_1\epsilon_1 C_u^{\epsilon_1-1} C_v^{\epsilon_2} & aa_1\epsilon_2 C_u^{\epsilon_1} C_v^{\epsilon_2-1} \\ a_2 C_u^{\epsilon_1} S_v^{\epsilon_2} & 0 & aC_u^{\epsilon_1} S_v^{\epsilon_2} & 0 & aa_2\epsilon_1 C_u^{\epsilon_1-1} S_v^{\epsilon_2} & aa_2\epsilon_2 C_u^{\epsilon_1} S_v^{\epsilon_2-1} \\ a_3 S_u^{\epsilon_1} & 0 & 0 & aS_u^{\epsilon_1} & aa_3\epsilon_1 S_u^{\epsilon_1-1} & 0 \end{pmatrix} \qquad (10)$$

These equations yield a model that has no inertia and comes to rest as soon as all the applied forces vanish or equilibrate.

Equation (14) is discretized in material coordinates u using nodal finite element basis functions. We carry out the discretization by tessellating the surface of the model into bilinear quadrilateral elements, except at the polar caps, where we use linear triangular elements (see Appendix B). The local (nodal) basis functions associated with these elements lead to a sparse K_{dd} [2].

The formulation of our model yields numerically stable equations of motion that may be integrated forward through time using explicit procedures. For fast interactive response, we employ a first-order Euler method to integrate (14). The Euler procedure updates the degrees of freedom q of the model at time $t + \Delta t$ according to the formula

$$q^{(t+\Delta t)} = q^{(t)} + \Delta t \left(C^{(t)}\right)^{-1}\left(f_q^{(t)} - Kq^{(t)}\right) \qquad (15)$$

where Δt is the time step size. Note that we need never assemble the large K_{dd} submatrix of K. Instead, we compute $\Sigma_j (k_{dd})_{ij} q_{dj}$ for each node i in an "element-by-element" fashion.

Taking time steps in q is straightforward, but the rotation component q_θ is a little delicate. We present q_θ using quaternions. Updating quaternions at each time step is easier than directly updating a rotation matrix and ensuring that it remains orthogonal. Quaternions also avoid problems with "gimbal lock" that may arise when Euler angles are used to represent rotations.

A quaternion $[s, v]$ with unit magnitude $\| [s, v] \| = s^2 + v^T v = 1$ specifies a rotation of the model from its reference position through an angle $\theta = 2\cos^{-1} s$ around an axis aligned with vector $v = [v_1, v_2, v_3]^T$. The rotation matrix corresponding to $[s, v]$ is

$$R = \begin{bmatrix} 1 - 2(v_2^2 + v_3^2) & 2(v_1 v_2 - sv_3) & 2(v_1 v_3 + sv_2) \\ 2(v_1 v_2 + sv_3) & 1 - 2(v_1^2 + v_3^2) & 2(v_2 v_3 - sv_1) \\ 2(v_1 v_3 - sv_2) & 2(v_2 v_3 + sv_1) & 1 - 2(v_1^2 + v_2^2) \end{bmatrix}. \qquad (16)$$

To obtain q_θ from (15), we use the generalized torque at time t given by $f_\theta^T = \int f^T B du$ (see (33)), with B

$$B(u) = -R\tilde{p}(u)G \qquad (17)$$

[16], where R represents the rotation matrix at time t, where $\tilde{p}(u)$ is the dual 3×3 matrix of the position vector $p(u) = (p_1, p_2, p_3)^T$ (see (3)) defined as

$$\tilde{p}(u) = \begin{bmatrix} 0 & -p_3 & p_2 \\ p_3 & 0 & -p_1 \\ -p_2 & p_1 & 0 \end{bmatrix} \qquad (18)$$

and where G is a 3×4 matrix whose definition is based on the value of the quaternion $q_\theta = [s, v]$ representing the rotation at time t:

$$G = 2 \begin{bmatrix} -v_1 & s & v_3 & -v_2 \\ -v_2 & -v_3 & s & v_1 \\ -v_3 & v_2 & -v_1 & s \end{bmatrix}. \qquad (19)$$

V. APPLIED FORCES

In the dynamic model fitting process, the data are transformed to an externally applied force distribution $f(u, t)$. Using (33), we convert the external forces to generalized forces f_q, which act on the degrees of freedom of the model. We employ two types of forces based on the structure of the input data—short-range forces obtained through gradients of potential functions and long-range forces based on distances between data points and the model's surface.

Techniques for generating suitable potential functions from monocular, binocular, and dynamic image sequences are described in [22]. For example, to attract a 3D model towards significant intensity gradients in a continuous image $I(x, y)$, we construct the potential function

$$P(x, y) = \| \nabla(G_\sigma * I) \| \qquad (20)$$

where G_σ denotes a Gaussian smoothing filter of characteristic width σ, which determines the extent of the region of attraction of the intensity gradient. Typically, the attraction has a relatively short range. The potential function applies a force

$$f = \beta \nabla P(\Pi x) \qquad (21)$$

to the model, where β controls the strength of the force, and Π is a suitable projection of points on the model into the image plane.

To compute the potential function in practice, we begin with a digital image $I(i, j)$, convolve it with a discrete filter G_σ, and compute at each pixel (i, j) the magnitude of the discrete gradient operator calculated from central finite differences of neighboring pixel values. To evaluate (21) at the location of a projected model point $\Pi x = (x, y)$, we first calculate using central finite differences the discrete gradients ∇P_k at the four pixels $k = 1, \cdots, 4$ that surround (x, y). We then consider these pixels as the nodes of the quadrilateral finite element of Fig. 10, with $a = b = 1$, in order to define a bilinear interpolant in the region between the pixels, i.e., using (48) and (49), the interpolant is given by $\nabla P(x, y) = \Sigma_{k=1}^4 N_k (2(x - x_c), 2(x - y_c)) \nabla P_k$, where (x_c, y_c) denotes the centroid of the four pixels.

Alternatively, we may define long-range forces

$$f(u_r) = \beta \| r - x(u_r) \| \qquad (22)$$

based on the separation between a datapoint r in space and the force's point of influence u_r on the model's surface. In general, $u_r = (u_r, v_r)$ will fall somewhere within an element on the surface of the model. We can compute $x(u_r)$ in the domain of a quadrilateral element, for instance, according to its bilinear local interpolant $x(u_r) = \Sigma_{i=1}^4 N_i (2(u_r - u_c)/a, 2(v_r - v_c)/b) x_i$, where the x_i are the nodal positions (see (48) and (49)). The equivalent forces on each of the four nodes is $f_i = N_i (2(u_r - u_c)/a, 2(v_r - v_c)/b) f(u_r)$. When u_r falls within the domain of a triangular element at the polar caps of the model, the computations proceed in an analogous fashion using the corresponding formulas given in Appendix B-2.

Usually, we want u_r to minimize the distance $d(u) = \| r - x(u) \|$. A closed-form analytic formula for u_r is unavailable for a discrete deformable superquadric. A brute-force

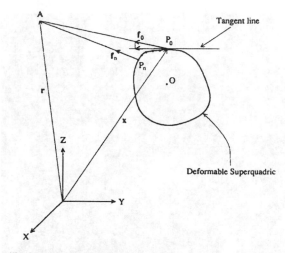

Fig. 3. Migration of data force point of influence over model surface.

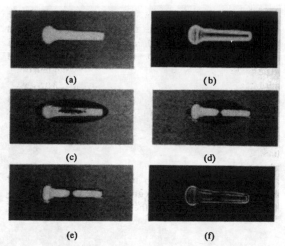

Fig. 4. Fitting deformable superquadric to pestle image (see text for (a)–(f)).

approach that works well in our experiments is to place u_r at a node of the model, which minimizes d. The complexity of this operation is high—$O(mn)$, where m is the number of datapoints and n is the number of nodes—but it need not be carried out at every time step. A more efficient approach (not used in the experiments) is to use a nonlinear optimization procedure. With a good starting point (from the previous time step), conjugate gradient or quasi-Newton methods will converge to a solution in a few steps, making such an approach linear in m. The minimization method must be applied within element domains using the nodal shape functions as an analytic representation of the model's surface. The bookkeeping in the minimization is complicated by the need to optimize across element boundaries.

We have experimented with an alternative approach that involves a dynamic procedure for migrating points of influence over the model's surface until they arrive at locations of minimal distance from the given datapoints. Starting from initial points of influence not necessarily at minimal distance (Fig. 3), we project the force at each time step onto the unit tangent vectors $(\partial x/\partial u)/\|\partial x/\partial u\|$ and $(\partial x/\partial v)/\|\partial x/\partial v\|$ to the surface at the current point of influence $P_0 = u_0$, and we migrate the point in the u plane by taking an Euler step in u and v proportional to the magnitude of the respective projections. Thus, the point of influence migrates to a point P_n of minimal distance, where the tangential components of the force vanish. The scheme works well, unless the surface is highly convoluted.

VI. EXPERIMENTS

We have evaluated our approach in simulations involving image and range data. Our experiments run at interactive rates on a Silicon Graphics Personal Iris 4D-25TG workstation including the real-time graphics.

A. 2D Image Data

Fig. 4 shows the various steps of fitting a deformable superquadric to a 120×128, 256-intensity monocular image

Fig. 4(a) of a 3D object—a pestle. The size of the image is rescaled to fit within the unit square on the $x - y$ plane. Fig. 4(b) shows the potential function $P(x, y)$ generated from the image by computing the magnitude of the intensity gradient.

Fig. 4(c) shows the initial state of the deformable superquadric displayed in wireframe projected onto the image. The surface of the model is discretized into 5043 nodes. The initialization consists of specifying the center of the model c, along with the major and minor axes, $a \cdot a_1$ and $a \cdot a_2$, by picking four points with the mouse. This initializes the translation q_c and rotation q_θ of the model. We also fix $\epsilon_1 = \epsilon_2 = 1.0$. In this and subsequent experiments, the local deformation q_d is initially set to zero. Note that the initialization step produces a very crude first approximation to the pestle.

Fig. 4(d) shows an intermediate step in the fitting process that simulates the equations of motion using stiffness parameters $w_0 = 1.0 \times 10^{-6}$ and $w_1 = 4.0 \times 10^{-2}$. Using an orthogonal projection Π, nodes of the model whose positions x in space lie near the image plane ($|x_3| < 0.2$) are subject to a force directed parallel to the image plane:

$$f = \beta \left(\frac{\partial P}{\partial x}, \frac{\partial P}{\partial y}, 0 \right)^T \qquad (23)$$

where the force strength factor is $\beta = 4.0 \times 10^{-6}$. The forces deform the model, and Figs. 4(e) and (f) show the final state of the model at equilibrium, superimposed on the image and the potential, respectively.

In the second experiment, we use the image of a doll shown in Fig. 5(a), whose potential is shown in Fig. 5(b). The specifics of this experiment are identical to those of the previous one, except that the discrete models consisted of 963 nodes, and their stiffness parameters were $w_0 = 0.001$ and $w_1 = 0.1$. Fig. 6(a) illustrates the results of the initialization phase for the doll image, which was carried out as described above, showing 11 crude approximations to the major body parts of the figure. The image forces deform the part models into the final shapes shown in Fig. 6(b).

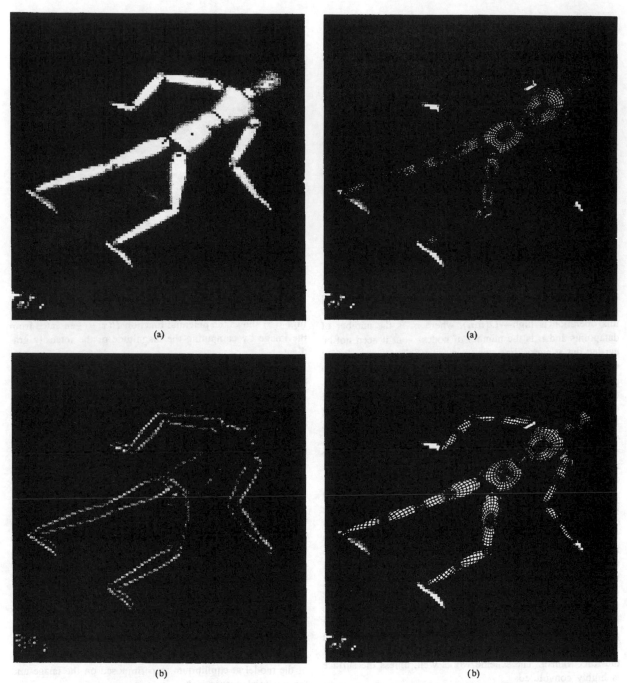

(a)

(a)

(b)

(b)

Fig. 5. (a) Doll image and (b) potential.

Fig. 6. Fitting deformable superquadrics to doll image (see text for (a)–(b)).

The above simulations did not require user intervention beyond the initialization phase. It is important to realize that initialization requires only a rough segmentation of the image into blobs corresponding to parts. We therefore expect that the initialization can be automated using available image segmentation techniques. The reaction-diffusion space segmentation process of Kimia *et al.* [9] appears promising for this purpose.

B. 3D Range Data

3D data generally provide greater constraint in the model fitting process than do 2D image projections. The following experiments utilize range data from the NRCC 3D image database [15]. We have experimented with the two force techniques for fitting the model to 3D data described in the previous section. In the following simulations, we have applied forces to the model using the brute-force nearest-node search method, updating the nodes of attachment for each datapoint every 200 iterations.

In the third experiment, we fit a deformable superquadric model with 2603 nodes to 3D data sparsely sampled from the upper "hemisphere" of an egg (from range map EGG 1 CAT # 233). Fig. 7(a) shows the 499 range datapoints. The stiffness parameters of the model were $w_0 = 1.0 \times 10^{-6}$ and $w_1 = 0.1$. We initialized the model to a sphere located at the center of gravity of the data ($a = 1.2, a_1 = a_2 = a_3 = 0.5$, $\epsilon_1 = \epsilon_2 = 1.0$). Fig. 7(b) shows the fitted deformable superquadric at equilibrium, and Fig. 7(c) shows a top view of the fitted model. Evidently, the fit is accurate over the portions of the surface covered by datapoints, but it begins to deteriorate at the boundary of the data near the "equator" because of the influence of the underside of the model, which remains too spherical due to the lack of datapoints.

In the fourth experiment, we fit a model with 1683 nodes to 3D data sparsely sampled from the upper part of a mug with a pitted surface (from range map MUG 1 CAT # 251). Fig. 8(a) shows the 651 range datapoints. The stiffness parameters of the model were $w_0 = 0.01$ and $w_1 = 0.1$. We initialized the model to a "tubular" shape ($a = 1.5, a_1 = a_2 = 0.3$, $a_3 = 0.8, \epsilon_1 = 0.7, \epsilon_2 = 1.0$). Fig. 8(b) shows the fitted deformable superquadric at equilibrium. The underside of the model is smooth due to the lack of data, but the pitted texture of the top surface has been accurately reconstructed by the local deformational degrees of freedom of the deformable superquadric.

VII. CONCLUDING REMARKS

We have developed deformable superquadrics, which are dynamic models with global and local deformation properties inherited from superquadric ellipsoids and membrane splines. These physically based models are governed by equations of motion. We are able to simulate and render simplified versions of the equations at interactive rates on a graphics workstation. The dynamic equations make deformable superquadrics responsive to forces derived from image or range data, which compels the model to conform to the data. The model is useful for reconstructing 3D objects or parts of objects with irregular, local shape features from such data. It also promises to be useful for abstracting global shape features of objects for the purposes of recognition.

In addition to specifying the stiffness parameters (w_0 and w_1) of the model along with a few parameters in the numerical simulation procedures, we must currently provide reasonable initial estimates for the translation, rotation, and global deformation variables of our model, especially when fitting them to 2D image data. Initial values may be estimated by rough segmentation and calculation of central moments of the data [17].

We are currently implementing the full, second-order equations of motion (12) and extending our formulation to accommodate other global deformations such as bends, shears, and tapers. Additional deformations of this sort may provide useful degrees of freedom to deformable superquadrics or to related

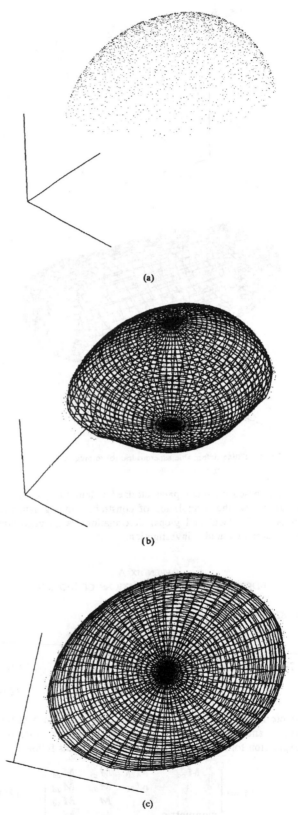

(a)

(b)

(c)

Fig. 7. Fitting deformable superquadric ((b),(c)) to egg range data (d).

113

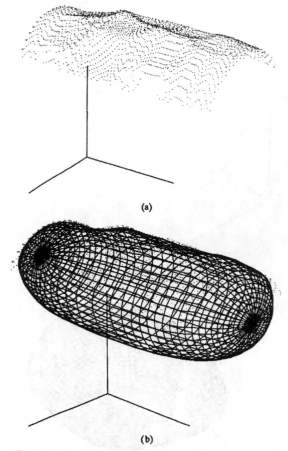

(a)

(b)

Fig. 8. Fitting deformable superquadric (b) to mug range data (a).

models based on other parameterized volumetric primitives. Additionally, the formulation of constraints among dynamic models with local and global deformations is an important topic currently under investigation.

Appendix A
Derivation of the Equations of Motion

1. Kinetic Energy: Mass Matrix

The kinetic energy of the model is given by

$$T = \frac{1}{2} \int \mu \dot{x}^T \dot{x} \, du = \frac{1}{2} \dot{q}^T \left[\int \mu L^T L \, du \right] \dot{q} = \frac{1}{2} \dot{q}^T M \dot{q} \tag{24}$$

where $M = \int \mu L^T L \, du$ is the symmetric mass matrix of the object, and $\mu(u)$ is the mass density of the object. Using the expression for L from (11), we can rewrite M as follows:

$$M = \begin{bmatrix} M_{cc} & M_{c\theta} & M_{cs} & M_{cd} \\ & M_{\theta\theta} & M_{\theta s} & M_{\theta d} \\ & & M_{ss} & M_{sd} \\ \text{symmetric} & & & M_{dd} \end{bmatrix} \tag{25}$$

where

$$
\begin{array}{ll}
M_{cc} = \int \mu I \, du & M_{\theta s} = \int \mu B^T R J \, du \\
M_{c\theta} = \int \mu B \, du & M_{\theta d} = \int \mu B^T R S \, du \\
M_{cs} = R \int \mu J \, du & M_{ss} = \int \mu J^T J \, du \\
M_{cd} = R \int \mu S \, du & M_{sd} = \int \mu J^T S \, du \\
M_{\theta\theta} = \int B^T B \, du & M_{dd} = \int \mu S^T S \, du.
\end{array}
\tag{26}
$$

2. Energy Dissipation: Damping Matrix

We assume velocity dependent kinetic energy dissipation, which can be expressed in terms of the (Raleigh) dissipation functional:

$$\mathcal{F} = \frac{1}{2} \int \gamma \dot{x}^T \dot{x} \, du \tag{27}$$

where $\gamma(u)$ is a damping density. Since it has the same form as (24), we can rewrite (27) as follows:

$$\mathcal{F} = \frac{1}{2} \dot{q}^T C \dot{q} \tag{28}$$

where the damping matrix C has the same form as M, except that γ replaces μ.

3. Strain Energy: Stiffness Matrix

We define the deformation characteristics of the model in terms of a deformation strain energy. We impose a strain energy of the general form

$$\mathcal{E}(x) = \frac{1}{2} q^T K q \tag{29}$$

where

$$K = \begin{pmatrix} 0 & 0 & 0 & 0 \\ & 0 & 0 & 0 \\ & & K_{ss} & K_{sd} \\ \text{symmetric} & & & K_{dd} \end{pmatrix} \tag{30}$$

is the stiffness matrix. The zero submatrices indicate that only the global q_s and local q_d deformational degrees of freedom can contribute to the strain energy.

4. External Forces and Virtual Work

The external forces $f(u, t)$ applied to the model do virtual work, which can be written as

$$\delta W_F = \int f^T L \delta q \, du = \int f_q \delta q \, du \tag{31}$$

where

$$f_q = f^T L = (f_c, f_\theta, f_s, f_d) \tag{32}$$

with

$$
\begin{array}{ll}
f_c^T = \int f^T \, du, & f_s^T = \int f^T R J \, du \\
f_\theta^T = \int f^T B \, du, & f_d^T = \int f^T R S \, du
\end{array}
\tag{33}
$$

is the vector of generalized external forces associated with the degrees of freedom of the model.

5. Lagrange Equations of Motion

The Lagrange equations of motion for the model take the form

$$\frac{d}{dt}\left(\frac{\partial T}{\partial \dot{q}}\right)^T - \left(\frac{\partial T}{\partial q}\right)^T + \left(\frac{\partial \mathcal{F}}{\partial \dot{q}}\right)^T + \delta_x \mathcal{E} = f_q. \quad (34)$$

The first two terms of (34) express inertial forces and can be written as

$$\frac{d}{dt}\left(\frac{\partial T}{\partial \dot{q}}\right)^T - \left(\frac{\partial T}{\partial q}\right)^T = M\ddot{q} - g_q \quad (35)$$

where

$$g_q = -\dot{M}\dot{q} + \frac{1}{2}\left[\frac{\partial}{\partial q}\left(\dot{q}^T M \dot{q}\right)\right]^T \quad (36)$$

gives the centrifugal and Coriolis forces [16]. The third term expresses the friction forces and takes the form

$$\frac{\partial \mathcal{F}}{\partial \dot{q}} = C\dot{q}. \quad (37)$$

The fourth term, the variational derivative of $\mathcal{E}$ with respect to x, expresses the elastic forces

$$\delta_x \mathcal{E} = Kq. \quad (38)$$

Substituting the above expressions into (34) yields the equations of motion (12).

APPENDIX B
DERIVATION OF K_{dd}

We discretize the model in material coordinates u using finite elements. We can derive K_{dd} as an assembly of the local stiffness matrices K_{dd}^j associated with each element domain $E_j \subset$ u. Since $d(\mathrm{u},t) = [d_1(\mathrm{u},t), d_2(\mathrm{u},t), d_3(\mathrm{u},t)]^T$, we can rewrite the membrane spline deformation energy (13) on E_j as the sum of component energies

$$\mathcal{E}^j(d) = \mathcal{E}^j(d_1) + \mathcal{E}^j(d_2) + \mathcal{E}^j(d_3) \quad (39)$$

where for $k = 1,2,3$

$$\mathcal{E}^j(d_k) = \int_{E_j} w_1^j\left(\left(\frac{\partial d_k}{\partial u}\right)^2 + \left(\frac{\partial d_k}{\partial v}\right)^2\right) + w_0^j d_k^2\, du. \quad (40)$$

In accordance to the theory of elasticity, (40) can be written in the form

$$\mathcal{E}^j(d_k) = \int_{E_j} \sigma_k^{jT} \epsilon_k^j\, du \quad (41)$$

where

$$\epsilon_k^j = \left[\frac{\partial d_k}{\partial u}, \frac{\partial d_k}{\partial v}, d_k\right]^T \quad (42)$$

is the strain vector and

$$\sigma_k^j = D_k^j \epsilon_k^j = \begin{pmatrix} w_1^j & 0 & 0 \\ 0 & w_1^j & 0 \\ 0 & 0 & w_0^j \end{pmatrix}\epsilon_k^j \quad (43)$$

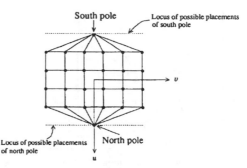

Fig. 9. Model tesselation in material coordinates.

is the stress vector associated with component k of d. Therefore, the element stress vector is

$$\sigma^j = D^j \epsilon^j = \begin{pmatrix} D_1^j & 0 & 0 \\ 0 & D_2^j & 0 \\ 0 & 0 & D_3^j \end{pmatrix}\begin{pmatrix} \epsilon_1^j \\ \epsilon_2^j \\ \epsilon_3^j \end{pmatrix} \quad (44)$$

where $D_1^j = D_2^j = D_3^j$.

We denote the finite element nodal shape functions by N_i^j, $i = 1, \cdots, n$, where n is the number of nodes associated with element E_j. Hence, we can write (42) as

$$\epsilon_k^j = \sum_{i=1}^n \gamma_i^j\left(q_{d_k}^j\right)_i = \Gamma_k^j q_{d_k}^j \quad (45)$$

where $\gamma_i^j = \left[\frac{\partial N_i^j}{\partial u}, \frac{\partial N_i^j}{\partial v}, 1\right]^T$, $\Gamma_k^j = \left(\gamma_1^j \gamma_2^j \cdots \gamma_n^j\right)$, and $q_{d_k}^j = \left[\left(q_{d_k}^j\right)_1, \left(q_{d_k}^j\right)_2, \cdots, \left(q_{d_k}^j\right)_n\right]^T$. We can write the element strain vector ϵ^j as

$$\epsilon^j = \begin{pmatrix} \epsilon_1^j \\ \epsilon_2^j \\ \epsilon_3^j \end{pmatrix} = \begin{pmatrix} \Gamma_1^j & 0 & 0 \\ 0 & \Gamma_2^j & 0 \\ 0 & 0 & \Gamma_3^j \end{pmatrix}\begin{pmatrix} q_{d_1}^j \\ q_{d_2}^j \\ q_{d_3}^j \end{pmatrix} = \Gamma^j q_d^j \quad (46)$$

where $\Gamma_1^j = \Gamma_2^j = \Gamma_3^j$. Thus, the element stiffness matrix is

$$K_{dd}^j = \int_{E_j} \Gamma^{jT} D^j \Gamma^j\, du = \mathrm{diag}\left(\int_{E_j} \Gamma_k^{jT} D_k^j \Gamma_k^j\, du\right). \quad (47)$$

Fig. 9 illustrates the tessellation of the material coordinate system $\mathrm{u} = (u, v)$ into finite element domains. The need for quadrilateral and triangular elements is evident. Equation (4) implies that the v material coordinate of both north ($u = \pi/2$) and south ($u = -\pi/2$) poles may be arbitrary. This is illustrated in the figure by the dotted lines. The next two sections describe the bilinear quadrilateral and linear triangular elements that we employ in our implementation.

1. Bilinear Quadrilateral Elements

The nodal shape functions of the bilinear quadrilateral element (Fig. 10) are

$$N_i(\xi, \eta) = \frac{1}{4}(1 + \xi\xi_i)(1 + \eta\eta_i) \quad (48)$$

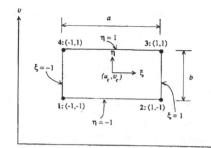

Fig. 10. Bilinear quadrilateral element. The four nodes are numbered.

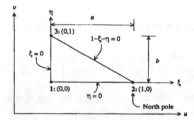

Fig. 11. North pole linear triangular element. The three nodes are numbered.

where (ξ_i, η_i) are the reference coordinates of node i shown in the figure. The relationship between the reference coordinates and material coordinates $u = (u, v)$ is given by

$$\xi = \frac{2}{a}(u - u_c), \qquad \eta = \frac{2}{b}(v - v_c) \qquad (49)$$

where (u_c, v_c) are the coordinates of the element center. The required derivatives of the shape functions may be computed as follows:

$$\frac{\partial N_i}{\partial u} = \frac{\partial N_i}{\partial \xi}\frac{\partial \xi}{\partial u} + \frac{\partial N_i}{\partial \eta}\frac{\partial \eta}{\partial u} = \frac{1}{2a}\xi_i(1 + \eta\eta_i) \qquad (50)$$

$$\frac{\partial N_i}{\partial v} = \frac{\partial N_i}{\partial \xi}\frac{\partial \xi}{\partial v} + \frac{\partial N_i}{\partial \eta}\frac{\partial \eta}{\partial v} = \frac{1}{2b}(1 + \xi\xi_i)\eta_i \qquad (51)$$

and we may integrate a function $f(u, v)$ over E_j by transforming to the reference coordinate system:

$$\iint\limits_{E_j} f(u, v)\, du\, dv = \int_{-1}^{1}\int_{-1}^{1} f(\xi, \eta)\frac{ab}{4}\, d\xi\, d\eta. \qquad (52)$$

We approximate such integrals using Gauss-Legendre quadrature rules.

Using the above formulas, we can compute the matrix $\int \Gamma_k^{j^T} D_k^j \Gamma_k^j\, du$ and, hence, the element stiffness matrix K_{dd}^j for the bilinear quadrilateral element.

2. Linear Triangular Elements

As we stated above, the v coordinates of the poles are arbitrary. Hence, we can use right triangular elements in which the v coordinate of the pole is set equal to the v coordinate of one of the other nodes in each triangle.

a) North Pole Linear Triangular Elements: The nodal shape functions for the north pole linear triangular element (Fig. 11) are

$$N_1(\xi, \eta) = 1 - \xi - \eta \qquad (53)$$
$$N_2(\xi, \eta) = \xi \qquad (54)$$
$$N_3(\xi, \eta) = \eta. \qquad (55)$$

The relationship between the uv and $\xi\eta$ coordinates is

$$\xi = \frac{1}{a}(u - u_1) \qquad (56)$$

$$\eta = \frac{1}{b}(v - v_1) \qquad (57)$$

where (u_1, v_1) are the coordinates of node 1 at which $(\xi_1, \eta_1) = (0, 0)$. Computing the derivatives of the shape functions as in (50) and (51) yields

$$\frac{\partial N_1}{\partial u} = -\frac{1}{a}; \quad \frac{\partial N_2}{\partial u} = \frac{1}{a}; \quad \frac{\partial N_3}{\partial u} = 0 \qquad (58)$$

$$\frac{\partial N_1}{\partial v} = -\frac{1}{b}; \quad \frac{\partial N_2}{\partial v} = 0; \quad \frac{\partial N_3}{\partial v} = \frac{1}{b} \qquad (59)$$

and we may integrate a function $f(u, v)$ over the E_j using

$$\iint\limits_{E_j} f(u, v)\, du\, dv = \int_0^1 \int_0^{(1-\eta)} f(\xi, \eta)ab\, d\xi\, d\eta. \qquad (60)$$

We approximate such integrals using Radau quadrature rules.

Using the above formulas, we can compute the matrix $\int \Gamma_k^{j^T} D_k^j \Gamma_k^j\, du$ and, hence, K_{dd}^j for the north pole linear triangular element.

b) South Pole Linear Triangular Elements: The nodal shape functions for the south pole linear triangular element (Fig. 12) are

$$N_1(\xi, \eta) = 1 - \xi \qquad (61)$$
$$N_2(\xi, \eta) = \xi - \eta \qquad (62)$$
$$N_3(\xi, \eta) = \eta. \qquad (63)$$

The relationship between the uv and $\xi\eta$ coordinates is

$$\xi = \frac{1}{a}(u - u_1) \qquad (64)$$

$$\eta = \frac{1}{b}(v - v_1) \qquad (65)$$

where (u_1, v_1) are the coordinates of node 1 at which $(\xi_1, \eta_1) = (0, 0)$. Computing the derivatives of the shape functions as in (50) and (51) yields

$$\frac{\partial N_1}{\partial u} = -\frac{1}{a}; \quad \frac{\partial N_2}{\partial u} = \frac{1}{a}; \quad \frac{\partial N_3}{\partial u} = 0 \qquad (66)$$

$$\frac{\partial N_1}{\partial v} = 0; \quad \frac{\partial N_2}{\partial v} = -\frac{1}{b}; \quad \frac{\partial N_3}{\partial v} = \frac{1}{b} \qquad (67)$$

and we may integrate a function $f(u, v)$ over the E_j using

$$\iint\limits_{E_j} f(u, v)\, du\, dv = \int_0^1 \int_0^{(1-\xi)} f(\xi, \eta)ab\, d\eta\, d\xi. \qquad (68)$$

We approximate such integrals using Radau quadrature rules.

Using the above formulas, we can compute the matrix $\int \Gamma_k^{j^T} D_k^j \Gamma_k^j\, du$ and, hence, K_{dd}^j for the south pole linear triangular element.

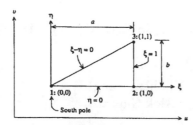

Fig. 12. South pole linear triangular element. The three nodes are numbered.

REFERENCES

[1] A. Barr, "Superquadrics and angle-preserving transformations," *IEEE Comput. Graphics Applications,* vol. 18, pp. 21–30, 1981.

[2] K.-J. Bathe and E. L. Wilson, *Numerical Methods in Finite Element Analysis.* Englewood Cliffs, NJ: Prentice-Hall, 1976.

[3] I. Biederman, "Human image understanding: Recent research and theory," *Comput. Vision Graphics Image Processing,* vol. 32, pp. 29–73, 1985.

[4] A. Blake and A. Zisserman, *Visual Reconstruction.* Cambridge, MA: MIT Press, 1987.

[5] R. Brooks, "Symbolic reasoning among 3D models and 2D images," *Art. Intell.,* vol. 17, pp. 285–348, 1981.

[6] M. Gardiner, "The superellipse: A curve between the ellipse and the rectangle," *Scientific Amer.,* vol. 213, pp. 222–234, 1965.

[7] A. D. Gross and T. E. Boult, "Error of fit measures for recovering parametric solids," in *Proc. Sec. Int. Conf. Comput. Vision,* 1988, pp. 690–694.

[8] A. Gupta and R. Bajcsy, "Part description and segmentation using contour, surface, and volumetric primitives," in *Sensing and Reconstruction of Three-Dimensional Objects and Scenes, Proc. SPIE 1260,* B. Girod (Ed.), 1990, pp. 203–214.

[9] B. B. Kimia, A. Tannenbaum, and S. W. Zucker, "Toward a computational theory of shape: An overview," Tech. Rep. TR-CIM-89-13, Comput. Vision Robotics Lab., 1989.

[10] D. Marr and H. K. Nishihara, "Representation and recognition of the spatial organization of three-dimensional shapes," *Proc. Roy. Soc. London B,* vol. 200, pp. 269–294, 1978.

[11] A. Pentland, "Perceptual organization and the representation of natural form," *Art. Intell.,* vol. 28, pp. 293–331, 1986.

[12] ____, "Automatic extraction of deformable part models," Tech. Rep. Vision-Sciences 104, MIT Media Lab., 1988.

[13] ____, "Canonical fitting of deformable part models," in *Sensing and Reconstruction of Three-Dimensional Objects and Scenes, Proc. SPIE 1260,* B. Girod (Ed.), 1990, pp. 216–228.

[14] T. Poggio. V. Torre, and C. Koch, "Computational Vision and regularization theory," *Nature,* vol. 317, pp. 314–319, 1985.

[15] M. Rioux and L. Cournoyer, "The NRCC three-dimensional image data files," Tech. Rep. CNRC 29077, Nat. Res. Council Canada, 1988.

[16] A. A. Shabana, *Dynamics of Multibody Systems.* New York: Wiley, 1989.

[17] F. Solina and R. Bajcsy, "Recovery of parametric models from range images: The case for superquadrics with global deformations," *IEEE Trans Patt. Anal. Mach. Intell.,* vol. 12, pp. 131–146, 1990.

[18] R. Szeliski, *Bayesian Modeling of Uncertainty in Low-Level Vision.* Boston: Kluwer, 1989.

[19] D. Terzopoulos, "Regularization of inverse visual problems involving discontinuities," *IEEE Trans. Patt. Anal. Mach. Intell.,* vol. PAMI-8, pp. 413–424, 1986.

[20] ____, "The computation of visible-surface representations," *IEEE Trans. Patt. Anal. Mach. Intell.,* vol. 10, pp. 417–438, 1988.

[21] D. Terzopoulos and A. Witkin, "Physically based models with rigid and deformable components," *IEEE Comput. Graphics Applications,* vol. 8, pp. 41–51, 1988.

[22] D. Terzopoulos, A. Witkin, and M. Kass, "Constraints on deformable models: Recovering 3D shape and nonrigid motion," *Art. Intell.,* vol. 36, pp. 91–123, 1988.

[23] A. Witkin and W. Welch, "Fast animation and control of nonrigid structures," *Comput. Graphics,* vol. 24, pp. 243–252, 1990.

Demetri Terzopoulos (S'78—M'85) was born in Krestena, Greece, in 1956. He received the B.Eng. degree with distinction in honors electrical engineering and the M.Eng. degree in electrical engineering from McGill University, Montreal, Canada, in 1978, and 1980, respectively, and the PhD degree in artificial intelligence from the Massachusetts Institute of Technology, Cambridge, MA, in 1984.

Since September 1989, he has been Associate Professor of Computer Science at the University of Toronto and Fellow of the Canadian Institute for Advanced Research, Toronto, Canada. Since 1985, he has been affiliated with Schlumberger, Inc., serving as Program Leader at the Laboratory for Computer Science, Austin, TX, and at the former Palo Alto Research Laboratory. During 1984–1985, he was a Research Scientist at the MIT Artificial Intelligence Laboratory, Cambridge, MA. Previously, he held summer positions at the National Research Council of Canada, Ottawa, (1977–1978) and Bell-Northern Research, Montreal (1980).

Dr. Terzopoulos has published research papers in computational vision, computer graphics, digital image and speech processing, and parallel numerical algorithms and has been invited to speak internationally on these topics. He has received several scholarships and awards, including a AAAI-87 Conference Best Paper Award from the American Association for Artificial Intelligence. He serves on the editorial boards of *CVGIP: Graphical Models and Image Processing* and the *Journal of Visualization and Computer Animation.* He is a member of the American Association for Artificial Intelligence, the New York Academy of Sciences, and Sigma Xi.

Dimitri Metaxas was born in Athens, Greece, in 1962. He received the Diploma in electrical engineering with highest honors from the National Technical University of Athens in 1986 and the M.Sc. degree in computer science from the University of Maryland, College Park, in 1988.

During the summer of 1985, he conducted research in artificial intelligence at NEC's research laboratories in Tokyo, Japan, and from June 1987–June 1988, he worked at the University of Maryland Center for Automation Research. Currently, he is pursuing the PhD degree in computer vision at the Department of Computer Science, University of Toronto, where he holds a University Open Fellowship. He has publications in the areas of computer vision, computer graphics, computer systems, databases, and artificial intelligence.

Mr. Metaxas is a member of the Technical Chamber of Greece.

The Extruded Generalized Cylinder: A Deformable Model for Object Recovery

Thomas O'Donnell[*†]
Terrence E. Boult[**]

Xi-Sheng Fang[*]
Alok Gupta[†]

[*] Dept. of Computer Science
Columbia University
New York, N.Y. 10027
Email: odonnell@cs.columbia.edu

[†] Siemens Corporate Research, Inc.
755 College Road East
Princeton, N.J. 08540
alok@scr.siemens.com

Abstract

There is increasing interest in the recovery of generalized cylinders (GCs) with curved spines. However, existing formulations of such GCs, for example those based on the Frenet-Serret frame or the tube model, suffer serious drawbacks: discontinuities, a lack of expressive power, "narrowing" in the plane normal to the spine, non-intuitive twisting behavior, and/or off-axis nonorthogonality of their local coordinate systems. We discuss some of the problems associated with the non-orthogonality of the coordinate system based on the Frenet-Serret frame. This non-orthogonality is induced by torsion effects and we show how to correct for it. We then introduce a new model, the extruded GC (EGC) model, which overcomes all the problems mentioned above. For complex axes, the EGC model is also simpler to understand and use than existing models. The EGC model is further extended by including local surface deformations. Recovery of the deformable EGC via a physically-motivated paradigm is demonstrated on pre-segmented data from a human carotid artery.

1 Introduction and Previous Work

Generalized cylinders (GCs) are the result of sweeping a possibly varying cross section along a path specified by a spine which may be an arbitrary space curve. Since GCs were first proposed as a general-purpose model for computer vision by Binford [1], their use has become widespread. A variant of GCs, straight homogeneous generalized cylinders (SHGCs) have the constraint that their cross-section functions be scaled versions of a reference curve and that their spines be linear. Due to their simple yet relatively powerful form, SHGCs are the most common variant of GCs found in the literature [10, 11, 3, 7]. More re-

cently, however, the lack of expressiveness of SHGCs has prompted researchers to contemplate more sophisticated variants [15, 4, 16, 9].

While allowing a GC's cross section to vary is a rather straightforward exercise, the relaxation of constraints on the spine introduces subtle and not-so-subtle complications in how to describe the GC. Two properties of the spine which may cause difficulties in formulating general-axis GCs are regions with non-zero torsion and points of inflection.

A handful of vision researchers have used the Frenet-Serret formulation as the basis of their GC. It is true that it defines a frame at each point along the curve, but these individual orthogonal frames do not extend to form an orthogonal frame field in 3 space. As pointed out by Koenderink [6, p. 141], "[moving frames]...only define the frame field on a piece of the submanifold *itself*, not on the surrounding space."[‡] We will look at this issue in more detail in sections 1.2 & 1.3.

Zerroug and Nevatia [16] allow a variable circular cross-section and a curved planar spine. They use the Frenet frame as the basis of their local coordinate system; however, they do not address the problem of using that formulation when the axis has inflection points or straight segments.

In this paper, we present some limitations of the Frenet-Serret based model and formulate an *extruded* generalized cylinder (EGC) that allows a *non-planar* spine and overcomes the problems resulting from spine inflection points and spine torsion. We then invoke a physically-motivated paradigm (based on an extension of [14]) for the recovery of a deformable EGC. Our model differs from the physically-based symmetry-seeking model proposed by Terzopoulos et al. [13] in that we aim to quantify as much global shape as possible by explicitly modeling the spine and the cross-section functions. Their symmetry-seeking model accounts for any deformation from the initial shape through local deformations only. The resulting large deformations place strong demands on getting the

[*] Supported in part by DARPA contract DACA-76-92-C-007, and by NSF PYI grant #IRI-90-57951, with industrial support from Texas Instruments, IBM and Siemens CRC.

[‡] The submanifold refers to the spine curve.

Reprinted from *Proc. IEEE Computer Vision and Pattern Recognition Conf.*, 1994, pp. 174–180.

"correct" material properties and forces for use in the deformation process. To keep deformations small, our local deformations manifest themselves after the gross global shape is accounted for by a handful of parameters. This work differs from the work of Terzopoulos & Metaxas [14] in that we consider a more general global shape function, an EGC, as opposed to a superellipsoid. This allows for the global model to account for much more of the underlying shape and provides a better match to our domain.

The next subsections will discuss the drawbacks of two existing general-axis GC formulations: the tube model [4], and a more commonly used model based on the Frenet-Serret frame. We then present a correction to some of the problems associated with the Frenet-Serret-based formulation. Our *extruded* GC (EGC) model, which overcomes deficiencies in existing formulations, is proposed in Section 2. Results of recovering the globally and locally deformable model from presegmented carotid artery data are presented in Section 3. Finally, we conclude with some observations about curved generalized cylinders and discuss future work.

1.1 The Tube Description

A GC with a general axis might also be viewed as a generalized tube. There are a few definitions of "tubular" surfaces, e.g.[6], which define the GC surface as an envelope of spheres centered on the spine. However, such formulations do not allow "general cross-sections" such as ellipses and parametric formulations of the surfaces (envelopes) are not given.

A recent variation of the general-axis GC, dubbed the "the tube description" was applied to the recovery of plant root structures [4]. The model sets up an object-centered coordinate frame uvw which is translated from the origin of the world coordinate system xyz by the vector $\vec{T}$. A cross-section function defined in $[uvw]$ is free to rotate with respect to the U axis by α, $\mathbf{R}_u(\alpha)$, and the new V axis by θ, $\mathbf{R}_v(\theta)$. The relationship between the world coordinate system and the local one is:

$$[xyz1]^\mathsf{T} = [uvw1]^\mathsf{T} \times \mathbf{R}_u(\alpha) \times \mathbf{R}_v(\theta) + \vec{T}$$

The tube model is elegant, but since "narrowing" of the tube may result (Figure 1) its use in recovery is limited. In the next subsection we examine a description which allows the cross-section to be kept at a constant angle with respect to the spine.

1.2 The Frenet-Serret Description

If we assume the cross-section maintains a fixed angle with respect to the spine, then to define a general-axis GC we need only to represent two things: the spine

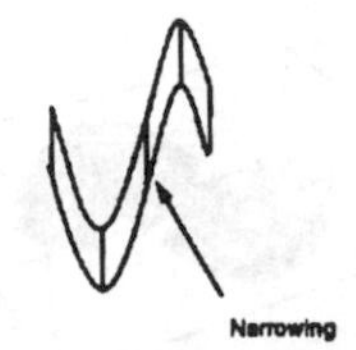

Narrowing

Figure 1: Profile of a generalized cylinder based on the tube description. Because a spine is not explicitly defined, it is possible to specify the cross section to lie in a plane other than the plane normal to the spine. Here the plane containing the cross section remains in a fixed orientation. This results in an unnatural narrowing of the cylinder and accompanying volume decrease where the cross section plane is at an angle from the normal plane.

and the cross-section shape. This type of formulation requires the cross-section function to be defined via a moving local coordinate frame which is attached to the spine. The Frenet-Serret formulae allow us to describe one such local coordinate frame.

For a space curve $\vec{r}(u)$ the Frenet-Serret formulae contain the equations for the unit tangent ($\vec{T}(u)$), unit normal ($\vec{N}(u)$), and unit binormal ($\vec{B}(u)$) vectors to the curve.

Let $s(u)$ be defined as the arc length along $\vec{r}(u)$, $\kappa(u)$ be the curvature and $\tau(u)$ the torsion . (In the remainder, we drop the explicit parameterization of terms with respect to u and denote differentiation with respect to u via $'$, e.g. $\vec{r}'$.) Then define:

$$\vec{T} = \vec{r}'/s'$$
$$\vec{B} = (\vec{r}' \times \vec{r}'')/((s')^3 \kappa)$$
$$\vec{N} = \vec{B} \times \vec{T}$$
$$\tau = \vec{r}' \cdot (\vec{r}'' \times \vec{r}''')/(s'^6 \kappa^2)$$
$$s' = |\vec{r}'|$$

The moving trihedron formed by $\vec{T}(u)$, $\vec{N}(u)$ and $\vec{B}(u)$, may be used as a local foundation for GCs. The $\vec{N}$ and $\vec{B}$ vectors in the plane normal to the curve serve as axes onto which the cross section function may be plotted. Thus we can define a GC with axis $r(u)$ and polar parametric cross-section function $a(u, \theta)$ as

$$\vec{r}(u) + a(u, \theta)(\cos \theta \vec{N} + \sin \theta \vec{B}) \qquad (1)$$

This formulation of a general-axis GC has three major drawbacks. The first, and simplest, is that it cannot describe a GC with a linear spine because the vector $\vec{N}$ is no longer well-defined. Following the formulae, if $\vec{r}$ is linear, the term $\vec{r}''$ becomes the zero vector and the $\vec{N}$ and $\vec{B}$ vectors both collapse into the zero vector. Thus, a special case description of a straight GC must be used in these situations.

The second drawback is related to the first. The formulation cannot describe GCs with $\vec{r}$ linear at *any*

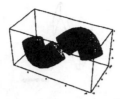

Figure 2: A discontinuity in the cylinder based on the Frenet-Serret description due to an inflection point in the spine function.

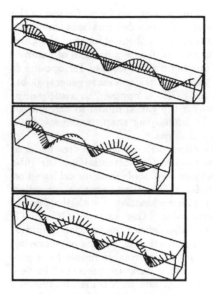

Figure 3: The Normal vectors of three coordinate frames on a simple helical spine. Note that a helix has constant non-zero torsion. Top: The standard frenet-frame exhibits extreme but intuitive twist along the spine. Middle: The orthogonal frenet frame twists less but the twist in non-intuitive. (Notice that it is not in sync with the period of the helix). Bottom: The EGC frame. The U vector always has a component in the up direction.

point along the spine; this includes inflection points where the spine is locally straight. At these points the same effect described above occurs resulting in a discontinuity in the GC (Figure 2). Even worse: if the curvature changes sign (i.e., $\vec{r}'' \neq \vec{0}$) the Frenet frame flips its orientation such that the positive $\vec{B}$ direction points in the formerly negative $\vec{B}$ direction (similarly for $\vec{N}$). This greatly complicates a simple scheme to interpolate over the discontinuity. In this case a cylinder with its cross section not centered on the axis will reappear on the opposite side of the spine after crossing the inflection point. Considering that inflection points appear frequently in common spine functions (e.g polynomials, trigonometric functions), this is a serious drawback.

Finally, the local coordinate system produced by the moving trihedron is nonorthogonal off the spine if $\vec{r}(u)$ exhibits torsion. (See [17] for a more complete description and proof). The intuition behind this nonorthogonality is that since the $\vec{N}, \vec{B}$ pair wind around the spine excessively in the presence of torsion (see Figure 3), the space surrounding the spine warps.

Initially we believed this warping would cause a major problem for performing vector calculus operations commonly employed in vision applications. However, after more careful consideration we have discovered that measures such as the surface gradient, when calculated as a cross product of the partial derivatives of the surface parameters, are off in magnitude, but their directions are correct. Therefore, equations depending only on the direction of these measures (e.g., limb equations) yield correct results. However, researchers making use of the magnitude of the results of such operations should beware.

Given the drawbacks listed above, the standard Frenet-Serret frame has limited applicability as a foundation for a generalized cylinder. However, it is adequate for cylinders with planar spines which are nowhere straight, e.g. sections of generalized torii.

1.3 Orthogonal Frenet-Serret Description

The nonorthogonality of the Frenet-Serret frame may be corrected following a scheme proposed by C.H. Tang [12]. The Frenet-Serret frame is explicitly unrotated at each point along the curve by a value $\Phi(s)$, based on the torsion exhibited along the curve:

$$\Phi(s) = \int_0^s -\tau(s)ds \qquad (2)$$

This performs what is called an attitude transformation.

We replace $\vec{N}$ and $\vec{B}$ by $\vec{M}$ and $\vec{Q}$ respectively according to:

$$\vec{M} = \cos\Phi\vec{N} + \sin\Phi\vec{B}$$
$$\vec{Q} = -\sin\Phi\vec{N} + \cos\Phi\vec{B}$$

to create the new coordinate system in the normal plane (see Figure 4). The resulting coordinate system for a helix is shown in Figure 3.

Replacing $\vec{M}$ with $\vec{N}$ and $\vec{Q}$ with $\vec{B}$ in (1) results in a GC with a potentially different shape. To create the same shaped GC with an orthogonal frame the rotation by Φ must be compensated for by substituting θ with $\theta - \Phi$ in the polar parametric representation of the cross-section.

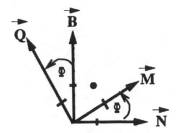

Figure 4: The winding of the $\vec{N}, \vec{B}$ axes due to torsion causes the space off the spine to warp. $\vec{Q}, \vec{M}$ represent the proper positions of the axes to create an orthogonal local coordinate system.

1.3.1 The issues associated with the Frenet based formulations

Unfortunately, for the orthogonal frame just described, a closed-form solution of equation (2) can only be computed for very simple curves. The general case requires a numerical solution to the integral, greatly hampering use of the corrected form.

More of a problem is the result that the amount of derotation (i.e., the frame's attitude transformation) at any point depends on the integral of torsion over the preceding section of the spine. Thus our "local" coordinate system is no longer local!

For another example of how the orthogonality of the frame might impact a vision application consider the work by Ulupinar and Nevatia [15] on the recovery of SHGCs from limbs. They define constraints on possible SHGC configurations based on the orthogonality of a mesh superimposed on the model surface and based on its underlying parameterization. If they were to extend their work to cylinders with curved spines exhibiting torsion and maintained this constraint they might find their results surprising. Notice that twist exhibited by the orthogonal Frenet frame is non-intuitive in the sense that its rotation around the spine is not in obvious sync with the period of the spine for even the simple case of the helix. (Figure 3). Applying the orthogonality constraint directly on this frame would cause the cross section function to twist in this fashion resulting in a rather odd looking cylinder in the case of a non circular cross section.

We now address issues associated with both the standard Frenet frame and its orthogonal variant. Note that both the frames seem to twist around the axis as they move along the curve (Figure 3). For the orthogonal frame, if the cross-section is symetric and centered on the spine, the overall object twist seems reasonable, albeit possibly hard to predict. However, when the axis is not contained within the cross-section the twist results in the cross-section sweeping out a

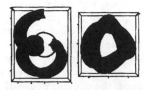

Figure 5: Left shows the the non-intuitive effect of the "natural" twist of the orthogonal Frenet-Serret frame on GC definition with an off-centered cross-section. The helical spine shown from this viewing angle almost forms a circle. On the right is the same offset cross-section and spine but using the EGC formulation described in the next section.

screw pattern around the axis (see figure 5). For the standard Frenet frame the twisting of the frame causes an off-center cross-section to rotate about spine. However, since the rotation is in sync with the period of the spine the screw pattern does not appear.

In addition, due to this twisting of the coordinate frame, small changes in the underlying spine can cause large changes in the shape of a cylinder with a non-circular cross section. This is especially true of the standard Frenet frame. Imagine a cylinder with an elliptic cross section sweeping out a planar curve with small constant curvature. The normal vector, $\vec{N}$, initially lies on one side of the curve. If the spine is then slightly perturbed to make it locally helical the frame will sweep around 360 degrees in that region. The resulting cylinder will exhibit a huge twist as a result of a small perturbation in the spine upon which it is defined. In this sense the Frenet based GCs are unstable.

Another problem with this twisting is that a point specified parametrically will rotate around the spine and within the normal plane. In the orthogonal formulation, the amount of rotation depends on the integral of the torsion along the spine. If, during a fitting process, the spine is changed, then the parametric location of all "later" points changes! That is: the twist propagates down the spine.

Combine these "twist" related problems with the difficulties with straight spines and discontinuities and we end up with a local coordinate system which can be very difficult to use. For these reasons we have abandoned the Frenet-Serret frame as a basis for our general-axis GC model.

2 The Extruded GC

This section presents a new model for general-axis GCs which we call the extruded GC model or EGC.

The intuitive description of an EGC is given by its

spine, its cross-section and its twist parameter. Imagine an extrusion process (e.g. for plastic piping, cake frosting or making pasta) with an aperture that can vary. Let us assume it is extruding a GC primarily along the $\vec{X}$ direction. As the tip of the extruder follows a prescribed space curve, it moves so as to keep the cross-section in the normal plane of the tip. The default behavior (no twist) is to keep the tip's reference mark in an "up" direction. If the user desires a twist, a rotation of this reference mark can be specified. This section details the mathematical development of a subclass of EGC's that is used in our experiments. For all their generality, EGC's will still be unable to model small surface perturbations which can be important in some applications. Thus we discuss adding local perturbations to them.

We begin with the definition of the spine/coordinate system. Like the Frenet-Serret form, our model makes use of an explicit spine, $\vec{r}(u)$, sitting in world coordinates (X,Y,Z). For simplicity we restrict our attention to spines where one component of $\vec{r}(u)$ is a linear function, though the idea can be extended assuming only the existence of a monotonic component. Without loss of generality, let $x(u)$ be linear and make the remaining components functions of $x(u)$. In this way the length, in the X-dimension of the spine and the initial starting point on the space curve $\vec{r}(u)$ are explicitly included in the formulation. The entire curve is spanned by $u : 0 \rightarrow 1$. Our experimentation used cubic polynomials to describe the spine:

$$
\begin{aligned}
x(u) &= Start + (Length)u \\
y(x(u)) &= b_0 + b_1 x(u) \\
&\quad + b_2 x(u)^2 + b_3 x(u)^3 \\
z(x(u)) &= c_0 + c_1 x(u) \\
&\quad + c_2 x(u)^2 + c_3 x(u)^3,
\end{aligned}
$$

however, any functions for y and z would be acceptable.

The unit tangent vector $\vec{T}$ to the the spine is calculated defining a normal plane to the spine in which the vectors $\vec{U}$ and $\vec{L}$ reside. $\vec{U}$ and $\vec{L}$ form the coordinate system upon which the cross section function is plotted. They perform the same function as $\vec{N}$ and $\vec{B}$ do in the Frenet-Serret from.

To avoid the complications of straightness, local and otherwise, $\vec{U}$ and $\vec{L}$ are not functions of the second derivative of $\vec{r}$. Rather, $\vec{U}$ (for Up) is chosen such that it always points in the direction of the world $\vec{Z}$ vector, and $\vec{L}$ (for Left) is calculated to be orthogonal to both $\vec{U}$ and $\vec{T}$. Given this construction method it should be noted that the EGC frame is non-orthogonal. This is acceptable, however, as we have already noted the difficulties of an orthogonal frame.

We desire that $\vec{U}$ remain on one side of the

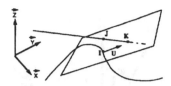

Figure 6: Calculation of the vector $\vec{U}$.

spine, never crossing it. Therefore a point $J = (x(u), y(x(u)), z(x(u)) + 1)$ is found directly "above" the point on the spine $I = (x(u), y(x(u)), z(x(u)))$ where the local coordinate frame is currently being calculated. K is the intersection of the line projecting J onto the normal plane in the direction of the tangent vector at I. We let $\vec{U}$ be the normalized vector extending from I in the direction of K (see Figure 6). $\vec{L}$ is then calculated via the cross product:

$$
\vec{U} = I\vec{K}/|I\vec{K}|, \qquad \vec{L} = \vec{U} \times \vec{T} \tag{3}
$$

K is calculated from the equation:

$$
K(t) = \begin{pmatrix} x(t) - T_x T_z \\ y(x(t)) - T_y T_z \\ z(x(t)) + T_x{}^2 + T_y{}^2 \end{pmatrix} \tag{4}
$$

This frame is intuitively easy to understand: we have a tangent and a "privileged" direction, called up. Bruce and Giblin [2] provide a sound (and independent) foundation for this approach to constructing a coordinate system: Given a space curve $\Gamma : \mathbf{I} \rightarrow \Re^3$, where $\mathbf{I}$ is an open connected subset of the unit circle S^1 (with increasing t corresponding to a counterclockwise orientation) it is possible choose a smooth family of unit vectors $\vec{V}(t)$ normal to the tangent of Γ, $\vec{T}(t)$ such that $\vec{V}(t) \cdot \vec{T}(t) = 0$ for all t. This may be done by considering the smooth map $T : I \rightarrow S^2$ which takes t to $\vec{T}$. From any vector $\vec{V}$ in $S^2 - T(\mathbf{I})$ the field $\vec{V}(t)$ may be obtained by orthogonally projecting V onto each of the normal planes to Γ and normalizing. By Sard's Theorem there are many such vectors. Of the many choices, we have simply chosen one which we felt would be easy to understand and manipulate.

Now that a suitable spine and coordinate frame have been developed, we proceed with the extruded cylinder construction. The cylinder's cross section is parameterized as a function of position along the the spine (i.e. a function of $x(u)$). The radii scaling parameters in the $\vec{U}$ and $\vec{L}$ directions are rad_1 and rad_2 respectively and the cylinder may twist according to the parameter ω.

In the experiments presented herein we have used a simple linear model for cross-section variations. The constant term determines the base value for the parameter and the coefficient term how the parameter will vary from the base value along the spine.

$$\begin{aligned}
rad_1(x(u)) &= URad_{coeff}(x(u) - Start) \\
&\quad + URad_{const} \\
rad_2(x(u)) &= LRad_{coeff}(x(u) - Start) \\
&\quad + LRad_{const} \\
\omega(x(u)) &= Twist_{coeff}(x(u) - Start) \\
&\quad + Twist_{const}
\end{aligned}$$

The use of *two independent* piecewise linear sweep rules has proven sufficient for the structures considered. They have added flexibility over homogeneous GCs by allowing the cross-section to vary from circular to elliptical.

The cross section γ itself is swept out via the parameter θ. Any twisting of the cross section is controlled by ω. For mathematical convenience we parameterize the 2D cross-section in a plane. For example, for a circular base cross-section, which is what we used in the experimental section, we have:

$$\gamma(\vec{\omega}, u) = \left[\begin{array}{cc} \cos\omega(x(u)) & -\sin\omega(x(u)) \\ \sin\omega(x(u)) & \cos\omega(x(u)) \end{array} \right]$$

$$\varrho(\vec{\theta}, u) = \left[\begin{array}{c} rad_1(x(u))\cos\theta \\ rad_2(x(u))\sin\theta \end{array} \right]$$

Note that after scaling in each direction these form ellipses. Other cross-section functions are, of course, allowed. For example, Figure 7 presents an EGC with super-quadratic cross-section.

Any point on the cross-section is then placed in the $[U\ L]$ frame via the attitude transformation $\mathcal{A}(u)$. (Recall that U and L both depend on the position u along the curve.) The transform is given by:

$$\mathbf{A}(u) = \left[\begin{array}{cc} U_x & L_x \\ U_y & L_y \\ U_z & L_z \end{array} \right] \tag{5}$$

Finally each surface point is translated according to the associated point $\vec{r}(u)$ on the spine. The envelope of all such points defines the surface of the cylinder.

$$\vec{r}(u) + \mathbf{A}(u)\gamma(\vec{\omega}, u)\varrho(\vec{\theta}, u) \tag{6}$$

2.1 Adding Local Deformations to the Extruded GC Model

Our GC model described above will form the foundation (a global model) upon which spline-like local deformations may take place. The composite deformable EGC is free to translate and rotate in space.

A point $\vec{x}$ on the model is expressed as

$$\vec{x} = \vec{t} + \mathbf{R}(\vec{c} + \vec{d}) \tag{7}$$

where $\vec{t}$ is the position of the starting end of the GC (i.e. u=0), $\vec{c}$ is a point on the global GC model, $\mathbf{R}$ is

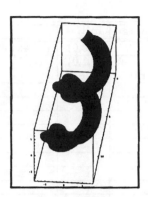

Figure 7: An EGC in the shape of a helix. The twisting artifact is no longer in evidence.

spatial the rotation matrix (on top of the GC's position) and $\vec{d}$ is the local deformation from the global model.

We represent the displacement as a linear combination of basis functions

$$\vec{d} = \mathbf{S}\vec{q_d} \tag{8}$$

where $\mathbf{S}$ is matrix of triangular finite element (FEM) shape functions and where the nodal positions, q_d, are expressed in generalized coordinates.

3 Experimental Results

The task of object recovery was performed using a physically-motivated approach roughly following [14]. The external forces driving the fitting process were a function of the distance from the datapoints to the closest points on the model.

The technique described above was applied to a pre-segmented left branch of a bifurcating human carotid artery. 328 datapoints were used and the entire process took 80 iterations. **

Table 1 shows the parameter settings before and after the fitting. Global deformations were prohibited (automatically) until the translation and rotation of the initial model had settled, i.e.:

$$(\|\vec{t}^i - \vec{t}^{i-1}\|_2 + \|\mathbf{R}^i - \mathbf{R}^{i-1}\|_2 < 0.1$$

Similarly local deformations were not permitted until the global parameters had reached a relatively stable state, i.e.

$$\sum_j^{parameters} |p_j^i - p_j^{i-1}| < .01.$$

The deformable aspects of the model used 120 nodes. The differential equation describing the fitting of the

---

**The computation took 3 minutes on a Sparc 10, but much of that time was used for graphics; we display the model/forces after each iteration.

parameter	initial	final
Trans	(0,0,0)	(.954,.449,.913)
Rot (quatern)	(0,1,0), .001	(0,.067,-.031), .997
b_0	0	.011
b_1	0	-.018
b_2	0	-.015
b_3	0	-.014
c_0	0	.025
c_1	0	-.084
c_2	0	.003
c_3	0	.009
Start	-1	-.968
Length	2.5	2.590
$URad_{const}$	0.15	.250
$URad_{coeff}$	0	.014
$LRad_{const}$	0.15	.283
$LRad_{coeff}$	0	.019
$Twist_{const}$	0	.000
$Twist_{coeff}$	0	.000

Table 1: Parameter values for the GC recovered for the carotid artery.

model was solved using simple Euler time stepping. The Euler coefficients, guiding the rigid body motion, global model deformations, and rigid body deformations were .3, .5 and 5 respectively. The Euler time step, Δt, was .0004. Figure 8 shows several points in the fitting process.

4 Conclusions and Future Work

We have presented four descriptions of generalized cylinders and outlined their deficiencies.

The EGC overcomes the drawbacks of these models. It has the ability to describe cylinders with (locally) straight as well as curved spines. The model also has an intuitively understandable "twisting" behavior – no twisting unless you request it. These two properties are quite useful when there is no a priori information about the curvature characteristics of the object under recovery. In addition, because we exploit an explicit spine, our model does not exhibit the narrowing effect of the tube model. In addition, the EGC can be made orthogonal if necessary by rotating its coordinate axis first to bring it in line with the Frenet frame and then by the integral of the torsion along the spine, Φ (from equation 2). The original shape can be recovered by a change of the variable θ by $\theta - \Phi$.

While our deformable EGC model is far more flexi-

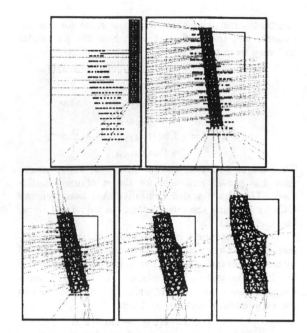

Figure 8: The fitting of the deformable cylinder to pre-segmented carotid artery data (selected iterations are shown left to right). The model is drawn as a black mesh, the dark gray points show the pre-segmented data, and the light gray lines represent the forces acting on the nodes of the model to produce the fitting. The magnitude of the force lines are proportional to the actual force strength and the directions are consistent with the true force directions.

ble then any existing GC model known to the authors, we continue work on extensions. In particular, we are currently extending our implementation of the EGC model to handle general splines as a spine. More experimentation with the recovery of the cylinder from 3D medical scanner images and 2D intensity images will further demonstrate the the utility of the model and is also being pursued. Work on segmenting 3D medical data is almost complete, and will be reported in a separate paper. Deriving constraints from 2D intensity images is far more difficult, and requires further research.

References

[1] T. O. Binford. Visual perception by computer. In *IEEE Conference on Systems and Control*, Miami, 1971.

[2] J. W. Bruce and P.J. Giblin. *Curves and Singularities*. Cambridge University Press, 1987.

[3] Ari D. Gross and Terrance E. Boult. Recovery of generalized cylinders from a single intensity view. In *Pro-*

ceedings of DARPA Image Understanding Workshop, pages 557–564, 1990.

[4] Q. Huang and G. C. Stockman. Generalized tube model: Recognizing 3D elongated objects from 2d intensity images. In *Proceedings of CVPR*, pages 104–109. IEEE, 1993.

[5] Koichi Kitamura, Jonathan M. Tobis, and Jack Sklansky. Estimating the 3-D skeletons and transverse areas of coronary arteries from biplane angiograms. *IEEE Transactions on Medical Imaging*, 7(3):173–187, 1988.

[6] Jan J. Koenderink *Solid Shape*. MIT Press, 1990.

[7] Takayuki Nakamura, Minoru Asada, and Yoshiaki Shirai. A qualitative approach to quantitative recovery of SHGC's shape and pose from shading and contour. In *Proceedings of the CVPR*, pages 116–121. IEEE, 1993.

[8] Thrasyvoulos N. Pappas and Jae S. Lim. A new method for estimation of coronary artery dimensions in angiograms. *IEEE Transactions on Acoustics, Speech, and Signal Processing*, 36(9):1501–1513, September 1988.

[9] Jean Ponce and David Chelberg. Finding the limbs and cusps of generalized cylinders. In *International Jounal of Computer Vision*, 9(3):195-209, 1987

[10] Jean Ponce, David Chelberg, and Wallace Mann. Invariant properties of the projections of straight homogeneous generalized cylinders. In *Proceedins of the International Conference on Computer Vision*, pages 631–635, 1987.

[11] K. Rao and R. Nevatia. Shape description from imperfect and incomplete data. In *Proceedings of International Conference on Pattern Recognition*, pages 125–129, 1990.

[12] C.H. Tang. An orthogonal coordinate system for curved pipes. *IEEE Trans. MTT* 19(1):69–70, 1969.

[13] D. Terzopoulos, A. Witkin, and M. Kass. Constraints on deformable models: Recovering 3D shape and nonrigid motion. *Artificial Intelligence*, pages 91–123, August 1988.

[14] Demetri Terzopoulos and Dimitri Metaxas. Dynamic 3D models with local and global deformations: Deformable superquadrics. In *Proceedings of the Third International Conference on Computer Vision*, pages 606–615, Osaka, Japan, December 1990. IEEE.

[15] Fatih Ulupinar and Ramakant Nevatia. Recovering shape from contour for SHGCs and CGCs. In *Proceedings of DARPA Image Understanding Workshop*, pages 544–556, 1990.

[16] Mourad Zerroug and Ramakant Nevatia. Quasi-invariant properties and 3-D shape recovery of nonstraight, non-constant generalized cylinders. In *Proceedings of CVPR*, pages 96–103, 1993.

[17] T O'Donnell, X-S. Fang, T. Boult and A. Gupta. On Generalized with Generalized Spines Columbia University Technical Report CUCS-009094.

Recovery of Nonrigid Motion and Structure

Alex Pentland and Bradley Horowitz

Abstract— The elastic properties of real materials provide constraint on the types of nonrigid motion that can occur, and thus allow overconstrained estimates of 3-D nonrigid motion from optical flow data. We show that by modeling and simulating the physics of nonrigid motion we can obtain good estimates of both object shape and velocity. Examples using grey scale and X-ray imagery are presented, including an example of tracking a complex articulated figure.

Index Terms—Deformable models, Finite element method, Kalman filtering, Modal analysis, Motion processing, Nonrigid motion, Physically based modeling, Shape representation, 3-D shape recovery, 3-D tracking.

I. INTRODUCTION

TO date, almost all research on recovering global, whole-body structure from optical flow has been based on rigid motion. Even schemes which address nonrigid motion, e.g., Ullman's incremental rigidity scheme [19], are usually based on minimizing the deviation from a rigid-body interpretation. Yet, nonrigid motion is everywhere: trees sway, flags flap, fish wriggle, arm and leg muscles bunch up, neck and body twist and bend, and cheeks bulge and stretch.

One way of coping with nonrigidity is to simply abandon the idea of recovering a whole-body description of the motion, and seek to recover structure on a patch-by-patch basis, perhaps allowing some limited form of nonrigidity [11], [17]. Unfortunately, using a local description requires that we limit ourselves to using only noise-sensitive local measurements and that we correctly and consistently match optical flow data to the same facets or patches. Consequently such patch-by-patch recovery of structure is not likely to be either very accurate or robust.

Moreover, we *want* more than a patch-by-patch description, because whole-body motions like bending, twisting, and the like are meaningful [12], especially when trying to interpret the actions and gestures of animals and people. To quote Gibson [8], "An elastic motion, including that of a walking man with his gestures and facial expressions, could be analyzed into a set of rigid motions of elementary particles if one wished to do so, but it is better thought of in terms of components like bending, flexing, stretching, skewing, expanding, and bulging." Several researchers have demonstrated recovery of limited global descriptions (e.g., symmetry axis shape) from

nonrigid motion [21]. The goal of this paper is to recover more nearly complete, but still overconstrained, global descriptions of nonrigid motion.

We suggest that the main limitation of previous approaches to recovering whole-body descriptions of nonrigid motion was that such motion was conceptualized as being mostly unstructured. As a consequence all one can say about it is how each point or patch is moving. To describe such completely unstructured motion requires three unknowns per object point, and as a consequence the problem of estimating nonrigid motions becomes badly underconstrained. In fact, however, most real objects are made of approximately elastic materials, and we will show this fact can be used to transform the nonrigid motion problem in to an *over*constrained problem with a reliable and efficient solution.

The key insight is that the coherent elastic behavior of real materials implies that nonrigid whole-body motion can be accurately described with relatively few parameters.[1] The optimal parameterization is obtained from the eigenvectors of the object's corresponding finite element method (FEM) model. These eigenvectors are often referred to as the 3-D object's *free vibration* or *deformation* modes. The parameterization is unique, and is obtained by a multiscale orthonormal linear transform (similar to the Fourier transform) that maps the object's point-by-point motion in Cartesian coordinates into a coordinate system based on the object's intrinsic deformation modes.

By describing object behavior using a truncated series of vibration/deformation modes one can obtain the best r.m.s. error description possible for a given number of parameters. By varying the number of parameters (often as a function of the number of sensor measurements available) one can smoothly make the transition from a coarse qualitative description to a finely detailed, accurate description—just as one can smoothly obtain more accuracy by adding more terms to a Fourier series. The important consequence for the problem of recovering nonrigid motion is that the problem can always be made overconstrained by reducing the number of vibration/deformation modes. The limiting case is rigid-body motion, which is equivalent to using only the lowest six vibration/deformation modes.

Because the modal representation is derived from the ideas of finite element analysis, we will begin by reviewing the finite element method.

II. THE FINITE ELEMENT METHOD

The finite element method (FEM) is the standard engineer-

Manuscript received September 17, 1990; revised February 28, 1991.

This work was supported in part by the National Science Foundation under Grant IRI-8719920, by the Rome Air Development Center of the Air Force Systems Command, and by the Defense Advanced Research Projects Agency under Contract F30602-89-C-0022.

The authors are with the Vision and Modeling Group, The Media Lab, Massachusetts Institute of Technology, Cambridge, MA 02139.

IEEE Log Number 9100891.

[1] Except in unusual cases, for example, an object being torn apart by a chaotic flow

Reprinted from *IEEE Trans. Pattern Analysis and Machine Intelligence*, Vol. 13, No. 7, July 1991, pp. 730–742.

ing technique for simulating the dynamic behavior of an object. Use of such techniques has become quite popular in machine vision, following the seminal work of Terzopoulos, Witkin, and Kass [18]. One motivation for using the FEM for vision is that vision is often concerned with estimating changes in position, orientation, and shape, quantities that the FEM accurately describes. Another motivation is that by allowing the user to specify forces that are a function of sensor measurements, the intrinsic dynamic behavior of the FEM can be used to solve fitting, interpolation, or correspondence problems.

In the FEM, interpolation functions are developed that allow continuous material properties, such as mass and stiffness, to be integrated across the region of interest. Note that this is quite different from the finite difference schemes commonly used in computer vision, although the resulting equations are quite similar. One major difference between the FEM and the finite difference schemes is that the FEM provides an analytic characterization of the surface between nodes or pixels, whereas finite difference methods do not. All of the results presented in this paper will be applicable to both the finite difference and finite element formulations.

Having formulated the appropriate FEM integrals, they are then combined into a description in terms of discrete *nodal points*. Energy functionals are then formulated in terms of nodal displacements $\mathbf{U}$, and the resulting set of simultaneous equations is iterated to solve for the nodal displacements as a function of impinging loads $\mathbf{R}$:

$$\mathbf{MU} + \mathbf{C\ddot{U}} + \mathbf{K\dot{U}} = \mathbf{R} \tag{1}$$

where $\mathbf{U}$ is a $3n \times 1$ vector of the $(\Delta x, \Delta y, \Delta z)$ displacements of the n nodal points relative to the object's center of mass, $\mathbf{M}$, $\mathbf{C}$, and $\mathbf{K}$ are $3n$ by $3n$ matrices describing the mass, damping, and material stiffness between each point within the body, and $\mathbf{R}$ is a $3n \times 1$ vector describing the x, y, and z components of the forces acting on the nodes.

Equation (1) is known as the *governing equation* in the finite element method, and may be interpreted as assigning a certain mass to each nodal point and a certain material stiffness between nodal points, with damping being accounted for by dashpots attached between the nodal points. Inertial and centrifugal effects are accounted for by adding appropriate off-diagonal terms to the mass matrix. For additional detail about the finite element formulation see reference [3] or [20].

The most obvious drawback of both the finite difference or finite element methods is the large computations expense. Such methods require roughly $3nm_k$ operations per time step, where $3n$ is the order of the stiffness matrix and m_k is its half bandwidth.[2] Normally $3n$ such time steps are required to obtain an equilibrium solution. A related drawback in vision applications is that the number of description parameters is often roughly equal to the number of sensor measurements, necessitating the use of heuristics such as symmetry and smoothness. This results in nonunique and unstable descriptions, with the consequence that it is difficult to determine whether or not two models are equivalent.

[2] See Bathe [3] Appendix A.2.2 for complete discussion on bandwidth of a stiffness matrix.

Perhaps the most important problem with using such physically based methods for vision, however, is that all of the degrees of freedom are coupled together. Consequently, closed-form solutions are impossible and solutions to the sort of inverse problems encountered in vision are very difficult.

Thus there is a need for a method which transforms (1) into a form which is not only less costly, but also admits of closed-form solutions. Since the number of operations is proportional to the half bandwidth m_k of the stiffness matrix, a reduction in m_k will greatly reduce the cost of step-by-step solution. Moreover, if we can actually diagonalize the system of equations, then the degrees of freedom will become uncoupled and we will be able to find closed-form solutions.

A. Modal Analysis

To accomplish the goal of diagonalizing the system of equations a linear transformation of the nodal point displacements $\mathbf{U}$ can be used

$$\mathbf{U} = \mathbf{P\tilde{U}} \tag{2}$$

where $\mathbf{P}$ is a square orthogonal transformation matrix, and $\tilde{\mathbf{U}}$ is a vector of generalized displacements. Substituting Equation 2 into Equation 1 and premultiplying by $\mathbf{P}^T$ yields:

$$\mathbf{\tilde{M}\ddot{\tilde{U}}} + \mathbf{\tilde{C}\dot{\tilde{U}}} + \mathbf{\tilde{K}\tilde{U}} = \mathbf{\tilde{R}} \tag{3}$$

where

$$\mathbf{\tilde{M}} = \mathbf{P}^T \mathbf{MP}; \qquad \mathbf{\tilde{C}} = \mathbf{P}^T \mathbf{CP};$$
$$\mathbf{\tilde{K}} = \mathbf{P}^T \mathbf{KP}; \qquad \mathbf{\tilde{R}} = \mathbf{P}^T \mathbf{R}. \tag{4}$$

With this transformation of basis set a new system of stiffness, mass and damping matrices can be obtained which has a smaller bandwidth then the original system.

A. Use of Free Vibration Modes

The optimal transformation matrix $\mathbf{P}$ is derived from the free vibration modes of the equilibrium equation. Beginning with the governing equation, an eigenvalue problem can be derived

$$\mathbf{K}\phi_i = \omega_i^2 \phi_i \mathbf{M} \tag{5}$$

which will determine an optimal transformation basis set.

The eigenvalue problem in (5) yields $3n$ eigensolutions.

$$(\omega_1^2, \phi_1), (\omega_2^2, \phi_2), \cdots, (\omega_{3n}^2, \phi_{3n})$$

where all the eigenvectors are $\mathbf{M}$-orthonormalized. Hence

$$\phi_i^T \mathbf{M} \phi_j = \begin{cases} 1; & i = j \\ 0; & i \neq j \end{cases} \tag{6}$$

and

$$0 \leq \omega_1^2 \leq \omega_2^2 \leq \omega_3^2 \leq \cdots \leq \omega_{3n}^2. \tag{7}$$

The eigenvector ϕ_i is called the ith mode's *shape vector* and ω_i is the corresponding frequency of vibration. Each eigenvector ϕ_i consists of the (x, y, z) displacements for each

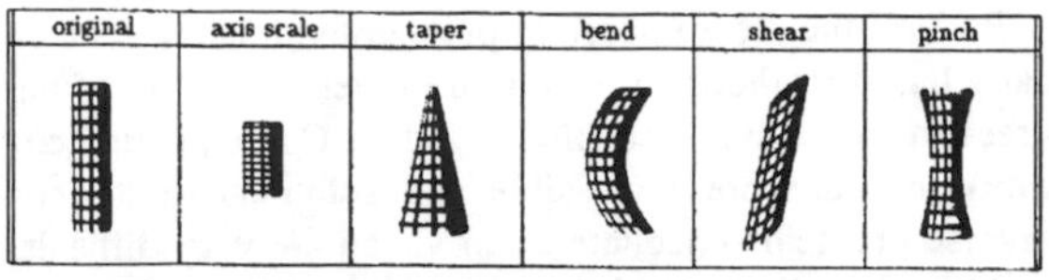

Fig. 1. Several of the lowest frequency vibrations modes of a cylinder. English labels are for descriptive purposes only.

node, that is, the $3j - 2$, $3j - 1$, and $3j$ elements are the x, y, and z displacements for node j, $1 \leq j \leq n$.

The lowest frequency modes are always the rigid-body modes of translation and rotation. The eigenvector corresponding to x-axis translation, for instance, has ones for each node's x-axis displacement element, with all other elements being zero. In the finite element formulation, rotational motion is linearized so that nodes on the opposite sides of the body have opposite directions of displacement.

The next lowest frequency modes are smooth whole-body deformations that leave the center of mass and rotation fixed. That is, the (x, y, z) displacements of the nodes are a low-order function of the node's position, and the nodal displacements balance out to zero net translational and rotational motion. Compact bodies (simple solids whose dimensions are within the same order of magnitude) normally have low-order modes that are similar to those shown in Fig. 1. Bodies with very dissimilar dimensions, or which have holes, etc., can have substantially more complex low-frequency modes.

Using these modes we can define a transformation matrix $\boldsymbol{\Phi}$, which has for its columns the eigenvectors ϕ_i and a diagonal matrix $\boldsymbol{\Omega}^2$, with the eigenvalues ω_i^2 on its diagonal

$$\boldsymbol{\Phi} = [\phi_1, \phi_2, \phi_3, \cdots, \phi_{3_n}] \tag{8}$$

$$\boldsymbol{\Omega}^2 = \begin{bmatrix} \omega_1^2 & & & & \\ & \omega_2^2 & & & \\ & & \cdot & & \\ & & & \cdot & \\ & & & & \cdot \\ & & & & & \omega_{3n}^2 \end{bmatrix}. \tag{9}$$

Using (9), (5) can now be written as

$$\mathbf{K}\boldsymbol{\Phi} = \boldsymbol{\Omega}^2\boldsymbol{\Phi}\mathbf{M} \tag{10}$$

and since the eigenvectors are $\mathbf{M}$-orthonormal

$$\boldsymbol{\Phi}^T\mathbf{K}\boldsymbol{\Phi} = \boldsymbol{\Omega}^2$$
$$\boldsymbol{\Phi}^T\mathbf{M}\boldsymbol{\Phi} = \mathbf{I}. \tag{11}$$

From the aforementioned formulations it becomes apparent that matrix $\boldsymbol{\Phi}$ is the optimal transformation matrix $\mathbf{P}$ for systems in which damping effects are negligible.

To also diagonalize the damping matrix $\mathbf{C}$ with the same transform, $\mathbf{C}$ must be restricted to a special form. The normal assumption is that the damping matrix is constructed by using the *Caughey series* [3]

$$\mathbf{C} = \mathbf{M} \sum_{k=0}^{p-1} a_k [\mathbf{M}^{-1}\mathbf{K}]^k. \tag{12}$$

Restriction to this form is equivalent to the assumption that damping, which describes the overall energy dissipation during the system response, is proportional to system response. At $p \leq 2$ (12) reduces to *Rayleigh damping* ($\mathbf{C} = a_0\mathbf{M} + a_1\mathbf{K}$), and $\mathbf{C}$ is diagonalized by $\boldsymbol{\Phi}$. Most finite element analyses assume Rayleigh damping [3].

In this case, the general governing equation (3) is reduced to

$$\ddot{\tilde{\mathbf{U}}} + \tilde{\mathbf{C}}\dot{\tilde{\mathbf{U}}} + \boldsymbol{\Omega}^2\tilde{\mathbf{U}} = \boldsymbol{\Phi}^T\mathbf{R}(t) \tag{13}$$

where $\tilde{\mathbf{C}} = a_0\mathbf{I} + a_1\boldsymbol{\Omega}^2$, or equivalently to $3n$ independent and individual equations of the form

$$\ddot{\tilde{u}}_i(t) + \tilde{c}_i\dot{\tilde{u}}_i(t) + \omega_i^2\tilde{u}_i(t) = \tilde{r}_i(t) \tag{14}$$

where $\tilde{c}_i$ are modal damping parameters and $\tilde{r}_i(t) = \phi_i^T\mathbf{R}(t)$ for $i = 1, 2, 3, \cdots, 3n$. Therefore, the matrix $\boldsymbol{\Phi}$ is the optimal transformation for both damped and undamped systems, given the Rayleigh damping is assumed.

In summary, we have shown that the general finite governing equation is decoupled when using a transformation matrix $\mathbf{P}$ whose columns are the free vibration mode shapes of the FEM system [3], [16], [13], [15]. These decoupled equations may then be integrated numerically (see [13]) or solved in closed form by use of a *Duhamel* integral (see [15]).

B. Accuracy and the Number of Modes Employed

The modal representation decouples the degrees of freedom within the nonrigid dynamic system of (1) but it does not by itself reduce the total number of degrees of freedom. However, modes associated with high resonance frequencies (large eigenvalues) normally have little effect on object shape. This is because, for a given excitation energy, the displacement amplitude for each mode is *inversely* proportional to the *square* of the mode's resonance frequency and because damping is proportional to a mode's frequency. The consequence of these combined effects is that high-frequency modes generally have very little amplitude.

We can therefore discard high-frequency modes with little loss of accuracy or generality, with the result that we have fewer equations in fewer unknowns and (because of Nyquist considerations) we can employ a much larger time step when performing a simulation. For a typical problem this approach can decrease computational cost by *two orders of magnitude* while maintaining good accuracy [13]. Moreover, for a fixed number of modes the computation scales as $O(n)$ rather than $O(n^2)$ or $O(n^3)$. For complex shapes this linear scaling behavior can be extremely important, and it is for this reason that this type of reduced-basis modal analysis has become the standard method for extremely large engineering problems, such as the analysis of airplane frames or large buildings.

Fig. 2 shows a sampling of shapes that can be achieved by elastically deforming an initial spherical shape using its 30 lowest frequency deformation modes (note that the first six modes are rigid-body translation and rotation). As can be seen, a wide range of nonrigid motions and their resulting shapes can be produced with relatively few deformation modes. As Fig. 2 illustrates, discarding high-frequency modes is *not* equivalent

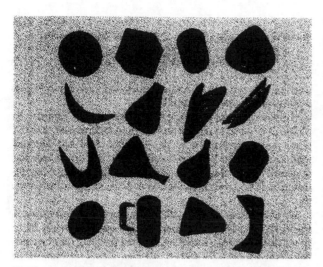

Fig. 2. A sampling of shapes produced by elastically deforming an initial spherical shape using its 30 lowest frequency deformation modes. As can be seen, a wide range nonrigid motions and their resulting shapes can be described by relatively few deformation modes.

to assuming that the surface is smooth, because we can still generate sharp bends, creases, and so forth.

As can be seen, besides decoupling the degrees of freedom, the modal representation also provides a natural hierarchy of scale so that we can smoothly vary the level of detail by adding in or discarding high-frequency modes. That is, the modal representation provides a natural multiscale representation for 3-D object shape in much the same manner that the Fourier transform provides a multiscale representation for images.

The ability to decouple the order the degrees of freedom has several important implications for machine vision applications. For instance, by matching the level of detail (the number of modes) to the number of sensor measurements the shape recovery process can be kept overconstrained. Similarly, because the degrees of freedom are orthogonal, shape and velocity descriptions are *unique* for an object in canonical position (the restriction to canonical position is necessary because rotations have been linearized). These properties contrast markedly to representations based on nodes, polynomials, or splines where descriptions are normally neither unique nor overconstrained.

III. RECOVERING NONRIGID MOTION

In this paper, we will analyze the case where the object geometry at time $t = 0$ is known, and where object motion is viewed under orthographic projection. Determination of initial object geometry and modal description can be accomplished as described in Pentland and Sclaroff [20]. The problem, then, is to find the rigid and nonrigid 3-D motions dU/dt that best account for the observed 2-D image velocities. The major difficulty in finding such a solution is that there are $3n$ unknown degrees of freedom in the model and at most $2n$ degrees of freedom in the observations. Thus, we must somehow reduce the number of unknowns to obtain a solution.

The modal representation offers a principled physically-based method for reducing the number of degrees of freedom.

Because we known that the elastic properties of real materials imply that the high-frequency modes are (almost always) of low amplitude, we can discard many of these modes without incurring significant error.

Further, because the modal representation is frequency-ordered, it has stability properties that are similar to those of a Fourier decomposition. Just as with the Fourier decomposition, an exact[3] subsampling of the data points points does not change the low-frequency modes. Similarly, irregularities in local sampling and measurement noise tend to primarily affect the high-frequency modes, leaving the low-frequency modes relatively unchanged.

Again, we note that discarding these high-frequency modes is *not* equivalent to a general smoothness constraint, because we can still generate sharp bends, creases, and so forth (see Fig. 2). What we cannot do with a reduced-basis modal representation is generate several sharp creases that are close together.

We will therefore pose our problem in the modal coordinate system: the problem is to find the set of 3-D *mode* velocities $d\tilde{U}/dt$ that best account for the observed 2-D image velocities. If we use the m lowest frequency modes, then there will be only m unknown degrees of freedom in the model and up to $2n$ degrees of freedom in the observations. Thus by appropriate choice of m, the problem can always be made overconstrained. Whenever the 3-D velocities of the individual nodes are required, we can convert $\tilde{U}$ back to the original space coordinates by multiplying by Φ.

A. Kinematic Solution

We first note that ϕ_i, the ith column of Φ, describes the *deformation* the object experiences as a consequence of the modal force $\tilde{r}_i$. Or perhaps more intuitively, ϕ_i describes how each of the n nodal points $(x_j, y_j, z_j)^T$ change as a function of $\tilde{u}_i$, the ith mode's amplitude

$$\phi_i = \left(\frac{dx_1}{d\tilde{u}_i}, \frac{dy_1}{d\tilde{u}_i}, \frac{dz_1}{d\tilde{u}_i}, \cdots, \frac{dx_n}{d\tilde{u}_i}, \frac{dy_n}{d\tilde{u}_i}, \frac{dz_n}{d\tilde{u}_i}\right)^T. \quad (15)$$

Letting V be the 3-D velocity of each node

$$V = \left(\frac{dx_1}{dt}, \frac{dy_1}{dt}, \frac{dz_1}{dt}, \cdots, \frac{dx_n}{dt}, \frac{dy_n}{dt}, \frac{dz_n}{dt}\right)^T \quad (16)$$

we then have that

$$V = \Phi\frac{d\tilde{U}}{dt} = \Phi\dot{\tilde{U}}. \quad (17)$$

Given the 3-D motions of each node, then we can solve for the modal velocities $\dot{\tilde{U}}$ as follows:

$$\dot{\tilde{U}} = \Phi^{-1}V. \quad (18)$$

Thus having observed 3-D nodal velocities V, the kinematic solution for the modal amplitudes $\tilde{U}^t$ at time t is simply

$$\tilde{U}^t = \dot{\tilde{U}}^t \Delta t + \tilde{U}^{t-1} = \Phi^{-1}V^t\Delta t \quad (19)$$

[3]E.g., if there are 2^k points a sampling of every 2^l points $(l < k)$ is an exact subsampling.

where at each time step, the object's resting shape is reset so that $\tilde{U}^{t-1} = 0$. The primary limitation of this solution stems from the finite element method's linearization of modes such as rotation. Because these modes are linearized, it is important to limit interframe motion to small rotations (less than $10°$) and deformations (less than 10% of the object size).

B. Estimation from 2-D Data

Given the kinematic solution of (19), the remaining problem is to obtain a generalization that uses 2-D measurements of optical flow as input data. More concretely, the problem is to estimate the rigid-body motion and nonrigid 3-D global deformation at each subsequent time t given only noisy estimates of 2-D (orthographically projected) optical flow (u_i^t, v_i^t) at m image points (x_i, y_i). The image points (x_i, y_i) are *not* assumed to be either dense or uniformly sampled.

This can be accomplished by allocating each of the available optical flow vectors (u_i, v_i) among the nodal points whose image projections are close to (x_i, y_i), the flow vector's image position. The most accurate method of accomplishing this allocation is to use the interpolation functions H used to define the finite element model, as described in [20], Appendix A. However, when the mesh of nodes is sufficiently dense that each optical flow vector projects near to some node, then we have found that it is sufficiently accurate to use simple bilinear interpolation of the flow vectors to the surrounding three nodes. An inexpensive method of accomplishing this is discussed in the Appendix.

This produces estimates of the projected 2-D nodal velocities.

$$\mathbf{V}_P = (u_1, v_1, u_2, v_2, \cdots, u_n, v_n)^T. \quad (20)$$

We define the matrix Φ_P similarly, by removing rows of Φ that correspond to z-axis displacements. Note that nodes without nearby optical flow may have no velocity estimate; therefore, rows of $\mathbf{V}_P$ and Φ_P corresponding to the x and y displacements of these nodes are undefined (contain no information) and must also be removed.

Some modes, including translation, scaling, and shearing along the z-axis, cannot be observed under orthographic projection. Therefore, columns of Φ_P and rows of $\tilde{U}$ corresponding to these modes must also be removed. Because the remaining mode shapes are orthogonal to the translation, scaling, and shearing modes, they remain unaffected. Similarly, in some cases the 2-D motions caused by a particular modal deformation are very small, so that the mode's amplitude cannot be reliably estimated. Such ill-conditioned estimates can be prevented by discarding modes for which the corresponding column of Φ_P has small magnitude.

With these definitions we may now generalize (19) to obtain an estimate of the object's 3-D shape $\tilde{U}^t$ at time t based on the optical flow data. The generalization is simply

$$\tilde{U}^t = \Phi_P^{-1} \mathbf{V}_P{}^t \Delta t. \quad (21)$$

Equation (21) is underconstrained if all of the modes are present in Φ_P; however, by discarding a sufficient number of the low-amplitude high-frequency modes, the estimate can always be made overconstrained.[4] Therefore, in practice, Φ_P^{-1} is calculated by use of a Moore–Penrose pseudoinverse

$$\tilde{U}^t = \left(\Phi_P^T \Phi_P\right)^{-1} \Phi_P^T \mathbf{V}_P^t \Delta t \quad (22)$$

with the columns of Φ_P and the rows of $\tilde{U}$ corresponding to high-frequency modes deleted.

Equation (22) provides us with a least-squares estimate of $\tilde{U}$, the object's rigid motion and nonrigid deformation. It is the best r.m.s. error estimate of the projected rigid and nonrigid motions given the observed optical flow vectors, where the projected mode shapes are described (analytically) by the columns of Φ_P and the finite element interpolation functions H.

We have found that 30 deformation modes are adequate to account for most rigid and nonrigid motions, so that only 15 or so independent flow vectors are required per body. In situations with very sparse flow vectors, we can reduce the number of deformation modes still further in order to keep the calculation overconstrained. In the limiting case, we require only three independent flow vectors in order to estimate the six rigid body motions, and four vectors to obtain an overconstrained estimate.[5]

IV. EXAMPLES USING SYNTHETIC DATA

A. An Illustrative Example

Fig. 3 illustrates how a complex sum of rigid and nonrigid motions can be decomposed into a sum of the object's free vibration modes. Fig. 3(a) shows a box, and Fig. 3(b) shows the complex optical flow field generated as the box undergoes both rigid and nonrigid motion. The general approach taken in this paper is to decompose such complex motions into a set of simpler orthogonal modal deformations. This is accomplished by using (22) to "explain" the complex flow field of (b) by use of a set of simpler "modal flow fields" illustrate in Figs. 3(c–f). The modal amplitudes that are required to obtain this "explanation" provides us with an estimate of the object's new 3-D shape, shown in Fig. 3(g).

More specifically, the estimation process starts by interpolating the 2-D flow vectors to the nearest nodes on the (assumed known) 3-D model of the box. Note that these flow vectors do *not* have to be dense or regularly sampled. Equation (22) is then used to decompose this flow field into a sum of the rigid and nonrigid deformations ("modal flow fields") described by the columns of Φ_P. These columns correspond to the free vibration modes of the box, as determined from its finite element description. In this case, (22) determines that three nonrigid and one rigid-body motion have occurred; the nonrigid motions are the pinching-, tapering-, and bending-like motions shown in Figs. 3(c), 3(d), and 3(e), and the rigid-body motion is the rotation shown in Fig. 3(f).

[4] Note that when there are many more optical flow vectors than degrees of freedom in the finite element model, the interpolation functions H act as filters to bandlimit the sensor data, thus reducing aliasing.

[5] Note that this is different than the normal "n views of m points" result in that we are assuming that the initial object geometry is known. Note also the restriction to small inter-frame rotations and deformations.

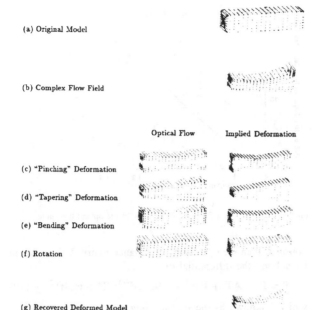

(a) Original Model

(b) Complex Flow Field

Optical Flow   Implied Deformation

(c) "Pinching" Deformation

(d) "Tapering" Deformation

(e) "Bending" Deformation

(f) Rotation

(g) Recovered Deformed Model

Fig. 3. All motions, including complex nonrigid motions, can be decomposed into the linear sum of a set of orthogonal basis motions. In our algorithm we use the free vibration modes of the object as the basis set. In this example, a complex flow field is decomposed into the sum of three nonrigid motions and a rigid-body rotation.

The combination of these motions, when applied to the original box shape, produces an estimate of object's new shape which is shown in Fig. 3(g). The result of this decomposition process, therefore, allows us to track, predict, and describe the global 3-D rigid and nonrigid motion using only sparse 2-D estimates of optical flow.

B. A Statistical Evaluation

To evaluate the stability and accuracy of the decomposition and estimation process, an experiment was conducted in which randomly selected forces were applied to an elastic spherical body to produce simulated rigid-body and nonrigid motions. A typical example is shown in Fig. 4. The resulting 2-D optical flow field was then observed, and the rigid and nonrigid motions estimated by use of (22). To make the experiment more realistic, various amounts of uniformly distributed noise was added to the optical flow field before (22) was applied. Each noise condition was repeated with 100 different randomly selected forces and consequent motions. The mean accuracy of the estimation process was then measured.

Fig. 5 shows the accuracy of the decomposition and estimation process. The signal-to-noise ratio (SNR) for the motion estimates were calculated by

$$dB = 10 * \log_{10} \left(\frac{\sum \left\| \tilde{U} \right\|^2}{\sum \left\| \hat{\tilde{U}} - \tilde{U} \right\|^2} \right) \qquad (23)$$

where $\hat{\tilde{U}}$ is the estimated motion, $\tilde{U}$ the true motion, and the sums are taken over the 100 experimental trials. This statistic

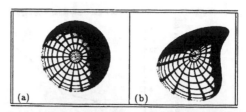

Fig. 4. Random forces were applied to an elastic spherical body in order to evaluate the accuracy of the kinematic solution. (a) Shape at frame zero. (b) Shape at frame one, after a randomly selected force was applied.

compares the variance (squared magnitude) of the estimation errors to the variance of the true motion.

The SNR of the optical flow field was calculated by

$$dB = 10 * \log_{10} \left(\frac{\sum \| V_P \|^2}{\sum \| \hat{V}_P - V_P \|^2} \right) \qquad (24)$$

where $\hat{V}_P$ is the noise-corrupted 2-D flow field, V_P the true 2-D flow field, and the sums are taken over the 100 experimental trials. This statistic compares the variance of the flow field noise to the variance of the true flow field.

In this experiment, both rigid and nonrigid motions were estimated simultaneously. Fig. 5(a) shows the accuracy at estimating rigid-body components of motion as a function of the signal-to-noise ration (SNR) of the optical field (i.e., only the first six elements of U, which are the rigid-body modes, were used to compute the SNR). It can be seen that the accuracy of estimation is linearly related to the SNR of the flow field. The most noisy conditions shown here (approximately 5 dB SNR) corresponds to approximately 56% added noise.

Fig. 5(b) shows the accuracy at estimating nonrigid components of motions as a function of the signal-to-noise ratio (SNR) of the optical flow field (i.e., elements 7 through 30 of U, which are the nonrigid motion modes, were used to compute the SNR). Again, it can be seen that the accuracy of estimation is linearly related to the SNR of the flow field up to at least 50% noise.

The major factor that permits the stability and noise-resistance shown here is the fact that data is integrated over the entire body rather than only over a small patch. It should be noted, however, that because Φ linearizes object rotation and deformation it is important that interimage rotations and deformations remain small. For larger rotations and deformations we have found that it is necessary to use an iterative estimation scheme.

V. Dynamic Estimation of Rigid and Non-Rigid Motion

In the previous sections we have addressed kinetmatic estimation, where velocity at only one instant is considered. For time sequences, however, it is necessary to also consider the *dynamic* properties of the body and of the data measurements. The Kalman filter [9], [10] is the standard technique for obtaining estimates of the state vectors of dynamic models, and for predicting the state vectors at some later time. Outputs

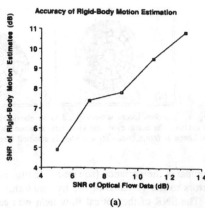

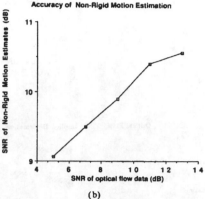

Fig. 5. (a) Rigid-body motion estimation error. (b) Nonrigid motion estimation error, both as a function of the SNR of the optical flow field.

from the Kalman filter are the optimal (weighted) least-squares estimate for non-Gaussian noises [1], [7].

The first use of Kalman filtering for motion estimation was by Brodia and Chellappa [4], who presented a careful evaluation of the approach. Work by Faugeras, Ayache, and their collegues, and more recently many others, has thoroughly developed the subject [6], [2]. In this section, we will develop a Kalman filter that estimates position and velocity for the finite element modal parameters. We will then show that this particular type of Kalman filter is mathematically equivalent to time integration of the FEM governing equation for appropriate choices of mass $\mathbf{M}$ and stiffness $\mathbf{K}$. That is, the Kalman filter may be viewed as a simulation of the model's behavior, with the observed optical flow acting as guiding "forces."

A. The Kalman Filter

Let us define a dynamic process

$$\dot{\mathbf{X}} = \mathbf{AX} + \mathbf{B}a \qquad (25)$$

and observations

$$\mathbf{Y} = \mathbf{CX} + n \qquad (26)$$

where a and n are white noise processes having known spectral density matrices. Then the *optimum observer* [9], [10] is given by the following *Kalman filter*

$$\dot{\hat{\mathbf{X}}} = \mathbf{A}\hat{\mathbf{X}} + \hat{\mathbf{K}}_f\left(\mathbf{Y} - \mathbf{C}\hat{\mathbf{X}}\right) \qquad (27)$$

provided that the Kalman gain matrix $\hat{\mathbf{K}}_f$ is chosen correctly.

1) The Kalman Gain Factor: The gain matrix $\hat{\mathbf{K}}_f$ in (27) minimizes the covariance matrix $\mathbf{P}$ of the error $e = \mathbf{X} - \hat{\mathbf{X}}$. Assuming that the cross variance between the system excitation noise a and the observation noise n is zero, then

$$\hat{\mathbf{K}}_f = \mathbf{PC}^T\mathcal{N}^{-1} \qquad (28)$$

where the observation noise spectral density matrix $\mathcal{N}$ must be nonsingular [7]. Assuming that the noise characteristics are

constant, then the optimizing covariance matrix $\mathbf{P}$ is obtained by solving the differential of $\mathbf{P}$

$$0 = \dot{\mathbf{P}} = \mathbf{AP} + \mathbf{PA}^T - \mathbf{PC}^T\mathcal{N}^{-1}\mathbf{CP} + \mathbf{B}\mathcal{A}\mathbf{B}^T \qquad (29)$$

which is known as the *Riccati equation*.

2) Estimation of Displacement and Velocity: In the current application, we are primarily interested in estimation of the modal amplitudes $\tilde{\mathbf{U}}$ and their velocities $\tilde{\mathbf{V}} = \dot{\tilde{\mathbf{U}}}$. $\hat{\mathbf{U}}$ and $\tilde{\mathbf{V}}$ are therefore the state variables of our dynamic system, and the governing equations are

$$\dot{\tilde{\mathbf{U}}} = \tilde{\mathbf{V}}$$
$$\dot{\tilde{\mathbf{V}}} = a \qquad (30)$$

where a is a vector of externally applied nodal accelerations, which will be considered to be noise. The observed variable will be $\mathbf{M} \times 1$ vector of the 2-D nodal velocities $\mathbf{V}_P$, and from (21) we have that

$$\mathbf{V}_P^t = \frac{\Phi_P}{\Delta t}\dot{\mathbf{U}}^t + n \qquad (31)$$

where n is a vector giving the observation noise. In this analysis, the object's resting state is reset at each time step so that $\hat{\mathbf{U}}^{t-1} = 0$. This coordinate transform allows traking across large rotations and deformations.

It is important to note that both rotational and nonrigid dynamics are inherently nonlinear. The finite element formulation, however, linearizes this behavior so that small times steps and small nodal displacements are required to obtain an accurate simulation using the FEM. Because we are employing the FEM's linearization of dynamic behavior for motion estimation, our formulation will be an *extended* Kalman filter. The behavior of such an extended Kalman filter is difficult to analyze mathematically, and so properties such as convergence and unbiased estimation must be evaluated experimentally or numerically. Such an evaluation will be presented in the following section.

In state-space notation, the system of equations is

$$\begin{bmatrix} \dot{\tilde{\mathbf{U}}} \\ \dot{\tilde{\mathbf{V}}} \end{bmatrix} = \begin{bmatrix} \mathbf{0} & \mathbf{I} \\ \mathbf{0} & \mathbf{0} \end{bmatrix} \begin{bmatrix} \tilde{\mathbf{U}} \\ \tilde{\mathbf{V}} \end{bmatrix} + \begin{bmatrix} \mathbf{0} \\ \mathbf{I} \end{bmatrix} a$$

where $\mathbf{I}$ is the $n \times n$ identity matrix.

Comparing with (25) and (26), we obtain

$$\mathbf{A} = \begin{bmatrix} 0 & \mathbf{I} \\ 0 & 0 \end{bmatrix}, \qquad \mathbf{B} = \begin{bmatrix} 0 \\ \mathbf{I} \end{bmatrix}, \qquad \mathbf{C}^T = \begin{bmatrix} \Phi_P/\Delta t \\ 0 \end{bmatrix}. \quad (32)$$

The Kalman filter is therefore

$$\begin{bmatrix} \dot{\tilde{U}} \\ \dot{\tilde{V}} \end{bmatrix} = \begin{bmatrix} 0 & \mathbf{I} \\ 0 & 0 \end{bmatrix} \begin{bmatrix} \tilde{U} \\ \tilde{V} \end{bmatrix} + \begin{bmatrix} \hat{K}_{f,1} \\ \hat{K}_{f,2} \end{bmatrix} \left(V_P - [\Phi_P/\Delta t \quad 0] \begin{bmatrix} \tilde{U} \\ \tilde{V} \end{bmatrix} \right) \quad (33)$$

where $\hat{K}_{f,1}$ and $\hat{K}_{f,2}$ are the Kalman gain matrices for velocity and acceleration, respectively. By collapsing terms, (33) become

$$\begin{bmatrix} \dot{\tilde{U}} \\ \ddot{\tilde{U}} \end{bmatrix} = \begin{bmatrix} \dot{\tilde{U}} + \hat{K}_{f,1}\left(V_P - \Phi_P\tilde{U}/\Delta t\right) \\ \hat{K}_{f,2}\left(V_P - \Phi_P\tilde{U}/\Delta t\right) \end{bmatrix}. \quad (34)$$

We may solve for the Kalman gain matrices by first using (28) to obtain

$$\begin{bmatrix} \hat{K}_{f,1} \\ \hat{K}_{f,2} \end{bmatrix} = \begin{bmatrix} P_{11} & P_{12} \\ P_{12} & P_{22} \end{bmatrix} \begin{bmatrix} \Phi_P/\Delta t \\ 0 \end{bmatrix} \mathcal{N}^{-1}$$

$$= \begin{bmatrix} P_{11}\Phi_P\mathcal{N}^{-1}/\Delta t \\ P_{12}\Phi_P\mathcal{N}^{-1}/\Delta t \end{bmatrix} \quad (35)$$

where the P_{ij} are $m \times m$ blocks of the error covariance matrix $\mathbf{P}$, and $\mathcal{N}$ is the $m \times m$ spectral density matrix of the observation noise n.

We will assume that n and a originate from independent noise. We have determined experimentally that it is reasonable to choose $\mathcal{N} = n^2\Phi_P^T\Phi_P/\Delta t^2$, i.e., that the error in estimating each mode value is independent and of equal variance. Using this spectral density matrix, the optimum covariance matrix $\mathbf{P}$ can be found by solving (29) for the $P_{i,j}$, which yields

$$\begin{bmatrix} 0 & 0 \\ 0 & 0 \end{bmatrix} = \begin{bmatrix} 2P_{12} - n^{-2}P_{11}^2 & P_{22} - n^{-2}P_{11}P_{12} \\ P_{22} - n^{-2} - P_{12}P_{11} & a^2\mathbf{I} - n^{-2}P_{12}^2 \end{bmatrix}. \quad (36)$$

Similarly, assuming that a is independent for each mode, then its spectral density matrix is $\mathcal{A} = a^2\mathbf{I}$ and thus

$$P_{11} = \left(2an^3\right)^{1/2}\mathbf{I}$$
$$P_{12} = an\mathbf{I}$$
$$P_{22} = \left(2a^3n\right)^{1/2}\mathbf{I}. \quad (37)$$

Finally, from (28), we can determine the Kalman gain matrices

$$\begin{bmatrix} \hat{K}_{f,1} \\ \hat{K}_{f,2} \end{bmatrix} = \begin{bmatrix} \left(\frac{2a}{n}\right)^{1/2}\Phi_P^{-1}\Delta t \\ \left(\frac{a}{n}\right)\Phi_P^{-1}\Delta t \end{bmatrix}. \quad (38)$$

Substituting this result into (34), we obtain

$$\begin{bmatrix} \dot{\tilde{U}} \\ \ddot{\tilde{U}} \end{bmatrix} = \begin{bmatrix} \dot{\tilde{U}} + \left(\frac{2a}{n}\right)^{1/2}\Phi_P^{-1}\Delta t\left(V_P - \Phi_P/\Delta t\tilde{U}\right) \\ \left(\frac{a}{n}\right)\Phi_P^{-1}\Delta t\left(V_P - \Phi_P/\Delta t\tilde{U}\right) \end{bmatrix}. \quad (39)$$

Letting $\tilde{V}_P = \Phi_P^{-1}V_P$, we obtain in the modal coordinate system

$$\begin{bmatrix} \dot{\tilde{U}} \\ \ddot{\tilde{U}} \end{bmatrix} = \begin{bmatrix} \dot{\tilde{U}} + \left(\frac{2a}{n}\right)^{1/2}\left(\tilde{V}_P\Delta t - \tilde{U}\right) \\ \left(\frac{a}{n}\right)\left(\tilde{V}_P\Delta t - \tilde{U}\right) \end{bmatrix}. \quad (40)$$

Each mode is independent within this system of equations, and so we may write the Kalman filter for each of the separate modes

$$\begin{bmatrix} \dot{\tilde{u}}_i \\ \ddot{\tilde{u}}_i \end{bmatrix} = \begin{bmatrix} \dot{\tilde{u}}_i + \left(\frac{2a}{n}\right)^{1/2}(\tilde{v}_i\Delta t - \tilde{u}_i) \\ \left(\frac{a}{n}\right)(\tilde{v}_i\Delta t - \tilde{u}_i) \end{bmatrix} \quad (41)$$

where $\tilde{v}_i$ is the ith element of $\tilde{V}_P$.

Having determined the optimal observer equations for mode amplitude and velocity, we can now formulate the displacement prediction at time $t + 1$. For mode i, this is

$$\tilde{u}_i^{t+1} = \tilde{u}_i^t + d_1\dot{\tilde{u}}_i^t + d_2\left(\tilde{r}_i^t - \tilde{u}_i^t\right) \quad (42)$$

which is exactly the central-difference update rule for direct time integration of the finite element governing equations, with "loads" $\tilde{r}_i^t = \tilde{v}_i^t\Delta t$, $d_1 = \Delta t$ and $d_2 = 2\Delta t^2/\bar{m}_i = (a/n)\Delta t^2 + (2a/n)^{1/2}\Delta t$.

The equivalence between these Kalman filter equations and time-integration of a finite-element governing equation provides an intuitive interpretation of the Kalman filter. In essence, it is smoothing the optical flow data over space by modeling it using the low-frequency whole-body mode shapes and smoothing over time by use of a mass matrix $\mathbf{M}$

$$\mathbf{M} = \frac{2\Delta t}{(a/n)\Delta t + (2a/n)^{1/2}}\mathbf{I}. \quad (43)$$

The effect of the mass matrix is to integrate information across time, thus providing a more accurate estimate than is possible from a single measurement of velocity. When the observation noise is large relative to the acceleration or excitation noise, the solution becomes similar to simple-time averaging. When the acceleration noise is large relative to the observation noise, the solution becomes similar to the single-measurement case.

VI. An Example Using Synthetic Data

In the kinematic case, our major concern was the behavior of the estimator with increasing levels of noise. In the dynamic case, our principal concern is the convergence and possible bias of the Kalman filter. There is reason for such concern, as both rotational dynamics and nonrigid dynamics are nonlinear problems that are linearized by the FEM. As a consequence, the Kalman filter developed here may be more properly considered an *extended* Kalman filter and despite the well-known stability and accuracy of the FEM, there is no proof

133

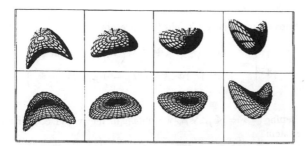

Fig. 6. Using the Kalman filter to track rigid and nonrigid motion. Top row: Input image sequence. Bottom row: estimated position and shape.

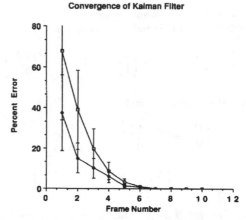

Fig. 7. Estimation error as a function of frame number, for two ratios of acceleration noise to optical flow field noise. Optical flow SNR is 10 dB.

of convergence and bias-free behavior. We therefore have evaluated the stability and accuracy of our formulation using synthetic data.

A. An Illustrative Example

Fig. 6 shows an example of tracking both rigid and nonrigid motion. The top row of Fig. 6 shows four frames from a 30 frame image sequence of a rotating, translating, and deforming solid. In this example, the initial position, shape, and (linearized) velocity of the object was assumed known. Exact optical flow data from this sequence was corrupted by uniform noise to produce a 16 dB SNR (approximately 15% noise). This noisy optical flow was used as input to the Kalman filter of (42), thus producing estimates of position, shape, and motion. The interframe time step was 0.1 s, and the parameters of the Kalman noise model were $(a/n) = 0.3$ (large accelerations are assumed to be relatively rare).

The bottom row of Fig. 6 shows the resulting estimates of shape and motion. In this example, the rigid-body modes were tracked with an error of 29.1 dB SNR (approximately 3.5% error). The error in both rigid-body and nonrigid modes was 18.5 dB SNR (approximately 11.9% error). The fact that object motion could be tracked with much less error than was present in the optical flow is attributable to the integration of information across the whole body and across time.

The major source of error in the nonrigid modes was introduced by a single ill-conditioned mode, i.e., a mode for which even large deformations cause only small 2-D motions. In Fig. 6, for instance, even though the amount of bending perpendicular to the image plane is almost 5% in error the tracking object appears nearly identical to the original object. Such ill-conditioned modes can be detected by examination of the columns of Φ, although this was not done in this experiment.

B. A Statistical Evaluation

The previous examples have shown that our formulation can produce accurate estimates of motion, but they do not allow evaluation of either convergence or stability. To evaluate these properties, we followed the methodology of Brodia and Chellappa [4], and constructed an experiment in which there were large errors in the initial velocity estimates. This condition is equivalent to the case in which a very large acceleration "spike" produces a large interframe change in

system velocities. Following this acceleration spike, the behavior of the Kalman filter over successive frames was observed to determine whether or not the Kalman estimates would converge rapidly to the correct value.

In our this experiment noisy motion estimates for 100 image sequences were used as input to (42). The motion estimate noise level averaged 20 dB (i.e., the noise magnitude was 10% of the flow vector magnitude). The mean velocity for each mode (including rigid-body modes) was approximately 5 cm/s. The interframe time interval was 0.25 s. In each trial the initial estimate of each mode's velocity was zero so that the mean initial error was 5 cm/s for each mode. This condition is equivalent to applying an acceleration of 20 cm/s^2 to a resting system between the 0th and 1st frames of the image sequence.

The Kalman filter's output was then observed over the next twelve image frames, as shown in Fig. 7. In this figure percent error was measured as

$$\text{Percent Error} = 100 * \left(\frac{\sum \|\hat{\mathbf{U}} - \tilde{\mathbf{U}}\|}{\sum \|\tilde{\mathbf{U}}\|} \right) \quad (44)$$

where $\hat{\mathbf{U}}$ is the estimated motion, $\tilde{\mathbf{U}}$ the true motion, and the sums are taken over the 100 experimental trials.

The experiment was repeated with two separate measurement/acceleration noise models, one with $a/n = 2$ (large accelerations are common) and one with $a/n = 0.5$ (large accelerations are uncommon). The upper curve in Fig. 7 shows the estimates convergence with the $a/n = 0.5$ model, the lower curve shows convergence with $a/n = 2.0$. The error bars show the standard deviation of the 100 separate estimates at each frame number. Note that although the mean error goes very nearly to zero, in individual trials the errors were in the range of ±1%.

As can be seen from Fig. 7, stable and accurate convergence was achieved in both cases. All modes, including rigid-body modes, behaved in a very similar manner. When the noise model was more appropriate to the large initial acceleration (the case where $a/n = 2.0$) convergence to approximately

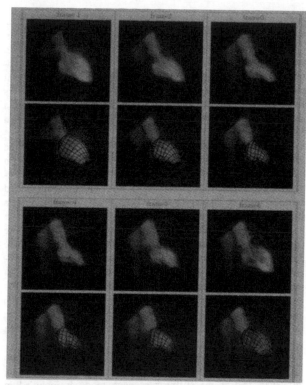

Fig. 8. Recovery of the rigid and nonrigid motion of a 3-D model of human heart ventricle; time proceeds from top left to bottom right.

10% error was achieved by frame 3. When the noise model was less appropriate (the case where $a/n = 0.5$) convergence to 10% error required 4 frames. In both cases, and for all modes, convergence was both stable and unbiased.

As in the kinematic estimation case, the major factor that permits the stability and noise-resistance shown here is the fact that data is integrated over the entire body rather than only over a small patch. As with the kinematic case, it must be noted that because Φ linearizes object motion, it is important that interimage rotations and deformations remain small.

VII. EXAMPLES USING REAL DATA

Fig. 8 shows an example of recovering nonrigid motion from optical flow data and (42). The upper image in each box shows six successive frames of transmission X-ray data, from which the rigid and nonrigid motions of the heart ventricle were estimated. Time increases from top left to bottom right; total elapsed time is approximately one second. Optical flow was computed by use of a block-wise version of the Horn–Shunck optical flow algorithm.

The 3-D shape and motion of the heart ventricle was tracked over time using this optical flow data. The computation started with an initial 3-D model of the ventricle, shown in wireframe at the top left of Fig. 8 (the bottom image in frame 1). The initial shape can be computed as described in Pentland and Sclaroff [20]. Equation (42) was used to estimate the 3-D rigid and nonrigid motion of the ventricle at each time step. The resulting rigid and nonrigid motions are shown

by the wireframe illustrations at the bottom of each frame, overlayed on the original X-ray imagery. Execution time was approximately one second per frame on a standard Sun 4/330.

It can be seen that the 3-D shape of the ventricle model is quite similar to the shape seen in the original imagery. The major defect appears near the top of the wireframe model in frames 3 and 4. Close examination showed that the tracking process became confused in this area because of the large deformations occurring between frames 2 and 3; as a consequence, the top edge of the model became "stuck" on edges in the surrounding volume.

Note that the estimated ventricle, shape is very nearly the same in the first and last frames, even though there was no constraint maintaining the position, rotation, or volume of the model during the estimation process. The fact that the 3-D model returned to its original shape, position, and volume at the point at which the real ventricle returned to its original shape and position is evidence of the stability of the Kalman filter solution.

A. Constrained Motion

In many cases the observed motion is known to be constrained, for example, by gravity or by a hinge or other attachment. Such constrained motion adds a *bias* or *control* term to (25), but as long as it varies sufficiently slow with respect to the Kalman filter's sampling rate, it does not otherwise affect the convergence or stability of the estimator [1], [7]. We may therefore hope to use the Kalman filter of (42) to track the rigid and nonrigid behavior of *constrained* objects as well as freely moving objects.

In the ThingWorld modeling and simulation system [13], [12], [15], [14], which provides the software base for the work described here, both gravity and spring-like constraints may be used to affect object behavior. To attach two objects to each other, for instance, a spring constraint is placed between a point on each object's surface, and this constraint exerts equal and opposite attractive forces on the two points of attachment. In the Kalman state equations such forces appear as a constant or slow varying acceleration bias, i.e., (30) becomes

$$\dot{\mathbf{U}} = \tilde{\mathbf{V}}$$
$$\dot{\mathbf{V}} = \mathbf{R}^c + a \qquad (45)$$

where $\mathbf{R}^c$ is a vector describing the load exerted on each nodal point by all active constraints (see [14] for additional details). The spring force is proportional to the square of the distance between the two constrained points.

Given *a priori* knowledge of such a motion constraint, we can compensate for the contribution of that constraint to the state equations and then estimate motion as previously. The simplest way to accomplish this is to modify (42) to account for this new term

$$\tilde{u}_i^{t+1} = \tilde{u}_i^t + d_1 \dot{\tilde{u}}_i^t + d_2 \left(\tilde{r}_i^t - \tilde{u}_i^t \right) + 2\Delta t^2 \tilde{r}_i^c / \tilde{m}_i \qquad (46)$$

where $\tilde{m}_i = \rho \sum_j |\phi_{i,j}|$ is an estimate of the ith mode's generalized mass, parameterized by ρ, an estimate of the object's density.

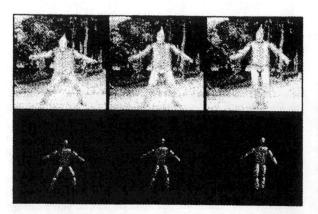

Fig. 9. Three frames from an image sequence showing tracking of a jumping man using an articulated, physically based model. Despite poor quality optical flow (due to pronounced highlights on thighs and other parts of the body) the overall tracking is reasonably accurate. This accuracy is in part due to the presence of articulation constraints between the various parts of the model.

Fig. 9 illustrates a relatively complex example of tracking an object in which motion is *a priori* known to be constrained to certain part junctions (joints). This figure shows three frames from a twelve image sequence of a well-known tin woodsman caught in the act of jumping. Despite the limited range of motion, this example is a difficult one because of the poor quality optical flow, due to pronounced highlights on thighs and other parts of the body.

In this example, an articulated 3-D model was constructed by hand, with the spring-like constraints described previously inserted between the various body parts. In this manner, the combined behavior of the various parts were constrained to be consistent with the articulation of the human body.

Optical flow estimates were than calculated by use of a block-wise Horn–Schunk algorithm, and (46) was used to estimate the constrained rigid-body motions of the various parts. In this case, only the six rigid body modes were employed because of the large amount of noise in the optical flow data. The estimates of constrained motion for this sequence are illustrated by the bottom row of Fig. 9.

As can be seen by comparing the 3-D motion of the model with that in the original image, the resulting tracking is reasonably accurate. To a substantial extent this accuracy is attributable to the articulation constraints, as without them errors due to moving surface highlights would have caused the "thigh" parts to fly off in wildly incorrect directions. The interpart connectivity enforced by these constraints allowed the stable motion estimates for the body and lower legs to counterbalance these erroneous motion estimates.

VIII. Conclusions

We have introduced a physically correct model of elastic nonrigid motion. This model is based on the finite element method, but decouples the degrees of freedom by breaking down object motion into rigid and nonrigid *vibration* or *deformation modes*. Because of the intrinsic elastic properties of real materials, it can be shown that the high-frequency modes in this representation rarely have significant amplitude, so that they may be discarded without introducing undue error.

The result is an accurate representation for both rigid and nonrigid motion that has greatly reduced dimensionality, capturing the intuition that nonrigid motion is normally coherent and not chaotic. Because of the small number of parameters involved, we have been able to use this representation to obtain accurate overconstrained estimates of both rigid and nonrigid global motion.

We have also shown that these estimates can be integrated over time by use of an extended Kalman filter, resulting in stable and accurate estimates of both 3-D shape and 3-D velocity. The formulation was then extended to include constrained nonrigid motion. Examples of tracking single nonrigid objects and multiple constrained objects were presented.

An inevitable limitation of our technique stems from the fact that certain rigid-body and nonrigid motions cannot be observed under orthographic projection. The inability to observe motions such as translation in z, shear along the z-axis, etc., means that errors in estimation of these motions are unavoidable. Further, the situation is exacerbated when observing extremely simple objects, such as planes or rods, as in these cases there is not enough data to distinguish between various of the modal deformations.

For instance, when observing a rod, rigid-body rotation cannot be distinguished from lengthwise contraction. Note, however, that if the stiffness of each mode is included in the calculation (by scaling each column of Φ proportional to the corresponding eigenvalue) then most of the observed 2-D motions will be accounted for by low-frequency modes such as rotation, and relatively little allocated to higher frequency modes such as nonrigid contraction. The preferential allocation of observed 2-D motion to the lower frequency modes (including the rigid-body modes) is similar to human observers' well-known bias toward the simplest motion interpretation.

Another limitation of our current technique stems from the use of optical flow, rather than feature points, as the input data. The use of optical flow data requires us to integrate object motion over time in order to determine the object's current position and shape; there is no way to "anchor" our estimates of position and shape to our current observations. As a result small biases in estimating rotation, etc., can grow over time and eventually destroy our ability to accurately track the object. We are therefore working on integrating feature point information into our motion and shape estimates so that we no longer have to rely completely on time integration to determine the object's current state.

Appendix
Programming Shortcuts

When presented with this approach, some researchers have expressed concern over the expense of calculating the mass and stiffness matrices $\mathbf{M}$ and $\mathbf{K}$, as well as the cost of calculating their low-order eigenvectors Φ. However, efficient FEM codes for producing $\mathbf{K}$ have been commercially available for over twenty years, and many are in the public domain. Similarly, given a stiffness matrix $\mathbf{K}$, the low-frequency eigenvectors can then be efficiently obtained (in ascending order) via the power method. Moreover, all of these calculations will typically be performed off-line as a precomputation step.

However, for many vision (and some graphics) applications even this level of effort is sometimes unnecessary. This is because 1) it is often unnecessary to have detailed estimates of the material properties, as these are either unknown or unimportant, and 2) the low-frequency eigenvectors are determined by the low-order moments of inertia, so that compact bodies of similar size have similar eigenvectors. Thus, for vision applications with relatively noise-free data, it appears that it is sufficient to use a single, extremely elastic FEM model of the base shape (in our case an ellipsoid) that is to be fit to sensor data.

The following sections explain how these two facts can be utilized to efficiently obtain rough-and-ready approximations to the Φ, $\widetilde{M}$, and $\widetilde{K}$ matrices for arbitrary samplings of an object's surface.

A. Calculating a Polynomial Characterization of the Modes

The modes of an object can be characterized by 3-D polynomial functions whose coefficients are determined by a linear regression of polynomials with m terms in appropriate powers of x, y, and z, against the n triples of x, y, and z that compose ϕ_{i*}, a $3n \times 1$ vector containing the elements of Φ

$$\alpha = \left(\beta^T \beta\right)^{-1} \beta^T \phi_{i*} \quad (47)$$

where α is an $m \times 1$ matrix of the coefficients of the desired deformation polynomial, β is an $3n \times m$ matrix whose first column contains the object-centered coordinates of the nodes $(x_1, y_1, z_1, x_2, y_2, z_2, \cdots, x_n, y_n, z_n)^T$, and whose remaining columns consist of the modified versions of the nodal coordinates where the x, y, and/or z components have been raised to various powers. See [13] for more details.

By linearly superimposing the various deformation mappings, one can obtain an accurate accounting of the object's nonrigid deformation. In the thing world modeling system [13], [14], the set of polynomial deformations is combined into a 3 by 3 matrix of polynomials, D that is referred to as the *modal deformation matrix*. This matrix transforms predeformation point positions $\mathbf{X} = (x, y, z)^T$ into the deformed positions

$$\mathbf{X}^* = \begin{pmatrix} d_{00} & d_{01} & d_{02} \\ d_{10} & d_{11} & d_{12} \\ d_{10} & d_{21} & d_{22} \end{pmatrix} \mathbf{X}. \quad (48)$$

A simple version of $\mathbf{D}$ that is derived from a 20 node element is given by the following:

$d_{00} = \tilde{u}_7 + y\tilde{u}_{13} + z\tilde{u}_{16} - (\tilde{u}_{14} + \tilde{u}_{17})\,\text{sgn}(x) - \tilde{u}_{15} - \tilde{u}_{18},$

$d_{01} = \tilde{u}_{12} + 2y(\tilde{u}_{14} + \text{sgn}(x)\tilde{u}_{15}),$

$d_{02} = \tilde{u}_{11} + 2z(\tilde{u}_{17} + \text{sgn}(x)\tilde{u}_{18}),$

$d_{10} = \tilde{u}_{12} + 2x(\tilde{u}_{20} + \text{sgn}(y)\tilde{u}_{21}),$

$d_{11} = \tilde{u}_8 + x\tilde{u}_{19} + z\tilde{u}_{22} - (\tilde{u}_{20} + \tilde{u}_{23})\,\text{sgn}(y) - \tilde{u}_{21} - \tilde{u}_{24},$

$d_{12} = \tilde{u}_{10} + 2z(\tilde{u}_{23} + \text{sgn}(y)\tilde{u}_{24}),$

$d_{20} = \tilde{u}_{11} + 2x(\tilde{u}_{26} + \text{sgn}(z)\tilde{u}_{27}),$

$d_{21} = \tilde{u}_{10} + 2y(\tilde{u}_{29} + \text{sgn}(z)\tilde{u}_{30}),$

$d_{22} = \tilde{u}_9 + x\tilde{u}_{25} + y\tilde{u}_{28} - (\tilde{u}_{26} + \tilde{u}_{29})\,\text{sgn}(z) - \tilde{u}_{27} - \tilde{u}_{30}.$

$$(49)$$

We have found that this characterization of mode shapes provides a reasonable description of the behavior of the ellipsoids used in our fitting process.

The modal amplitudes $\tilde{u}_i$ have intuitive meanings: $\tilde{u}_1 - \tilde{u}_6$ are the rigid body modes (translation and rotation), $\tilde{u}_7 - \tilde{u}_9$ are the x, y, and z radius, $\tilde{u}_{10} - \tilde{u}_{12}$ are shears about the x, y, and z axes, and $\tilde{u}_{13+3j} - \tilde{u}_{13+3j+2}$ may be described as tapering, bending, and pinching around the jth pairwise combination of the x, y, and z axes. Note that because the rigid body modes are calculated in the object's coordinate system, they must be rotated to global coordinates before being integrated with the remainder of any dynamical simulation.

B. Approximate Calculation of Φ, $\widetilde{M}$, and $\widetilde{K}$

We can make use of the aforementioned mode characterization to numerically approximate the matrix Φ for any point sampling of the surface. In essence, we are precalculating how energy in each of the various modes displaces of a set of points on the surface. We then store this mode-displacement relationship into the Φ matrix, thus approximating how these points distribute load to the original nodal points and the various vibration modes.

This numerical approximation is accomplished by noting that ϕ_{i*} (the ith column of Φ) describes how the n nodal points $\mathbf{X}^w = \left(x_j^w, y_j^w, z_j^w\right)^T$ change with u_i, the ith mode's amplitude

$$\phi_{i*} = \left(\frac{\partial x_1^w}{\partial u_i}, \frac{\partial y_1^w}{\partial u_i}, \frac{\partial z_1^w}{\partial u_1}, \cdots, \frac{\partial x_n^w}{\partial u_i}, \frac{\partial y_n^w}{\partial u_i}, \frac{\partial z_n^w}{\partial u_i}\right)^T. \quad (50)$$

Thus, by applying small amounts of each deformation $\tilde{u}_i$ and measuring the resulting change in the coordinates of each surface points as it is passed through (71), we obtain finite difference approximations to the $(j+1, i)$, $(j+2, i)$ and $(j+3, i)$ entries of Φ for any sampling of surface points.

We can use this method to efficiently obtain a sampling of the surface that matches the projection of the sensor data onto the surface, thus considerably simplifying the fitting process. Even when iterating the solution to find better virtual spring attachment points, the distances between nodes and projected data positions will be small, and so simple bilinear interpolation can be used to distribute the data forces to the surrounding three surface points without incurring significant error.

Given a Φ with nodes evenly sampled throughout the body, we can use the common assumption that the object's mass is distributed equally among the sampled points to obtain

$$\widetilde{M} = \Phi^T M \Phi = \Phi^T m I \Phi \quad (51)$$

where m is the mass assigned to each sample point. The modal stiffnesses $\tilde{k}_i$ are more difficult to estimate; however, given that detailed material properties are unimportant, one may simply assign a stiffness proportional to $\tilde{m}_i$ for the nonrigid modes $\tilde{u}_i$, and a stiffness of 0.0 for the rigid-body modes $\tilde{k}_i$, $1 \leq i \leq 6$.

C. Efficiency Considerations for Motion Estimation

When an object rotates the intrinsic (object-centered) and global coordinate systems are no longer identical. Because Φ is calculated in the intrinsic coordinate system, (22) must be generalized to allow rotations. This is accomplished by rotating the (x, y, z) triplets in the columns of Φ from the object coordinate system to the global coordinate system by use of the object's current (estimated) rotation matrix R:

$$\left(\phi^*_{i,3*j}, \phi^*_{i,3*j+1}, \phi^*_{i,3*j+2}\right)^T =$$
$$R^{-1}(\phi_{i,3*j}, \phi_{i,3*j+1}, \phi_{i,3*j+2})^T \quad (52)$$

for $i = 1, 2, 3, \cdots, 3n$ and $j = 1, 2, 3, \cdots, n$, and then applying (22). This rotation also makes the problem of detecting modes that do not affect the optical flow field easier, because the corresponding column of Φ will contain no x and y components.

D. Surface Detail Description

In the ThingWorld system [13], [14], the low-order modal representation is augmented by a surface mesh description of the surface's detailed structure, in order to obtain a more general shape representation. This spline description can be either a physically based mesh or a simple spline. The basic idea is to replace the implicit function description $f(x, y, z) = d = 1$ with the more general implicit function $f(x, y, z) = d(x, y, z)$. This allows us to capture more detailed structure than is possible with any fixed number of modes without losing the advantages of an implicit function representation. The surface details are normally treated as error residuals relative to the model's dynamic behavior, although they are used in point, ray, or surface intersection calculations.

ACKNOWLEDGMENT

The authors would like to thank I. Essa for his summary of Bathe and Segerlind [5], from which Section II-A was derived.

REFERENCES

[1] M. Aoki, *Optimization of Stochastic Systems: Topics in Discrete-Time Dynamics*, 2nd ed. New York: Academic, 1989.
[2] N. Ayache, O. D. Faugeras, "Maintaining representations of the environment of a mobile robot," *IEEE Trans. Robot. Automation*, vol. 5, no. 6, pp. 804–819, 1989.
[3] K.-J. Bathe, *Finite Element Procedures in Engineering Analysis*. Englewood Cliffs, NJ: Prentice-Hall, 1982.
[4] T. J. Broida and R. Chellappa, "Estimation of object motion parameters from noisy images," *IEEE Trans. Patt. Anal. Mach. Intell.*, vol. 8, no. 1, pp. 90–99, Jan. 1986.
[5] I. Essa, "Contact detection, collision forces and friction for physically-based virtual world modeling," M.S. thesis, Dep. Civil Eng., M.I.T., Cambridge, MA, 1990.
[6] O. D. Faugeras, N. Ayache, and B. Faverjon, "Building visual maps by combining noisy stereo measurements," in *Proc. IEEE Conf. Robot. Automation*, San Francisco, CA., Apr. 1986.
[7] B. Friedland, *Control System Design*. New York: McGraw-Hill, 1986.
[8] J. J. Gibson, *The Senses Considered as Perceptual Systems*. New York: Houghton Mifflin, 1966.
[9] R. E. Kalman, "A new approach to linear filtering and prediction problems," *Trans. ASME, J. Basic Eng.*, vol. 82D no. 1, pp. 35–45, 1960.
[10] R. E. Kalman and R. S. Bucy, "New results in linear filtering and prediction theory," *Trans. ASME, J. Basic Eng.*, vol. 83D, no. 1, pp. 95–108, 1961.
[11] P. Werkhoven, A. Toet, and J. J. Koenderink, "Displacement estimates through adaptive affinities," *IEEE Trans. Patt. Anal. Mach. Intell.*, vol. 12, no. 7, pp. 658–662, July 1990.
[12] A. Pentland and J. Williams, "The perception of non-rigid motion: Inference of material properties and force," in *Proc. Int. Joint Conf. Artificial Intell.*, Aug. 1989.
[13] A. P. Pentland and J. R. Williams, "Good vibrations: Modal dynamics for graphics and animation," in *Proc. ACM SIGGRAPH Conf.*, vol. 23, no. 4, pp. 215–222, 1989.
[14] A. Pentland, I. Essa, M. Freidmann, B. Horowitz, and S. Sclaroff, "The thingworld modeling system: Virtual sculpting by modal forces," *Computer Graphics*, vol. 24, no. 2, pp. 143–144, 1990.
[15] A. P. Pentland, "Automatic extraction of part deformable models," *Int. J. Computer Vision*, vol. 4, pp. 107–126, 1990.
[16] L. J. Segerlind, *Applied Finite Element Analysis*. New York: Wiley, 1984.
[17] M. Subbarro. Interpretation of Image Flow: A Spatio-Temporal Approach," *IEEE Trans. Patt. Anal. Mach. Intell.*, vol. 11, no. 3, pp. 266–278, Mar. 1989.
[18] D. Terzopoulos, A. Witkin, and M. Kass, "Symmetry-seeking models for 3-D object reconstruction," *Int. J. Comput. Vision*, vol. 1. no. 3, pp. 211–221, 1987.
[19] S. Ullman, "Maximizing the rigidity: The incremental recovery of 3-D structure from rigid and rubbery motion," *Perception*, vol. 13, pp. 255–274, 1984.
[20] A. Pentland and S. Scarloff, "Closed form solutions to physically based shape modeling and recognition," *IEEE Trans. Patt. Anal. Machine Intell.*, this issue, pp. 715–729.
[21] D. Terzopolous, A. Witkin, and M. Kass, "Constraints on deformable models: Recovering 3–D shape and nonrigid motion," *Artificial Intell.*, vol. 36, no. 1, pp. 91–123, 1988.

Alex Pentland, for a photograph and biography, see this issue, p. 729.

Bradley Horowitz received the BS degree in computer science from the University of Michigan, Ann Arbor, in 1988; he is expected to receive the MS degree from the Massachusetts Institute of Technology, Cambridge, MA, in May 1991, and is currently a PhD candidate and Research Assistant in the Vision and Modeling Group at the M.I.T. Media Laboratory.

At the University of Michigan, he was a member of the Artificial Intelligence Lab, where he worked on autonomous robot navigation. His research interests include computer vision and graphic, and image compression.

SECTION II

Segmentation and Reconstruction

A Review of Biomedical Image Segmentation Techniques

Raj Acharya and Raghu P. Menon
Biomedical Imaging Group (BMIG)
Department of Electrical and Computer Engineering
State University of New York
Buffalo, NY 14260

Abstract

Image segmentation is an important aspect of biomedical image analysis. Grouping a generalized image into units that are homogeneous with respect to one or more characteristic results in a segmented image. Image segmentation can be classified on the basis of methods and application areas. Here we discuss the various methods of image segmentation and classify them on the basis of the approaches adopted and their applications to specific segmentation needs. On the basis of segmentation methods, we classify them into boundary-, region-, and texture-based approaches. We further classify segmentation into low-, medium-, and high-level segmentation methods and discuss a number of methods that come under the above classifications. The discussion is aimed at providing an introduction to the recent techniques in biomedical image segmentation and their applications.

1. Introduction

Image segmentation has its roots in work based on preferences exhibited by human beings in grouping or organizing sets of shapes arranged in a visual field. Grouping preferences could be based on features such as proximity, similarity, and continuity or on figure/ground discrimination. Grouping of segmentation results in the organization of a scene into meaningful units that is a significant step toward image understanding.

Grouping parts of a generalized image into units that are homogeneous with respect to one or more characteristics results in a segmented image. The segmented image extends the generalized image into the beginnings of domain-dependent information. Hence image segmentation is a crucial step in the process of image understanding. In this discussion, we first give a brief review of early, essentially low-level segmentation techniques, then proceed to review some of the recent techniques in biomedical image segmentation.

There have been various methods proposed for image segmentation. These schemes can be conveniently grouped into boundary-based and region-based techniques.

- Boundaries of images are an important part of the hierarchy of structures that link raw image data with their interpretation [1]. The goal of such techniques is to perform a level of segmentation, that is, to make a coherent feature to form many individual local edge elements. Boundary-based schemes proceed in two steps:

  1. Detection of local edges by some type of differentiation.
  2. Grouping of these local edges into boundary contours that separate object voxels from background voxels.

  A number of edge operators have been proposed for this purpose. Zucker [2] proposed an optimal 3-dimensional edge operator, essentially a Sobel operator for this purpose. Liu [3] developed a 3D surface detection algorithm that extends the classical Robert's operator into 3D space. Herman and Liu [4] have further extended this algorithm to 4D. In our discussion we will review a few boundary based techniques, namely deformable models and morphology-based approaches.

- The goal of region–based techniques is to use image characteristics to map individual pixels in an input image to sets of pixels called regions. We review region-based approaches based on neural networks and graph theoretic approaches.

In addition, texture-based segmentation is of importance, especially in detecting information where defects and abnormalities in biomedical structures show up as differences in texture. Fractal-based methods are useful for this.

Biomedical image segmentation methods can also be grouped into the following broad categories.

1. Low-level segmentation
2. Medium-level segmentation
3. High-level segmentation

In our discussion we shall treat the problem of biomedical image segmentation as being classified into these three broad categories and review methods in each. We shall discuss the following *low-level segmentation* techniques.

1. Feature clustering
2. Split and merge techniques

Under *medium-level segmentation* techniques we will review the following.

1. Fuzzy clustering-based image segmentation
2. Segmentation using fractal dimensions
3. Graph theoretic image segmentation
4. Segmentation using deformable models
5. Morphological image segmentation methods
6. Neural network-based image segmentation

Under *high-level segmentation* methods we will discuss the following.

1. Pyramid-based image segmentation
2. Expert system-based image segmentation

2. Low-Level Segmentation

Image segmentation involves the extraction of the desired object from the background. Most of the existing low-level segmentation techniques can be broadly classified into two classes: feature clustering and region-based segmentation. Feature-clustering techniques range from simple pixel classification based on intensity (for example, thresholding) to clustering multidimensional feature vectors. Region-based segmentation techniques are either based on uniformity of regions (region growing and/or splitting) or the discontinuity of neighboring regions (boundary detection).

2.1 Feature Clustering

For each pixel, a number of local properties, such as edge magnitudes, busyness, texture measures and spectral characteristics, are used to form an N-dimensional feature vector V_{xy}. Each class of region is assumed to form a distinct cluster in the N-dimensional feature space and a suitable clustering algorithm, such as K-means clustering,

leader clustering algorithm, or spatial clustering [5], is then used to group points into distinct clusters. These clusters are then remapped to spatial domains to generate the desired regions.

Thresholding is a special case of feature clustering where $N = 1$. In the case of intensity thresholding,

$$s(x, y, z) = I_k \text{ for } t_{k-1} \leq f(x, y, z) \leq t_k, \, k = 0, 1, \ldots M$$

where $f(x, y, z)$ and $s(x, y, z)$ are the input and output image intensities at (x, y, z), respectively, and t_k, $k = 0, 1 \ldots M$ are the threshold values ($t_k > t_{k-1}$). Thresholding can be defined as applying an operator T at (x, y, z) where T is a function of the form

$$T((x, y, x), f_v(x, y, z), f(x, y, z))$$

where f_v is a function over the region v centered around (x, y, z) and $f(x, y, z)$ is the intensity at (x, y, z).

2.2 Split and Merge Techniques

To use this algorithm, the image pixels need to be organized into a pyramidal grid structure of regions. In this grid structure, regions are organized in groups of four [1]. Any region can be split into four subregions and the appropriate four can be merged into a single larger region. The algorithm can be formulated as follows. [1]

1. Pick a grid structure and homogeneity property H. If for a region R in the structure, $H(R)$=false, split into four subregions. If for four regions, $R_{k1}, R_{k2}, \ldots, R_{k4}$, $H(R_{k1} \cup R_{k2} \cup R_{k3} \cup R_{k4}) = true$, merge into single region. When no regions can be merged, stop.
2. If there are neighboring regions R_i and R_j such that $H(R_i \cup R_j) = true$, merge these regions.

3. Medium-Level Segmentation

In this section, we discuss the methods of obtaining scene domain cues from picture domain cues. The important aspects of this stage are (1) recognizing suitable representation schemes for scene domain cues and (2) forming high-level data structures from the segmented image.

The process of forming high-level data structures from the segmented image can be divided into two main classes: forming boundaries (or surfaces in 3D) and forming regions (or solids in 3D). A few of the boundary-based techniques are deformable model-based techniques and morphology-based approaches which we will discuss in the following sections. When the shape of the boundary is not known, available techniques for boundary forming consists of graph-searching algorithms. Also fuzzy-clustering methods are useful where the partitions between clusters in the desired segmented image are not well defined. In graph-searching algorithms, edge elements of the image are represented as a graph and the algorithm tries to find the lowest-cost path between two nodes of the graph using a search algorithm such as A * [6, 7] or F* [8]. We shall review the F* algorithm first in this section as it is used extensively in medium-level segmentation problems. In addition, we shall review a texture based segmentation method, namely fractal-dimension-based image segmentation, as texture-based methods are important where defects show up as differences in texture.

3.1 Boundary Forming with F* Algorithm

As the F* algorithm [9] is used extensively in medium-level segmentation of biomedical images, we shall discuss this algorithm briefly before moving on to other methods of medium-level segmentation.

The F* algorithm principle is the same as that of A* where a minimum-cost path from the starting point (s) to the goal point (g) is iteratively constructed by extending the best partial path available at each iteration. This is done by selecting the point v that has the minimum-cost path from s to g via v where the cost is the sum of the lowest-cost path found so far from s to v and the estimate of a minimum-cost path from v to g. This algorithm requires an order of N^2 operations (for a simple implementation). The F* algorithm finds the optimum path from s to g using a cost array C by iteratively updating a path array P. This array (P) is initialized to infinity except at s, which is set to $C(s)$. The first step in updating consists of adjusting all the elements of the yth row from left to right using the rule,

$$P(x, y) = \mathbf{min} \{P(x - 1, y - 1) + C(x, y), P (x, y - 1) + C(x, y),$$
$$P(x + 1, y - 1) + C(x, y), P(x - 1, y) + C(x, y),$$
$$P(x, y)\}$$

and then adjusting all the elements in the yth row from right to left, using

$$P(x, y) = \mathbf{min} \{P(x + 1, y) + c(x, y), P(x, y)\}$$

Each additional pass involves a bottom-to-top pass followed by a top-to-bottom pass using the above two rules. When all the changes in P are such that the new value is greater than $P(g)$, the algorithm terminates and the optimum path can be found by backtracking from g and moving along the minimum value of P at each neighborhood until s is reached. Since it is shown that the number of iterations required is the number of "row" index rever-

sals along the optimal path, this algorithm performs better than A* in general.

The initial points are found by a crude local maxima detection method where each point which is a local maxima and the difference of maximum and minimum is greater that a given value is selected. Each end point of the resulting curve segments are then used as a starting point. For each starting point s, the best path is found for all candidate points that are r distance from s and within $\pm\theta$ of the current direction. The next point along the path with the least cost out of all candidates is selected as the new starting point and the process is repeated until the accumulated cost exceeds a predetermined value or it finds an existing curve.

Another approach is to find an initial estimate of the boundary using a simple thresholding followed by boundary tracking. An active contour model [9] is then used to refine the initial estimate.

Forming regions from the segmented images can be accomplished by using a connected component labeling algorithm [1, 10] to label each region (that is, assign a different value for each separate region). For 3D images, we can use the above algorithm to label each of the 2D slices of the image and to form a list of overlapping regions for the entire image. This list can then be used to assign a unique number for every solid object.

Boundary (or surface) representations can be easily converted into regions (or solids) by using a filling algorithm [11], and the reverse can be accomplished using a boundary-tracking algorithm [12] or a surface-tracking algorithm [13, 14]. Once the surface and volumetric representations are obtained, we can use these to find various basic parameters of the objects such as surface area, perimeter, bounding box, and other qualitative measures such as eccentricity, Euler number, and shape number. There are number of algorithms that compute these properties from various boundary and region representations [1, 15, 16].

3.2 Fuzzy Clustering

A large number of clustering algorithms are based on objective function minimization to generate partitions in data. These are square error algorithms where the weighted distances of points from the cluster prototypes is minimized. When the partitions are fuzzy as in fuzzy c-means algorithms, they are called fuzzy-clustering techniques. Clarke et al. employed fuzzy clustering techniques for segmentation of MRI brain images. The algorithm for the generation of fuzzy clusters is discussed below.

3.2.1 Fuzzy clustering algorithm

The fuzzy-clustering technique is unsupervised; that is, it does not need to be trained to perform the classification [17]. It takes a finite data set $X = x_1; x_2, ..., x_n$ as input, each $x_i \in X$ is a feature vector ;$x_i = (x_{i1}, x_{i2}, ..., x_{is})$ where

x_{ij} is the jth feature of subset x_i, and s is the dimensionality of x_i. A function $u : X \rightarrow [0, 1]$ is defined, which assigns to each x_i in X its grade of membership in the fuzzy set u. The function u is called a fuzzy subset of X. The goal is to partition X by means of fuzzy sets. A fuzzy c-partition is defined as $c \times n$ matrix U such that

1. Each row U_i represents the ith fuzzy subset of X.
2. Each column U^j exhibits the membership grades of datum j in every fuzzy subset.
3. The membership grades of each datum in all fuzzy subsets ads up to 1.
4. No fuzzy subset is empty.
5. No fuzzy subset is all of X.

Let M_{fc} denote the fuzzy c-partitions of X, then $U \in M_{fc}$. The fuzzy c-means algorithm uses iterative optimization to approximate minima of an objective function J_m. [18]

$$J_m(U, v) = \sum_{k=1}^{n} \sum_{i=1}^{c} (U_{ik})^m (d_{ik})^2$$

where $v = (v_1, v-2, ..., v_c)$ with v_i being the cluster center of class i; $1 \leq i \leq c$ and $d_{ik}^2 = \|x_k - v_i\|^2$.

3.3 Segmentation Using Fractal Dimensions

Fractal dimension estimation as a means of segmentation of medical images has found widespread application in the case of texture segmentation of images. A considerable amount of work has been done in this area. Pentland [19] suggested the estimation of Fourier transform of the image over a finite window and used it for texture classification. Peleg et al. [21] found 48 features using fractal dimension of the original and smoothed versions of the image. Keller et al. [21] used fractal dimension estimated by box counting and a lacunarity measure for texture segmentation. Chaudhuri et al. [22] used four texture features derived using fractal geometry of images. This method will be examined n more detail in the following sections.

3.3.1 Fractal dimensions for texture segmentation
Texture is used extensively by the human visual perception system to understand a scene. Textured regions give different interpretations depending on distances and degrees of visual attention. This makes tonal segmentation techniques, which are normally suited for edge detection within an image, unsuitable for texture segmentation as the so-called "edges" are in the interior of textured regions.

Fractal dimensions (FD) of an image is relatively insensitive to image scaling and shows a strong correlation to the human judgment of surface roughness [22]. The FD of an image can be computed using various methods of which the box-counting method will be discussed in this section. The FDs of the original as well as the high- and low-gray-level-valued versions of the image are used as features. The fourth feature is based on the concept of multifractals, computed by a higher moment of box-counting [23] [24].

3.3.2 Estimation of fractal dimension
Manderboldt [25] stated that a criterion of a surface being a fractal is self similarity. Self-similarity can be explained as follows. A bounded set A in Euclidian space is said to be self similar when A is the union of N_r-distinct copies of itself, each of which is similar to A scaled down by a ratio r. The fractal dimension D of A can be derived from the equation [22]

$$1 = N_r r^d \; or \; D = \frac{\log(N_r)}{\log(1/r)} \tag{1}$$

N_r can be counted in the following manner. Consider an image of size $M \times M$ pixels that has been scaled down to size $s \times s$ where s is an integer and $M/2 \geq s > 1$. Thus scaling ratio $r = s/M$. Now consider the image as a 3D space with (x, y) denoting the 2D position and the third coordinate (z) specifying the gray level. The (x, y) space is partitioned into grids of size $s \times s \times s$. Assign numbers 1, 2, ... to the boxes as shown in Figure 1. Here $s = 3$.

If the minimum and maximum gray level of the image in the (i, j)th grid fall in the boxes k and l respectively, then

$$n_r(i, j) = l - k + 1 \tag{2}$$

is the contribution of N_r in the (i, j)th grid. For example, in Figure 1 $n_r(i, j) = 3 - 1 + 1$. For all grids,

$$N_r = \sum_{i,j} n_r(i, j) \tag{3}$$

N_r is calculated for different values of r and then using Equation 1, the fractal dimension D is estimated. This method is called the differential-box-counting (DBC) method [22].

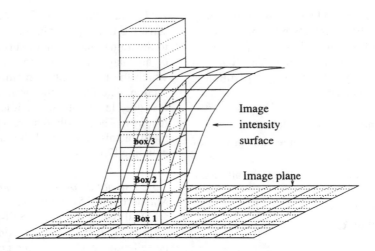

Figure 1. Determination of n_r.

3.3.3 Feature selection

Four fractal-based features are used for texture segmentation. They are as follows:

1. FD of original image
2. FD of high-gray-level image
3. FD of low-gray-level image
4. Multifractal FD

All features are normalized to lie in [0, 1].

Feature 1

FD of the original image I_1 is computed on overlapping windows of size $(2W+1) \times (2W+1)$ with 50 percent horizontal overlap. Thus at (i, j) the first feature value $F_1(i, j)$ is defined as

$$F_1(i, j) = FD \{I_1(i + l, j + k); \quad -W \le l, k \le W\} \quad (4)$$

Since $2{:}0 \le F_1(i, j) \le 3{:}0$, the normalized feature can be defined as

$$f_1(i, j) = F_1(i, j) - 2 \text{ so that } 0 \le f_1(i, j) \le 1$$

Features 2 and 3

The high- and low-gray-valued images are defined as, respectively

$$I_2(i, j) = \begin{cases} I_1(i, j) - L_1 & \text{if} \quad I_1(i, j) > L_1 \\ 0 & \textit{otherwise} \end{cases} \quad (5)$$

$$I_3(i, j) = \begin{cases} 255 - L_1 & \text{if} \quad I_1(i, j) > (255 - L_{1)} \\ I_3(i, j) & \textit{otherwise} \end{cases} \quad (6)$$

where $L_1 = g_{min} + av/2$; $L_2 = g_{max} - av/2$ while g_{max}, g_{min}, and av denote the maximum, minimum, and average gray value in I_1, respectively. The FDs are computed and the normalized features are computed in a similar manner to that of f_1.

Feature 4

The fourth feature is the multifractal with an exponent of order two. The basics of multifractals are as follows.

For a distribution $\mu(\epsilon)$ defined within a certain volume, the pointwise dimension α is defined as

$$\lim_{r \to 0} \mu_x(r) \sim r^\alpha \quad (7)$$

where $\mu_x(r)$ is the total measure contained in a sphere of radius r around the point x. The difference between this and the box method is that α fluctuates widely as a function of position x. Thus the distribution may be described by several singularities of type α together with the FD of the set in which the singularity is defined. In order to define the FD a partition function $\chi(q, r)$ may be defined as follows.

$$\chi(q,r) = \sum_x \left[n'_r \right]^q \simeq r^{\tau(q)}$$

where r is the scaling ratio and $n'_r = n_r / N_r$, n_r and N_r are given by equations 2 and 3, respectively. This function evaluates all possible singularities of the distribution by studying all the q moments of the coarse-grained distribution for different sizes of coarse graining. $\tau(q)$ defines the small r behavior of $\chi(q, r)$. The generalized FD $D(q)$ is then given as

$$(q-1)D(q) = r(q) = \lim_{r \to 0} \frac{\ln \chi(q,r)}{\ln r} \quad q \neq 1$$

Then for $q = 2$

$$D(2) = \lim_{r \to 0} \frac{\ln \sum_x [n_r']^2}{\ln r} \qquad (8)$$

Thus the normalized feature f_4 is defined as

$$f_4 = TD - D(2)$$

where TD is the topological dimension, which is two in the case of images.

3.3.4 Feature space smoothing
When these features are directly used for segmentation, considerable misclassification can occur in the interior and the border of the region. There are several edge-preserving smoothing techniques that can be used which will not be discussed here.

3.3.5 Unsupervised segmentation
In this approach it is assumed that only the number of texture classes K is known. Here at first the histogram of each feature computed over the whole region is examined. If f_i is the ith feature and H_i is its histogram, let N_i denote the number of peaks in H_i and let the peaks occur at $f_{i1}, f_{i2}, \ldots, f_{iN_i}$. Thus initially,

$$k_0 = \prod_{i=1}^{4} N_i$$

The data are distributed among the K_0 clusters using the nearest-neighbor rule. If a seed point does not obtain the data, then it is disregarded. At each iteration, the cluster with the least number of data is deleted by redistributing its data to other more-populated clusters. The redistribution is done by the nearest-neighbor rule. Thus the number of clusters is reduced with each iteration. The algorithm terminates when K clusters are reached. The classified data are mapped back into image space.

3.4 Graph-Theoretic Approach

Data clustering is an important part of data analysis. Graph-theoretic approaches have been proposed for data clustering. A few of these methods are

- Single link and complete link hierarchical algorithms formulated and implemented using a threshold graph as proposed by Hubert and Matula [26] [27].

- Forming clusters by breaking inconsistent arcs in the minimum spanning tree of the proximity graph as proposed by Zahn [28] or graphs constructed based on limited neighborhood sets as suggested by Urquhart [29].

- Detecting clusters using directed trees as proposed by Koontz et al. [30].

- Cluster detection based on network ow theory as proposed by Leahy [31].

The last method as applied to the image segmentation problem will be investigated in this section.

3.4.1 Data clustering through graph theory
The data to be clustered are represented by an undirected adjacency graph G: Each vertex of G corresponds to a data point, and an arc links two vertices in G if the corresponding data points are neighbors according to a given neighborhood system. A flow capacity is then assigned to each arc in G. This is chosen to reflect the feature similarity between the pair of inked vertices. The clustering is achieved by removing arcs of G to form mutually exclusive subgraphs. For the case of an unconstrained optimal K-subgraph partition of G, the arcs selected for removal are those in a set of $K-1$ minimum cuts with the smallest $K-1$ values among all possible minimum cuts separating all pairs of vertices. The method minimizes the largest inter-subgraph maximum flow among all possible K partitions of G, hence minimizing the similarity between subgraphs, which in this case are clusters. The reason for this method of minimization can be explained as follows.

The purpose of the clustering algorithm is to group together components into a minimal number of clusters. This can be formulated in terms of the adjacency graph G formed from the components. G can be divided into a number of unconnected subgraphs by removal of the arcs connecting the subgraphs. The set of vertices in each subgraph then represents a single cluster. Each of the remaining subgraphs contains a set of connected vertices or components whose union represents a spatially connected region of the image. Since arc capacities are a measure of the similarity between connected neighbors, partitioning a graph G into two subgraphs with as dissimilar features as possible would involve minimizing the maximum flow between the two subgraphs [31].

3.4.2 Image segmentation using graph theory
The graph-theoretic approach has been applied to the image segmentation problem successfully. In the method described below, the segmentation is achieved by searching for closed contours of edge elements. The edge elements are computed prior to construction of the graph. The edge strength is computed as a function of intensity differences between the pixel pair and between pixels in the vicinity by using masks similar to those shown in Figure 2.

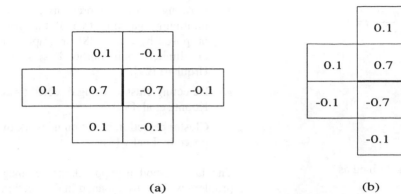

Figure 2. Edge strength masks. (a)Horizontal edges. (b)Vertical edges.

If $x_{i,j}$ is the grey scale intensity of the pixel at the coordinates (i, j), and if $D_{i,j}^{H}$ and $D_{i,j}^{V}$ are the edge elements defined by the pixel pairs $(x_{i,j}, x_{i,j+1})$ and $(x_{i,j}, x_{i+1,j})$, respectively, then

$$D_{i,j}^{H} = \left| \begin{matrix} \delta.(x_{i,j} - x_{i,j+1}) + (x_{i-1,j} - x_{i-1,j+1}) \\ +(x_{i+1,j} - x_{i+1,j+1}) + (x_{i,j-1} - x_{i,j+2}) \end{matrix} \middle/ (\delta+3).\sigma \right| \quad (9)$$

$$D_{i,j}^{V} = \left| \begin{matrix} \delta.(x_{i,j} - x_{i+1,}) + (x_{i,j-1} - x_{i+1,j-1}) \\ +(x_{i,j+1} - x_{i+1,j+1}) + (x_{i-1,j} - x_{i+2,j}) \end{matrix} \middle/ (\delta+3).\sigma \right| \quad (10)$$

where δ and σ are control parameters. δ controls the smoothing effect of the edge masks. σ is proportional to the smallest intensity difference that indicates the potential presence of a region boundary in the image. For a cut in the graph G that partitions G into two subgraphs, the edge elements corresponding to the arcs belonging to the cut form a close edge contour. The value of the cut is equal to the sum of the capacities of its arcs. If a small capacity is assigned to strong edge element and vice versa, then the cuts with small value correspond to closed contours with strong edge elements. Conversely, isolated strong edges will not produce boundaries in the segmented image, since there is a high cost associated with the inclusion of weak edges, necessary to form a closed boundary through these isolated edges. An appropriate arc capacity function to achieve this goal is as follows:

$$C_{i,j}^{P} = \begin{cases} e^{-(D_{i,j}^{P})^{2}}, & \text{if } 3 > D_{i,j}^{P}, \ p = HorV \\ e^{-3D_{i,j}^{P}}, & \text{if } D_{i,j}^{P} \geq 3 \end{cases} \quad (11)$$

Here $C_{i,j}^{H}$ and $C_{i,j}^{V}$ are the capacities of the arcs connecting $v_{i,j}$ to $v_{i,j+1}$ and $v_{i+1,j}$, respectively, where $v_{i,j}$ is the vertex corresponding to pixel $x_{i,j}$. The minimum cuts of G are computed from a flow-and-cut-equivalent tree T^* of G, which can be constructed using the Gomory-Hu algorithm [32]. The optimal K-partition can be equivalently obtained by disconnecting the $K - 1$ arcs in T^* with the smallest $K - 1$ arc capacities.

3.5 Deformable Models

There are a number of methods using deformable models for image segmentation, such as:

1. Parametrically deformable models, which are essentially 2D in nature and aid in the segmentation of image slices. The approach is based on elliptic Fourier decomposition as proposed by Staib et al. [33].

2. Energy minimizing snakes that are attracted to image features such as lines and edges, whereas internal spline forces impose a smoothness constraint, as described by Kass et al. [9].

3. 3D deformable surfaces, used by Cohen et al. [34] where deformable models that deform under the action of internal forces, such as the elastic properties of the surface, and external forces attracting the surface toward detected edge elements.

4. Deformable superquadrics, proposed by Terzopoulos et al. [35] and deformable generalized cylinders, proposed by O'Donnell and Gupta [36], which incorporate global shape parameters of a superellipsoid and generalized cylinder, respectively, and local degrees of freedom based on elastic properties and action of external forces. These models can be used to extract gross shape features from visual data, which can be used for indexing onto a database of stored models to provide shape recognition. Local deformations help in reconstructing the details of complex shapes to provide shape reconstruction.

Additional work in the area of image segmentation using deformable templates has been done. A few of these approaches are listed below. Widrow [37] used parameterized templates called rubber masks to model objects. The parameters are sizes and relationships between subparts. Yuille et al. [38] used a parameterized template for an eye consisting of a circle bounded by two parabolas. The template was deformed to the image by optimizing a cost function based on morphological features. Deformable models based on Markov models of 2D boundaries incorporating knowledge from statistical features have been used by Chow et al. [39]. Fischler and Elschlager [40] used models where components of an object are held together by spring forces. Schudy [1] used spherical harmonic parameterization for boundary finding. Gritton and Parrish [41] used a flexible bead chain where the beads are putative boundary points. Cooper [42] formulated boundary estimation using maximum likelihood.

The techniques summarized above, as well as many variants of them, have been used for a variety of segmentation tasks in medical image analysis. Some representative examples are included in Chapters 12 through 19. In the rest of this section, we examine one of the techniques mentioned above, using deformable superquadrics, in more detail. The basis shape of a deformable superquadric is the superquadric ellipsoid, which is formulated below.

3.5.1 Superquadric ellipsoid

The reference shape is a superquadric ellipsoid which is formulated as

$$s = a \begin{pmatrix} a_1 & C_u^{\epsilon_1} C_v^{\epsilon_2} \\ a_2 & C_u^{\epsilon_1} S_v^{\epsilon_2} \\ a_3 & S_u^{\epsilon_1} \end{pmatrix}$$

Here a_1, a_2, $a_3 \leq 1$ are aspect ratios, ϵ_1, ϵ_2 are squareness parameters, $a \geq 0$ is a scale parameter. Also, $-\frac{\pi}{2} \leq v \leq \frac{\pi}{2}$ and $-\pi \leq u \leq \pi$, $S_\omega^\epsilon = \mathrm{sgn}(\sin \omega)|\sin \omega|^\epsilon$ and $C_\omega^\epsilon = \mathrm{sgn}(\cos \omega)|\cos \omega|^\epsilon$.

The superquadric parameters can be grouped together into a parameter vector denoted as

$$q_s = (a, a_1, a_2, a_3, \epsilon_1, \epsilon_2)^T$$

3.5.2 Geometry of the deformable superquadric

The reference shape for the deformable superquadric is the superquadric as formulated above. The position of points on the model relative to an inertial frame of reference ϕ in space is given by u=(u,v) where u is the intrinsic coordinates of the model.

$$x(u, t) = (x_1(u, t), x_2(u, t), x_3(u, t))^T$$

The position can be expressed in terms of a noninertial-model-centered frame of reference φ as

$$x = c + R_p$$

where the orientation of φ is given by the rotation matrix $R(t)$. The positions of the points on the model relative to the model frame $p(u, t)$ can be expressed as the sum of the reference shape $s(u, t)$ and a displacement function $d(u, t)$.

$$p = s + d$$

d can be expressed as a linear combination of basis functions $b_i(u)$.

$$d = \sum_i \mathrm{diag}(b_i) q_i$$

This can be written as

$$d = S q_d$$

where S is the shape matrix whose entries are the basis functions and $q_d = (..., q_l, ...)^T$ are the degrees of freedom of the vector d.

3.5.3 Kinematics

The velocity of the points on the model is given by

$$\dot{x} = \dot{c} + B\dot{\theta} + R\dot{s} + RS\dot{q}_d$$

where $\dot{\theta} = (..., \theta_i, ...)^T$ is the vector of rotational coordinates of the model. $B = \left[... \frac{\partial(R_p)}{\partial \theta_i} ... \right]$.

Thus

$$\dot{x} = [I \ B \ RJ \ RS]\dot{q} = L\dot{q}$$
$$q = (q_c^T, q_\theta^T, q_s^T, q_d^T)^T$$

J is the Jacobian of the superquadric. I is the identity matrix.

Degrees of freedom q.

The degrees of freedom of the model are as follows.

1. $q_c = c$: Global rigid motion coordinate that specifies the position of the model with respect to the inertial frame of reference.

147

2. $q_\theta = \theta$: Global rotational motion coordinate that specifies the rotational orientation of the model with respect to the inertial frame of reference.

3. q_s : Global deformation coordinate of the model.

4. q_d : Local deformation coordinates of the model.

The goal is to recover q, which is the vector of degrees of freedom. This vector gives a complete description of position of points on the model. The model is made dynamic in q by introducing mass damping and deformation strain energy. Thus the equations of motion of the model take the form

$$M\ddot{q} + C\dot{q} + Kq = g_q + f_q$$

where $M = \int \mu L^T L du$ is the mass matrix of the object and $\mu(u)$ is the mass density of the object. $C = \int \gamma L^T L du$ is the damping matrix and $\gamma(u)$ is the damping density. g_q are inertial forces and $f_q(u, t)$ are external forces associated with the degrees of freedom of the model.

$$K = \begin{bmatrix} 0 & 0 & 0 & 0 \\ & 0 & 0 & 0 \\ & & K_{ss} & K_{sd} \\ symmetric & & & K_{dd} \end{bmatrix}$$

is the stiffness matrix.

3.5.4 Elasticity
The stiffness matrix K determines the elastic properties of the model. K_{ss} and K_{dd} are set to zero and a generalized spline deformation is imposed on q_d.

$$\varepsilon(d) = \int \omega_1((\frac{\partial d}{\partial u})^2 + (\frac{\partial d}{\partial v})^2) + \omega_0 d^2 du$$

where ω_1 and ω_0 are stiffness parameters. $\varepsilon(d)$ is a membrane energy and it gives a small and continuous deformation function.

3.5.5 External forces

• **Short-range forces**
Potential function $P(x, y)$ is used to attract a 3D model toward intensity gradients in an image. This is given as

$$P(x, y) = \|\nabla(G_\sigma * I)\|$$

where G_σ denotes a Gaussian smoothing filter and $I(x, y)$ is the image.

The force applied due to the potential function is

$$f = \beta \nabla P(\Pi x)$$

where β controls the strength of the force and Π is a suitable projection of points on the model onto the image plane.

• **Computation of potential function**
Convolve a digital image with a discrete filter G_σ. Calculate discrete gradients ∇P_k for each pixel using the four neighboring pixels, that is, $k = 1, \ldots 4$. Consider these pixels as the nodes of a bilinear quadrilateral finite element. The potential gradient for the element is then given by

$$\nabla P(\Pi x) = \sum_{k=1}^{4} N_k(2x - xc), 2(y - y_c)) \nabla P_k$$

where N_k denotes the nodal shape function of the finite element and (x_c, y_c) denotes the centroid of the four pixels.

• **Long-range forces**
Long-range forces may be defined as

$$f(u_r) = \beta \| r - x(u_r) \|$$

where r is a data point in space and u_r is the point of influence of the force on the model's surface.

$x(u_r)$ can be computed for each element as in a bilinear quadrilateral element

$$x(u_r) = \sum_{i=1}^{4} N_i(2(u_r - u_c)/a, 2(v_r - v_c)/b) x_i$$

where x_i are the nodal positions.

The equivalent forces for each of the four nodes are

$$f_i = N_i(2(u_r - u_c)/a, 2(v_r - v_c)/b) f(u_r)$$

• **Minimizing u_r**
u_r should be so chosen as to minimize the distance $d(u) = \| r - x(u) \|$. This can be achieved by moving points of influence over the model surface until they arrive at locations of minimal distance. Starting from initial points of influence, the force is projected at each time step onto unit tangent-vectors $(\partial x/\partial u)/ \| (\partial x/\partial u) \|$ and $(\partial x/\partial v)/ \| (\partial x/\partial v) \|$ to the surface of influence $P_0 = u_0$ (Figure 3).

The point is migrated in the u plane by taking steps in *u* and *v* proportional to the magnitude of the respective projections. At P_n there is no tangential component and minimum is achieved.

3.5.6 Finite element approach

The deformable superquadric can be modeled and the various forces computed with the help of finite element methods. The stiffness matrices have to be formulated in finite-elements to apply the finite-element methods. The conversion of the model into finite elements is as described below.

- **Discretization into finite elements**

Figure 4 shows tessellation of the model in material coordinates into finite-element domains. The model is tessellated into bilinear quadrilateral and linear triangular elements.

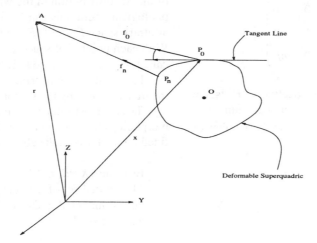

Figure 3. Migration of point of influence over model surface.

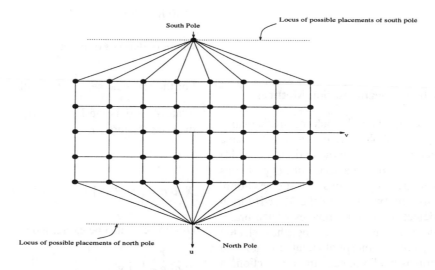

Figure 4. Model tessellation in material coordinates.

149

- **Stiffness matrices K_{dd} in finite elements**

The membrane spline deformation can be written as a combination of component energies

$$\varepsilon^j(d) = \varepsilon^j(d_1) + \varepsilon^j(d_2) + \varepsilon^j(d_3)$$

This can be written in the form

$$\varepsilon^j(d_k) = \int_{E_k} \sigma_k^{j^T} \varepsilon_k^j \, du$$

where

$$\varepsilon_k^j = \left[\frac{\partial d_k}{\partial u}, \frac{d_k}{\partial v} d_k\right]^T \quad \sigma_k^j \varepsilon_k^j = \begin{pmatrix} \omega_1^j & 0 & 0 \\ 0 & \omega_1^j & 0 \\ 0 & 0 & \omega_0^j \end{pmatrix} \varepsilon_k^j$$

are the strain and stress vectors respectively. E_j is the element domain. The finite-element nodal-shape functions are denoted by N_i^J $i = 1 \ldots n$, where n is the number of nodes in element E_j. Hence

$$\in_k^j = \sum_{i=1}^n \gamma_i^j(q_{d_k}^j) = \Gamma_k^j q_{d_k}^j$$

where $\gamma_i^j = \left[\frac{\partial N_i^j}{\partial u}, \frac{N_i^j}{\partial v}, 1\right]^T$ is the strain vector for each node in the element. Γ_k^j is the sum of the strain vectors over all nodes of the element. Thus the element stiffness matrix is given as

$$K_{dd}^{j=} \int_{E_j} \Gamma^{j^T} D_k^j \Gamma^j \, du.$$

3.6 Morphological Image Segmentation Methods

Mathematical morphology is a branch of mathematics based on set theory. Morphological operators [43] have been used for biomedical image segmentation. Vogt [44] breaks down the 3D problem into a series of 2D problems when using morphological operations for segmentation. Bomans et al. [45] use an extension of the Marr-Hildreth operator for edge detection in MRI images of the brain. They use morphological filters to refine the selected edges. Acharya [46] applies morphological operators to segmenting multidimensional images. In this section, a brief review of morphological operators is followed by their application to medical image segmentation. The spe-cific case of cardiac computed tomography scans are discussed in this section [46].

3.6.1 Mathematical morphology

Mathematical morphology [43] [47] uses set transformations for image analysis. It extracts the impact of a particular shape on images via the concept of structuring element (SE). The SE encodes the primitive shape information. The shape is described as a set of vectors referenced to a particular point, the center. During morphological transformation, the center scans the whole image and the matching shape information is used to define the transformation. The transformed image is thus a function of the SE distribution in the whole image. The basic morphological operations can be described on the basis of an arbitrary space E. Let $P(E)$ be the set of all subsets $X \in E$. With each point X of space E, a spatially varying set $B(X)$ called the SE is associated. The set $X \in P(E)$ can be modified based on set transformation of X by E. Let B_x denote the translate of B by the vector x (Figure 5).

The two most fundamental transforms in mathematical morphology are erosion and dilation. These can be defined on the basis of the above assumptions as

1. Erosion: $\{X : B_x \subset X\}$

   The eroded set of X is the locus of centers x of translate B_x included in the set X. This is denoted as $X \theta B$ and is given by

$$X \theta B = \bigcap_{b \in B} X_b$$

2. Dilation

   Dilation is a dual transform of erosion and can be expressed as

$$X^C \oplus B = (X \theta B)^C$$

where $\oplus$ denotes dilation.

For the reflected set $\check{B}$ of B with respect to the origin, the dilate $X \oplus \check{B}$ is the locus of B_x which hit (denoted by $\Uparrow$) the set X (Figure 5).

$$X \oplus \check{B} = \left\{x : B_x \bigcap X \neq \phi\right\} = \left\{x : B_x \Uparrow X\right\}$$

Dilation can also be expressed as

$$X \oplus \check{B} = \bigcup_{y \in \check{B}} X_y$$

150

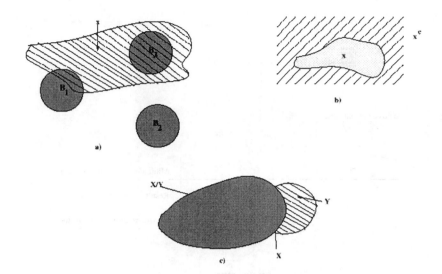

Figure 5. a) B_1 hits X ($B_1 \Uparrow X$);B_2 misses X ($B_2 \subset X^c$); B_3 is included in X ($B_3 \subset X$). (b) Complement X^c of set X. (c) Difference X / Y of the two sets X and Y.

The next two important operators are opening and closing. These can be defined as

1. Opening

$$X_B = (X \theta B) \oplus \overset{\vee}{B}$$

2. Closing

$$X^B = [(X^C)_B]^C = (X \oplus B) \theta B$$

As can be seen, these operators can be expressed in terms of dilation and erosion.

Gray Scale Operators

For purposes of segmentation, these operators need to be extended to gray scale images [43]. The concept of *surface* of a set and its *umbra* help in solving this problem. The gray-scale image is viewed as a 3D entity, two dimensions being the spatial coordinates of the image, the third being the intensity of the image. The intensity is interpreted as a surface over the E^2 plane. The umbra provides the means to express the surface as a set in order to perform morphological operations. If $B = B_r$ is the SE and $B(r)$ denotes the gray-level value of the rth vector, the Erosion $E_i(X, B)$ and Dilation $D_i(X, B)$ of X by B can be defined as

$$E_i(X, B) = \inf(X(i + r) - B(r)), r \in B$$

$$D_i(X, B) = \sup(X(i + r) + B(r)), r \in B$$

Signed morphological operators

All the above operators used positive elements in the definition of the SE. This can be extended to signed morphological operators, which are useful in edge detection operators. This can be done as follows. Let the set of SEs be partitioned into $B = B_P, B_N$ where B_P represents nonnegative vectors and B_N represent negative vectors. Then the signed operators (Figure 6 and Figure 7) can be defined as

$$se(X, B) = \inf(X(i + r) - B_P(r)) - \sup(X(i + r) + B_N(r))$$

$$sd(X, B) = \sup(X(i + r) + B_P(r)) - \inf(X(i + r) - B_N(r))$$

where *se* stands for signed erosion and *sd* stands for signed dilation. The fast implementation of these signed operators can be achieved through generalized operators.

Generalized morphological operators

Generalized erosion and dilation operators are used to effectively use morphological operators in multiple dimensions. These can be defined as follows. Let B be a structuring element and $B_i; i \in I$ be a finite set of points from B such that

$$B_i = b, b \in B_i \bigcup C$$

where C is the center of the SE. Then generalized erosion is

$$ge = \bigcup_{i \in I} \bigcap_{b \in B_i} X_b = \bigcup_{i \in I} ERO(X_i B_i)$$

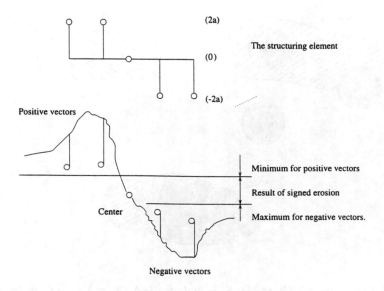

A signed erosion on a real edge with a complex structuring element. The result is the difference between the minmum obtained from the positive vectors and the maximum obtained from the negative vectors. In this case, positive and negative vectors are on a line (1D), and each subset is located on one side of the Center. This is always the case for oriented edge detection.

Figure 6. Signed erosion.

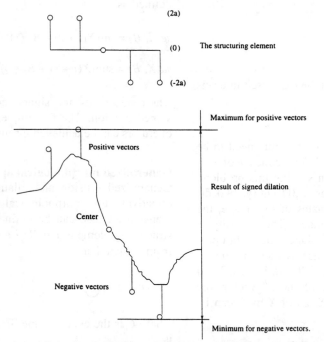

A signed dilation on a real edge with a complex structuring element. The result is the difference between the maximum obtained from the positive vectors and the minimum from the negative vectors.

Figure 7. Signed dilation.

where b_i is the ith partition vector of the SE and $ERO(X, B_i)$ is the erosion of set X by the SE B_i. Similarly generalized dilation is

$$gd = \bigcap_{i \in I} \bigcup_{b \in B_i} X_b = \bigcap_{i \in I} DIL(X, B_i)$$

where DIL is the dilation of set X by SE B_i. On the basis of the above definitions of generalized operators, cross-opening and cross-closing can be defined as follows.

$$ERO\ (DIL(X, B_j), B_i) = E_i D_j(X)$$

is the cross-closing at (i, j) of X where B_i and B_j are two subsets of B, and

$$DIL\ (ERO((X, B_j), B_i)) = D_i E_j(X)$$

is the cross-opening of X at (i, j). These can be extended into generalized opening and closing as follows.

$$go(X, B, I) = gd\big(ge(X, B, I), B, I\big) = \bigcap_{i \in I} \bigcup_{j \in I} D_i E_j(X)$$

where go is the generalized opening operator and

$$gc(X, B, I) = ge\big(gd(X, B, I), B, I\big) = \bigcup_{i \in I} \bigcap_{j \in I} E_i D_j(X)$$

where gc is the generalized closing operator.

For application to segmentation problems, generalized gray-level operators are defined. If $B = B_j = B_1; B_2, \dots$ represent a partitioned set of SEs, each member being itself a set of vectors $B_j = r$, with a gray value associated with each vector, the generalized gray-level erosion (ge) and dilation (gd) can now be defined as

$$ge(X, B, j) = \sup_j (\inf(X((i+r)) - B_j(r))), \quad r \in B_j$$

$$gd(X, B, j) = \sup_j (\inf(X((i+r)) - B_j(r))), \quad r \in B_j$$

The generalized signed operators are defined as

$$gse(X, B, I) = max(se(X, B_i)), \quad i \in I$$

$$gsd(X, B, I) = min(sd(X, B_i)), \quad i \in I$$

The desired edges can be extracted by designing the appropriate structuring elements. An example is as shown below.

$$B_j = (cU, a)$$

where U is a unit vector in the desired direction, and c is a scaling parameter.

3.6.2 Segmentation

The segmentation algorithm using the above mathematical morphology techniques can be split into the following important steps.

1. Search space definition
2. Surface candidate elements
3. Surface candidate element linkage
4. Surface Construction

Search space definition

The search space is important for the segmentation procedure as it constrains the space in which the algorithm looks for the surface. This reduces the computation time for feature detection. The search space $S(Y)$ of an object Y is defined as

$$S(\ ) = (\partial Y\ (gd)B)$$

where $\partial Y = \overline{Y} \cap \overline{Y}^C$ is the boundary of Y. Search space definition results in definition of constrained feasible set for surface candidate elements. This defines the subset of voxels in the multidimensional volume in which the surface candidate elements are located. This can be specified in terms of constraint propagation and projection information.

- **Constraint propagation**

This is in two forms, namely spatial and temporal. The two forms can be explained as follows.

  - **Spatial Constraint Propagation** If the object Y is partitioned into $Y = Y_1, Y_2, \dots, Y_n$ where each Y_k corresponds to a contiguous block of slices, the search space is defined as

$$S(Y_k) = (\partial Y_{k-1}(gd)B) \bigcup \partial Y_{k+1}(gd)B$$

This uses the features (∂Y) computed in one block to be propagated as constraints into adjacent blocks in order to define search space.

  - **Temporal Constraint Propagation** If $Y^t = Y^1, Y^2, \dots Y^T$ is a set of objects at different times t, the search space for the object y at instance l is defined as

$$S(Y^l) = \partial Y^{t=l-1}(gd)B \bigcup \partial Y^{t=l+1}(gd)B$$

153

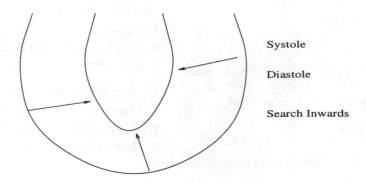

Systole

Diastole

Search Inwards

Figure 8. Systole and Diastole Phase of the heart.

where times $l - 1$ and l could be two successive instances of the diastolic phase of the heart cycle. As shown in Figure 8, consider the diastolic and systolic phase of the heart. The search space for the systolic phase of the heart cycle can be obtained with the knowledge of the diastolic phase by using the erosion operator [48, 49] as shown below.

$$S(Y)_{systole} = (\partial Y_{diastole} \; \theta \, B(Y, \lambda))$$

where $B(Y, \lambda)$ is the SE with radius λ.

- **Projection information**

For images obtained with projection information (for example, CT scan images), the projection information is useful for defining search space (Figure 9).

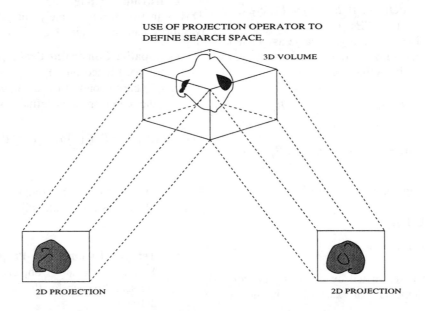

USE OF PROJECTION OPERATOR TO
DEFINE SEARCH SPACE.

3D VOLUME

2D PROJECTION

2D PROJECTION

Figure 9. Projection Information as obtained with a CT scan.

The projections can be represented as

$$p(l, m) = \int_a^b f(x, y, z)dq$$

where $p(l, m)$ is the projection of $f(x, y, z)$ along the direction q. By the use of 2D operators in properly selected projections, borders of the object can be obtained. These contours in the projections along with the anatomical knowledge specify the search space in 3D volume.

Surface candidate elements
The generalized signed operators as defined in the section on morphology can be used as structuring elements $B_j = (cU, a)$ for scale space edge detection [50].

Surface candidate element linkage
This is achieved by using the F* algorithm [8].

Surface construction
The goal is recovery of a good approximation of the true surface given the set of noisy candidate elements. The surface candidate elements can be obtained with the aid of 3D edge operators. The true surface is defined as a partition between regions of different properties.

3D surface definition can be described in the following manner. Consider a surface in 3D with parametric form given by the equation

$$S(\alpha, \beta) = [x(\alpha, \beta), y(\alpha, \beta), z(\alpha, \beta)]$$

The surface construction can be expressed as

$$Q(\alpha, \beta) = \Phi_{\alpha, \beta}S(\alpha, \beta)$$

where $S(\alpha, \beta)$ represents the data from which the filtered estimates $Q(\alpha, \beta)$ is obtained and $\Phi_{\alpha, \beta}$ is the filtering function. The operator $\Phi_{\alpha, \beta}$ can be simplified by expressing it as a combination of two univariate operators, leading to the surface approximation

$$Q(\alpha, \beta) = \Phi_\alpha \Phi_\beta S(\alpha, \beta)$$

This means that Φ_α operates on $S(\alpha, \beta_n)$ while Φ_β operates on $S(\alpha_m, \beta)$. For mn discrete values of $S(\alpha_m, \beta_n)$, Q is given by

$$Q(\partial, \beta) = \sum_{n=0}^{b} \sum_{m=0}^{a} S(\alpha_m, \beta_n) R_{m,a}(r) G_{n,b}(g)$$

where $R_{m,a}(r)$ and $G_{n,b}(g)$ are filter functions. In matrix form,

$$Q(\alpha, \beta) = RSG^T$$

where R and G are the filter functions

$$R = [R_{0,a}(r), R_{1,a}(r), ..., R_{a,a}(r)]R = [G_{0,b}(g), g_{1,b}(g), ..., G_{b,b}(g)]$$

and S is the matrix of coefficients,

$$S = \begin{pmatrix} S(\alpha_0, \beta_0) & S(\alpha_0, \beta_1) & \cdots & S(\alpha_0, \beta_n) \\ S(\alpha_1, \beta_0) & S(\alpha_1, \beta 1) & \cdots & S(\alpha_1, \beta_n) \\ \vdots & \vdots & \ddots & \vdots \\ S(\alpha_\alpha, \beta_0) & S(\alpha_\alpha, \beta_1) & \cdots & S(\alpha_\alpha, \beta_n) \end{pmatrix}$$

3.7 Neural Networks

Artificial neural networks have been used for image segmentation techniques based on the notion that neural networks may reduce requirements for user expertise in segmentation problems, which has been the case with most segmentation schemes. Neural network approaches are essentially shape-based approaches that make use of shape-based feature extraction. Lin et al. [51] segment X-ray CT, MRI, and PET images using a neural network algorithm. The image segmentation is formulated as a constraint satisfaction problem and a constraint satisfaction neural network is used to perform the segmentation. Neural net-based approaches have been adopted by Veronin et al. [52] for optical image segmentation. They used texture discrimination and employed biologically based orientation-specific filters as the main component coupled with a neural network to achieve segmentation. Sundaramoorthy et al. [53] use a shape-based feature space for segmenting medical images using neural networks. The following sections describe the approach followed by them.

The segmentation method described below consists of two important steps, feature extraction and the actual segmentation using a neural network [35].

3.7.1 Feature extraction
The feature extraction step is necessary in deciding what would be the input to the segmentation algorithm. *Features* are extracted from the input image and fed to the segmentation stage to be processed further. The feature extraction step is extremely important for the segmentation problem as the features selected should be appropriate for the segmentation algorithm. Correctly chosen features can reduce computational complexity as well as improve overall performance of the segmentation method. The feature extraction step proposed by Sundaramoorthy [53] is described below.

The algorithm generates n-dimensional vectors called RSVs (regional shape vectors) on a pixel-by-pixel basis. For each pixel, the corresponding RSV characterizes the distance from that pixel to the boundary of the object containing the pixel in each of the n directions. As typical biomedical images are essentially discrete in nature, any pixel can be defined by 8 neighborhoods. The RSV is determined by

$$RSV_{k,l}(i)\Big|_{o}^{n-1} =$$

$$\frac{\text{Distance to object boundary in direction } i \text{ from pixel } (k,l)}{\sqrt{M \cdot N}}$$

where $I(x, y)$ is the image with dimensions $M \times N$. (k, l) is a pixel position in the image.

The boundaries are determined by selecting a suitable threshold and then identifying the desired object based on the threshold. The RSV represents a particular pixel's position with respect to the edges of the object containing it. For objects with reasonably smooth boundaries, the RSVs of pixels forming the object tend to form a cluster in n-dimensional feature space. If objects with distinctly different shapes form clusters in n-D space, a classifier can be designed to take advantage of this fact and segment the desired objects. This property will be used in the design of the segmentation method using an artificial neural network.

3.7.2 Segmentation using an artificial neural network
The RSV algorithm produces feature spaces with highly nonlinear cluster boundaries. An artificial neural network can be used to segment the feature spaces. Sundaramoorthy [53] used a three-layer perceptron network with a supervised back-propagation training algorithm capable of forming arbitrarily nonlinear decision boundaries in feature space to handle the complex feature space. The procedure for training and segmentation are described below.

The inputs to the network were

- $I_{in}(x, y)$, the input image
- $I_d(x, y)$ which is the ideal or desired image
- T_l and T_h, the minimum and maximum threshold values used to define object boundaries

The algorithm proceeds as follows.

1. Initialize the network with random weights.
2. Check whether $I_{in}(x, y)$ lies within limits of T_l and T_h. If true, compute RSV for (x, y).
3. Input RSV to compute neural network output.
4. Compare output with desired output $I_d(x, y)$ and adjust weights.

5. Repeat from step 2 for all (x, y)
6. Compute classification error maps using actual and desired outputs.

The classification error maps aid in evaluating the performance of the neural network. The performance of the neural network, however, depends on other factors too. During training as the back-propagation algorithm is used, there is the possibility of being influenced by local minima. Also, if the training set is very large, individual feature contribution to the global learning process can be affected with each iteration, losing information gained in another region of the image. To alleviate this problem, the image can be sparsely sampled during each iteration. Thus the training algorithm can be made to cycle through all image pixels skipping a fixed number of iteration. This facilitates samples from different regions of the image to be presented to the network more rapidly, thus providing the means for the network to learn more rapidly.

4. High Level Segmentation

So far we have discussed individual components of the image understanding system, starting from obtaining picture domain cues from the image to forming scene domain cues, model instantiation, and refining picture cues using the instantiated model. The next component of an image segmentation system is the control strategy that supervises the overall activity of the components and directs the interpretation process. Knowledge-based systems are used for this stage of image segmentation. Here we discuss the expert-system-based model and also the pyramid-based method of segmentation as high level image segmentation methods.

In addition, data structures formed during medium-level processing can be used for the task of shape analysis, interpretation, and labeling (forming and matching a scene model). Concavity checking tools can aid in this process, forming yet another high-level image segmentation tool.

4.1 Pyramidal Segmentation

A pyramid is a general structure for representing copies of the image at multiple resolutions. Pyramidal image data structures involve searching for objects at low resolution and then refining the areas of interest with increasing resolutions until the highest resolution of interest is reached. The need for such a method of image segmentation arose because of the following reasons. First, the number of computations is fewer with this method because of decreased resolution. Second, unwanted detail present in the image are less prominent in images with reduced resolution.

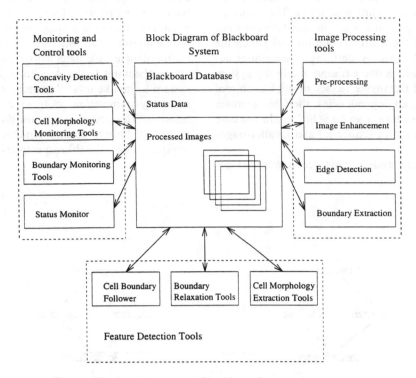

Figure 10. Organization of blackboard control structure.

Pyramidal methods have been applied to various fields, and image segmentation is an area where these methods have found extensive application. One of the problems associated with this approach is due to the decomposition of the image into subimages which results in ease of detection of certain images and rejection of other images. Bister [54] proved that thin elongated objects cannot be detected using pyramidal methods. On the other hand, compact forms can be successfully delineated using this method as suggested by Rosenfeld [55] and Baugher [56]. An approach suggested by Meer [57] to tackle this problem involves a scheme based on graph theory. A short summary of this method is given below.

4.1.1 Stochastic pyramid

The approach suggested by Meer [57] involved the *stochastic pyramid*, which can be explained as follows. The image is transformed into a graph with every vertex corresponding to a pixel and every link to a neighboring relationship. The pyramid is then built up by iterative contractions of the graph into smaller stable graphs. The contraction of the graph into an upper stable one is a stochastic process. The stochastic pyramid is not reproducible and therefore leads to varying regions of segmentation. Its efficiency is established only if sharp regions of the image are correctly delineated, independent of the realization of the pyramid. An optimal stochastic pyramid has been proposed by Mathieu et al. [58]. Mathieu et al. [58] have applied the concept of stochastic pyramids to segmenta-

tion of MRI heart images. They rely on the concept of the optimal stochastic pyramid, which was developed by them for this purpose.

4.2 Expert-System-Based Approaches

Expert systems mimic the reasoning process of an expert to divide a medical image into semantically meaningful entities. The entities can then be related to fundamental biomedical processes, both in health and in disease, that are of interest to health care research. These kinds of systems have been used by Chen et al. [59] for image segmentation of tomographic brain images. Raya et al. [60] have used this method for segmentation of multidimensional images. Botto et al. [61] have used expert-system-based segmentation methods for extraction of biomedical structures in microscopic images. Efford [62] uses knowledge-based segmentation for hand and wrist radiographic images. Here we discuss the blackboard model of problem solving applied to segmentation of confocal microscopic images as proposed by Samarabandu et al. [63], which supervises the overall activity of components in the image segmentation problem and directs the interpretation process.

4.2.1 Blackboard model of problem solving

The blackboard model (Figure 10) is an *opportunistic reasoning* model that arrives at a solution in an incremental fashion. Each knowledge source looks at the in-

157

termediate solution that is stored in the blackboard data structure and updates it toward a solution. The sequence in which the knowledge sources are invoked depends entirely on the state of the current solution and hence the term "opportunistic." Thus by defining a sequential dependency, we can achieve one extreme where the system acts as a pipeline and the image passes through each tool in turn. By abolishing all dependencies, the other extreme of parallel execution of tools can be achieved. In the case illustrated, a combination of sequential and parallel stages are used.

Initially, the preprocessing tools are applied in se-

quence to generate the enhanced image. The simplest boundary extraction tools such as thresholding and boundary tracing are then applied to obtain a primary segmentation. The bottom-up cycle terminates when no inconsistencies are detected by the shape, size, and concavity-checking tools. Any inconsistency will cause the system to invoke a combination of feature extraction and boundary completion tools to correct the object under scrutiny. The control structure during a bottom-up only phase and bottom-up and top-down phase are illustrated in Figure 11(a) and (b) respectively.

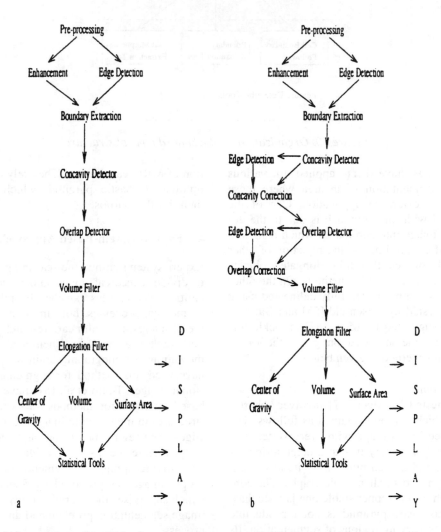

Figure 11. (a) Sample invocation of tools for bottom-up operation. (b) Using both bottom-up and top-down approaches.

4.3 Concavity Detector and Shape Analysis Tools

The data structures formed during medium-level processing can be used for the task of shape analysis, interpretation, and labeling (forming and matching a scene model). High-level processing tools consist of shape and size analysis tools and concavity checking tools. These tools contain 3D and 2D shape and size information of common objects to enable them to detect irregular objects. A modified form of chain code which eliminates the discontinuities at $0° \rightarrow 359°$ and $359° \rightarrow 0°$ transitions, is used in the concavity checking tool. The shape analysis tool finds the major and minor axes of each object and the size analysis tools find the area within each 2D object and the volume of 3D objects. Another tool of interest finds the center of gravity of individual cellular structures and hence reduces the amount of data to be processed and displayed. This is very useful when studying a large number of cells whose shapes and sizes are not important.

5. Summary and Conclusions

We have reviewed a variety of biomedical image segmentation techniques in the above discussion. The objective of this exercise was to provide a general overview of these techniques and provide the reader with references to the techniques involved for more detailed study. There are a number of other techniques for image segmentation that were not discussed because of space constraints. A few of these methods are listed in the references for readers interested in a more detailed study of biomedical image segmentation methods. An attempt has been made through this discussion to classify the problem of image segmentation into broad categories and to treat individual methods as belonging to one of the categories. Additional methods continue to be developed for image segmentation that can be included in future review discussions on this problem.

References

[1] D.H. Ballard and C.M. Brown, *Computer Vision*, Prentice Hall, Englewood Cliffs, N.J., 1982.

[2] S.W. Zucker and R.A. Hummel, "An Optimal Three-Dimensional Edge Operator," Report 79-10, McGill University, Toronto, Ontario, Canada, Apr. 1979.

[3] H.K. Liu, "Two and Three Dimensional Boundary Detection," *Computer Graphics and Image Processing*, Vol. 6, Apr. 1977, pp. 123–134.

[4] G.T. Herman and H.K. Liu, "Dynamic Boundary Surface Detection," *Computer Graphics and Image Processing*, Vol. 7, 1978, pp. 130–138.

[5] J.A. Hartington, *Clustering Algorithms*, John Wiley and Sons, New York, N.Y., 1975.

[6] A. Martelli, "Edge Detection Using Heuristic Search Methods," *Computer Graphics and Image Processing*, Vol. 25, Aug. 1972, pp. 169–182.

[7] R.O. Duda and P.E. Hart, *Pattern Classification and Scene Analysis*, John Wiley and Sons, New York, N.Y., 1973.

[8] M.A. Fischler, J.M. Tenenbaum, and H.C. Wolf, "Detection of Roads and Linear Structures in Low Resolution Aerial Imagery Using a Multi-Source Knowledge Integration Technique," *Computer Graphics and Image Processing*, Vol. 15, Mar. 1981, pp. 201–203.

[9] J.K. Samarabandu, R.S. Acharya, and P.C. Cheng, "Analysis and Presentation of Three Dimensional Data Sets," in *Multidimensional Microscopy*, P.C. Cheng, ed., Springer Verlag, Berlin, 1993, pp. 231–250.

[10] J. Hequard and R.S. Acharya, "Connected Component Labeling Using Linear Octree," *Pattern Recognition*, 1990.

[11] T. Pavlidis, "Segmentation of Pictures and Maps Through Functional Approximation," *Computer Graphics and Image Processing*, Vol. 1, 1972, pp. 360–372.

[12] S. Papert, "Use of Technology to Enhance Education," Technical Report 298, AI Lab, MIT, 1973.

[13] M.L. Rhodes, "An Algorithmic Approach to Controlling Search in Three Dimensional Image Data," *Proc. SIGGRAPH*, ACM Press, New York, N.Y., 1979, pp. 134–142.

[14] E. Artzy, G. Frider, and G.T. Herman, "The Theory, Design Implementation, and Evaluation of a Three-Dimensional Surface Detection Algorithm," Technical Report MIPG43, State Univ. of New York at Buffalo, Mar. 1980.

[15] A. Rosenfeld and A. Kak, *Digital Picture Processing*, Academic Press, New York, N.Y., 1976.

[16] J.K. Udupa, "Determination of 3-D Shape Parameters from Boundary Information," Technical Report MIPG42, State Univ. of New York at Buffalo, Jan. 1980.

[17] L.P. Clarke et al., "Comparison of Supervised Pattern Recognition Techniques and Unsupervised Methods for MRI Segmentation," *SPIE Image Processing*, Vol. 1652, 1992, pp. 668–677.

[18] L. Biduet, "Composite PET and MRI for Accurate Localization and Metabolic Modeling," *SPIE, Image Processing*, Vol. 1445, 1991, p. 67.

[19] A.P. Pentland, "Fractal Based Description of Natural Scenes," *IEEE Trans. Pattern Analysis and Machine Intelligence*, Vol. 6, 1984, pp. 661–674.

[20] S. Peleg, et al., "Multiple Resolution Texture Analysis and Classification," *IEEE Trans. Pattern Analysis and Machine Intelligence*, Vol. 6., 1984, pp. 518–523.

[21] J. Keller, R. Crownover, and S. Chen, "Texture Description and Segmentation through Fractal Geometry," *Computer Vision Graphics and Image Processing*, Vol. 22, pp. 150–160.

[22] B.B. Chaudhuri, N. Sarkar, and P. Kundu, "Improved Fractal Geometry Based Texture Segmentation Technique," *IEE Proceedings-E*, Vol. 140, No. 5, Sept. 1993, pp. 233–241.

[23] J.J. Gangepain and C. Roques-Carmes, "Fractal Approach to Two dimensional and Three dimensional Surface Roughness," *Wear,* Vol. 109, pp. 119-126.

[24] P. Grassberger, "Generalized Dimension and Strange Attractors," *Phys. Lett.* A, Vol. 97, 1983, pp. 227–230.

[25] B. B.Manderboldt, *Fractal Geometry of Nature*, Freeman Press, San Francisco, Calif., 1982.

[26] L.J. Hubert, "Some Applications of Graph Theory to Clustering," *Psychometrika*, Vol. 38, 1974, pp 435–475.

[27] D.W. Matula, "Graph Theoretic Techniques for Cluster Analysis Algorithms," in *Classification and Clustering*, J. Van Ryzin, ed., Academic Press, New York, N.Y., 1977, pp. 95–129.

[28] C.T. Zahn, "Graph Theoretic Methods for Detecting and Describing Gestalt Clusters," *IEEE Trans. Computer*, Vol. 20, 1971, pp. 68–86.

[29] R. Urquhart, "Graph Theoretical Clustering Based on Limited Neighborhood Sets," *Pattern Recognition*, Vol. 15, 1982, pp. 173–187.

[30] W.L. Koontz, P.M. Narendra, and K. Fukunaga, "A Graph-Theoretic Approach to Nonparameter Cluster Analysis," *IEEE Trans. Computers.*, Vol. 24, Sept. 1976, pp. 936–944.

[31] Z. Wu and R. Leahy, "An Optimal Graph Theoretic Approach to Data Clustering: Theory and its Application to Image Segmentation," *IEEE Trans. Pattern Analysis And Machine Intelligence*, Vol. 15, Nov. 1993, pp. 1101–1113.

[32] R.E. Gomory and T.C. Hu, "Multi-terminal Network Flows," *SIAM J. Appl. Math.*, Vol. 9, 1961, pp. 551–570.

[33] L.H. Staib and J.S. Duncan, "Boundary Finding With Parametrically Deformable Models," *IEEE Trans. Pattern Analysis and Machine Intelligence*, Vol. 14, 1992, pp. 1061–1075.

[34] I. Cohen, L.D. Cohen, and N. Ayache, "Using Deformable Surfaces to Segment 3-D Images and Infer Differential Structures," *CVGIP: Image Understanding*, Vol. 56, No. 2, 1992, pp. 242–263.

[35] D. Terzopoulos and D. Metaxas, "Dynamic 3D Models with Local and Global Deformations: Deformable Superquadrics," *IEEE Trans. Pattern Analysis and Machine Intelligence*, Vol. 13, No. 7, July 1991, pp. 703–714.

[36] T. O'Donnell, et al., "Extruded generalized Cylinder: A Deformable Model for Object Recovery," *Proc. CVPR*, IEEE Computer Society Press, Los Alamitos, Calif., 1994.

[37] B. Widrow, "The "Rubber Mask" technique-i and ii," *Pattern Recognition*, Vol. 5, 1973, pp. 175–211.

[38] A.L. Yuille, D.S. Cohen, and Hallinan, "Feature Extraction from Faces Using Deformable Templates," *Proc. IEEE Conf. Computer Vision and Pattern Recognition*, IEEE Computer Society Press, Los Alamitos, Calif., 1989, pp. 104–109.

[39] Y. Chow, U. Grenander, and D.M. Keenan, "Hands: A Pattern Theoretic Study of Biological Shapes," Monograph, Div. Applied Math., Brown University., Providence, RI, 1989.

[40] M.A. Fischler and R.A. Elschlager, "The Representation and Matching of Pictorial Structures," *IEEE Trans. Computers*, Vol. C-22, Jan. 1973, pp. 67–92.

[41] C.W.K. Gritton and E.A. Parrish, "Boundary Location Form an Initial Plan: The Bead Chain Algorithm," *IEEE Trans. Pattern Analysis and Machine Intelligence*, Vol. PAMI-5, Jan 1983, pp. 8–13.

[42] D.B. Cooper, "Maximum Likelihood estimation of Markov-Process Blob Boundaries in Noisy Images," *IEEE Trans. Pattern Analysis and Machine Intelligence*, Vol. PAMI-1, No. 4, Oct. 1979, pp. 372–284.

[43] J. Serra, *Image Analysis and Mathematical Morphology*, Academic Press, New York, N.Y., 1982.

[44] R. Vogt, "Precise Extraction of Bones from CT Scans," *Advances in Mathematical Morphology,* Vol 2.

[45] M. Bomans et al., "3D Segmentation of MR Images of the Head for 3D Display," *IEEE Trans. Medical Imaging,* Vol. 9, No. 2, June 1990.

[46] R. Acharya, "Segmentation of Multidimensional Cardiac Images," to appear in *J. Computerized Medical Imaging and Analysis.*

[47] P. Maragos and R.W. Shafer, "Morphological Systems for Multidimensional Signal Processing," *Proc. IEEE,* Vol. 78, Apr. 1990, pp. 690–710.

[48] J. Samarabandu et al., "Analysis of Multi-Dimensional Confocal Images," in *Biomedical Image Processing II*, Vol. 1450 of *Electronic Imaging: Science and Technology*, SPIE, 1991.

[49] R.S. Acharya, "Surface Representation Using Geodesic Morphology," *Proc. IEEE Int'l Conf. System Eng.*, IEEE Computer Society Press, Los Alamitos, Calif., 1991, pp. 257–260.

[50] A. Morales and R. Acharya, "Nonlinear Multiscale Filtering Using Mathematical Morphology," *SPIE Proc. Nonlinear Image Processing*, 1990.

[51] W. Lin et al., "Neural Networks for Medical Image Segmentation," Northwestern University, Electrical Engineering and Computer Science, 1991.

[52] C.P. Veronin et al., "Optical Image Segmentation Using Neural-Based Wavelet Filtering Techniques," *Optical Engineering*, Vol. 3, No. 2, Feb. 1992, pp. 287–293.

[53] G. Sundaramoorthy, J.D. Hoford, and E. Hoffman, "Regional Shape Based Feature Space for Segmenting Biomedical Images Using Neural Networks," *Proc. SPIE, Biomedical Image Processing and Biomedical Visualization*, Vol. 1905, Part 1, 1993, pp. 64–74.

[54] M. Bister, J. Cornelis, and A. Rosenfeld, "A Critical View of Pyramidal Segmentation Algorithms," *Pattern Recognition Letters*, Vol. 11, 1990, pp. 605–617.

[55] A. Rosenfeld and A. Sher, "Detection and Delineation of Compact objects Using Intensity Pyramids," *Pattern Recognition*, Vol. 21, 1990, pp. 147–151.

[56] E.S. Baugher and A. Rosenfeld, "Boundary Localization in an Image Pyramid," *Pattern Recognition* Vol. 19, 1986, pp. 373–395.

[57] P. Meer, "Stochastic Image Pyramids," *Computer Vision, Graphics and Image Processing*, Vol. 45, 1989, pp. 269–294.

[58] C. Mathieu, I.E. Magnin, and C. Baldy-Porcher, "Optimal Stochastic Pyramid: Segmentation of MRI Data," *Medical Imaging VI: Image Processing. Proc. SPIE*, Vol. 1652, 1992, pp. 14–22.

[59] S.Y. Chen and W.C. Lin, "An Expert System for Medical Image Segmentation," *SPIE: Medical Imaging III: Image Processing*, Vol. 1092, 1989, pp. 162–172.

[60] S.P. Raya and G. Herman, "Low Level Segmentation of Multidimensional Images," *Proc. SPIE*, Vol. 1199, 1989, pp. 913–919.

[61] A. Botto et al., "Expert Segmentation for the Extraction of Biomedical Structures in Microscopical Images," *SPIE: Medical Imaging III: Image Processing*, Vol. 1092, 1989, pp. 194–198.

[62] N.D. Efford, "Knowledge Based Segmentation and Feature Analysis of Hand and Wrist Radiographs," *Proc. SPIE*, Vol. 1905, 1993, pp. 596–607.

[63] J.K. Samarabandu, R.S. Acharya, and P.C. Cheng, "Visualization and Interactive Exploration of md Confocal Images," *Computerized Medical Imaging and Graphics*, Vol. 17, No. 3, 1993, pp. 183–188.

[64] R.S. Acharya, "Mathematical Morphology for MD Image Analysis," in *Image Processing* Vol. 1092, *Medical Imaging III*, SPIE, 1989, pp. 338–350.

[65] R.S. Acharya et al., "Multi-Dimensional Image Analysis of Confocal Images," *Trans. Royal Microscopical Society*, Vol. 1, July 1990, pp. 289–292.

[66] R.S. Acharya, "3D Segmentation Algorithms, in *Signal Processing and Pattern Recognition in Nondestructive Evaluation of Materials*, C. H. Chen, ed., Springer-Verlag, Berlin, 1987, pp. 255–291.

[67] D.H. Ballard, "Strip Trees: A Hierarchical Representation for Curves," *Comm. ACM*, Vol. 24, May 1981, pp. 310–321.

[68] R.C. Gonzales and P. Wintz, *Digital Image Processing*, Addison Wesley, Reading, Mass., 1977.

[69] A.K. Jain, *Fundamentals of Digital Signal Processing*, Prentice Hall, Englewood Cliffs, N.J., 1989.

[70] M. Kass and A. Witkin, "Snakes: Active Contour Models," *Proc. IEEE 1st Int'l Conf. Computer Vision*, IEEE Computer Society Press, Los Alamitos, Calif., 1987, pp. 259–268.

[71] H.P. Nii, "Blackboard Systems: The Blackboard Model of Problem Solving and the Evolution of Blackboard Architecture," *The AI Magazine*, Summer 1986, pp. 38–53.

[72] S.K. Pal and R.A. King, "Image Enhancement Using Smoothing with Fuzzy Sets," *IEEE Trans. Systems, Man, and Cybernetics*, Vol. 11, July 1981, pp. 494–501.

[73] S.M. Pizer et al., "Adaptive Histogram Equalization and its Variations," *Computer Vision, Graphics and Image Processing*, Vol. 39, 1987, pp. 355–368.

[74] J. Samarabandu et al., *3D Structural Analysis from Biological Confocal Images*, SPIE, 1991.

[75] J.S. Weszka, "A Survey of Threshold Selection Methods," *Computer Graphics and Image Processing*, Vol. 7, 1978, pp. 259–265.

[76] J.S. Weszka and A. Rosenfeld, Threshold Evaluation Techniques," *IEEE Trans. Systems Man and Cybernetics*" Vol. 8, 1978, pp. 622–629.

[77] L.A. Zadeh, et al., *Fuzzy Sets and their Application to Cognitive and Decision Processes*, Academic Press, New York, N.Y., 1975.

[78] J.B. Zimmerman, "Effectiveness of Adaptive Contrast Enhancement," PhD thesis, Dept. of Computer Science, Univ. of North Carolina, 1985.

[79] S.W. Zucker, "Region Growing: Childhood and Adolescence," *Computer Vision, Graphics, and Image Processing*, 1976, pp. 382–399.

[80] Y.F. Wang, "Characterzing Three-Dimensional Surface Structures form Visual Images," *IEEE Trans. Pattern Analysis and Machine Intelligence*, Vol. 13, No. 1, 1991, pp. 52–60.

[81] P.C. Cheng et al., "Visualization in Biomedical Microscopies," *Chapter 3-D Image Visualization in Light Microscopy and X-ray Micro-Tomography*, Andres Kriete, ed., VCH, Weinheim, Federal Republic of Germany, 1992, pp. 361–398.

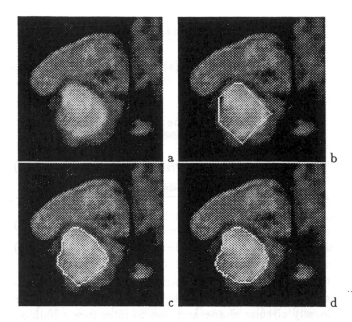

Figure 2: The energy minimization process: (a) original slice, (b) initial contour, (c) contour after two iterations, and (d) final contour.

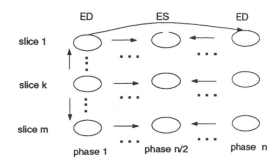

Figure 3: Spatial and temporal propagation in a cardiac study.

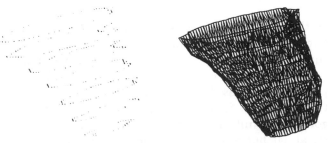

Figure 4: Left: slices are stacked together in 3D space. Right: polyhedral surface made by triangulated slices.

their uncertainty windows. For a closed contour, we run DP twice (two-loop DP), once with one point fixed and the second time by fixing another point. This recovers a closed contour by moving all the given points. Propagation through space is trivial to do by sampling the input contour, and running DP to recover the final contour. However, the DP algorithm is slow due to the larger search space and the global optimization. We use multiscale analysis, where DP is run on the coarse level to reduce the search space by a quarter. The results from the coarse scale are brought down the multiscale pyramid by running DP in smaller search windows. Although the result is no longer guaranteed to be optimal, we have found that it's very close to the optimal result. The speed up achieved by multiscale analysis makes the two-loop DP feasible in our system.

3   Cardiac Study Analysis

Having described the individual segmentation algorithms (SD and DP), we now describe the overall analysis of a cardiac study. We have incorporated the two algorithms into a user interface that allows the user to interactively specify starting contours and invoke various propagation schemes. Figure 5(*top*) shows a snapshot of the user interface with all the pop up windows. A summary of the complete process is shown in

Figure 1. As explained before, the user draws a contour on an ED slice and presses the spatial propagation button. This invokes the multiscale DP algorithm for the inner wall and the SD algorithm for the outer wall. The resulting contour is then propagated above and below the starting slice. The propagation scheme is shown in Figure 3.

After the ED phase is segmented, the contours from each slice position are propagated in time, always proceeding from ED to ES. Thus propagation proceeds in opposite direction during diastole (see Figure 3). The temporal propagation uses the SD algorithm and segments the entire study. Contours from the segmented study can be stacked together and triangulated to obtain 3-D surfaces corresponding to inner and outer walls (see Figure 4). The polyhedral surface can be displayed in a continued loop to generate 3-D visualization of the beating heart. It can also be directly used to compute volume enclosed by the surface. Alternately, voxels in the image can be counted to approximate the volume. We computed volumes using both methods and the results were found to tally closely. The ejection fraction and myocardial mass were computed from the volume measurements.

4 Results on a Patient Study

We have analyzed seven patient studies with our system and obtained very encouraging results. We now present the results of analyzing a patient study having 12 phases with 10 slices per phase. The results from ED to ES (6 phases) and the volume graph are shown in Figure 5. The diagnostic quantities for the patient were: myocardial mass: 216.53 g, ED volume: 100 ml, ES volume: 25 ml, and ejection fraction: 75.46.

5 Conclusions and future work

We presented a complete cardiac MR segmentation system using deformable models. We are currently testing a method for automatic initialization of the ventricular boundary. Our long term plans include using a 3-D physically based deformable model to segment 2-D slices. With respect to wall motion analysis, we are looking at both local and global approaches. Computation of stress and other motion parameters seem to be very promising from SPAMM data.

References

[1] A.A. Amini, S. Tehrani, and T. Weymouth. Using dynamic programming for minimizing the energy of active contours in the presence of hard constraints. In *Proc. of the 3rd Int. Conf. on Computer Vision*, 1990.

[2] D. Geiger, A. Gupta, L. A. Costa, and J. Vlontzos. Dynamic programming for detecting, tracking and matching deformable contours. Tech. Report SCR-93-TR-443, Siemens Corporate Research, Princeton, NJ, 1993.

[3] W.E. Higgins, N. Chung, and E.L. Ritman. Extraction of left ventricular chamber from 3-d ct images of the heart. *IEEE Trans. Med. Imaging*, 9:384–395, 1990.

[4] M. Kass, A. Witkin, and D. Terzopolous. Snakes: Active contour models. In *Proc. First Int. Conf. Computer Vision, London, U.K.*, 1987.

[5] D.R. Thedens, D.J. Skorton, and S.R. Fleagle. A 3D graph searching technique for cardiac border detection in sequential images and its application to magnetic resonance data. In *Computers in Cardiology*, 1991.

[6] L. von Kurowski, A. Singh, and M-Y. Chiu. Cardiac mr image segmentation using deformable models. In *Proc. of the SPIE Conference on Biomedical Image Processing and Biomedical Visualization*, 1992.

Address for correspondence:

Dr. Alok Gupta
Siemens Corporate Research, Inc.
755 College Road East, Princeton, NJ 08540. USA.
Email: alok@scr.siemens.com

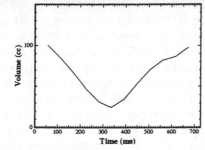

Figure 5: Snapshot of user interface (top). ED to ES Segmentation (middle) and volume graph (bottom).

Features Extraction and Analysis Methods for Sequences of Ultrasound Images

Isabelle L. Herlin and Nicholas Ayache[*]

Our principal motivation is to study time sequences of echocardiographic raw data to track specific anatomical structures. First, we show that the image processing can make direct use of the audio signal data, avoiding loss of information and yielding optimal results. Second, we develop a strategy which takes a time sequence of raw data as input, computes edges, initiates a segmentation of a pre-selected anatomical structure, and uses a deformable model for its temporal tracking. This approach is validated in a real-time sequence of ultrasound images of the heart to track the left auricle and the mitral valve.

Keywords: feature extraction, image processing, ultrasound, edge detection, segmentation, tracking

There is a continuously increasing demand in the automated analysis of 2D and 3D medical images in hospitals[1]. Among these, ultrasound images play a crucial role, because they can be produced at video-rate and therefore allow a dynamic analysis of moving structures. Moreover, the acquisition of these images is non-invasive, and the cost of acquisition is relatively low compared to other medical imaging techniques.

On the other hand, the automated analysis of ultrasound images is a real challenge for active vision, because it combines most of the difficult problems encountered in computer vision in addition to some specific ones related to the acquisition mode:

- images are usually provided in polar geometry instead of cartesian geometry
- images are degraded by a very high level of corrupting noise
- observed objects usually correspond to non-static, non-polyhedric and non-rigid structures.

The geometric transformation (called *scan correction*) which transforms the data from a polar representation to the correct cartesian representation is usually applied through a bilinear interpolation.

We show in this paper the limitations of this scheme, which does not account for the varying resolution of the data, and we propose a new method, called *sonar-space filtering*, which consists of computing the scan conversion with a low-pass filtering of the cartesian image applied directly to the available polar data, and which can be used to optimally reconstruct the data with a chosen level of spatial linear filtering.

Furthermore, we develop a methodology to automatically track a physiological structure on an echocardiographic sequence. Interactivity is used to initiate the process on the first image of the sequence. Then edges are computed, and an approximative segmentation of the structure is obtained by using deterministic algorithms. This information is finally combined with a deformable model to obtain the temporal tracking of the pre-selected structure.

Finally, to further demonstrate the efficiency of our approach, we apply it to difficult time sequence of ultrasound images of the heart to track the left auricle and the mitral valve.

PREVIOUS WORK

Our approach is different from previous work because we directly study the ultrasonic data. More commonly, feature extraction is applied to the cartesian video data. To our knowledge, there is only one study where all processing is performed on sector scans in polar coordinate form. This was published by Taxt[2], and reports noise reduction and segmentation in time-varying ultrasound images. But a comparative study of scan correction methods to obtain cartesian images has apparently

INRIA, B.P. 105, 78153 Le Chesnay, France
Paper received: 26 May 1992

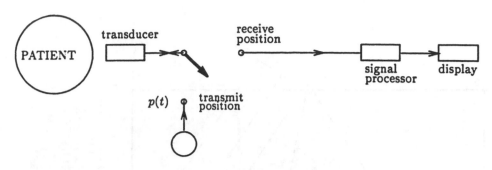

Figure 1. Elementary pulsed ultrasonic system

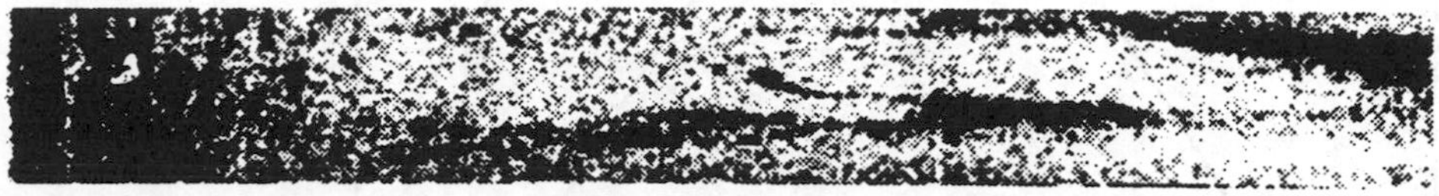

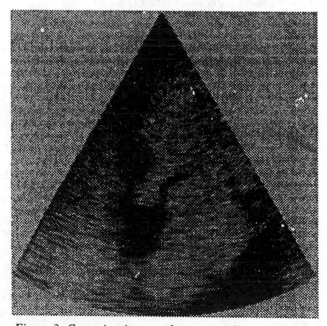

Figure 2. Ultrasound image on raw data

not been pursued yet. For cartesian images, the most commonly used approach to obtain the contour of left ventricle (in echocardiography) is radical search[3-5]: the procedure starts from a point inside the heart chamber and searches along different radial lines for edge points. The best-known dynamic approach is that of Zhang and Geiser[6], who compute temporal cooccurrences to obtain both stationary points and moving points. The temporal information has also been used to filter images obtained at the same instant of the cardiac cycle[7].

ACQUISITION OF AN ECHOGRAPHIC IMAGES

The purpose of this section is to present some primary characteristics of image formation using echographic technologies.

A basic imaging system, called a pulsed system, is illustrated in Figure 1. When the switch is in the transmit position, the pulse waveform $p(t)$ excites the transducer[8].* This results in a wavefront that is propagated in the body. The transducer produces a relatively narrow beam of propagation whose angular direction of propagation into the body is known. Immediately following the transmission, the system switches to the receive position, using the same transducer. The pulse is attenuated when it propagates through the body. When the wavefront hits a discontinuity, a scattered wave is produced. This scattered wave is received by the transducer, and the resultant signal is processed and displayed along a line representing the direction of the beam.

IMAGE REPRESENTATION IN CARTESIAN COORDINATES

The process of converting from the polar coordinates

___

* Other types of echographs using pseudo-random correlation are studied in the literature.[9]

representation to the cartesian coordinates representation is necessary for the convenience of the users. Physicians are accustomed to viewing images in Cartesian data, and it would be difficult for them to interpret polar data. Moreover, visualization hardware and image processing algorithms are designed for data in cartesian coordinates.

Let us suppose that M different orientations are used to obtain an echocardiographic image, and that each return signal is digitized to L points. Figure 2 shows an echographic image, with M rows and L columns, obtained with a commercial echographic machine, providing an image represented in polar coordinates. Figure 3 shows the cartesian image corresponding to the same data.

Figure 3. Cartesian image after conversion

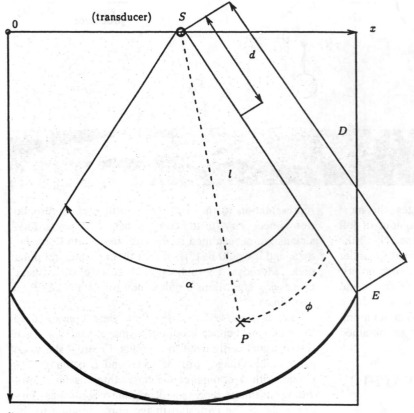

(transducer) *S*

0   *x*

Figure 4. Parameters of the conversion process

Scan conversion requires the knowledge of the following set of parameters (see Figure 4):

- the angular extent of data acquisition wedge α
- minimal distance d for data acquisition
- total distance D for data acquisition (these distances being calculated from the skin)
- the number of rows N desired in the ouput cartesian image (The number of columns will be related to α, and will assume square pixels).

Several methods may be used for the conversion process. Usually, the video image on the echographic machine is obtained by assigning to a cartesian point the grey level of the nearest available point in polar coordinates, or the value of the bilinear interpolation of its four nearest points. In fact, we found that these methods do not make an optimal use of the available original data, and we introduced a new method, called *sonar-space filtering*, which can be used to optimally reconstruct the data with a chosen level of spatial linear filtering.

Conversion by sonar-space filtering

We assume that it is desired that the continuous input cartesian image $I(x, y)$ be filtered by the impulse response filter $f(x, y)$. The resulting image $R(x, y)$, in continuous space, is given by the convolution product:

$$R(x,y) = \int_{-x}^{x} \int_{-x}^{x} f(x-u, y-v) \cdot I(u,v)\mathrm{d}u\, \mathrm{d}v \qquad (1)$$

However, the input is only available in the polar coordinate space. We thus apply the following change of variables:

$$\theta = \left(\arctan\left(\frac{y}{x-x_0} \right) - \left(\frac{\pi-\alpha}{2} \right) \right) / \Delta_\alpha$$

$$\rho = \left(\sqrt{(x-x_0)^2 + y^2} \right) * e - \Delta_N$$

168

where $\Delta_N = d * (L - l) / (D - d)$ represents the distance from the surface of the skin where the acquisition process begins, measured in pixel units along a scan line of the raw data, $\Delta_\alpha = \alpha/(M - 1)$ is the angular difference between two successive angular positions of the probe, and $e = D/(D - d)\ (L - 1)/(N - 1)$ performs the change of pixel sampling rates along the axial direction of the beam, according to the desired height N of the cartesian image.

We obtain:

$$R(x, y) = \int_0^{2\pi} \int_0^x f(x - u(\rho, \theta), y - v(\rho, \theta)) \cdot$$
$$I(\rho, \theta) \cdot |J(\rho, \theta)| \mathrm{d}\rho\, \mathrm{d}\theta \qquad (2)$$

Here $|J(\rho, \theta)|$ is the determinant of the Jacobian matrix corresponding to the inverse transformation of variables:

$$x = \left(\frac{\rho + \Delta_N}{e}\right) \cos\left(\theta \Delta_\alpha + \frac{\pi - \alpha}{2}\right) + x_0$$
$$y = \left(\frac{\rho + \Delta_N}{e}\right) \sin\left(\theta \Delta_\alpha + \frac{\pi - \alpha}{2}\right)$$

It is easily seen that

$$|J(\rho, \theta)| = \frac{(\rho + \Delta_N) * \Delta_\alpha}{e^2}$$

We have transformed the convolution in the cartesian coordinates to an infinite integral in polar coordinates, corresponding to the domain of the raw data.

Once the two-dimensional convolution filter f is chosen, we define its rectangle of essential support: say a rectangular window of width $2X$ and $2Y$. Outside this region of support the absolute value of the impulse response must be lower than a pre-selected a threshold s, i.e.,

$$|f(u, v)| < s \quad \text{if } ((|u| \geq X) \text{ OR } (|v| \geq Y))$$

Therefore the integral is approximated by a finite integral over the domain

$$(x - X \leq u \leq x + X) \text{ AND } (y - Y \leq v \leq y + Y)$$

The filter is also sampled in this domain to approximate the integral by a discrete summation. Filtered numerical outputs are evaluated at original data point locations within the continuous domain.

We thus obtain the following equation:

$$R(x, y) = C \sum_k f(x - u(\rho_k, \theta_k) y - v(\rho_k, \theta_k)) \cdot$$
$$I(\rho_k, \theta_k) \cdot |\text{Jac}(\rho_k, \theta_k)|. \qquad (3)$$

where the summation is over the discrete collection of point (ρ_k, θ_k) in polar coordinates, where C is used to normalize the data, and:

$$|J(\rho_k + \theta_k)| = \frac{(\rho_k + \Delta_N) * \Delta_N}{e^2}$$

We have transformed the computation of $R(x, y)$ into a discrete summation on a window of size $2X$ by $2Y$, making use of image data only at points where it is defined in the polar coordinate domain. Note that for the raw data, or more generally for any sonar-like data, the sampling of the filter is not regular along the x and y axes, but it rather conforms to the sampling density of raw data. In this formula, the $|J(\rho_k, \theta_k)|$ value represents the surface area of the polar pixel patch in the cartesian domain. We present in the following subsections the different values that we have chosen for the function f for different processing of the echocardiographic raw data.

Visualization application

In practice, the convolution filter $f(x, y)$ is typically separable, and is denoted by $f(x)g(y)$. Then, classical 1D smoothing and derivation filters can be used.

For visualization applications of sonar-space filtering, we used the Deriche's smoothing function[10] with $f(x) = g(x) = L(x)$:

$$L(x) = k_2(\alpha \sin(\omega|x|) + \omega \cos(\omega|x|))^{-\alpha|x|} \qquad (4)$$

The conversion algorithm simultaneously performs a conversion to cartesian coordinates and a smoothing of the data (whose amplitude can be adjusted with α), thus producing a cartesian image with a reduced speckle. Other smoothing functions could be used instead.

It will be noted that the visualization quality is not significantly different, or better, with sonar-space filtering than with classical bi-linear interpolation method. But our objective is not to improve visualization, but rather to improve automatic analysis of echocardiographic sequences.

169

Edge detection application

For further automatic boundary tracking, our goal is to use spatio-temporal approaches[11]. A time-varying edge may be represented as a surface in 3D space, in which x and y are two spatial dimensions (in the cartesian coordinates space) and t is the temporal dimension. We modify Deriche's edge detector for this goal. Another approach could be to generalize Deriche's detector with spatio-temporal functions as in Hwang and Clark[12]. We denote by G_x and G_y the two spatial components of the gradient vector, and $I(x, y, t)$ the 3D grey-level function. Let D be the Deriche differentiation filter and L the associated smoothing filter:

$$L(x) = k(\alpha \sin(\omega|x|) + \omega \cos(\omega|x|))^{-\alpha|x|} \qquad (5)$$

$$D(x) = k \sin(\omega|x|)^{-\alpha|x|} \qquad (6)$$

The two components of the gradient vector have the following expression:

$$G_x = (D_x L_y L_t) \otimes I(x, y, t)$$

$$Gy = (L_x D_y L_t) \otimes I(x, y, t)$$

where the subscripts are used to explain along which axis the corresponding filter is applied. Each component is obtained by differentiation in the associated direction and filtering in the other spatial direction and temporal directions.

The norm of the gradient is defined by:

$$N(x,y,t) = \sqrt{G_x^2 + G_y^2}$$

The edges are obtained as local maxima of the gradient norm in the direction of the 2D gradient vector. The temporal dimension is only used to smooth the result. This produces a significant image enhancement in regions that are not moving too fast.

We denote by α_x, α_y, and α_t the filtering parameters of the Deriche filters (cf. equations (5) and (6)) for the respective axes x, y and t. Since the 2D space is homogeneous, we can choose $\alpha_x = \alpha_y$. The value of α_t is independent, and must be chosen according to the temporal resolution.

TEMPORAL TRACKING

At this stage we assume that we will work on ultrasound cartesian images and on edges represented in a cartesian space, whatever the methods used to obtain this information.

Our objective is to perform temporal tracking of a pre-selected anatomical structure by combining different kinds of information. First, we want to obtain an approximate segmentation of the structure by using simple deterministic processing. Second, we want to use the edges computed directly on the raw data. These will be combined by a regularization process that takes an initial segmentation and deforms it from its initial position to make it better conform to the pre-detected edges. This approach is the idea behind the use of deformable models.

Estimation of the boundaries of the anatomical structure

To obtain a crude estimation of the boundaries of anatomical structures, we use techniques from mathematical morphology. The model of a cardiac cavity is very simple. This is an ovoid region with low intensity. These regioris cannot be obtained by simple thresholding because of the speckle noise. But the fine structures of the speckle may be easily suppressed by the following morphological operations[13]:

- A first order opening eliminates the small bright structures on dark background.
- The dual operation (first order closing) suppresses the small dark structures.

After these operations, a simple thresholding gives an image C where all the cardiac cavities are represented in white. This detection can be refined by the use of higher level information. The specialist points out, using a computer mouse, the chosen cavity on the first image of the sequence. The whole cavity is then obtained by a conditional dilatation which begins at this point.

Use of a deformable model

The previous operations usually provide an approximately-correct but locally-inaccurate positioning of the structure boundaries. In order to improve this crude segmentation to an accurate determination of the boundaries, we use the deformable models of Cohen and Cohen[14], in the spirit of Kass et al.[15]

The deformable model is initialized in the first image by the crude approximation of the structure boundary. It evolves under the action of image forces, which are counter-balanced by its own internal forces to preserve its regularity. Image forces are computed as the derivative of an attraction potential related to the previously computed spatio-temporal edges. Typically, the potential is inversely proportional to the distance of the nearest edge point.

Deformable models may be used independently on each frame or iteratively on the sequence: once the model has converged in the first frame, its final position is used as the initial one in the next frame, and the process is repeated.

EXPERIMENTAL RESULTS FOR SONAR-SPACE FILTERING

This section gives the results obtained by bilinear interpolation and sonar-space filtering evaluated in terms of the visualization and edge detection capabilities of the methods.

The simple example concerns polar scanning of a thin dark structure (represented by horizontal lines in polar data) in a white background. Figure 5 presents the polar data: 512 rays of 128 pixels. The dark structure has a width of three rays. Figure 6 presents edges obtained on cartesian images reconstructed by bilinear interpolation and sonar-space filtering.

Because bilinear interpolation does not make use of all available polar data, information is lost which can never be retrieved by further processing such as edge detection or segmentation.

To conclude this section with ultrasound data, one can see in Figure 7 the reconstructed image using sonar-space filtering with $\alpha = 1$, and the same image with the detected edges superimposed. The value of the parameter α is determined experimentally, but is the same for all ultrasound images provided by an echographic machine.

EXPERIMENTAL RESULTS FOR TEMPORAL TRACKING

We first note that temporal smoothing reduces some local distortions on the deeper edges of the left auricle (compare the bottom right cavity of Figure 8). Simultaneously, temporal smoothing can cause a problem for the mitral valve (middle thin structure of Figure 8), which is moving fast with respect to the temporal resolution. The strategy is thus to use temporal smoothing only to study cavities, and to apply spatial gradient techniques to study fast moving structures like the valves.

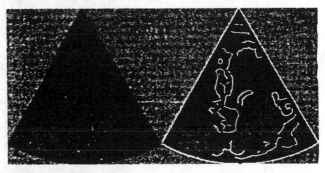

Figure 7. Cartesian image and best edges obtained by sonar-space filtering

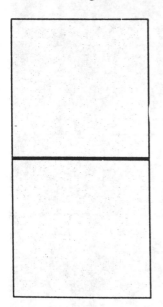

Figure 5. Polar data

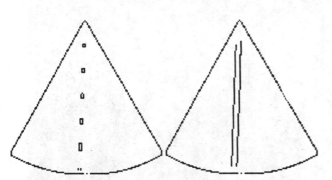

Figure 6. Left: edges on bilinear interpolation image; right: sonar-space filtering

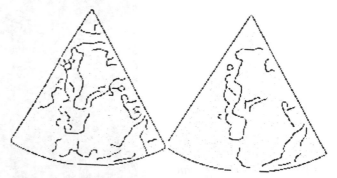

Figure 8. Left: no temporal smoothing of edges; right: temporal smoothing of edges

171

Second, we present the use of deformable models to analyze echocardiographic data after the scan-correction process has been applied.

For structures moving slowly (heart cavities), deformable models may be applied iteratively using an initialization process and the results of edge detection. The software of Cohen and Cohen[14] requires three parameters. The elasticity and rigidity coefficients model the properties of the cavity boundary curve. The third coefficient is a weight representing the attraction of the edges. The results of this application of the deformable model may be seen in the first frame of Figure 12 for the segmentation of left auricle. The result is then used to initialize the second frame. The parameters are the same and the process is repeated sequentially through all frames, as it can be seen in Figure 12.

For structures moving fast (mitral valve), deformable models are applied independently on each frame and results of these applications may be seen in Figure 11.

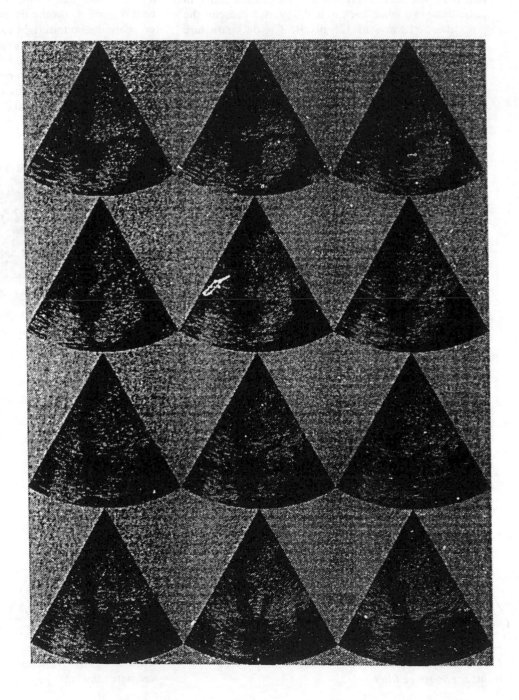

Figure 9: Data after scan-correction

172

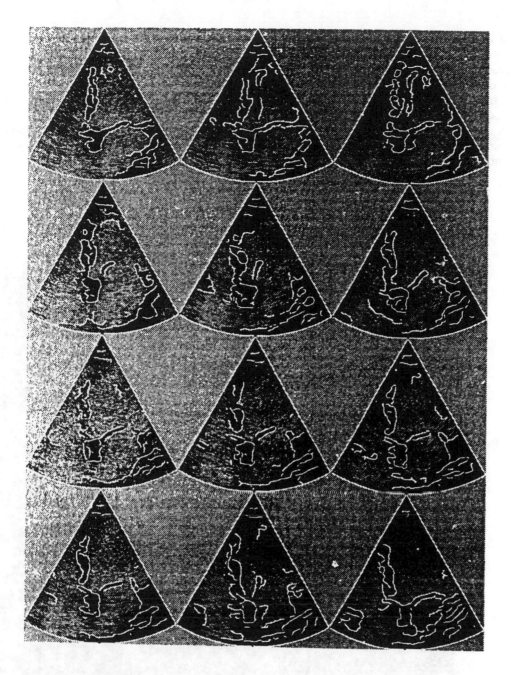

Figure 10: Edges

We summarize the advantages of using deformable models to analyze echocardiographic data:

- Deformable models allow a compromise between an initial segmentation based on grey levels and texture properties, and an edge detection process performed directly on raw data.

- The values of the parameters required by the deformable model are the same for both the regularization application on a single frame and for the tracking application on a sequence. They can be chosen interactively on the first image of the sequence.

The methods presented in this paper were applied to four different sequences obtained from two different echographs. The data presented here were obtained in a polar coordinate form on a VIGMED echograph at Henri Mondor hospital in Creteil, France. A sequence contains 38 images from a cardiac cycle. Figure 9 shows a cartesian representation of the original data. (Only one image in four is displayed.) The left heart cavities (auricle and ventricle) and the mitral valve are visible in a typical image. Our aim is to track them. Tracking of the latter structure is successfully achieved in this example due to the fact that the edges were obtained from sonar-space filtering. Other methods (bilinear interpolation followed by edge detection) generally do not give accurate edges for the deep structures, and cannot therefore be used for further temporal tracking. Edges are shown in Figure 10, and temporal tracking is presented in Figures 11 and 12.

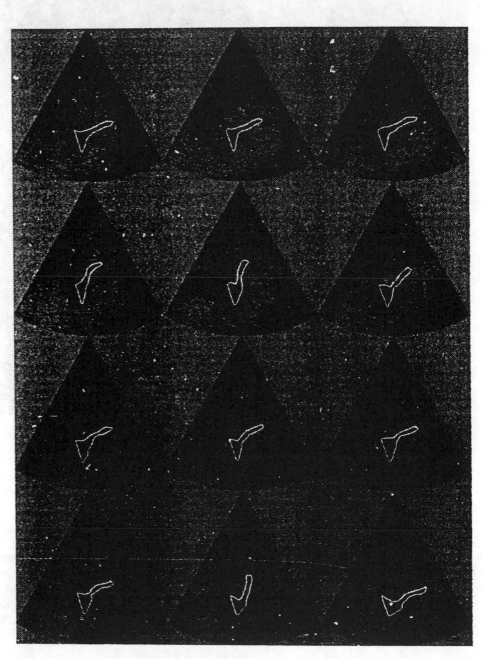

Figure 11. Temporal tracking of the mitral valve

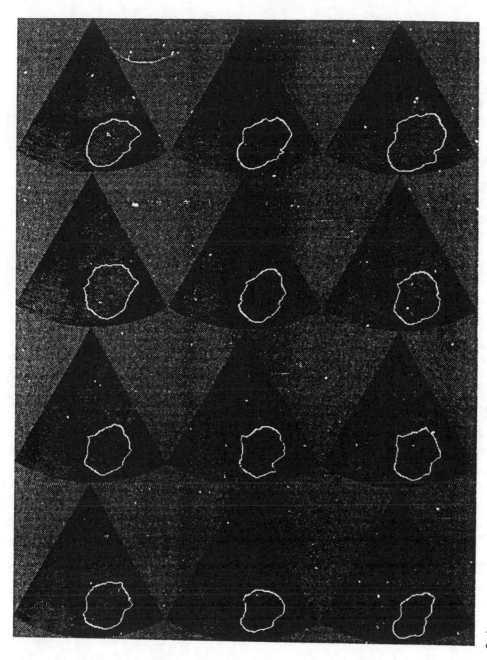

Figure 12. Temporal tracking of the left auricle

CONCLUSIONS

We have showed in this paper the importance of using an appropriate conversion method when dealing with images produced in polar coordinates. We introduced a new method which computes both the conversion and a convolution of the polar data with a smoothing filter in a single process. Using this approach, the quality of the edges and features that are extracted can be enhanced. This approach is more flexible because it allows a vari-

able level of smoothing to be chosen according to the actual resolution of the original data. This is not the case when an additional smoothing is required after a conversion by other algorithms. We showed the enhancement produced on edge detection by our approach.

Finally, we demonstrated the effectiveness of this approach by solving a complete application. We used morphological operators to initialize a deformable model in the first image of a time sequence. Then we applied our edge detector and we let the deformable

175

model converge toward the detected edges. Using the solution as an initialization in the following image, we tracked the left auricle boundary in a sequence of 38 images.

Our future research will concentrate on the generalization of these methods to be applied to 3D ultrasound images produced in spherical coordinates

ACKNOWLEDGEMENTS

We gratefully acknowledge Gabriel Pelle (INSERM, CHU Henri MONDOR, FRANCE) for providing the data and for helpful discussions, and Robert Hummel for a significant improvement of the final manuscript.

This work was partially supported by MATRA Espace and Digital Equipment Corporation.

REFERENCES

1. Ayache, N., Boissonnat, J.D., Cohen, L., Geiger, B., Levy-Vehel, J., Monga O., and Sander, P., "Steps toward the automatic interpretation of 3-D images," in H. Fuchs, K. Hohne, and S. Pizer, (eds), *3D Imaging in Medicine*, Springer-Verlag, Berlin, (1990), pp 107–120.

2. Taxt, T., Lundervold, A., and Angelsen, B., "Noise reduction and segmentation in time-varying ultrasound images," *Proc. 10th Int'l Conf. Pattern Recognition*, Atlantic City, New Jersey, USA, June 1990.

3. Faure, F., Gambotto, J.P., Montserrat, G., and Patat F., "Space medical facility study," Technical report, ESQ, final report, 6961/86/NL/PB, 1988.

4. Buda, A.J., Delp, E.J., Meyer, J.M., Jenkins J.M., Smith, D.N., Bookstein, F.L., and Pitt, B., "Automatic computer processing of digital 2-dimensional echocardiograms," *Amer. J. Cardiol.*, Vol. 51, (1983), pp 383–389.

5. Jenkins, J.M., Qian, O., Besozzi, M., Delp, E.J., and Buda, A.J., "Computer processing of echocardiographic images for automated edge detection of left ventricular boundaries," *Proc. Computers in Cardiology*, Vol. 8, 1981.

6. Zhang, L.F. and Geiser, E.A., "An approach to optimal threshold selection on a sequence of two-dimensional echocardiographic images, *IEEE Trans. Biomedical Engineering*, Vol. 29, August 1982.

7. Unser, M., Dong L., Pelle, G., Brun, P., and Eden, M., "Restoration on echocardiagrams using time warping and periodic averaging on a normalized time scale," *Medical Imaging*, Newport Beach, Calif, 1989.

8. Macovski, A., *Medical Imaging Systems*, Prentice Hall, N.J., 1983.

9. Newhouse, V.L., *Progress in Medical Imaging*, Springer Verlag, Berlin, 1988.

10. Deriche, R. "Using Canny's criteria to derive a recursively implemented optimal edge detector," *Int'l J. Computer Vision*, Vol. 1, No. 2, May 1987.

11. Monga, O. and Deriche R., "3D edge detection using recursive filtering: application to scanner images," Technical Report 930, INRIA, November 1988.

12. Hwang T. and Clark J.J., "A spatio~temporal generalization of Canny's edge detector," *Proc. 10th Int'l Conf. Pattern Recognition*, Atlantic City, New Jersey, June 1990.

13. Serra, J., *Progress in Medical Imaging*, Springer-Verlag, Berlin, 1988.

14. Cohen, L.D. and Cohen, I., "A finite element method applied to new active contour models and 3D reconstruction from cross sections," *Proc. Int'l Conf. Computer Vision*, Osaka, Japan, December 1990.

15. Kass, M., Witkin, A., and Terzopoulos, D., "Snakes: Active contour models, *Proc. 1st Int'l Conf. Computer Vision*, UK, 1987, pp 259–268.

Using Deformable Surfaces to Segment 3-D Images and Infer Differential Structures

Isaac Cohen,* Laurent D. Cohen,§ and Nicholas Ayache*

*INRIA, Domaine de Voluceau, Rocquencourt, B.P. 105, 78153 Le Chesnay Cedex, France; and § CEREMADE, U.R.A. CNRS 749, Université Paris IX–Dauphine, Place du Marechal de Lattre de Tassigny, 75775 Paris Cedex, France

Received August 7, 1991; accepted February 20, 1992

In this paper, we use a 3-D deformable model, which evolves in 3-D images, under the action of internal forces (describing some elasticity properties of the surface), and external forces attracting the surface toward some detected edgels. Our formalism leads to the minimization of an energy which is expressed as a functional. We use a variational approach and a conforming finite element method to actually express the surface in a discrete basis of continuous functions. This leads to reduced computational complexity and better numerical stability. The power of the approach to segmenting 3-D images is demonstrated by a set of experimental results on various complex medical 3-D images. Another contribution of this approach is the possibility to infer easily the differential structure of the segmented surface. As we end up with an analytical description of class $\mathscr{C}^\infty$ of the surface almost everywhere, this allows us to compute, for instance, its first and second fundamental forms. From this, one can extract a curvature primal sketch of the surface, including some intrinsic features which can be used as landmarks for 3-D image interpretation. © 1992 Academic Press, Inc.

1. INTRODUCTION

We propose a deformable 3-D shape model which can be used to extract reliable surfaces in 3-D images and infer a differential structure on them.

Usually, 3-D images are given as a set of intensity voxels (volume elements). A 3-D edge detector, after a *local* image analysis [27, 36], provides a set of 3-D edgels (edge elements). These edgels can be considered as the trace of a certain number of surfaces. One is then confronted with a dual problem:

1. Select edgels belonging to the same surface trace; this is the segmentation problem.

2. Recover a continuous and differentiable description of each surface; this yields a path between the original sparse discrete data and the ability to compute a differential structure useful for interpretation [1, 19, 20].

Both questions were analyzed by Sander and Zucker [31], who proposed solving (1) by a connectivity analysis and (2) by the fitting of a set of local quadratic models. But difficulties arise when the connectivity analysis fails because edges are too sparse and also when the model is too local to reliably describe a complex shape.

Another approach to solving a similar problem in 2-D consists of introducing an active deformable model [22], which solves the segmentation problem (1) assuming that an initial estimate is provided (an initial solution might be provided by several means, including user interactivity, which is usually encouraged in medical applications), and the interpolation problem (2) when the curve is expressed in a basis of continuous functions [14, 28]. Such models were generalized in 2½-D and 3-D [34, 33], where the deformable surface is evolving under the forces computed on a 2-D image or a set of 2-D images.

In contrast with the methods of reconstruction based on a 2-D slice-by-slice approach [6, 13, 14], we use, in this paper, a 3-D deformable model, which evolves in 3-D images, under the action of internal forces (describing some elasticity properties of the surface), and external forces attracting the surface toward some detected edgels. This formalism leads to the minimization of an energy which is expressed as a functional. We use a variational approach and a conforming finite element method to express the surface in a discrete basis of continuous functions. This method allows us to perform an "adaptive subdivision" of the parametrization domain without adding nodal points and consequently without increasing the size of the linear system we solve. This leads to reduced computational complexity and better numerical stability than those of a classical finite difference method.

The power of the approach to segment 3-D images is demonstrated by a set of experimental results on complex medical 3-D images (see also [11]).

Another contribution of this approach is the ability to easily infer the differential structure of the segmented surface. As we end up with an analytical description of class $\mathscr{C}^\infty$ of the surface almost everywhere (except between two finite element patches, where the representation is only of class $\mathcal{C}^1$; i.e., the tangent plane is continuous), we can compute for instance, its first and second fundamental forms [17]. From this, one can extract a curvature primal sketch of the surface [30, 8], including some intrinsic features which can be used as landmarks for 3-D image interpretation [2, 19].

Last but not least, a careful analysis of our external forces (those which attract the deformable surface toward the edges) shows some intriguing connections with the properties of minimal surfaces: if the deformable surface is a minimal surface (i.e., a surface whose mean curvature is everywhere zero), then it satisfies also the definition of an edge surface.

The paper is organized as follows: We first define the 3-D deformable model (Section 2) and then give an appropriate external force (Section 3) and its relationship with 3-D edge points (Section 4). We show then how to solve this minimization problem by a conforming finite element method (Section 5) and give a correct choice of the regularization parameters (Section 6). An algorithmic complexity comparison between the conforming finite element method and the finite difference method is given in Section 7. Section 8 indicate how to infer the differential structure of the 3-D images from the obtained surface. Finally Section 9 describes a set of experimental results on synthetical and complex medical 3-D images.

2. ENERGY-MINIMIZING SURFACES

A 3-D image is given by a set of intensity voxels, or as a set of successive 2-D cross sections. In our first work [13, 14] we processed 3-D images as a set of successives 2-D images. This is a familiar approach which is also used in tracking methods [3, 12, 21], but this method is not effective and cannot take into account the spatial homogeneity of the data. In the following we consider the 3-D image data as a set of pixel and the boundaries of a 3-D image are described by a set of surfaces.

A deformable surface model allows us to characterize these surfaces [33, 34]. This characterization consists of determining the location and the shape of the surface.

In the following we restrict ourselves to parameterized surfaces, since any 3-D surface has a local parameterization [17].

This model is defined by a space of admissible deformations Ad and a functional E to minimize. This functional E represents the energy of the model. A surface v is defined by the mapping

$$\Omega = [0, 1] \times [0, 1] \to R^3$$

$$(s, r) \longmapsto v(s, r) = (x(s, r), y(s, r), z(s, r))$$

and the associated energy E is given by

$$E: \mathrm{Ad} \to R$$

$$v \longmapsto E(v) = \int_\Omega w_{10} \left| \frac{\partial v}{\partial s} \right|^2 + w_{01} \left| \frac{\partial v}{\partial r} \right|^2 + 2 w_{11} \left| \frac{\partial^2 v}{\partial s \partial r} \right|^2$$

$$+ w_{20} \left| \frac{\partial^2 v}{\partial s^2} \right|^2 + w_{02} \left| \frac{\partial^2 v}{\partial r^2} \right|^2 + P(v(s, r)) ds\, dr,$$

where P is the potential associated with the external forces. The external forces refer to the forces which allow the surface to localize the image attributes. So, if we want the surface to be attracted by 3-D edge points, the potential P is expressed in terms of a 3-D gradient image. The internal forces acting on the shape of the surface depend on the coefficients w_{ij} such that the elasticity is determined by (w_{10}, w_{01}), the rigidity by (w_{20}, w_{02}), and the resistance to twist by w_{11}. Therefore the coefficients w_{ij} determine the mechanical properties of the surface. These coefficients are also called regularization parameters. We can also constrain the surface structure by adjusting boundary conditions (for instance, to create a cylinder or a torus).

A local minimum v of E satisfies the associated Euler–Lagrange equation

$$- \frac{\partial}{\partial s} \left(w_{10} \frac{\partial v}{\partial s} \right) - \frac{\partial}{\partial r} \left(w_{01} \frac{\partial v}{\partial r} \right) + 2 \frac{\partial^2}{\partial s \partial r} \left(w_{11} \frac{\partial^2 v}{\partial s \partial r} \right)$$

$$+ \frac{\partial^2}{\partial s^2} \left(w_{20} \frac{\partial^2 v}{\partial s^2} \right) + \frac{\partial^2}{\partial r^2} \left(w_{02} \frac{\partial^2 v}{\partial r^2} \right) = -\nabla P(v) \qquad (1)$$

$$+ \text{ boundary conditions},$$

which represents the necessary condition for a minimum $(E'(v) = 0)$. A solution of Eq. (1) can be seen as either realizing the equilibrium between internal (or regularizing) and external forces or reaching a minimum of the energy E.

The boundary conditions constrain the surface structure by specifying different properties of the surface at the boundaries of the parameterization domain $\Omega = [0, 1] \times [0, 1]$. For example, setting $v(s, 0) = v(s, 1)$, $\forall s \in [0, 1]$, or $v(0, r) = v(1, r)$, $\forall r \in [0, 1]$, constrains the surface v to have a cylindrical structure. The other structures such torus or sphere can be obtained in a similar way.

Since the energy function is not convex, there may be many local minima of E. The Euler–Lagrange equation (1) may characterize any such local minimum. But as we are interested in finding a 3-D contour in a given area, we assume in fact that we have a rough *prior* estimation of the surface. This estimate is used as initial data for the associated evolution equation in which we add a temporal parameter t:

$$\frac{\partial v}{\partial t} - \frac{\partial}{\partial s}\left(w_{10}\frac{\partial v}{\partial s}\right) - \frac{\partial}{\partial r}\left(w_{01}\frac{\partial v}{\partial r}\right) + 2\frac{\partial^2}{\partial s\,\partial r}\left(w_{11}\frac{\partial^2 v}{\partial s\,\partial r}\right)$$

$$+ \frac{\partial^2}{\partial s^2}\left(w_{20}\frac{\partial^2 v}{\partial s^2}\right) + \frac{\partial^2}{\partial r^2}\left(w_{02}\frac{\partial^2 v}{\partial r^2}\right) = -\nabla P(v) \qquad (2)$$

$v(0, s, r) = v_0(s, r)$ initial estimation
+ boundary conditions.

A solution to the static problem is found when the solution $v(t, s, r)$ converges as t tends to infinity; then the term $\partial v/\partial t$ vanishes, providing a solution of the static problem.

This evolution equation can also be seen as a gradient descent algorithm starting with the initial estimate v_0 (see Section 5.3).

3. DEFINING THE POTENTIAL P

The potential P is such that the force $F(v) = -\nabla P(v)$ must attract the surface to the image attributes that we are looking for. Our main goal is the extraction of "good" edge points (i.e., to be able to remove spurious edge points, while ensuring connected contours). Thus the surface must be attracted by edge points and minimize the energy

$$E_{\text{ext}} = \int\int_\Omega P(v(s, r))ds\,dr. \qquad (3)$$

For this purpose the authors of [22] set the potential $P = -|\nabla\mathcal{I}|^2$ so that edge points will minimize E_{ext}, where $\mathcal{I}$ is the 3-D image convolved with a Gaussian function. For numerical stability (a complete discussion is given in [13, 14]) we normalize the force

$$F(v) = -k\frac{\nabla P}{\|\nabla P\|},$$

where k is a parameter which allows us to tune the attraction force. Now, all the edge points including spurious ones have the same ability to attract the surface. But spurious points generally form small connected components in 3-D images; consequently, when the surface converges toward the real contours, all these points first attract the surface and then are ignored by the regularization effect of the algorithm.

Another way to make the edge points attract the surface is by using a Chamfer distance [7] or an Euclidean distance [16] image. The distance image is obtained by computing at each image point (pixel) the distance to the nearest edge point (these points are obtained by a local edge detector). These distances allow us to compute at each image point the attraction force to the nearest edgels. This force can be computed in different ways,

allowing us to test different forces according to the rate of convergence of the algorithm. For instance,

$$P(v(s, r)) = -e^{-d(v(s,r))^2}$$

produces a slow convergence whereas

$$P(v(s, r)) = \frac{-1}{d(v(s, r))} \quad \text{and} \quad P \equiv -1 \text{ if } d(v(s, r)) = 0$$

produces a faster convergence [$d(v(s, r))$ denotes the distance between $v(s, r)$ and the nearest edge whereas the smallest distance between two distinct points is one pixel]. The use of such attraction potentials is detailed in [15].

4. MINIMIZING SURFACES AND 3-D IMAGE EDGE POINTS

In the previous section we showed how to choose correctly the potential P such that the surface will localize accurately the edge points. Here we comment on the relationship between the surface minimizing the energy of external forces E_{ext} and 3-D edge points. This is a generalization to 3-D surfaces of the result given by Fua and Leclerc [18] for 2-D curves. We use the following definition of the 3-D edges, as proposed by Canny [9].

DEFINITION. A 3-D edge is a surface $\mathcal{S}$ whose points have a maximal gradient magnitude in the direction normal to the surface. All points along the surface $\mathcal{S}$ (called Canny's edge points) satisfy

$$\frac{d|\nabla\mathcal{I}(x(s, r))|}{dN(x(s, r))} = 0, \qquad (4)$$

where $N(x(s, r))$ is the normal to the surface $\mathcal{S}$ parameterized by the application $x(s, r)$ and $\mathcal{I}$ denotes the image $I(x, y, z)$ convolved with a Gaussian.

As in [18], to establish the relation between the energy-minimizing surfaces and this definition, let us define the energy associated to the external forces as

$$E_P(\mathcal{S}) = -\frac{1}{|\mathcal{S}|}\int_\Omega |\nabla\mathcal{I}(x(s, r))|dA, \qquad (5)$$

where $|\mathcal{S}| = \int\int_\Omega |x_s \times x_r|\,ds\,dr$ is the surface area and $dA = \sqrt{EG - F^2}\,ds\,dr$ is the standard surface area measure.

In Appendix A we show that a surface $\mathcal{S}$ is a local minimum of E_P, with respect to infinitesimal deformation, if

$$\frac{d|\nabla \mathcal{I}(x(s, r))|}{dN(x(s, r))} = \frac{eG - 2fF + gE}{EG - F^2}$$

$$\left(|\nabla \mathcal{I}(x(s, r))| - \frac{1}{|\mathcal{S}|} \int_\Omega |\nabla \mathcal{I}(x(s, r))| dA\right), \tag{6}$$

where $E(s, r)$, $F(s, r)$, $G(s, r)$, $e(s, r)$, $f(s, r)$, and $g(s, r)$ are the coefficients of the first and second fundamental forms in the basis $\{x_s, x_r, N\}$ (using the same notations as that in [17]). A remarkable result is that the quotient $(1/2)$ $[(eG - 2fF + gE)/(EG - F^2)]$ is the mean curvature of the surface $\mathcal{S}$.

Equation (6) shows that there exists two very interesting special cases:

1. minimal surfaces (i.e., surfaces with a mean curvature which is everywhere zero) and

2. surfaces whose trace is made of edgels with constant gradient magnitude (then the term within parentheses in Eq. (6) vanishes).

Indeed, in both cases, the second member of Eq. (6) vanishes to zero, which means that Canny's edge points coincide with the minimal external energy of a deformable model.

In practice these are interesting but exceptional academic situations, and the deformable model simply converges toward a solution which is an equilibrium between the applied external forces (corresponding to the energy E_P) and the internal forces, parameterized by the elasticity coefficients w_{ij}.

5. NUMERICAL SOLUTION BY A CONFORMING FINITE ELEMENT METHOD

We consider the same evolution equation as that in Section 2:

$$\frac{\partial v}{\partial t} - \frac{\partial}{\partial s}\left(w_{10}\frac{\partial v}{\partial s}\right) - \frac{\partial}{\partial r}\left(w_{01}\frac{\partial v}{\partial r}\right) + 2\frac{\partial^2}{\partial s \partial r}\left(w_{11}\frac{\partial^2 v}{\partial s \partial r}\right)$$

$$+ \frac{\partial^2}{\partial s^2}\left(w_{20}\frac{\partial^2 v}{\partial s^2}\right) + \frac{\partial^2}{\partial r^2}\left(w_{02}\frac{\partial^2 v}{\partial r^2}\right) = -\nabla P(v) \tag{7}$$

$v(0, s, r) = v_0(s, r)$ initial estimation

+ boundary conditions.

The boundary conditions allow us to constrain the topology of the surface (for instance, to consider the topology of a cylinder, a torus, or a sphere). In the following, to simplify the notation, we consider Eq. (7) with zero-boundary conditions (more general cases can be handled by a simple change of variables). In our case, we consider deformable models of fixed topology. One could refer to [24, 25] to find varying topology models.

The solution of Eq. (7) is performed in two steps. First

we solve the static problem (1) with a conform Finite Element Method (FEM) [10] and then solve the evolution problem with a finite difference method. This can be done since the space variables (s, r) and the temporal variable t are independent.

5.1. Solution of the Static Problem: The Variational Problem

The solution of Eq. (1) is performed through a variational method. This consists of defining a bilinear form $a(u, v)$ and a linear form $L(v)$ such that solving Eq. (1) is equivalent to solving the associated variational problem: Find a function v in the Sobolev space $H_0^2(\Omega)$ such that

$$a(v, u) = L_v(u), \quad \forall u \in H_0^2(\Omega), \tag{8}$$

where $H_0^2(\Omega)$ is the space of functions such that $\int_\Omega |D^m v|^2 < +\infty$ for $m = 0, 1, 2$, where $D^m v$ is the mth-order derivative of function v.

One can easily remark that solving the variational problem (8) is equivalent to minimizing the functional

$$J(u) = \tfrac{1}{2} a(u, u) - L_v(u).$$

Thus, by setting

$$a(u, v) = \int_\Omega w_{10}\frac{\partial u}{\partial s}\frac{\partial v}{\partial s} + w_{01}\frac{\partial u}{\partial r}\frac{\partial v}{\partial r} + w_{20}\frac{\partial^2 u}{\partial^2 s}\frac{\partial^2 v}{\partial s^2}$$

$$+ 2w_{11}\frac{\partial^2 u}{\partial s \partial r}\frac{\partial^2 v}{\partial s \partial r} + w_{02}\frac{\partial^2 u}{\partial r^2}\frac{\partial^2 v}{\partial r^2} ds\, dr$$

(remark that $a(u, v)$ is defined only for $u, v \in H_0^2(\Omega)$) and

$$L_v(u) = -\int_\Omega \nabla P(v)\, u\, ds\, dr,$$

solving (8) is equivalent to solving the Euler–Lagrange equation (1). We can further show that the problem (8) has a unique solution as long as the bilinear form $a(u, v)$ is symmetric and positive definite provided that the parameters w_{ij} are positive.

5.2. Discretizing the Variational Problem: The Conforming FEM

So far, we have dealt with the continuous form of the variational problem to show the existence and the uniqueness of the solution of (8). In the following we define an approximate problem of (8) which is called the discrete variational problem. This allows us to search for an approximate solution v_h of (8) in a finite-dimensional space $V_h \subset H_0^2(\Omega)$ (the solution v_h is such that $\|v - v_h\|_{H^2} \to 0$ as $h \to 0$; furthermore, for the FEM used in the following the order of convergence of $\|v - v_h\|_{H^2}$ is $O(h^2)$).

These two conditions ensure good numerical properties of the discretization schemes and are the basis of the *conforming* FEM [10]. This is different from the FEM mentioned by Terzopoulos [32, 33] or Pentland and Sclaroff [29], who refer in general to a nonconforming discretization scheme of a set of differential equations, such as that of Bathe [4] for instance.

A well-known approach to approximating such problems is Galerkin's method [10], which consists of defining a similar discrete problem, over a finite-dimensional subspace V_h of the Sobolev space $H_0^2(\Omega)$. The associated discrete problem for (8) is

$$\text{find } v_h \in V_h \text{ such that } a(v_h, u_h) = L_v(u_h), \quad \forall u_h \in V_h, \quad (9)$$

which leads to solving a linear system over the space V_h. The conforming finite element method provides an efficient tool for defining the space V_h. It is characterized by three aspects:

- A tessellation is established over the parameterization set $\Omega = [0, 1] \times [0, 1]$.

- The functions $v_h \in V_h$ are piecewise polynomials.

- There exists a basis in the space V_h whose functions have small support.

This last feature is very important since it defines the structure of the linear system that we solve. Choosing functions with small support induces a very sparse linear system and leads to a reduced computational complexity.

Details on the tessellation of the domain Ω and the construction of the subspace V_h with the Bogner–Fox–Schmit (BFS) elements [5] are given in Appendix B.

Expressing $v_h \in V_h$ in the BFS basis leads to the identity

$$
v_h = \sum_{i,j=0}^{N_s-1, N_r-1} v_h(a_{ij})\varphi_{ij} + \frac{\partial v_h}{\partial s}(a_{ij})\psi_{ij} \\
+ \frac{\partial v_h}{\partial r}(a_{ij})\eta_{ij} + \frac{\partial^2 v_h}{\partial s \partial r}(a_{ij})\zeta_{ij}, \quad (10)
$$

where $a_{ij} = (ih_s, jh_r)$ are the nodal points. Equation (10) gives us a $\mathscr{C}^1$ analytic solution over the set Ω.

Finally the solution of the discrete problem associated with Eq. (1) is equivalent to a solution of the linear system

$$A \cdot V = L, \quad (11)$$

where the matrix A is symmetric, definite positive, and tridiagonal per bloc. The reader can find all details on the variational problem and linear system (11) in Appendix B.

The FEM described above is a *conform* FEM. Some other numerical methods for solving this kind of partial differential equations are often used: the Finite Difference Method (FDM) and the *nonconforming* FEM. The FDM is easy to implement but has some drawbacks:

- the solution is known only at the nodal points and

- the applied forces are taken into account only at nodal points, and consequently, one must have a large number of nodal points to compute accurately the applied forces. This leads to a larger numerical complexity (see Section 7).

In the nonconforming FEM, the finite-dimensional space V_h does not belong to the space $H_0^2(\Omega)$; this may alter the smoothness of the solution. These methods do not propagate the stress and the strain correctly [35] and do not provide a decomposition of the solution in a discrete basis of continuous functions.

5.3. Solution of the Evolution Problem

In the previous section we showed that solving Eq. (1) can be done by solving a linear system $A \cdot V = L$; consequently the discrete form of the evolution of Eq. (7) is

$$\frac{\partial V}{\partial t} + A \cdot V = L_V.$$

This equation is solved by an implicit scheme,

$$
\frac{V^t - V^{t-1}}{\tau} + A \cdot V^t = L_{V^t} \quad (12)
$$
$$V^0 = v_0 \text{ initial estimation,}$$

where τ is the time step.

This scheme is difficult to solve since the term L is complex. Thus we have chosen an implicit scheme for V^t and an explicit scheme for the forces L. This leads to the solution of the linear system

$$(Id + \tau A) \cdot V^t = V^{t-1} + \tau L_{V^{t-1}}. \quad (13)$$

Finally to find a solution to Eq. (7) we must solve the linear system $M \cdot V = N$ at each time step, for which the matrix $M = (Id + \tau A)$ is banded, symmetric, and positive definite. This linear system is solved with a Conjugate Gradient (CG) method, in which the solution V^{t-1} is taken as an initial guess at time t. At each time step, the CG method converges in a few iterations (3 to 10 iterations). This approach appears to have a convergence faster than that of a Cholesky factorization and take less memory for storage.

5.4. Computation of the Vector L

The vector L, where

$$L_v(e_{ij}) = -\int_\Omega \nabla P(v_{t-1}(s, r))e_{ij}(s, r)\,ds\,dr$$

($e_{ij} = (\varphi_{ij}, \psi_{ij}, \eta_{ij}, \zeta_{ij})$ and $\varphi_{ij}, \psi_{ij}, \eta_{ij}$, and ζ_{ij} are the basis functions of the BFS element), represents the contribution of the external forces (which attract the surface toward the edges) in the linear system that we solve at each iteration. Thus, the more we weight the potential P the more accurate the result and the faster the convergence.

Since the potential P is known only at integer values (discrete image data) we must compute the $L_v(e_{ij})$ with a numerical integration. Consequently we compute ∇P at any point $(x, y, z) \in R^3$ by a trilinear interpolation of its eight neighbors.

To take into account all the contributions of the external forces, we modified the numerical integration formula such that every image point in the set $v([(i - 1)h_s, (i + 1)h_s] \times [(j - 1)h_r, (j + 1)h_r])$ is taken into account in the computation of each term $L_v(e_{ij})$. Let $F(s, r) = -\nabla P(v(s, r))$, and for each rectangle $K_{ij} = [ih_s, (i + 1)h_s] \times [jh_r, (j + 1)h_r]$,

$$d_1 = \text{Sup}[d(v(ih_s, jh_r), v((i + 1)h_s, jh_r)),$$
$$d(v(ih_s, (j + 1)h_r), v((i + 1)h_s, (j + 1)h_r))]$$

and

$$d_2 = \text{Sup}[d(v(ih_s, jh_r), v(ih_s, (j + 1)h_r)),$$
$$d(v((i + 1)h_s, jh_r), v((i + 1)h_s, (j + 1)h_r))],$$

where $d(\cdot, \cdot)$ denotes the 3-D Euclidean distance. Thus

$$\int_{K_{ij}} F(s, r)\,ds\,dr = \sum_{l=0}^{d_1} \sum_{m=0}^{d_2} \int_{lh_s}^{(l+1)h_s} \int_{mh_r}^{(m+1)h_r} F(s, r)\,ds\,dr$$

$$= \frac{h_s h_r}{d_1 d_2} \sum_{l=0}^{d_1} \sum_{m=0}^{d_2} F\left(ih_s + \frac{2l + 1}{2d_1} h_s, jh_r + \frac{2m + 1}{2d_2} h_r\right).$$

This method allows us to perform an adaptive subdivision of the rectangle K_{ij} without adding nodal points and consequently without increasing the size of the linear system that we solve. This method significantly reduces algorithmic complexity while increasing accuracy and convergence speed.

6. REGULARIZATION PARAMETERS

The elasticity and rigidity coefficients w_{ij} play an important role in the convergence process of the surface toward the image edges [11]. These coefficients must be chosen in a correct way such that the internal forces generated by the energy

$$E_{int}(v) = \int_\Omega w_{10} \left|\frac{\partial v}{\partial s}\right|^2 + w_{01} \left|\frac{\partial v}{\partial r}\right|^2 + 2w_{11} \left|\frac{\partial^2 v}{\partial s\, \partial r}\right|^2$$
$$+ w_{20} \left|\frac{\partial^2 v}{\partial s^2}\right|^2 + w_{02} \left|\frac{\partial^2 v}{\partial r^2}\right|^2 \, ds\, dr$$

have the same magnitude as the external forces $F(v)$. In this case a minimum of the energy E will be a trade-off between the internal and external energy, and the obtained surface will fit the edge points while being smooth and regular. If the internal energy is preponderant, the surface will tend to collapse on itself without detecting image edges, whereas if the external energy predominates, the surface will converge along the image edges with any degree of smoothing.

To ensure that both internal and external energy have the same order of magnitude we have found it sufficient to choose the coefficients w_{ij} such that the linear system of Eq. (7) is well conditioned. This leads to

$$w_{10} = w_{01} = h_s^2 h_r^2 \quad \text{and} \quad w_{20} = w_{11} = w_{02} = h_s^3 h_r^3,$$

where h_s and h_r are the discretization step of Ω.

We set $w_{10} = w_{01}$ and $w_{20} = w_{11} = w_{02}$ since the 3-D image data were isotropic and consequently all directions have the same weight.

7. NUMERICAL COMPLEXITY

In the following we compare the algorithmic complexity of the conforming FEM and the FDM. In both cases the discretization of the evolution equation (2) leads to the solution of the linear system (13), but the number of unknowns is different. In the conforming FEM at each nodal point a_{ij} ($i = 0 \cdots N_s - 1$ and $j = 0 \cdots N_r - 1$), we must compute $v_h(a_{ij})$, $(\partial v_h/\partial s)(a_{ij})$, $(\partial v_h/\partial r)(a_{ij})$, and $(\partial^2 v_h/\partial s\,\partial r)(a_{ij})$; consequently the matrix A is $4 \times N_s \times N_r$ and it has a tridiagonal per bloc structure (its bandwidth is $2N_s - 1$; see Appendix B.3).

In the FDM, the matrix A has a pentadiagonal per bloc structure (its bandwidth is $4N_s - 1$) and its size is $N_s \times N_r$ since at each nodal point a_{ij} ($i = 0 \cdots N_s - 1$ and $j = 0 \cdots N_r - 1$) we must determine $v_h(a_{ij})$.

The linear system is solved by a CG method. This method is an iterative method. At each CG iteration we must perform (44 *additions* + 42 *multiplications* + 1 *division*) $\times 4 \times N_s \times N_r$ for the conforming FEM and (18 additions + 16 multiplications + 1 division) $\times N_s \times N_r$ for the FDM.

Consequently, if we consider the same number of nodal points a_{ij} and that the necessary number of CG iterations is the same for both matrices, the numerical complexity of the conforming FEM is approximatively 12 times larger than that of the FDM. In practice, it appears [13, 14] that for 2-D deformable curves the number of points in the FDM must be at least equal to the length l, in pixels, of the initial guess, to compute accurately the attraction force. With the FEM, the number of points can typically be reduced to the order of $l/6$. If we assume that this result is still valid for the deformable surfaces (we have not implemented the FDM for deformable surfaces), we must consider, for the FDM, a number of discretizations points 36 times larger than that of the conforming FEM. In this case, the numerical complexity is $36/12 = 3$ times greater than the complexity of the conforming FEM.

This advantage is due to the computation of the vector $L_{V^{t-1}}$ in (13) and the nature of the method. In the classical FDM, we follow the evolution of a set of points. In the conform FEM, we actually deform the surface which is between the points of the grid, and the image forces between the grid points are also considered since the numerical integration is made at the pixel size so that no information is lost (see Section 5.4).

8. INFERRING THE DIFFERENTIAL STRUCTURE FROM 3-D IMAGES

8.1. *With the Previous Active Model*

In the previous sections we showed how to use the deformable surface to segment and fit some 3-D image edge points. In the following we assume that the surface has localized accurately the 3-D image edges, which means that we have reached a minimum of E. We now use this surface to compute the differential characteristics of the 3-D image surface boundary. This computation can be done analytically at each point of the surface since the use of conform FEM gives an analytic representation of the surface $v(s, r)$,

$$
v = \sum_{i,j=0}^{N_s-1, N_r-1} v_h(a_{ij})\varphi_{ij} + \frac{\partial v_h}{\partial s}(a_{ij})\psi_{ij} + \frac{\partial v_h}{\partial r}(a_{ij})\eta_{ij}
$$
$$
+ \frac{\partial^2 v_h}{\partial s\, \partial r}(a_{ij})\zeta_{ij}, \tag{14}
$$

where φ_{ij}, ψ_{ij}, η_{ij}, and ζ_{ij} are the basis functions and the coefficients $v_h(a_{ij})$, $(\partial v_h/\partial s)(a_{ij})$, $(\partial v_h/\partial r)(a_{ij})$, and $(\partial^2 v_h/\partial s\, \partial r)(a_{ij})$ are computed by solving the linear system (12) (Fig. 1). Another major contribution of the analytic repre-

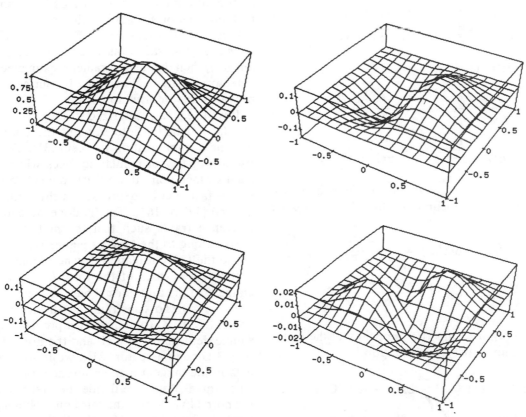

FIG. 1. Surface plots of the four basis functions φ, ψ, η, and ζ.

183

sentation is that at each point of the surface, the tangent plane is given by the vectors $v_s = \partial v/\partial s$ and $v_r = \partial v/\partial r$ (in the following the subscripts s, r, ss, rr, and sr denote the first and second derivatives). This allows us to compute all the differential characteristics in local coordinates and consequently handle more general situations.

Let us consider the basis $\{v_s, v_r, N\}$, where $N = (v_s \times v_r)/|v_s \times v_r|$, and let $T_p(\mathcal{S})$ denote the tangent plane to $\mathcal{S}$ at the point $p \in R^3$. Since N_s and N_r belong to $T_p(\mathcal{S})$ we can write

$$N_s = a_{11}v_s + a_{12}v_r$$

$$N_r = a_{21}v_s + a_{22}v_r,$$

and therefore dN_p, which denotes the differential of N computed at point p, is given by the matrix $(a_{ij})_{i,j=1\cdots 2}$ in the basis $\{v_s, v_r, N\}$. This matrix can be expressed in terms of the first and second fundamental forms of $\mathcal{S}$ as [17]

$$\begin{pmatrix} a_{11} & a_{12} \\ a_{21} & a_{22} \end{pmatrix} = \frac{-1}{EG - F^2} \begin{pmatrix} e & f \\ f & g \end{pmatrix} \begin{pmatrix} G & -F \\ -F & E \end{pmatrix},$$

where E, F, G, e, f, and g are the coefficients of the first and second fundamental forms in the basis $\{v_s, v_r, N\}$ defined by

$$E = \langle v_s, v_s \rangle, \quad F = \langle v_s, v_r \rangle, \quad G = \langle v_r, v_r \rangle,$$

$$e = \langle N, v_{ss} \rangle, \quad f = \langle N, v_{sr} \rangle, \quad g = \langle N, v_{rr} \rangle.$$

This gives the relations

$$a_{11} = \frac{fF - eG}{EG - F^2}, \quad a_{12} = \frac{gF - fG}{EG - F^2},$$

$$a_{21} = \frac{eF - fE}{EG - F^2}, \quad a_{22} = \frac{fF - gE}{EG - F^2},$$

known as the *equations of Weingarten*. Thus the Gaussian curvature K and the mean curvature H of $\mathcal{S}$ at p are

$$K = \det(dN_p) = \det(a_{ij}) = \frac{eg - f^2}{EG - F^2},$$

$$H = -\frac{1}{2}(a_{11} + a_{22}) = \frac{1}{2}\frac{eG - 2fF + gE}{EG - F^2}.$$

The principal curvatures are the opposites of the eigenvalues of dN_p; they satisfy the equation

$$\det(dN_p + kI) = k^2 - 2Hk + K = 0$$

and therefore $k = H \pm \sqrt{H^2 - K}$.

The principal curvature field can be used to extract the maxima of the larger curvature in the direction of the larger curvature [26]. This yields the ridges of the surface, which are very useful for matching. In Fig. 16, one can visualize the value of the larger principal curvature. The result appears to be qualitatively correct and can be compared to those obtained in [26] by another method, consisting of fitting locally a quadratic surface model. Our results are a little more noisy, but the advantage is that the segmentation and curvature are computed simultaneously. Also, our approach appears to be computationally much less expensive.

8.2. Using the Surface Normals to Improve the Model

In the previous example, the computation of the curvatures was based only on the location of the surface (i.e., the sole data given were the 3-D points (X, Y, Z), which are the 3-D image edge points) and the obtained curvatures are qualitatively correct, but the curvature does not vary smoothly. We believe that the use of additional information such as the normals of the surface improves the result of the computation of the curvatures. Monga *et al.* already used this property in [26] to fit local quadrics models to 3-D edgels. Lee [23] used positions and normals to fit surfaces fusing binocular stereo and photometric informations. Terzopoulos [32] also used the normal information for surface fitting.

Indeed, if we assume that the sought surfaces are noisy *isointensity* surfaces (as is usually the case in medical images), then the image gradient (estimated by a 3-D edge detector [27]) is colinear to the surface normal $\mathcal{N}$ and provides this information.

If we use a parameterized surface $v(s, r) = (x(s, r), y(s, r), z(s, r))$, taking into account the normals leads to a nonlinear minimization problem [31]. To avoid this, we use a property of regular surfaces which states that for each surface point there exists a neighborhood such that the surface can be expressed in the form $v(s, r) = (s, r, g(s, r))$ [17, p. 164]. This is done by choosing locally a reference frame such that the first two vectors of the basis belong to the tangent plane. We call this reference frame the tangent plane reference frame.

If v is a surface of the form $(s, r, v(s, r))$, a vector colinear to the unit normal has the simple form $N(s, r) = (-v_s, v_r, 1)$. To constrain the surface v to fit the data points (X, Y, Z) (obtained by a previous application of a simple deformable model) and the normals $\mathcal{N}$ (estimated by a 3-D edge detector [27]), we transform locally these data in the tangent plane reference frame of the surface. Once this is done, we divide the first two coordinates of the normal vector by the third one, obtaining a measured normal of the form $(N_1, N_2, 1)$ (this is always possible within a neighborhood of a regular surface point in the tangent plane reference frame).

We can now define a new energy given by $E = E_{\text{smooth}} + E_{\text{location}}$, where

$$E_{\text{location}}(v) = \frac{1}{2} C_1 \int_\Omega |v(s, r) - z|^2 \, ds \, dr$$

$$+ \frac{1}{2} C_2 \left(\int_\Omega |v_s(s, r) + N_1|^2 \, ds \, dr \quad (15) \right.$$

$$\left. + \int_\Omega |v_r(s, r) - N_2|^2 \, ds \, dr \right),$$

where z represent the third component of the projection of the data point (X, Y, Z) in the tangent plane reference frame.

Here, once again, the energy E_{smooth} constrains the surface to be smooth the E_{location} measures the discrepancy between the data and the surface. The coefficients C_1 and C_2 allow us to weigh differently the data points and the normals. This allows us to choose the coefficients C_1 and C_2 depending on the reliability of the data points or the normals (up to now we set $C_1 = C_2 = 1$).

A minimum of E is obtained by solving the equation

$$- \frac{\partial}{\partial s} \left(w_{10} \frac{\partial v}{\partial s} \right) - \frac{\partial}{\partial r} \left(w_{01} \frac{\partial v}{\partial r} \right) + 2 \frac{\partial^2}{\partial s \partial r} \left(w_{11} \frac{\partial^2 v}{\partial s \partial r} \right)$$

$$+ \frac{\partial^2}{\partial s^2} \left(w_{20} \frac{\partial^2 v}{\partial s^2} \right) + \frac{\partial^2}{\partial r^2} \left(w_{02} \frac{\partial^2 v}{\partial r^2} \right)$$

(16)

$$= -C_1(v - z) - C_2 \frac{\partial}{\partial s} (v_s + N_1) - C_2 \frac{\partial}{\partial r} (v_r - N_2)$$

+ boundary conditions.

This equation is solved with a conforming FEM as described in Section 5.

9. EXPERIMENTAL RESULTS

We now give results of the algorithms presented so far. Using a 3-D deformable model to segment a 3-D image provides better results than the iterated application of a 2-D deformable model to successive 2-D cross sections [14]. Indeed, the 3-D model easily bridges edge gaps in 3-D, i.e. not only within a cross section, but also between cross sections, ensuring that the result is globally a smooth surface and not only a collection of smooth planar curves. This significantly improves the robustness of the segmentation; for instance, it is even possible to remove all the edges of a single cross section (assuming that the edges are correctly detected in the other ones) without degrading the final result too much.

We present in Fig. 2 an example with artificial data. This figure represents overlays of some horizontal cross sections of the initial surface with the original data. The 3-D image here is a cylinder where we have removed some edges in three successive cross sections to compare the results obtained by a 2-D model applied to successive cross sections with those of a full 3-D deformable model. With the deformable surface we can restore the lost edges and obtain a perfect reconstruction of the cylinder (Fig. 3), whereas a 2-D model [14] cannot restore the lost edges even if we use the same attraction force as that for the 3-D model.

The deformable model can also handle noisy data. In Fig. 4, we have added Gaussian noise ($\sigma^2 = 0.8$) to the edge locations of a cylinder with an elliptic base. This figure shows some cross sections of the obtained surface with the data and a representation of the surface. We have also conducted some experiments on the accuracy of the model and its ability to handle noisy data. We have considered a set of data points (a surface plot is given in Fig. 17) obtained by sampling the analytical function $(s, r, z = \sqrt{1.0 - (s - 50.0)^2/2500.0})$ and corrupting by a

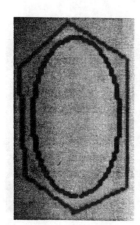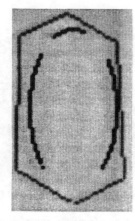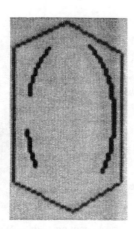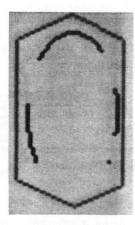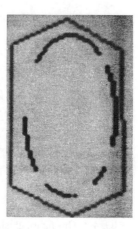

FIG. 2. Some successive cross sections of image edges (in black) and initial surface (in gray) given by the user.

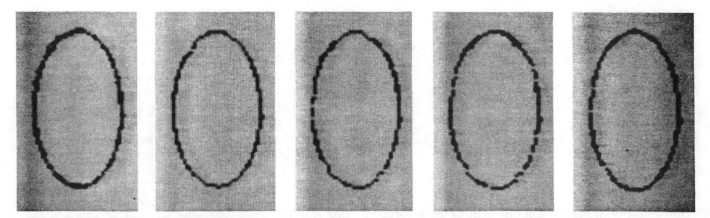

FIG. 3. Here we show how the deformable surface (in gray) can reconstruct the lost edges while having a 3-D homogeneity. In this example, a 2-D model cannot reconstruct the missing edges even if we use a 3-D potential.

Gaussian noise of variance $\sigma^2 = 0.01$, $\sigma^2 = 0.05$, and $\sigma^2 = 0.1$. Table 1 represents the obtained values, at six different points, of the surface approximating the function z. The mean error and the variance error are computed over the whole data set (these data vary between 0 and 1).

Figure 5 shows a set of cross sections of a vertebra (out of a total of 50 cross sections), obtained with an X-ray scanner and the initial segmentation provided by the user (the external curves show the intersection of the given surface with the corresponding cross sections).

Figure 6 shows the resulting surface obtained after 40 iterations, in the same set of cross sections. It is interesting to note the remarkable accuracy of the segmentation, although the detected contours were often incomplete (due to noise effect). Figure 7 shows a wire-frame representation of the resulting surface.

Figure 8 represents some cross sections of the 3-D edge image of a human heart (obtained with Magnetic Resonance Imaging (MRI)) with the initial surface (in gray). Figure 9 shows some cross sections of the surface, once it has reached the minimum of E. We can note the good localization of the surface on the 3-D edge points. Figure 10 gives a 3-D representation of the inside cavity of the left ventricle.

Figure 11 represents some cross sections of a human head (out of 70) obtained with MRI. Figure 12 shows some cross sections of the surface with the 2-D images. A representation of the surface is given in Fig. 13. Figure 14 shows the cross sections of the surface obtained on another set of MRI images and Fig. 15 a rendered representation of the surface.

We now present the results of the computation of curvature on the face surface. Figure 16 shows the computation of the larger value of the two principal curvatures, without using the normal information (the black areas correspond to high-curvature regions and the light gray areas to low-curvature regions). We can easily remark that the black areas tend to characterize the structures of the surface. These characteristics could be used to recog-

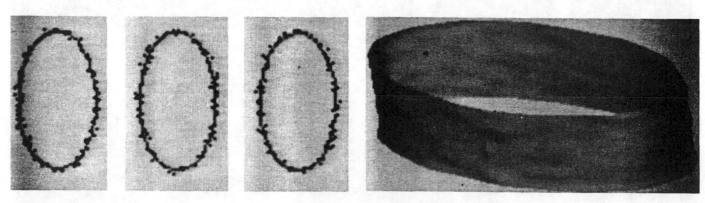

FIG. 4. This figure illustrate the use of deformable surface to segment noisy data. We added a Gaussian noise ($\sigma^2 = 0.8$) to the edge location of a cylinder with an elliptic base. This figure represents some cross sections of the solution (in gray) with the image plane and the complete surface.

186

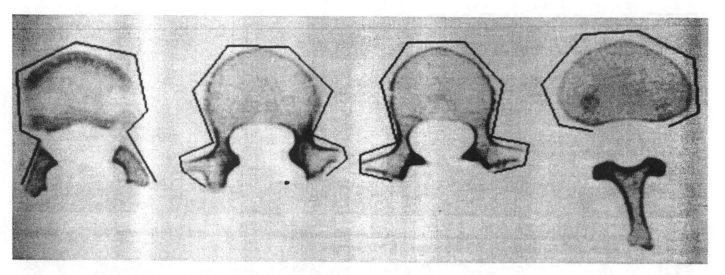

FIG. 5.   Some cross sections of the initial surface given by the user.

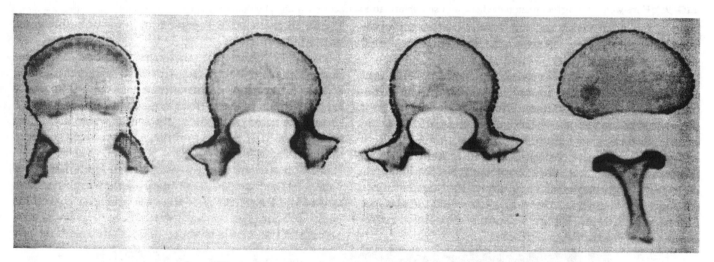

FIG. 6.   The corresponding cross sections of the solution.

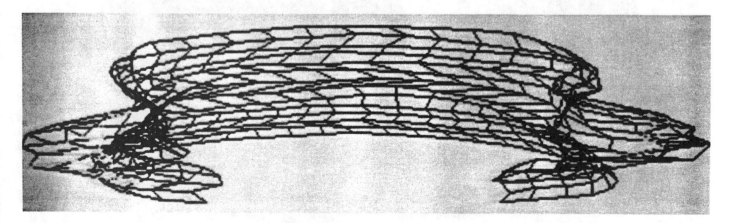

FIG. 7.   A wire-frame representation of the vertebra.

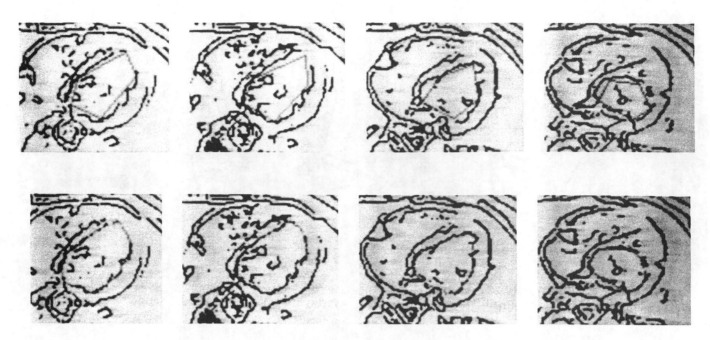

FIG. 9. Here we give a further example where we use a deformable surface constrained by boundary conditions (cylinder type) to segment the inside cavity of the left ventricle. Overlays of some cross sections of the surface (in gray) are shown with the contour image to show the accurate localization of the surface.

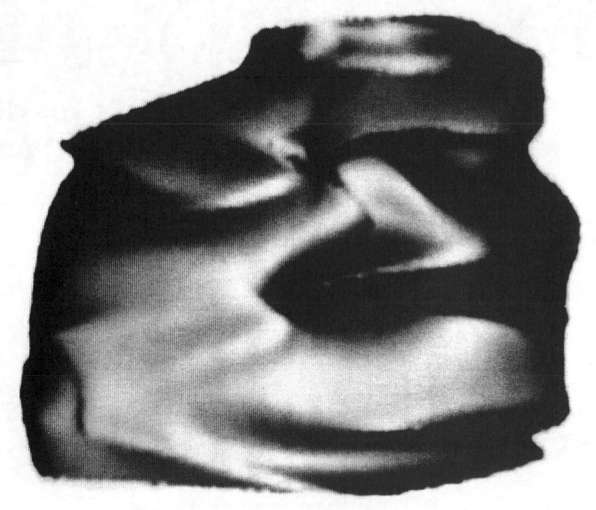

FIG. 10. A representation of the inside surface of the left ventricle.

188

TABLE 1
Results Obtained on Some Points of the Computed Surface on Noisy Data for Three Different Values of σ

Points	Theoretical value z_t	$\sigma^2 = 0.01$		$\sigma^2 = 0.05$		$\sigma^2 = 0.1$	
		Compued value z_c	Relative error $\|z_t - z_c\|$	Computed value z_c	Relative error $\|z_t - z_c\|$	Computed value z_c	Relative error $\|z_t - z_c\|$
(0.375, 0.5)	0.9682	0.8870	0.0812	0.8609	0.1073	0.8333	0.1349
(0.5, 0.5)	1.0000	0.9183	0.0817	0.8973	0.1027	0.8513	0.1487
(0.75, 0.5)	0.8660	0.8090	0.0570	0.7690	0.0970	0.6805	0.1855
(0.75, 0.5)	0.9682	0.8796	0.0886	0.8302	0.1380	0.7803	0.1879
(0.5, 0.25)	1.0000	0.9077	0.0923	0.8445	0.1555	0.7598	0.2402
(0.75, 0.75)	0.8660	0.8243	0.0417	0.8313	0.0347	0.7981	0.0679
Mean error		0.0658		0.0878		0.1409	
Variance error		0.0175		0.0316		0.0820	

nize anatomical structures from the 3-D images. Nevertheless, as discussed before, the results are qualitatively correct, but noisy.

To validate the use of the normal, we conducted a series of experiments on synthetic data. In Fig. 17 a rendered representation of the data and the theoretical value of the larger value of the two principal curvatures are shown. We have added Gaussian noise ($\sigma^2 = 0.01$) to

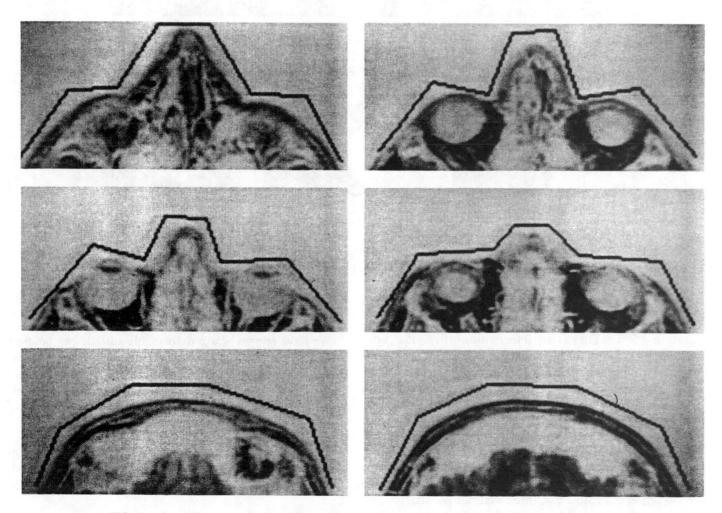

FIG. 11. Overlays of some cross sections of the initial surface given by the user with the original data.

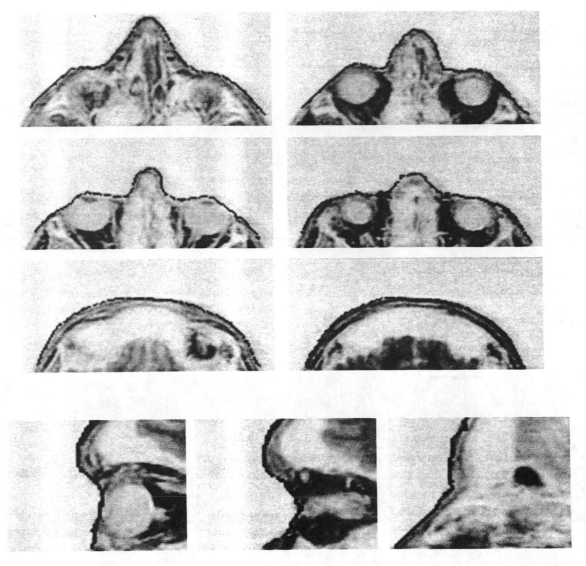

FIG. 12. Overlays of some horizontal and vertical cross sections of the surface obtained by the algorithm with the original data.

these data (Fig. 18). Figure 19 (left) shows the result of approximating the surface to the noisy data and the computation of the curvature information (Fig. 19, right) without the use of the normals. Figure 20 (right) shows the same quantities computed with the information of the surface normals and demonstrates the importance of this information for regularizing the result. This visual qualitative improvement is confirmed by a qualitative comparison of the computed second-order derivatives at different points on the surface. Typically, a gain of 10% in the accuracy of the second-order derivatives is provided by the normal information. Table 2 shows the larger value of the principal curvatures at three distinct points.

10. CONCLUSION AND FUTURE RESEARCH

We have shown how a deformable surface can be used to segment 3-D images by minimizing an appropriate energy. The minimization process is done by a variational method with a conforming finite element. Our method, including the use of an adaptive subdivision for force computation, has the following advantages:

1. it requires less discretization points and consequently produces a smaller linear system to be solved, thus reducing significantly the algorithmic complexity, and

190

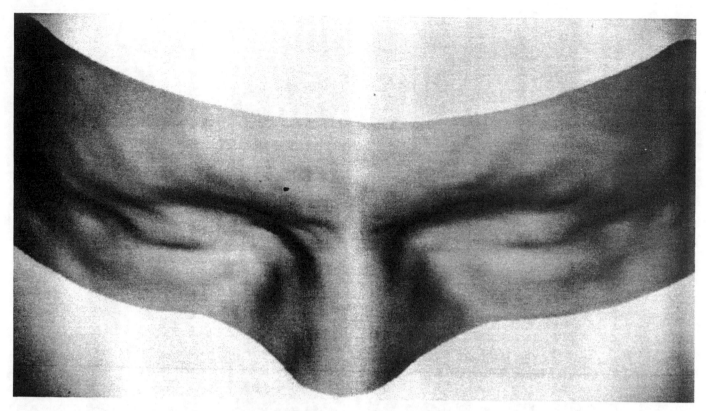

FIG. 13. A 3-D representation of the surface.

2. it provides an analytical representation of the surface.

This last feature is the most important one for inferring differential structures of the surface, and we showed how to compute the first and second fundamental forms of the deformable model. These characteristics provide a helpful tool for recognizing 3-D objects. They will be used soon to match the deformable surface to an anatomical atlas [2].

APPENDIX A: SURFACE AND 3-D EDGE POINTS

In this first appendix we give a necessary and sufficient condition for a surface to produce a local extremum of the energy

$$E_P(\mathcal{S}) = -\frac{1}{|\mathcal{S}|} \int_{\Omega} |\nabla \mathcal{I}(x(s, r))| dA,$$

where $|\mathcal{S}| = \int \int_{\Omega} |x_s \times x_r| \, dsdr$ and $dA = \sqrt{EG - F^2} \, dsdr$ is the standard surface area measure. A necessary and sufficient condition for the surface $\mathcal{S}$ to produce a local extremum of E_P with respect to infinitesimal deformations is

$$\frac{d|\nabla \mathcal{I}(x(s, r))|}{dN(x(s, r))} = \frac{eG - 2fF + gE}{EG - F^2}$$

$$\left(|\nabla \mathcal{I}(x(s, r))| - \frac{1}{|\mathcal{S}|} \int \int_{\Omega} |\nabla \mathcal{I}(x(s, r))| \, dsdr \right), \quad (17)$$

TABLE 2

The Comparison between the Larger Value of the Principal Curvature Computed on Noisy Data with and without the Use of Normals

| Points | Theoretical κ_t | Perfect data | Noisy data | | | |
		Computed curvature κ_c	Without normal κ_c	$\|\kappa_t - \kappa_c\|$	With normals κ_c	$\|\kappa_t - \kappa_c\|$
(0.25, 0.5)	2.658	2.418	1.846	0.812	1.924	0.734
(0.5, 0.75)	1.609	1.687	1.627	0.018	1.605	0.004
(0.65, 0.5)	2.141	1.276	1.746	0.409	1.802	0.340

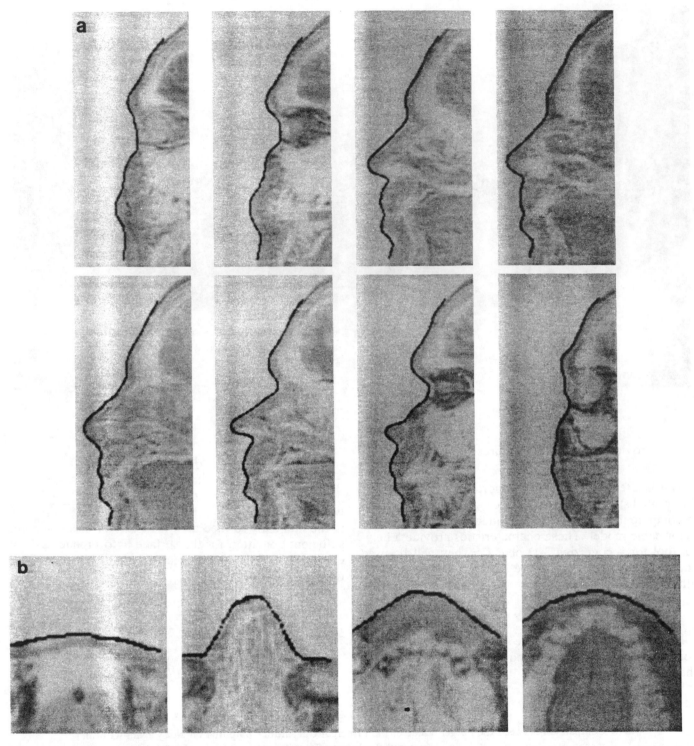

FIG. 14. Another example of the segmentation of the human face from MR images. Overlays of some vertical cross sections of the surface obtained by the algorithm with the original data.

where $E(s, r)$, $F(s, r)$, $G(s, r)$, $e(s, r)$, $f(s, r)$, and $g(s, r)$ are the coefficients of the first and second fundamental form in the basis $\{x_s, x_r, N\}$ (see [17] for details about the notations), $\Omega = [0, L] \times [0, M]$, and $P = |\nabla \mathcal{I}|$.

Let us consider $\mathcal{S}_\lambda$, a small deformation of the surface $\mathcal{S}$ such that the parametrization of $\mathcal{S}_\lambda$ is

$$x^\lambda = x + \lambda(\alpha x_s + \beta x_r + \gamma N), \qquad (18)$$

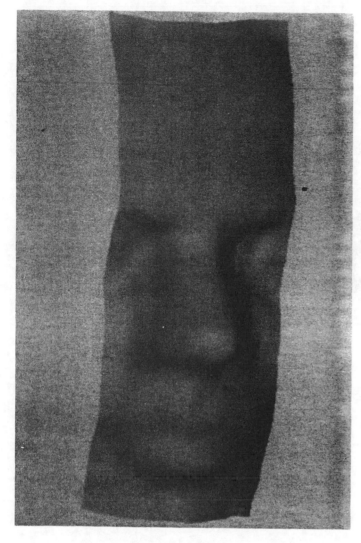

FIG. 15. A 3-D representation of the surface.

where $\alpha(s, r)$, $\beta(s, r)$, and $\gamma(s, r)$ are arbitrary continuous and differentiable functions and x_s, x_r, and N are the derivatives of x and the normal to the surface.

$\mathscr{S}$ is a local extremum of E_P if and only if

$$\left.\frac{dE_P(\mathscr{S}_\lambda)}{d\lambda}\right|_{\lambda=0} = 0, \qquad (19)$$

for all α, β, and γ.

We show that (19) holds if and only if (17) is satisfied. By definition

$$\begin{aligned}
E_P(\mathscr{S}_\lambda) &= -\frac{\int_\Omega P(x^\lambda(s, r))dA}{\int_\Omega dA} \\
&= -\frac{\int\int_\Omega P(x^\lambda(s, r))\sqrt{EG - F^2}\,dsdr}{\int\int_\Omega \sqrt{EG - F^2}\,dsdr}, \qquad (20)
\end{aligned}$$

where E, F, and G are the coefficients of the first fundamental form of $\mathscr{S}_\lambda$.

To compute the derivative $(dE_P(\mathscr{S}_\lambda)/d\lambda)|_{\lambda=0}$, we need to compute the derivatives of the vectors x_s, x_r, and N. For this purpose we use the equations [17, Sect. 4.3, p. 231]

$$\begin{aligned}
x_{ss} &= \Gamma^1_{11}x_s + \Gamma^2_{11}x_r + eN, \\
x_{sr} &= x_{rs} = \Gamma^1_{12}x_s + \Gamma^2_{12}x_r + fN, \\
x_{rr} &= \Gamma^1_{22}x_s + \Gamma^2_{22}x_r + gN,
\end{aligned}$$

where the coefficients Γ^k_{ij} are the Christoffel symbols of $\mathscr{S}$ in the parametrization x, and e, f, g are the coefficients of the second fundamental form of $\mathscr{S}$. In the following the Christoffel symbols Γ^k_{ij} have been replaced in terms of the coefficients of the first fundamental form E, F, G and their derivatives.

Thus computing $dE_P(\mathscr{S}_\lambda)/d\lambda$ and evaluating it at $\lambda = 0$ leads to

$$\begin{aligned}
|\mathscr{S}|\left.\frac{dE_P(\mathscr{S}_\lambda)}{d\lambda}\right|_{\lambda=0} = 0 &= \int\int_\Omega \sqrt{EG - F^2}\,\alpha\left[|\mathscr{S}|\frac{dP}{dx_s}\right. \\
&\quad \left. + (|\mathscr{S}|\,P - P_m)(\Gamma^1_{11} + \Gamma^2_{12})\right]dsdr \\
&\quad + \int\int_\Omega \alpha_s\sqrt{EG - F^2}(|\mathscr{S}|\,P - P_m)dsdr \\
&\quad + \int\int_\Omega \sqrt{EG - F^2}\,\beta\left[|\mathscr{S}|\frac{dP}{dx_r}\right. \\
&\quad \left. + (|\mathscr{S}|\,P - P_m)(\Gamma^1_{12} + \Gamma^2_{22})\right]dsdr \\
&\quad + \int\int_\Omega \beta_r\sqrt{EG - F^2}(|\mathscr{S}|\,P - P_m)dsdr \\
&\quad + \int\int_\Omega \gamma\left[\sqrt{EG - F^2}|\mathscr{S}|\frac{dP}{dN}\right. \\
&\quad \left. - (|\mathscr{S}|\,P - P_m)\frac{eG - 2fF + gE}{\sqrt{EG - F^2}}\right]dsdr
\end{aligned}$$

where $P_m = \int_\Omega P\,dA$.

Integrating by parts the integral (except the last one) yields (17) as a necessary and sufficient condition for (19) to be satisfied for all α, β, and γ.

APPENDIX B: DETAILS ON THE NUMERICAL SOLUTION

B.1. Variational Formulation

Let $\varphi \in H^2_0(\Omega)$ be a smooth function. If v is a solution of Eq. (7), we have

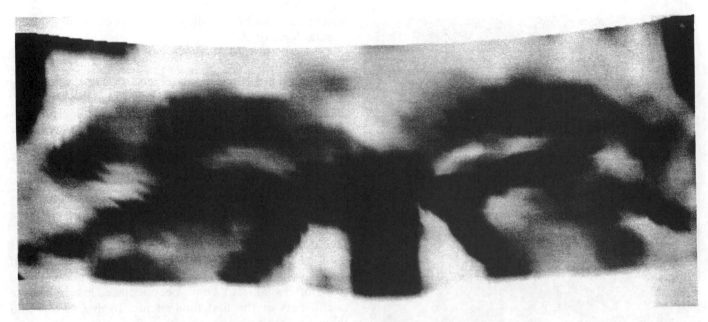

FIG. 16. A representation of the larger value of the principal curvatures. The high values are in black and the low values are in light gray. These values characterize some structures of the human face such as the eyebrows and the nose.

$$\int_\Omega \frac{\partial v}{\partial t} \varphi \, ds dr - \int_\Omega \frac{\partial}{\partial s}\left(w_{10}\frac{\partial v}{\partial s}\right)\varphi \, ds dr$$

$$- \int_\Omega \frac{\partial}{\partial r}\left(w_{01}\frac{\partial v}{\partial r}\right)\varphi \, ds dr$$

$$+ 2\int_\Omega \frac{\partial^2}{\partial s \partial r}\left(w_{11}\frac{\partial^2 v}{\partial s \partial r}\right)\varphi \, ds dr$$

$$+ \int_\Omega \frac{\partial^2}{\partial s^2}\left(w_{20}\frac{\partial^2 v}{\partial s^2}\right)\varphi \, ds dr$$

$$+ \int_\Omega \frac{\partial^2}{\partial r^2}\left(w_{02}\frac{\partial^2 v}{\partial r^2}\right)\varphi \, ds dr = - \int_\Omega \nabla P(v)\varphi \, ds dr,$$

where the function v depends on t, s, and r. We remark

that the variables (s, r) and t are independent; we can separate them (for more details see [10]). Green's formula yields

$$\frac{d}{dt}\int_\Omega v\varphi \, ds dr + \int_\Omega w_{10}\frac{\partial v}{\partial s}\frac{\partial \varphi}{\partial s}\, ds dr + \int_\Omega w_{01}\frac{\partial v}{\partial r}\frac{\partial \varphi}{\partial r}\, ds dr$$

$$+ 2\int_\Omega w_{11}\frac{\partial^2 v}{\partial s \partial r}\frac{\partial^2 \varphi}{\partial s \partial r}\, ds dr + \int_\Omega w_{20}\frac{\partial^2 v}{\partial s^2}\frac{\partial^2 \varphi}{\partial s^2}\, ds dr$$

$$+ \int_\Omega w_{02}\frac{\partial^2 v}{\partial r^2}\frac{\partial^2 \varphi}{\partial r^2}\, ds dr = - \int_\Omega \nabla P(v)\varphi \, ds dr.$$

Let us set

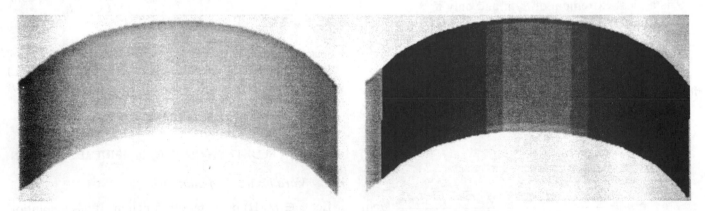

FIG. 17. A rendered representation of the theoretical data (left) and the value of the larger of the two principal curvatures (right).

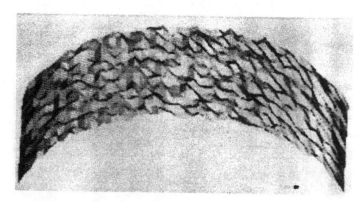

FIG. 18. A rendered representation of the noisy data ($\sigma^2 = 0.01$).

$$a(u, v) = \int_\Omega w_{10} \frac{\partial u}{\partial s} \frac{\partial v}{\partial s} + w_{01} \frac{\partial u}{\partial r} \frac{\partial v}{\partial r} + w_{20} \frac{\partial^2 u}{\partial s^2} \frac{\partial^2 v}{\partial s^2}$$

$$+ 2w_{11} \frac{\partial^2 u}{\partial s \partial r} \frac{\partial^2 v}{\partial s \partial r} + w_{02} \frac{\partial^2 u}{\partial r^2} \frac{\partial^2 v}{\partial r^2} \, ds dr$$

and

$$L_v(u) = - \int_\Omega \nabla P(v) u \, ds dr.$$

This leads to a new formulation of the problem given $v_0 \in L^2(\Omega)$ and $\nabla P \in L^2(0, T, L^2(\Omega))$, find a function $v \in L^2(0, T, H_0^2(\Omega)) \cap \mathscr{C}^1(0, T, L^2(\Omega))$ satisfying

$$\frac{d}{dt}(v(t), u) + a(v(t), u) = L_v(u), \quad \forall u \in H_0^2(\Omega),$$

$$v(0) = v_0(s, r) \tag{21}$$

$$w_{ij} \in L^\infty(\Omega) \quad \text{and} \quad w_{ij}(s) \geq \alpha > 0.$$

Since the variables, s, r, and t are independent, we can solve Eq. (21) in two steps. First solve the static equation

find $v \in H_0^2(\Omega)$ such that

$$a(v, u) = L_v(u), \quad \forall u \in H_0^2(\Omega), \tag{22}$$

where L_v is not supposed to depend on v (we remind the reader that there exists a unique solution to this equation, since the bilinear form $a(u, v)$ is symmetric and positive definite as long as $w_{ij} > 0$), and then solve the evolution equation (21). This yields Eq. (13).

B.2. Tessellation of Ω and the Basis Functions

Given the numbers of discretization points in the two axes of parametrization N_s, $N_r > 1$, we set $h_s = 1/(N_s - 1)$, $h_r = 1/(N_r - 1)$ and consider a uniform subdivision of Ω of step size h_s and h_r, composed of the nodes $a_{i,j} = (x_i, y_j) = (ih_s, jh_r)$, $0 \leq i \leq N_s - 1$, $0 \leq j \leq N_r - 1$. Thus

$$\Omega = [0, 1] \times [0, 1] = \bigcup_{i,j=0}^{N_s-1,N_r-1} K_{i,j}$$

$$= \bigcup_{i,j=0}^{N_s-1,N_r-1} [ih_s, (i+1)h_s] \times [jh_r, (j+1)h_r].$$

Since the higher derivatives appearing in Eq. (1) are of fourth order, the conform finite element space V_h must satisfy $V_h \subset \mathscr{C}^1 \cap H_0^2(\Omega)$ (for details see [10]). For this purpose the space $H_0^2(\Omega)$ is approximated with the Bogner–Fox–Schmit elements [5, 10] defined by

• The rectangles K_{ij}, defined by the vertices c_k, $1 \leq k \leq 4$,
• The set $P_{K_{ij}}$ of polynomials containing the basis functions

$$P_{K_{ij}} = Q_3(R^2) = \left\{ p, \, p(s, r) = \sum_{0 \leq k,l \leq 3} \gamma_{k,l} s^k r^l \right\},$$

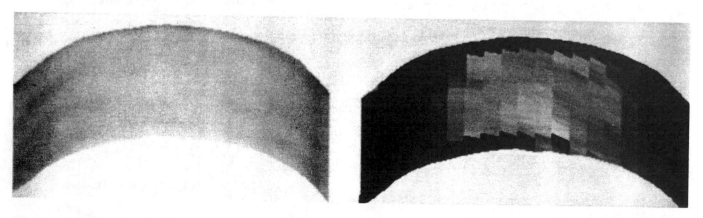

FIG. 19. A rendered representation of the surface fitted to the noisy data ($\sigma^2 = 0.01$) without normals (left) and the value of the larger of the two principal curvatures (right).

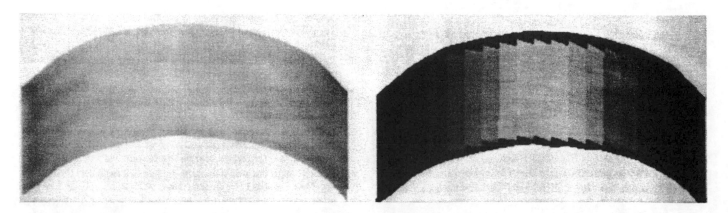

FIG. 20. A rendered representation of the surface fitted to the noisy data ($\sigma^2 = 0.01$) with taking into account the normals (left) and the value of the larger of the two principal curvatures (right).

- The set $\Sigma_{K_{ij}} = \{p(c_k), \partial p(c_k)/\partial s, \partial p(c_k)/\partial r, \partial^2 p(c_k)/\partial s \partial r, 1 \le k \le 4\}$, which allows us to define in a unique way the basis functions over each rectangles K_{ij}.

The subspace V_h is then defined by

$$V_h = \{v \in \mathscr{C}^1(\Omega), v_{|K_{ij}} \in Q_3(K_{ij})\},$$

where $Q_k(I)$ is the vector space of the restrictions to an interval $I \subset R^2$ of the polynomials whose degree is less than k for each variable, and $v_{|I}$ is the restriction of the function v to the subset I. The basis functions of the finite element subspace V_h are φ_{ij}, ψ_{ij}, η_{ij}, and ζ_{ij}, and they are defined in a unique way over each rectangle K_{ij} by

$$\varphi_{ij}(a_{kl}) = \delta_{ij,kl}, \quad \frac{\partial \varphi_{ij}}{\partial s}(a_{kl}) = \frac{\partial \varphi_{ij}}{\partial r}(a_{kl}) = \frac{\partial^2 \varphi_{ij}}{\partial s \partial r}(a_{kl}) = 0,$$

$$\frac{\partial \psi_{ij}}{\partial s}(a_{kl}) = \delta_{ij,kl}, \quad \psi_{ij}(a_{kl}) = \frac{\partial \psi_{ij}}{\partial r}(a_{kl}) = \frac{\partial^2 \psi_{ij}}{\partial s \partial r}(a_{kl}) = 0,$$

$$\frac{\partial \eta_{ij}}{\partial r}(a_{kl}) = \delta_{ij,kl}, \quad \eta_{ij}(a_{kl}) = \frac{\partial \eta_{ij}}{\partial s}(a_{kl}) = \frac{\partial^2 \eta_{ij}}{\partial s \partial r}(a_{kl}) = 0,$$

$$\frac{\partial^2 \zeta_{ij}}{\partial s \partial r}(a_{kl}) = \delta_{ij,kl}, \quad \zeta_{ij}(a_{kl}) = \frac{\partial \zeta_{ij}}{\partial s}(a_{kl}) = \frac{\partial \zeta_{ij}}{\partial r}(a_{kl}) = 0,$$

$$(23)$$

where

$$\delta_{ij,kl} = \begin{cases} 1 & \text{if } i = k \text{ and } j = l \\ 0 & \text{otherwise.} \end{cases}$$

Thus $\forall v_h \in V_h$ we have the identity

$$v_h = \sum_{i,j=0}^{N_s-1, N_r-1} v_h(a_{ij})\varphi_{ij} + \frac{\partial v_h}{\partial s}(a_{ij})\psi_{ij}$$
$$+ \frac{\partial v_h}{\partial r}(a_{ij})\eta_{ij} + \frac{\partial^2 v_h}{\partial s \partial r}(a_{ij})\zeta_{ij},$$

providing a continuous representation of the solution over the space Ω.

Equation (23) gives the expressions of the basis functions φ_{ij}, ψ_{ij}, η_{ij}, and ζ_{ij}. This leads to analytical expressions which are too long to be reported here. Instead, we give a graphical representation of the four basis functions (Fig. 1).

B.3. Discrete Problem and Linear System

Rewriting the discrete problem associated with Eq. (22) with the basis functions gives us the equations $\forall i, j = 0, \ldots, N_s - 1, N_r - 1$,

$$a(v_h, \varphi_{ij}) = L_v(\varphi_{ij})$$
$$a(v_h, \psi_{ij}) = L_v(\psi_{ij})$$
$$a(v_h, \eta_{ij}) = L_v(\eta_{ij}) \qquad (24)$$
$$a(v_h, \zeta_{ij}) = L_v(\zeta_{ij})$$

and, using identity (10), $\forall i, j = 0, \ldots, N_s - 1, N_r - 1$,

$$\sum_{k,l=0}^{N_s-1, N_r-1} v_h(a_{kl})a(\varphi_{kl}, \varphi_{ij}) + \frac{\partial v_h}{\partial s}(a_{kl})a(\varphi_{kl}, \psi_{ij})$$
$$+ \frac{\partial v_h}{\partial r}(a_{kl})a(\varphi_{kl}, \eta_{ij}) + \frac{\partial^2 v_h}{\partial s \partial r}(a_{kl})a(\varphi_{kl}, \zeta_{ij}) = L_v(\varphi_{ij})$$

$$\sum_{k,l=0}^{N_s-1, N_r-1} v_h(a_{kl})a(\psi_{kl}, \varphi_{ij}) + \frac{\partial v_h}{\partial s}(a_{kl})a(\psi_{kl}, \psi_{ij})$$
$$+ \frac{\partial v_h}{\partial r}(a_{kl})a(\psi_{kl}, \eta_{ij}) + \frac{\partial^2 v_h}{\partial s \partial r}(a_{kl})a(\psi_{kl}, \zeta_{ij}) = L_v(\psi_{ij})$$

$$\sum_{k,l=0}^{N_s-1, N_r-1} v_h(a_{kl})a(\eta_{kl}, \varphi_{ij}) + \frac{\partial v_h}{\partial s}(a_{kl})a(\eta_{kl}, \psi_{ij})$$
$$+ \frac{\partial v_h}{\partial r}(a_{kl})a(\eta_{kl}, \eta_{ij}) + \frac{\partial^2 v_h}{\partial s \partial r}(a_{kl})a(\eta_{kl}, \zeta_{ij}) = L_v(\eta_{ij})$$

196

$$\sum_{k,l=0}^{N_s-1,N_r-1} v_h(a_{kl})a(\zeta_{kl},\varphi_{ij}) + \frac{\partial v_h}{\partial s}(a_{kl})a(\zeta_{kl},\psi_{ij})$$

$$+ \frac{\partial v_h}{\partial r}(a_{kl})a(\zeta_{kl},\eta_{ij}) + \frac{\partial^2 v_h}{\partial s\partial r}(a_{kl})a(\zeta_{kl},\zeta_{ij}) = L_v(\zeta_{ij}).$$

$$(25)$$

Equation (25) is a linear system where the unknowns are $v_h(a_{kl})$, $(\partial v_h/\partial r)(a_{kl})$, $(\partial v_h/\partial s)(a_{kl})$, and $(\partial^2 v_h/\partial s\partial r)(a_{kl})$.

Finally the solution of the discrete problem associated with (22) leads to the solution of the linear system $A \cdot V = L$, where $A = (\tilde{A}_{ij,kl})_{i,k=0,\dots,Ns-1;j,l=0\dots Nr-1}$ is a tridiagonal bloc array,

$$\tilde{A}_{ij,kl} = \begin{pmatrix} a(\varphi_{ij},\varphi_{kl}) & a(\varphi_{ij},\psi_{kl}) & a(\varphi_{ij},\eta_{kl}) & a(\varphi_{ij},\zeta_{kl}) \\ a(\psi_{ij},\varphi_{kl}) & a(\psi_{ij},\psi_{kl}) & a(\psi_{ij},\eta_{kl}) & a(\psi_{ij},\zeta_{kl}) \\ a(\eta_{ij},\varphi_{kl}) & a(\eta_{ij},\psi_{kl}) & a(\eta_{ij},\eta_{kl}) & a(\eta_{ij},\zeta_{kl}) \\ a(\zeta_{ij},\varphi_{kl}) & a(\zeta_{ij},\psi_{kl}) & a(\zeta_{ij},\eta_{kl}) & a(\zeta_{ij},\zeta_{kl}) \end{pmatrix},$$

the $\tilde{A}_{ij,kl}$ array elements depending on the elasticity and rigidity coefficients.

ACKNOWLEDGMENT

This work was partially supported by Digital Equipment Corp.

REFERENCES

1. N. Ayache, J. D. Boissonnat, E. Brunet, L. Cohen, J. P. Chièze, B. Geiger, O. Monga, J. M. Rocchisani, and P. Sander. Building highly structured volume representations in 3-D medical images, in *Proceedings, Computer Aided Radiology, Berlin, West Germany 1989*.

2. N. Ayache, J. D. Boissonnat, L. Cohen, B. Geiger, J. Levy-Vehel, O. Monga, and P. Sander, Steps toward the automatic interpretations of 3-D images, in *3-D Imaging in Medicine* (H. Fuchs, K. Hohne and S. Pizer, Eds.), pp. 107–120, NATO ASI Series, Springer-Verlag, New York/Berlin, 1990.

3. N. Ayache, I. Cohen, and I. Herlin, Medical image tracking, in *Active Vision* (A. Blake and A. Yuille, Eds.), Chap. 20, MIT Press, Cambridge, MA, to appear.

4. K.-J. Bathe, *Finite Element Procedures in Engineering Analysis*, Prentice–Hall, Englewood Cliffs, NJ, 1982.

5. F. K. Bogner, R. L. Fox, and L. A. Schmit, The generation of interelement-compatible stiffness and mass matrices by the use of interpolation formulae, in *Proceedings, Conference on Matrix Methods in Structural Mechanics, Air Force Institute of Technology, Wright Patterson A.F. Base, OH, Oct. 1965*.

6. J. D. Boissonnat, Shape reconstruction from planar cross-sections, *Comput. Vision Graphics Image Process.* **44**, 1988, 1–29.

7. G. Borgefors, Distance transformations in arbitrary dimensions, *Comput. Vision Graphics Image Process.* **27**, 1984, 321–345.

8. M. Brady, J. Ponce, A. Yuille, and H. Asada, Describing surfaces, in *Proceedings, Second International Symposium on Robotics Research* (H. Hanafusa and H. Inoue, Eds.), pp. 5–16, MIT Press, Cambridge, MA, 1985.

9. J. Canny, A computational approach to edge detection, *IEEE Trans. Pattern Anal. Mach. Intelligence*, **PAMI-8**(6), Nov. 1986, 679–698.

10. P. G. Ciarlet, *The Finite Element Methods for Elliptic Problems*, North-Holland, Amsterdam, 1987.

11. I. Cohen, *Modèles deformables 2-D et 3-D: Application à la segmentation d'images médicales*, PhD thesis, Université Paris-IX Dauphine, June 1992.

12. I. Cohen, N. Ayache, and P. Sulger, Tracking points on deformables objects, in *Proceedings, Second European Conference on Computer Vision, Santa Margherita Ligure, Italy, May 1992*.

13. L. D. Cohen, On active contour models and balloons, *CVGIP Image Understanding* **53**(2), Mar. 1991, 211–218.

14. L. D. Cohen and I. Cohen, A finite element method applied to new active contour models and 3-D reconstruction from cross sections, in *Proceedings, Third International Conference on Computer Vision, IEEE Computer Society Conference, Osaka, Japan, Dec. 1990*, pp. 587–591.

15. L. D. Cohen and I. Cohen, *Finite Element Methods for Active Contour Models and Balloons from 2-D to 3-D*, Tech. Rep. 9124, CEREMADE, U.R.A. CNRS 749, Université Paris IX—Dauphine, Cahiers de Mathematiques de la Decision, Nov. 1991.

16. P. E. Danielsson, Euclidean distance mapping, *Comput. Vision Graphics Image Process.* **14**, 1980, 227–248.

17. M. P. do Carmo, *Differential Geometry of Curves and Surfaces*, Prentice–Hall, Englewood Cliffs, NJ, 1976.

18. P. Fua and Y. G. Leclerc, Model driven edge detection, in *Proceedings, DARPA Image Understanding Workshop, 1988*.

19. G. G. Gordon, Face recognition from depth and curvature, in *Proceedings, SPIE Conference on Geometric Methods in Computer Vision, San Diego, CA, July 1991*.

20. A. Guéziec and N. Ayache, Smoothing and matching of 3D-space curves, in *Proceedings, Second European Conference on Computer Vision (ECCV), Santa Margherita Ligure, Italy, May 1992*.

21. I. L. Herlin and N. Ayache, Features extraction and analysis methods for sequences of ultrasound images, in *Proceedings, Second European Conference on Computer Vision (ECCV), Santa Margherita Ligure, Italy, May 1992*.

22. M. Kass, A. Witkin, and D. Terzopoulos, Snakes: Active contour models, in *Proceedings, First International Conference on Computer Vision, London, June 1987*, pp. 259–268.

23. S. Lee, *Visual Monitoring of Glaucoma*, PhD thesis, Robotics Research Group, Department of Engineering Science, University of Oxford, 1991.

24. F. Leitner and P. Cinquin, Dynamic segmentation: Detecting complex topology 3D-object, in *Proceedings, International Conference of the IEEE Engineering in Medicine and Biology Society, Orlando, FL, Nov. 1991*, pp. 295–296.

25. F. Leitner, I. Marque, S. Lavallée, and P. Cinquin, Dynamic segmentation: Finding the edge with snake-splines, in *Proceedings, International Conference on Curves and Surfaces, Chamonix, France, June 1990*, pp. 1–4, Academic Press, San Diego, CA, 1990.

26. O. Monga, N. Ayache, and P. Sander, From voxel to curvature, in *Proceedings, Computer Vision and Pattern Recognition, IEEE Computer Society Conference, Lahaina, Maui, HI, June 1991*, pp. 644–649.

27. O. Monga and R. Deriche, 3-D edge detection using recursive filtering, in *Proceedings, IEEE Conference on Vision and Pattern Recognition, San Diego, CA, June 1989*.

28. J. A. Noble. Finding corners, in *Proceedings, Alvey Vision Conference, June 1987*, pp. 267–274.

29. A. Pentland and S. Sclaroff, Closed-form solutions for physically based shape modelling and recognition, *IEEE Trans. Pattern Anal. Mach. Intelligence* **PAMI-13**(7), July 1991, 715–729.

30. J. Ponce and M. Brady, Toward a surface primal sketch, in *Proceedings, IJCAI, 1985*.

31. P. T. Sander and S. W. Zucker, Inferring surface trace and differential structure from 3-D images, *IEEE Trans. Pattern Anal. Mach. Intelligence*, in press; a shortened version is available as Charting surface structure, in *Proceedings, First European Conference on Computer Vision, Antibes, Apr. 23–27*.

32. D. Terzopoulos, The computation of visible-surface representations, *IEEE Trans. Pattern Anal. Mach. Intelligence* **PAMI-10**(4), July 1988, 417–438.

33. D. Terzopoulos, A. Witkin, and M. Kass, Constraints on deformable models: Recovering 3-D shape and nonrigid motion, *AI J.* **36**, 1988, 91–123.

34. D. Terzopoulos, A. Witkin, and M. Kass, Symmetry-seeking models for 3-D object reconstruction, in *Proceedings, First International Conference on Computer Vision, June 1987*, pp. 269–276.

35. O. C. Zienkiewicz, *The Finite Element Method*. McGraw–Hill, 3rd ed., New York, 1977.

36. S. W. Zucker and R. M. Hummel, A three-dimensional edge operator, *IEEE Trans. Pattern Anal. Mach. Intelligence* **PAMI-3**(3), May 1981, 324–331.

Segmentation and Tracking of Cine Cardiac MR and CT Images Using a 3-D Deformable Model

A Gupta, T O'Donnell, and A Singh

Siemens Corporate Research, Princeton, USA

Abstract

Multi-slice multi-phase MR and EBT (Ultrafast CT) imaging is increasingly being used as a method for analyzing and diagnosing cardiac function. Segmentation of heart chambers facilitates computation of volume based quantities, as well as ventricular motion analysis. We present a 3D physically-based deformable model based approach to segmenting anisotropic cine MR and EBT images. The model has both rigid as well as nonrigid motion components. Past approaches have used deformable models without rigid components or used isotropic CT data. Our model adaptively subdivides the mesh in response to the forces extracted from image data. Additionally, the local mesh of the model encodes surface orientation to align the model with the desired edge directions, a crucial constraint for distinguishing close anatomical structures. We present results of segmenting multi-slice multi-phase cardiac MR and EBT studies with interslice resolution of 8 mm/slice, and intraslice resolution of 1mm/pixel.

1 Introduction

Multi-slice multi-phase MR and EBT (CT) imaging modalities are increasingly being used as a method for analyzing and diagnosing cardiac function. Segmentation of the heart chambers facilitates volume computation, as well as ventricular motion analysis. Successful techniques have been developed for segmentation of individual 2-D slices. However, these methods use 2-D models which limits the description of a 3-D phenomenon to two dimensions and uses only 2-D constraints. The resulting model lacks interslice coherency, making interslice interpolation necessary. In addition, the model is more susceptible to corruption due to noise local to one or more slices. We present an approach to segmenting cine MR and EBT images using a 3-D deformable model with rigid and nonrigid components. While other researchers have performed ventricular segmentation and tracking using 3-D models, either the model had no rigid component [1, 2] or the image modality was isotropic CT (DSR) data [5]. The 3D cine imaging modalities have interslice resolutions of 4 to 8 mm/slice, much larger than the intraslice resolution (1mm/pixel). Also, we choose not

to incorporate balloon forces since cardiac MR images have flow voids in the blood pool, which renders the balloon energy used by [5] ineffective in model fitting. Additionally, our model adaptively subdivides the mesh in response to the forces extracted from image data [8, 10]. Also, the local mesh of the model encodes surface orientation to align the model with the desired edge directions, a crucial constraint for distinguishing close anatomical structures. In the remainder of the paper we discuss the following issues: the shape model and its physically-based recovery formulation, incorporating smoothing, adaptive subdivision in the presence of image forces, local surface orientation and its preservation during subdivision. We show results for segmenting and tracking multi-slice multi-phase MR and EBT studies. Due to limitation of space, the reader is referred to [4] for details.

2 The Shape Model

Modeling, segmenting, and tracking a nonrigid object like the heart requires globally and locally deformable models capable of conforming to the object's shape while quantifying its global motion and shape parameters. We use a nonrigid extension of superquadrics [6] for representing and recovering global motion and global deformations like tapering, bending, twisting, etc.:

$$s = \begin{array}{l} sc\, a_1(\cos u)^{e_1}(\cos v)^{e_2} \\ sc\, a_2(\cos u)^{e_1}(\sin v)^{e_2} \\ sc\, a_3(\sin u)^{e_1} \end{array} \quad (1)$$

where a_1, a_2 and a_3 control the radius in the x, y, and z directions respectively while sc controls the overall scaling. Shape is determined by e_1, and e_2. Tapering, bending and twisting are introduced as parametric deformations on s. The local deformations, which are not amenable to compact parametric representations, are added to the rigid superquadric models as displacements on discretized surface [6, 3]:

$$\vec{x} = \vec{t} + \mathbf{R}(\vec{s} + \vec{d}) \quad \text{where} \quad \vec{d} = \sum_{i=1}^{3} N_i \vec{q_d} \quad (2)$$

where $\vec{t}$ is the position of the center of the global model, $\vec{s}$ is a point on the global model, and $\mathbf{R}$ is spatial the rotation matrix (on top of the superellipsoid's position). $\vec{d}$ is represented in the finite element (FEM) framework, which allows the surface properties to be interpolated and integrated over the entire surface, where N_i are the FEM shape functions and q_d, the displacements at nodes. Because we wish the local deformations to take place in a natural way, without points of high curvature, we introduce a membrane-like smoothing penalty into the fitting process.

$$E_{smooth} = \int_{Element} w_0(\frac{\partial d}{\partial \xi})^2 + w_1(\frac{\partial d}{\partial \eta})^2 d\xi d\eta \quad (3)$$

3 Mesh Tessellation & Subdivision

The model is initially tessellated such that the nodes are evenly distributed over the surface. Subdivision is invoked during model recovery to insure that the object being recovered is described with adequate resolution. Subdivision is initiated when the length of the longest edge of an element becomes "too long". This is in contrast to Metaxas & Koh [10], who use a measure of distance between the data and its closest point to the model as a subdivision condition, which is is appropriate for segmented data. Image data creates a force *field*, and there is no concept of being "close" to it. Our criterion for initiating the subdivision based on element length is indirectly adaptive: if the data causes large internodal distances to be formed, subdivision will be initiated.

We adapted the algorithm by [8] for subdivision in the presence of image forces and extended it to preserve element orientation during subdivision. The algorithm ensures *non-degeneracy* (i.e, new elements have vertex angles greater than or equal to half the smallest angle of the original element), and a *conforming* mesh (i.e, the intersection of two non-disjoint, non-identical elements consists either of a common node or common edge). An example of subdividing when the neighboring element has a different longest edge from the element being subdivided is shown in Figure 1. Our subdivision algorithm incorporates a novel technique of maintaining the orientation of element normals during subdivision. The reader is referred to [4] for the detailed orientation-preserving adaptive subdivision algorithm.

4 The Recovery Process

Model deformations mimic actual physical deformations through the simulation of Lagrangian dynamics [7]. The model has translational, rotational, global, and local

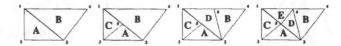

Figure 1: a) Element A is selected for subdivision. b) The subdivision results in element C and a new element A c) Element B is selected for subdivision and a recursive call of the algorithm is made. The result is element D and a new element B. d) The initial non-conformality is resolved by subdividing element D into element E and a new element D.

degrees of freedom, denoted as a row vector $\vec{q} = (\vec{q_t}^\top, \vec{q_\theta}^\top, \vec{q_s}^\top, \vec{q_d}^\top)^\top$ with $\vec{q_s} = \vec{s}$ and with a comma (,) representing the concatenation of row vectors. To solve for these, the model is made dynamic in $\vec{q}$ by introducing pseudo-mass, $\mathbf{M}$, pseudo-damping, $\mathbf{D}$, and pseudo-stiffness $\mathbf{K}$ terms. The apparatus of Lagrangian dynamics is applied to solve the above system of equations under the influence of external forces "emanating" from data.

$$\mathbf{M}\ddot{\vec{q}} + \mathbf{C}\dot{\vec{q}} + \mathbf{K}\vec{q} = \vec{f_q} \quad (4)$$

We simplify the above equations by setting the mass term to the zero and solve using Euler time stepping:

$$\vec{q}^{(t+\Delta t)} = \vec{q}^{(t)} + k_{Euler\_Coeff}\Delta t(\mathbf{C}^{(t)})^{-1}\vec{f_q}^{(t)} \quad (5)$$

where $k_{Euler\ Coeff}$ is the Euler Coefficient and Δt the time step.

5 Image Forces

The image forces attract the model to edges in the image and are calculated using the formula:

$$F = \nabla|(\nabla(I * G_\sigma))|$$

where I is the original image and G_σ represents a gaussian smoothing filter. Edges correspond to zero-crossings in the force vectors. Ideally the force calculation would involve the application of 3-D filters resulting in an image of 3D forces. Unfortunately the low resolution in the z-direction causes artifacts to appear and prohibits this approach. The artifacts are a result of the large change in edge position compared to window size in the z-direction. Figure 2 illustrates this problem by applying a 3x3x3 gradient filter on three consecutive 128 x 128 slices of an ellipsoidal object. Therefore we extract only x,y forces from each of the image slices using 2D filters. The results are interpolated both inter- and intra-slice to create a continuous 3D field of 2D forces in which the model sits. In addition to image forces, orientation forces aid in the fitting process by aligning the surface normals of the model with the edge normals

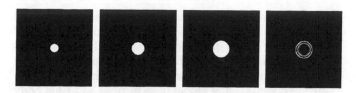

Figure 2: Anisotropic 3-D filtering artifact: the three input slices, and the resulting edges.

of nearby edges. If the dot product of the two normals is greater than 0.5, the vector difference between the two is applied as a force to the node. This reduces the influence of right ventricle (RV) edges when recovering the left ventricle (LV). RV edges have the appropriate normal direction but are opposite in orientation and the dot products with the model surface normals will be less than 0.5.

6   Segmentation & Tracking

Segmentation requires a good initial placement of the model for two reasons. First, image forces are short range (i.e., they trail off rapidly from edges). If they are too far away, the model will not be drawn to an edge. To some extent, however, this may be compensated for by blurring the gradient image before applying the second gradient filter to extract the forces (see equation 5). Second, nearby noisy edges are capable of distracting the model. The model must be placed beyond their sphere of influence. We call the starting state the "rest state" of the model.   Rigid-body and global deformations of the model are significantly effected by these concerns. These deformations must be severely damped since slight changes might easily cause the model to escape the sphere of influence of the appropriate edges. An increase of the a_1 parameter, for instance, might be necessary in the region of the model that initiates it; however, it might cause other regions to escape from the edges they should be near.   Tracking is done by segmenting the first phase using the technique described above. The resulting model is then placed in the image force field created by the next phase in the cardiac cycle, and so on. Clinical protocols allow sufficient sampling in time such that the model fit to phase n data is within the appropriate edges' spheres of influence in phase $n + 1$ data.

7   Results

We present three sets of results demonstrating the segmenting and tracking capabilities of the superquadric-based deformable model. Figure 3 shows a segmentation of the ED phase of a 3D cardiac study with 1mm × 1mm × 4mm resolution. No subdivision was allowed and the model was tessellated with 500 nodes.   Stiffness values $w0$ and $w1$

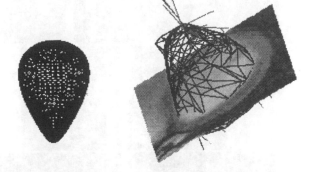

Figure 3: Segmentation results for the ED phase of a 3-D study: The initial superquadric model is shown on top left. The final recovered model is shown in the image space. Forces are shown in grey.

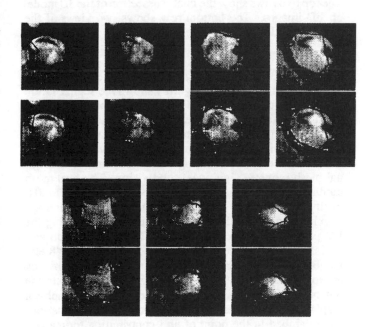

Figure 4: Segmentation of the first phase of 1mm × 1mm × 8mm cine cardiac study. The "rest state" of the model is shown above and the result below for each of the seven slices in the two rows. the model is the black wire mesh and the white lines attached to model nodes represent force vectors.

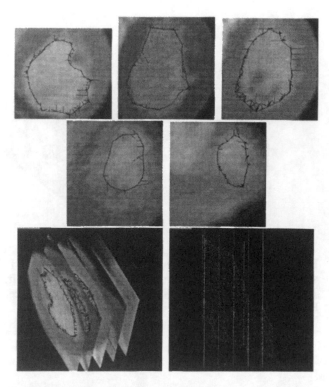

Figure 5: Segmentation of the ED phase of an EBT study. The top two rows show the final crossection of the 3D model on ED images. The bottom row shows two views of the final 3D model.

were set to .01 and the fitting required 300 iterations taking 2 minutes on a Sparc 10. Figure 4 shows the segmentation results on a cine cardiac MR study with 1mm × 1mm × 8mm resolution. The segmentation of phase 1 data along with the start state is presented. The model was originally tessellated with 112 nodes and subdivision was set to occur when edge lengths were longer than .15 mm. The original mesh required significant subdivision. The final mesh contained 804 nodes. The stiffness values were set to .01. Fitting took only 50 iterations due to the close initial approximation. Figure5 shows the results of segmenting the ED phase of a 5 level EBT study. The segmentation was initialized with 96 elements and subdivided into 1548 elements in 136 iterations of the algorithm. The algorithm took approximately 3 minutes to run on a SGI INdigo 2 Extreme but most of the processing time went into the graphical display. In both cases rigid-body and global deformations were damped to the point of non-contribution for reasons mentioned in the segmentation and tracking section.

8 Conclusions

We described a method for segmenting and tracking of multi-slice, multi-phase anisotropic cardiac MR and EBT data. The method described above has the advantage of operating in the clinically-used protocols for MR and EBT acquisition. Our results, however are still in the preliminary stages. The major challenges confronting effective segmentation and tracking include creating image forces for effectively producing global deformations and rigid body transformations, and additional constraints for reducing the attraction of the model to the epicardium. We are currently exploring a technique that combines the advantages of segmented data forces (the force emanating from a data point is proportional to the distance from the data point to the model [9]) and image forces as described above. It involves extracting edgels from the image and allowing the edgels to attract portions of the model with certain characteristics (e.g., expected orientation of surface normal) within some range of distance.

References

[1] I. Cohen, L. D. Cohen, and N. Ayache. Using deformable surfaces to segment 3-D images and infer differential structures. *CVGIP: IU*, 56(2):242–263, 1992.

[2] L. Cohen and I. D. Cohen. Finite Element Methods for Active Contour Models and Balloon for 2-D and 3-D Images. *IEEE PAMI*, 15(11):1131-1147, Nov. 1993.

[3] A. Gupta and C.-C. Liang. 3-D model-data correspondence and nonrigid deformation. In *Procs. of the Conf. on CVPR*, June 1993.

[4] A. Gupta, T. O'Donnell and A. Singh. A 3-D Deformable Model for Segmentation and Tracking of Anisotropic Cine Cardiac MR Images. In *SPIE Image Processing Conference*, Vol. 2167, 1994.

[5] T. McInerney and D. Terzopoulos. A finite element model for 3d shape reconstruction and nonrigid motion tracking. In *ICCV*, 518–523, 1993.

[6] D. Terzopoulos and D. Metaxas. Dynamic 3D models with local and global deformations: Deformable superquadrics. *Trans. PAMI*, 13(7):703–714, 1991.

[7] Demetri Terzopoulos and Dimitri Metaxas. Dynamic 3d models with local and global deformations: Deformable superquadrics. In *Procs of ICCV*, Dec 1990.

[8] M.C. Rivara. Algorithms for Refining triangular grids suitable for adaptive and multigrid techniques. In *International Journal for Numerical Methods in Engineering*, 20, pp. 745-756, 1984.

[9] T. O'Donnell, X.S. Fang, A. Gupta, T Boult. The Deformable Extruded Generalized Cylinder *Procs of CVPR Conference*, June 1994.

[10] Dimitri Metaxas and Eunyoung Koh. Efficient Shape Representation Using Deformable Models with Locally Adaptive Finite Elements In *Geometric Methods in Computer Vision II, SPIE 2031*, pp. 160-171, 1993.

Address for correspondence:

Dr. Alok Gupta
Siemens Corporate Research, Inc.
755 College Road East, Princeton, NJ 08540. USA.
Email: alok@scr.siemens.com

A DYNAMIC FINITE ELEMENT SURFACE MODEL FOR SEGMENTATION AND TRACKING IN MULTIDIMENSIONAL MEDICAL IMAGES WITH APPLICATION TO CARDIAC 4D IMAGE ANALYSIS

Tim McInerney and Demetri Terzopoulos

Department of Computer Science, University of Toronto, Toronto, ON, Canada M5S 1A4

(Received 9 May 1994)

Abstract—This paper presents a physics-based approach to anatomical surface segmentation, reconstruction, and tracking in multidimensional medical images. The approach makes use of a dynamic "balloon" model—a spherical thin-plate under tension surface spline which deforms elastically to fit the image data. The fitting process is mediated by internal forces stemming from the elastic properties of the spline and external forces which are produced from the data. The forces interact in accordance with Lagrangian equations of motion that adjust the model's deformational degrees of freedom to fit the data. We employ the finite element method to represent the continuous surface in the form of weighted sums of local polynomial basis functions. We use a quintic triangular finite element whose nodal variables include positions as well as the first and second partial derivatives of the surface. We describe a system, implemented on a high performance graphics workstation, which applies the model fitting technique to the segmentation of the cardiac LV surface in volume (3D) CT images and LV tracking in dynamic volume (4D) CT images to estimate its nonrigid motion over the cardiac cycle. The system features a graphical user interface which minimizes error by affording specialist users interactive control over the dynamic model fitting process.

Key Words: 3D/4D medical image analysis, Deformable models, Finite elements, Dynamics, Cardiac LV segmentation, Nonrigid motion tracking, Visualization, Interaction

1 INTRODUCTION

CT, MRI, PET and other noninvasive medical imaging technologies can provide exceptional views of internal anatomical structures, but the computer aided visualization, manipulation, and quantitative analysis of the multidimensional image data they produce is still limited. State-of-the-art medical imagers generate massive databases of static volume (3D) and dynamic volume (4D) images. These data sets, which usually suffer from sampling artifacts, spatial aliasing, and noise, are essentially "blocks of granite" with meaningful embedded structures. An important problem is to extract the surface elements belonging to an anatomical structure (the segmentation step) and to integrate these surface elements into a globally coherent surface model of the structure (the reconstruction step). Certain diagnostic procedures also require the tracking and deformation analysis of nonrigidly moving anatomical surfaces (e.g., the stretching of the left ventricle (LV) during the cardiac cycle is directly related to heart condition). The ease and accuracy of such procedures can be critically dependent upon the model used. Dynamic models are needed which are robust against noise-corrupted data and which are capable of accurately representing the complex geometries of anatomical surfaces while permitting the quantitative measurement of highly nonrigid tissue kinematics.

This paper describes a physics-based modeling approach that addresses the surface segmentation and reconstruction problems, as well as the geometric analysis and nonrigid motion estimation problems. We develop a dynamic, elastically deformable surface model whose deformation is governed by basic laws of nonrigid motion. The formulation of the motion equations includes a strain energy, simulated forces, and other physical quantities. The surface strain energy stems from a thin-plate under tension variational spline. Deformation results from the action of internal spline forces which impose surface continuity constraints and external forces which fit the surface to the image data. The inherently dynamic formulation of the model makes it suitable both for static anatomical surface reconstruction and for problems involving the reconstruction and tracking of nonrigidly moving organs.

To deal with closed anatomical surfaces, we formulate a deformable "balloon" model that is topologically isomorphic to a sphere. We employ the finite element method to spatially discretize the balloon, uniformly tessellating it into a set of connected triangular element domains. The finite element method provides an analytic, piecewise polynomial surface representation that is (C^1) continuous across triangles. We use a quintic finite element whose nodal variables include not only the nodal positions, but also the first and second parametric partial derivatives of the surface. The element is naturally suited to the surface energy functional because these same partial derivatives occur in the thin-plate under tension energy expression. The existence of parametric derivative nodal variables facilitates the computation of the differential properties of the modeled surface. In particular, the nodal variables and their time derivatives can be useful for computing the surface curvature, enclosed volume, and motion properties of anatomical surfaces.

We have implemented a system on a high performance graphics workstation which applies the dynamic model fitting technique to the segmentation of the LV surface in cardiac volume (3D) CT images and LV tracking in dynamic volume (4D) CT images in order to estimate nonrigid LV motion over the cardiac cycle. The system includes a graphical user interface which provides interactive visualization and affords control over the model fitting process. The interface allows a user to select the initial size and location of the model and to exert interactive forces on the model as it deforms to fit the data. This type of interactive control is desirable in medical image analysis applications where there is low tolerance for inaccuracy, because it allows specialist users to exploit their knowledge to correct model fitting errors.

2 BACKGROUND

The literature on segmentation and surface reconstruction in 3D medical images includes both manual and automatic techniques. The dominant manual method is slice-editing. In manual slice-editing a skilled operator, using a computer mouse, pen, or trackball traces the region of interest on each slice of the volume. This labor intensive method suffers from many drawbacks, such as difficulties in achieving reproducible segmentation results, difficulties in comparing measurements from different operators, and difficulties deducing 3D structure from 2D slices. The technique can be speeded up and made more reproducible, however, through the use of contour extraction methods such as interactive snakes (1, 31).

The traditional automatic segmentation methods, such as density thresholding and the application of (2D or 3D) edge operators, have many well-known problems. Edge detection and the more recent marching cube (2) technique reduce volume data into something that is more readily displayed through 3D

graphics, such as surface elements. However, they employ only the local properties of the image data; hence, they raise the difficult problem of establishing the connectivity of surface trace elements in order to assemble sensible global surface structures (3). These difficulties have prompted some researchers to settle for merely visualizing the volume data in its original form using morphology (4) or volume rendering techniques (5). Unlike global surface models, however, these voxel-display representations do not attempt to capture the geometric structure of anatomical structures; hence, they do not treat the data in a manner consistent with the physical properties of the imaged objects.

Deformable surface models are a promising approach to extracting anatomically meaningful structures from volume data. The dynamic form of the deformable model fitting technique described in this paper was first introduced by Terzopoulos, Witkin, and Kass (6). They proposed a dynamic deformable cylinder model constructed from generalized splines, along with force field techniques to fit the model to image data. This dynamic approach is being pursued by several researchers in computational vision (7–13). The use of finite element representations for variational problems in vision was first explored in (14). Our formulation applies the finite element method to the thin-plate under tension spline proposed in (15) in order to derive discrete nonrigid dynamics equations. The finite element representation yields piecewise continuous deformable surface models that generally require fewer variables for similar accuracy compared to finite difference approaches.

Our work is related to that of Young (16, 17) and Cohen and Cohen (18, 19) who also develop 3D deformable surface models which are based on the thin-plate under tension spline. Young fits an open bicubic Hermitian finite element based surface to the 3D locations of the coronary arteries at diastasis. The parameters of the time-varying displacement field were then fitted to the tracked displacements of the bifurcation points of the coronary arteries. Cohen and Cohen fit a cylindrical, bicubic Hermitian finite element based surface to MRI images of the LV. Another relevant deformable model is the discrete model developed by Miller et al. (20), which is subdivided and fitted to CT volume images by a relaxation process that minimizes a set of constraints such as the distance to the data or the local curvature of the model.

In our work we develop a closed 3D surface model based on a quintic triangular finite element with position and derivative nodal variables. The model begins as a uniformly tessellated icosahedron which may subdivide repeatedly to attain the desired geometric resolution. Our model is dynamic in the sense that it undergoes deformations that are governed by nonrigid Lagrangian mechanics. Note, however, that although these dynamics equations serve well in model fitting and tracking using multidimensional data sets, we make no attempt to model the actual biomechanical properties of the anatomical structure under consideration [such as the cardiac LV; see, e.g., (21)].

3 DYNAMIC DEFORMABLE BALLOON MODEL

The balloon model that we develop in this paper is constructed of the simulated thin-plate material under tension. The deformation energy of the material serves as a constraint which compels the model to vary smoothly almost everywhere. The balloon is represented as a vector-valued parametric function $\mathbf{x}(u, v) = [x(u, v), y(u, v), z(u, v)]^\top$ where vector $\mathbf{x}$ represents the positions of material points (u, v) relative to a reference frame in Euclidean 3-space.

The deformation energy of the thin-plate under tension material is given by the energy functional

$$\mathcal{E}_p(\mathbf{x}) = \iint \alpha_{10} \left| \frac{\partial \mathbf{x}}{\partial u} \right|^2 + \alpha_{01} \left| \frac{\partial \mathbf{x}}{\partial v} \right|^2$$
$$+ \beta_{20} \left| \frac{\partial^2 \mathbf{x}}{\partial u^2} \right|^2 + \beta_{11} \left| \frac{\partial^2 \mathbf{x}}{\partial u \partial v} \right|^2 + \beta_{02} \left| \frac{\partial^2 \mathbf{x}}{\partial v^2} \right|^2 \, du \, dv. \quad (1)$$

$\mathcal{E}_p$ is a controlled-continuity spline defined in (15). The nonnegative weighting functions $\alpha_{ij}(u, v)$ and $\beta_{ij}(u, v)$ control the elasticity of the material. The α_{10} and α_{01} functions control the tensions in the u and v directions, respectively, while the β_{02} and β_{20} functions control the corresponding bending rigidities, and the β_{11} function controls the twisting rigidity. Increasing the α_{ij} has a tendency to decrease the surface area of the material, while increasing the β_{ij} tends to make it less flexible. In general, the weighting functions may be used to introduce depth and orientation discontinuities in the material. In this paper, however, we do not make use of this capability and set the functions to constant values $\alpha_{ij}(u, v) = \alpha_{ij}$ and $\beta_{ij}(u, v) = \beta_{ij}$. Figure 1 shows the thin plate under tension balloon pulled radially by a spring point force (in (a) $\alpha_{ij} = 0.8$ and $\beta_{ij} = 0$, in (b) $\alpha_{ij} = \beta_{ij} = 0.5$, and in (c) $\alpha_{ij} = 0$ and $\beta_{ij} = 0.8$):

A general and elegant approach to fitting deformable surface models to data, especially when the data are time-varying, is to make the models dynamic. A dynamic formulation imposes a natural temporal continuity on the model, thereby permitting a smoothly animated display of the data fitting process. It also allows a user to interact with the model by applying constraint forces to pull it out of local minima towards the correct solution.

In a Lagrangian dynamics formulation, the positions of material points becomes a time-dependent function $\mathbf{x}(u, v, t)$ and we imbue the simulated material with mass and damping densities. The deformation energy yields internal elastic forces, and $\mathcal{E}_p(\mathbf{x})$ is minimized when these forces equilibrate against externally applied forces and the model stabilizes: $\partial \mathbf{x}/\partial t = \partial^2 \mathbf{x}/\partial t^2 = \mathbf{0}$.

The dynamic behavior of the balloon model during the fitting process is governed by the second-order partial differential equations

$$\mu \frac{\partial^2 \mathbf{x}}{\partial t^2} + \gamma \frac{\partial \mathbf{x}}{\partial t} + \delta_x \mathcal{E}_p = \mathbf{f}, \quad (2)$$

where the first term represents the inertial forces due to the mass density $\mu(u, v)$, the second term represents the damping forces due to the damping density $\gamma(u, v)$, the third term represents the elastic forces which resist deformation, and finally $\mathbf{f}(u, v, t)$ represents the external forces derived from the image data. The (generally nonlinear) data forces may be formalized as stemming from a data functional

$$\mathcal{E}_d(\mathbf{x}) = - \iint \mathbf{x}^\top \mathbf{f} \, du \, dv. \quad (3)$$

4 FINITE ELEMENT REPRESENTATION

The finite difference method or the finite element method are applicable to computing numerical solutions to the function $\mathbf{x}(u, v, t)$. Finite difference solutions approximate the continuous function $\mathbf{x}$ as a set of discrete nodes in space. A disadvantage of the finite difference approach is that the continuity of the solution between nodes is not made explicit. The finite element method, on the other hand, provides continuous surface approximations; that is, the method approximates the unknown function $\mathbf{x}$ in terms of combinations of local basis functions (22).

To apply the finite element method to our models, we tessellate the continuous material domain (u, v) into a mesh of M element subdomains E_j. We approximate $\mathbf{x}$ as a weighted sum of piecewise polynomial basis functions $\mathbf{N}_i$:

$$\mathbf{x}(u, v, t) \approx \hat{\mathbf{x}}(u, v, t) = \sum_{i=1}^{n} \mathbf{N}_i(u, v) \mathbf{q}_i(t), \quad (4)$$

where $\mathbf{q}_i$ is a vector of nodal variables associated with mesh node i.

Substituting (4) into (2) yields the discrete equations of motion

$$\mathbf{M}\ddot{\mathbf{q}} + \mathbf{C}\dot{\mathbf{q}} + \mathbf{K}\mathbf{q} = \mathbf{f}_q, \quad (5)$$

with $\mathbf{q} = [\mathbf{q}_1^\top, \ldots, \mathbf{q}_i^\top, \ldots, \mathbf{q}_n^\top]^\top$, where the mass matrix $\mathbf{M}$, damping matrix $\mathbf{C}$, and stiffness matrix $\mathbf{K}$

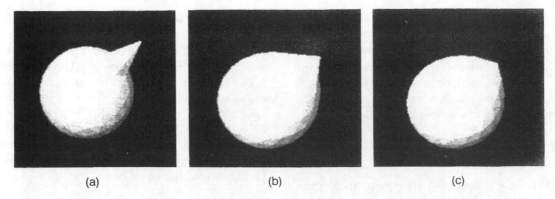

(a)　　　　　　　　(b)　　　　　　　　(c)

Fig. 1. Balloon models with varying elasticity and pulled by a spring point force.

are sparse, symmetric matrices and vector $\mathbf{f}_q$ are nodal data forces. These *global* matrices may be assembled from their associated local element matrices by expanding each element matrix appropriately into a $q \times q$ matrix and then summing:

$$\mathbf{M} = \sum_{j=1}^{M} \mathbf{M}_{q\times q}^j; \; \mathbf{C} = \sum_{j=1}^{M} \mathbf{C}_{q\times q}^j; \; \mathbf{K} = \sum_{j=1}^{M} \mathbf{K}_{q\times q}^j; \; \mathbf{f}_q = \sum_{j=1}^{M} \mathbf{f}_q^j, \quad (6)$$

where $\mathbf{M}^j$, $\mathbf{C}^j$, $\mathbf{K}^j$, and $\mathbf{f}_q^j$ are element mass, damping, and stiffness matrices, and nodal data forces associated with element E_j, $j = 1, \ldots, M$.

We now derive expressions for $\mathbf{M}^j$, $\mathbf{C}^j$, $\mathbf{K}^j$, and $\mathbf{f}_q^j$ from element kinetic and potential energy functionals. Let $\mathbf{x}^j(u, v, t)$ be the position of material point (u, v) within E_j, and let $\mathbf{q}^j$ denote the concatenation of nodal variables for all the nodes of E_j. Following (4), we write the element trial function

$$\hat{\mathbf{x}}^j(u, v, t) = \mathbf{N}^j(u, v)\mathbf{q}^j(t) \approx \mathbf{x}^j(u, v, t), \quad (7)$$

where $\mathbf{N}^j$ are the element shape functions. Recall that the basis functions $\mathbf{N}_i$ are obtained by superposing the shape functions associated with node i. The element velocity is $\partial\hat{\mathbf{x}}^j/\partial t = \mathbf{N}^j\dot{\mathbf{q}}^j$, where $\dot{\mathbf{q}}^j(t)$ is the rate of change of the nodal variables.

The kinetic energy associated with element E_j is

$$\frac{1}{2}\iint_{E_j} \mu \frac{\partial\hat{\mathbf{x}}^{j^\mathrm{T}}}{\partial t} \frac{\partial\hat{\mathbf{x}}^j}{\partial t} \, du \, dv = \frac{1}{2} \dot{\mathbf{q}}^{j^\mathrm{T}} \left[\iint_{E_j} \mu\mathbf{N}^{j^\mathrm{T}}\mathbf{N}^j \, du \, dv\right] \dot{\mathbf{q}}^j$$

$$= \frac{1}{2} \dot{\mathbf{q}}^{j^\mathrm{T}}\mathbf{M}^j\dot{\mathbf{q}}^j, \quad (8)$$

where the element mass matrix is given by

$$\mathbf{M}^j = \iint_{E_j} \mu\mathbf{N}^{j^\mathrm{T}}\mathbf{N}^j \, du \, dv. \quad (9)$$

We introduce a simple velocity-proportional kinetic energy dissipation according to the (Raleigh) dissipation functional

$$\frac{1}{2}\iint_{E_j} \gamma \frac{\partial\hat{\mathbf{x}}^{j\mathrm{T}}}{\partial t} \frac{\partial\hat{\mathbf{x}}^j}{\partial t} \, du \, dv = \frac{1}{2} \dot{\mathbf{q}}^{j\mathrm{T}}\mathbf{C}^j\dot{\mathbf{q}}^j. \quad (10)$$

The element damping matrix is proportional to the mass matrix and is given by

$$\mathbf{C}^j = \iint_{E_j} \gamma\mathbf{N}^{j^\mathrm{T}}\mathbf{N}^j \, du \, dv. \quad (11)$$

According to Eqn. (1) the element deformation matrix may be expressed as

$$\mathcal{E}_p^j(\mathbf{x}) = \iint_{E_j} \boldsymbol{\sigma}^{j^\mathrm{T}}\boldsymbol{\epsilon}^j \, du \, dv, \quad (12)$$

where the strain vector is

$$\boldsymbol{\epsilon}^j = \left[\frac{\partial\mathbf{x}^{j^\mathrm{T}}}{\partial u}, \frac{\partial\mathbf{x}^{j^\mathrm{T}}}{\partial v}, \frac{\partial^2\mathbf{x}^{j^\mathrm{T}}}{\partial u^2}, \frac{\partial^2\mathbf{x}^{j^\mathrm{T}}}{\partial u\partial v}, \frac{\partial^2\mathbf{x}^{j^\mathrm{T}}}{\partial v^2}\right]^\mathrm{T} = \mathbf{Lx}^j \quad (13)$$

and the stress vector is

$$\boldsymbol{\sigma}^j = \begin{bmatrix} \alpha_{10}^j\mathbf{I} & \mathbf{0} & \mathbf{0} & \mathbf{0} & \mathbf{0} \\ \mathbf{0} & \alpha_{01}^j\mathbf{I} & \mathbf{0} & \mathbf{0} & \mathbf{0} \\ \mathbf{0} & \mathbf{0} & \beta_{20}^j\mathbf{I} & \mathbf{0} & \mathbf{0} \\ \mathbf{0} & \mathbf{0} & \mathbf{0} & \beta_{11}^j\mathbf{I} & \mathbf{0} \\ \mathbf{0} & \mathbf{0} & \mathbf{0} & \mathbf{0} & \beta_{02}^j\mathbf{I} \end{bmatrix} \boldsymbol{\epsilon}^j = \mathbf{D}^j\boldsymbol{\epsilon}^j, \quad (14)$$

with $\mathbf{I}$ a 3×3 unit matrix. Using Eqn. (7), we can write

$$\boldsymbol{\epsilon}^j = \mathbf{LN}^j\mathbf{q}^j = \mathbf{B}^j\mathbf{q}^j, \quad (15)$$

where $\mathbf{B}^j$ is the element strain matrix. Inserting the expressions for $\boldsymbol{\epsilon}^j$ and $\boldsymbol{\sigma}^j$ into (12) yields

$$\mathcal{E}_p^j(\mathbf{x}) = \mathbf{q}^{j^\mathrm{T}}\mathbf{K}^j\mathbf{q}^j, \quad (16)$$

where the element stiffness matrix is given by

$$\mathbf{K}^j = \iint_{E_j} \mathbf{B}^{j^\mathrm{T}}\mathbf{D}^j\mathbf{B}^j \, du \, dv. \quad (17)$$

Finally, according to Eqn. (3), the potential energy in element E_j due to data forces $\mathbf{f}^j(u, v, t)$ is

$$-\iint\limits_{E_j} \hat{\mathbf{x}}^{jT}\mathbf{f}^j \, du \, dv = -\mathbf{q}^{j^1}\iint\limits_{E_j} \mathbf{N}^{j^1}\mathbf{f}^j \, du \, dv = -Q^{j^1}F_q^j, \quad (18)$$

where the nodal data forces are given by

$$\mathbf{f}_q^j = \iint\limits_{E_j} \mathbf{N}^{j^1}\mathbf{f}^j \, du \, dv. \quad (19)$$

5 MODEL STRUCTURE

The balloon model is a closed surface in Euclidean 3-space which is topologically isomorphic to a sphere. We initially discretize the balloon in the material coordinates (u, v) by tessellating it into a set of 20 triangular elements to form an icosahedron. We chose the icosahedron because it has a simple representation in material coordinates and it has a regular structure in Euclidean 3-space, with each of its 12 nodes connected to five neighboring nodes.

The parametric equation which initially maps the material (u_i, v_i) coordinates of the 12 icosahedron nodes into 3-space is given by

$$\mathbf{x}(u_i, v_i) = a \begin{pmatrix} \cos u_i \ \cos v_i \\ \cos u_i \ \sin v_i \\ \sin u_i \end{pmatrix}, \quad (20)$$

where $-\pi/2 \le v \le \pi/2$ and $-\pi \le u < \pi$ and $a \ge 0$ is a radius parameter.

5.1 Triangular C^1 finite element

We use a fifth-order triangular finite element to implement the balloon model (22). In view of the form of the deformation energy (1) which leads to the strain vector (13), it is natural to choose as nodal variables $\mathbf{x}$, along with its first and second parametric partial derivatives evaluated at each node i. The nodal variable vector for the balloon is therefore

$$\mathbf{q}_i(t)$$
$$= \left[\mathbf{x}_i^T, \left(\frac{\partial \mathbf{x}}{\partial u}\right)_i^T, \left(\frac{\partial \mathbf{x}}{\partial v}\right)_i^T, \left(\frac{\partial^2 \mathbf{x}}{\partial u^2}\right)_i^T, \left(\frac{\partial^2 \mathbf{x}}{\partial u \partial v}\right)_i^T, \left(\frac{\partial^2 \mathbf{x}}{\partial v^2}\right)_i^T\right]^T.$$
$$(21)$$

Figure 2 shows the C^1 continuous element defined locally in the dimensionless oblique coordinates (ξ, η). In this local coordinate system the material coordinates (u, v) can be expressed as

$$u = (1 - \xi - \eta)u_1 + \xi u_2 + \eta u_3,$$
$$v = (1 - \xi - \eta)v_1 + \xi v_2 + \eta v_3, \quad (22)$$

where (u_i, v_i) are the material coordinates at the nodes (as numbered in the figure), and the local nodal variable vector becomes

$$\mathbf{q}_{i_\xi}(t) = [\mathbf{x}_i^T, (\mathbf{x}_\xi)_i^T, (\mathbf{x}_\eta)_i^T, (\mathbf{x}_{\xi\xi})_i^T, (\mathbf{x}_{\xi\eta})_i^T, (\mathbf{x}_{\eta\eta})_i^T]^T. \quad (23)$$

The transformation from global to local coordinates is

$$\mathbf{q}_i = \mathbf{T}_i \mathbf{q}_{i_\xi} \quad (24)$$

where the transformation matrix $\mathbf{T}_i$ is specified in (22) (pp. 100–101).

Concatenating the $\mathbf{q}_{i_\xi}$ at each of the three nodes of element j, we obtain the 18-dimensional element nodal vector $\mathbf{q}_\xi^j = [\mathbf{q}_{1_\xi}^T, \mathbf{q}_{2_\xi}^T, \mathbf{q}_{3_\xi}^T]^T$. According to (7), we can write the local trial function as

$$\hat{\mathbf{x}}^j(\xi, \eta, t) = \mathbf{N}^j(\xi, \eta)\mathbf{q}_\xi^j(t). \quad (25)$$

The nodal shape functions $\mathbf{N}_i(\xi, \eta)$ which are contained in the 18×18 matrix $\mathbf{N}^j$ are, for node 1

$$\mathbf{N}_1 = \lambda^2(10\lambda - 15\lambda^2 + 6\lambda^3 + 30\xi\eta(\xi + \eta)),$$

$$\mathbf{N}_2 = \xi\lambda^2(3 - 2\lambda - 3\xi^2 + 6\xi\eta)$$

$$\mathbf{N}_3 = \eta\lambda^2(3 - 2\lambda - 3\eta^2 + 6\xi\eta),$$

$$\mathbf{N}_4 = \tfrac{1}{2}\xi^2\lambda^2(1 - \xi + 2\eta)$$

$$\mathbf{N}_5 = \xi\eta\lambda^2, \quad \mathbf{N}_6 = \tfrac{1}{2}\eta^2\lambda^2(1 + 2\xi - \eta),$$

for node 2,

$$\mathbf{N}_7 = \xi^2(10\xi - 15\xi^2 + 6\xi^3 + 15\eta^2\lambda),$$

$$\mathbf{N}_8 = \frac{\xi^2}{2}(-8\xi + 14\xi^2 - 6\xi^3 - 15\eta^2\lambda)$$

$$\mathbf{N}_9 = \frac{\xi^2\eta}{2}(6 - 4\xi - 3\eta - 3\eta^2 + 3\xi\eta),$$

$$\mathbf{N}_{10} = \frac{\eta^2}{4}(2\xi(1 - \xi)^2 + 5\eta^2\lambda)$$

$$\mathbf{N}_{11} = \frac{\xi^2\eta}{2}(-2 + 2\xi + \eta + \eta^2 - \xi\eta),$$

$$\mathbf{N}_{12} = \frac{\xi^2\eta^2\lambda}{4} + \frac{\xi^3\eta^2}{2},$$

and for node 3,

$$\mathbf{N}_{13} = \eta^2(10\eta - 15\eta^2 + 6\eta^3 + 15\xi^2\lambda),$$

$$\mathbf{N}_{14} = \frac{\xi\eta^2}{2}(6 - 3\xi - 4\eta - 3\xi^2 + 3\xi\eta)$$

$$\mathbf{N}_{15} = \frac{\eta^2}{2}(-8\eta + 14\eta^2 - 6\eta^3 - 15\xi^2\lambda),$$

$$\mathbf{N}_{16} = \frac{\xi^2\eta^2\lambda}{4} + \frac{\xi^2\eta^3}{2}$$

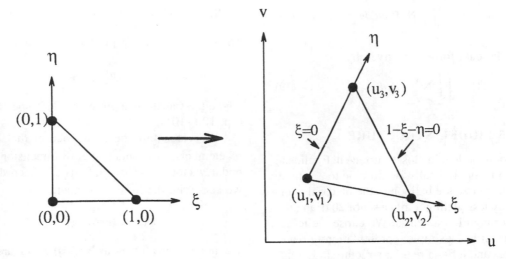

Fig. 2. C^1 continuous triangular element.

$$N_{17} = \frac{\xi \eta^2}{2} (-2 + \xi + 2\eta + \xi^2 - \xi\eta),$$

$$N_{18} = \frac{\eta^2}{4} (2\eta(1 - \eta)^2 + 5\xi^2\lambda),$$

where $\lambda = 1 - \xi - \eta$.

Note that the polynomial basis of the element is complete up to fourth-order terms and contains three fifth-order terms (22). The trial functions are C^∞ within elements and they ensure C^1 continuity between elements. Since Eqn. (1) contains up to second order derivatives, the element is conforming.

The shape functions are expressed in terms of the local coordinates (ξ, η) and it is convenient to work with these coordinates. Thus, the required derivatives of the shape functions in the strain matrix **B** are computed using repeated applications of the chain rule and Eqn. (23). Also, a function $f(u, v)$ may be integrated over E_j by transforming to the local coordinate system as follows:

$$\iint_{E_j} f(u, v) \, du \, dv = \iint_{E_j} f(u(\xi, \eta), v(\xi, \eta)) \det \mathbf{J} \, d\xi \, d\eta, \quad (26)$$

where

$$\mathbf{J} = \begin{bmatrix} \dfrac{\partial u}{\partial \xi} & \dfrac{\partial v}{\partial \xi} \\[2mm] \dfrac{\partial u}{\partial \eta} & \dfrac{\partial v}{\partial \eta} \end{bmatrix} \quad (27)$$

is the Jacobian matrix. These integrals are approximated using Gauss-Legendre quadrature rules (22).

5.2 Model refinement

Our implementation allows the balloon model to be refined during the fitting process by subdividing the triangular elements. Each element spawns 4 child elements by connecting the midpoints of its 3 edges (Fig. 3). This process may be applied recursively to each child element. The connectivity of all new vertices formed in this fashion is six, while the original 12 vertices of the icosahedron remain five-connected. Thus a low resolution model may be initially fit to the data, efficiently reconstructing the rough overall shape, and subsequently refined in steps as necessary to capture the detail. This approach greatly reduces the overall computation time required for reconstruction (Fig. 4).

Since each global subdivision of the balloon model increases the number of element nodes by approximately fourfold, this scheme has its limits. A better scheme is to locally subdivide the model in areas where the shape implied by the data varies considerably. Local subdivision is not pursued in this paper.

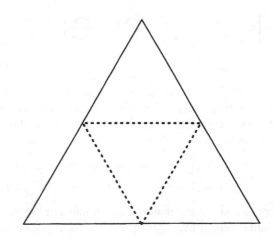

Fig. 3. Subdividing an equilateral triangular element.

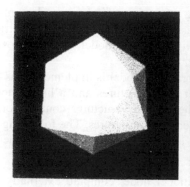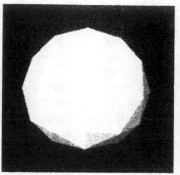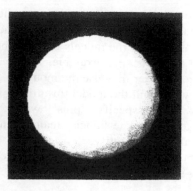

Fig. 4. Balloon model mesh in Euclidean 3-space at three subdivision levels.

6 APPLIED FORCES

Our dynamic model fitting paradigm applies data constraints to the model as external force distributions $\mathbf{f}(u, v, t)$. The contribution of the force distribution to each element E_j is converted through (19) to generalized forces $\mathbf{f}_q^j$ associated with the nodal variables of the element. Two types of data forces are applied to the balloon model-forces obtained through gradients of image potential functions and forces based on distances between data points and the model surface.

6.1 3D image forces

When extracting and reconstructing surfaces from 3D image data, we design forces that localize salient image features. For example, to attract our model towards significant 3D intensity edges (gradients) in some region of an image function $I(x, y, z)$ we construct a 3D potential function

$$P(x, y, z) = \lambda_1\|\nabla(G_\sigma * I)\| + \lambda_2\|O_{MD} * I\| \tag{28}$$

whose potential valleys (minima) coincide with the object surface (6). In the first term on the right hand side of (28), G_σ denotes a 3D Gaussian smoothing filter of characteristic width σ. This filter broadens or narrows the potential valleys of this term thus determining the extent of the region of attraction of the intensity gradient. Typically, the attraction has a relatively short range. In the second term, a 3D edge detector, the 3D Monga-Deriche (MD) operator (23), is applied to the image data to produce a 3D intensity edge field. The potential valleys of this term tend to be narrow and deep, complementing (and coinciding with) the wider but more shallow valleys produced by the first term. A weighted combination of these terms is formed so the model will ''slide down'' the shallow valleys and then drop into the deeper valleys thus locking onto image edges.

The potential function produces a force distribution

$$\mathbf{f}(\mathbf{x}) = \kappa \frac{\nabla P(\mathbf{x})}{\|\nabla P(\mathbf{x})\|} \tag{29}$$

on the model, where κ controls the strength of the force. We normalize the image force as for better numerical stability (9). Consequently, all significant edge voxels, including spurious edges, will attract the model equally. However, once the model converges towards the true 3D edges of the object, the smoothing effect of the model will give it a tendency to ignore spurious 3D edges.

Note that to compute ∇P at any model point $\mathbf{x}(u, v)$ from a discrete 3D image data set $I(i, j, k)$, we tri-linearly interpolate $I(\mathbf{x})$ using values at the eight surrounding pixels.

6.2 Balloon inflation force

When extracting object surfaces from 3D image data, the balloon model must first be initialized within the object. If the model is not close enough to the surface of the object, the short-range image forces defined previously may not attract it. For this reason, an internal pressure force is used to ''inflate'' the balloon model towards the object surface (6, 9). The force takes the form

$$\mathbf{f} = \kappa_1 \mathbf{n}(u, v), \tag{30}$$

where $\mathbf{n}(u, v)$ is the unit normal vector to the model surface at the point $\mathbf{x}(u, v)$, and κ_1 is the amplitude of this force. If κ_1 is negative, the force will deflate the balloon. We usually set the image force scale parameter κ and κ_1 to be of the same order, with κ slightly larger than κ_1 so that a significant 3D edge will stop the inflation, but with κ_1 large enough for the model to pass through weak or spurious edges.

6.3 User and constraint forces

Accurate measurement of medical image structures is important in a clinical setting. For this and other reasons, visualization and manual interaction are likely to remain essential in 3D biomedical image scenarios. Our dynamic modeling approach provides a facile interface to the models through the use of force interaction tools. For example, as the model is deforming, the user may use the mouse to specify spring forces which pull the model towards significant image features, or to specify "pins" which constrain the model to interpolate fiducial features in the data that a specialist can identify.

Both the mouse and pin forces are implemented as long-range spring-like point forces

$$\mathbf{f}(u, v) = \kappa \|\mathbf{p} - \mathbf{x}(u_p, v_p)\| \qquad (31)$$

proportional to the separation between the mouse or pin point $\mathbf{p}$ in space and the point of influence (u_p, v_p) of the force on the model's surface.

We approximate (u_p, v_p) as the model node with minimal distance to the point $\mathbf{p}$, using a heuristic local neighborhood search to find the nearest model node.

6.4 Parallel numerical integration

Our dynamic surface model is easiest to manipulate interactively during the fitting process if its motion is critically damped to minimize vibrations. Critical damping can be achieved by appropriately balancing the mass and damping distributions. Another way of eliminating vibration while preserving useful dynamics is to set the mass density $\mu(u, v)$ to zero, thus reducing (5) to

$$\mathbf{C}\dot{\mathbf{q}} + \mathbf{K}\mathbf{q} = \mathbf{f}_q. \qquad (32)$$

This first-order dynamical system governs a model which has no inertia and comes to rest as soon as all the forces equilibrate. Although (32) is simpler to implement and numerically more efficient, a model lacking inertia can experience difficulty tracking moving objects if external forces are not persistently reliable due to weak, noisy, or missing data. Nonetheless, we have successfully employed the first-order dynamic model (32) in our cardiac reconstruction and tracking system which is presented in the next section.

We integrate equation (32) forward through time using an explicit first-order Euler method. This method approximates the temporal derivatives with forward finite differences. It updates the degrees of freedom $\mathbf{q}$ of the model from time t to time $t + \Delta t$ according to the formula

$$\mathbf{q}^{(t+\Delta t)} = \mathbf{q}^{(t)} + \Delta t (\mathbf{C}^{(t)})^{-1} (\mathbf{f}_q^{(t)} - \mathbf{K}\mathbf{q}^{(t)}). \qquad (33)$$

In our implementation, we do not explicitly assemble and factorize a global stiffness matrix $\mathbf{K}$ as is common practice in applied finite element analysis. Instead, we update the nodal vectors $\mathbf{q}_i^{(t+\Delta t)}$ iteratively by computing the product $\mathbf{K}^j \mathbf{q}^j$ on an element-by-element basis using the element stiffness matrices $\mathbf{K}^j$. This approach makes the model fitting process easily parallelizable.

The deformable model is implemented as a list of finite element data structures and a list of node data structures. The element structures contain pointers to their associated node structures. The following actions are repeated at each time step of the model fitting process:

- For each model node, compute externally applied forces $\mathbf{f}_q$.
- For each element, accumulate the internal forces on the element nodal vectors $\mathbf{q}^j$ by computing the product $\mathbf{K}^j \mathbf{q}^j$.
- For each model node, update the position based on the applied and internal forces on the node using Euler time integration.

These operations can be readily parallelized on a shared memory multiprocessor (such as our 4 processor Silicon Graphics Iris 4D/340VGX workstation) by partitioning the element and node lists into equal sized sublists according to the number of processors available. Each processor then independently executes the loops using its assigned lists of elements and nodes.

7 A SYSTEM FOR 3D/4D MEDICAL IMAGE ANALYSIS

This section describes an interactive system, implemented on a Silicon Graphics Iris 4D/340 VGX workstation, that uses the deformable balloon model to extract (segment), reconstruct, and track surfaces of biological structures in volume images. The design of this experimental system is geared towards cardiac image analysis.

The system provides views of the data and model in separate windows to facilitate the interactive initialization and visualization of the data and the balloon model. One window displays a 3D view of the model embedded in three orthogonal image slices of the volume data (Fig. 5b), which are $118 \times 128 \times 128$ pixel CT images of a canine heart. The user can interactively rotate this 3D view in any direction as well as change the image slice of any image plane. In addition, the user may translate the model in any of the (x, y, z) directions, or scale the model. This capability is useful in initializing the balloon. The other window displays a 2D image slice of one of the three orthogonal image planes overlaid with the corresponding cross section of the balloon model (Fig. 5a). Note that our finite element surface representation makes it possible to compute any cross section of the balloon model to

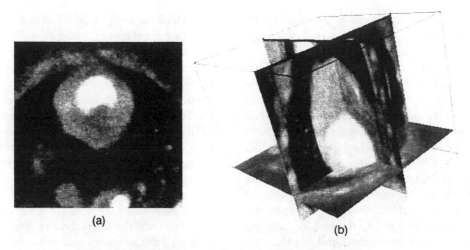

Fig. 5. (a) Image slice window. (b) Image volume window.

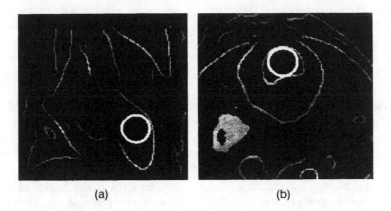

Fig. 6. *YZ* and *XY* view edge detected image slices showing initial cross sections of the balloon model. The edge maps are generated by the application of the 3D Monga-Deriche (MD) operator.

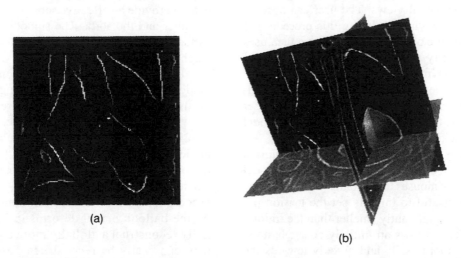

Fig. 7. Segmentation of LV. (a) Cross section of balloon model deforming towards LV edges, influenced by ''pin'' constraints and a ''spring'' pulling the model towards an edge. (b) Balloon model embedded in volume image deforming towards LV edges.

obtain a continuous planar contour. The user can quickly change or scan through the image slices of this orthogonal view or change to another orthogonal view.

The user can interact with the 3D model in the 2D image slice window by applying forces to a cross-sectional contour as if it were a deformable contour [i.e., a snake (1)]. By positioning the mouse at some point in the window and depressing a mouse button, the mouse position is determined and the closest model point on the cross-sectional contour is calculated. A spring force is then applied to the balloon model along the vector from the model point to the mouse position. The force is applied while the mouse button is depressed, and its direction can be changed by dragging the mouse to a new position in the window. The user can also interact with the model by positioning the mouse and depressing a mouse button to specify a pin point. Pin constraints apply a sustained spring force to the closest model point on the cross-sectional contour, forcing the model to adhere closely to the pin. This mechanism allows the user to reinforce or create an object edge. Furthermore, the user may interactively alter the surface tension and rigidity parameters α_{ij} and β_{ij} as well as alter the time step, alter the balloon and image forces, and initiate a global subdivision of the model. Once the model has been fitted to the object surface, the user may choose menu items which compute and display surface curvature, perform enclosed volume calculations, etc.

7.1 The segmentation/reconstruction process

To initiate the surface extraction/reconstruction process, the user scans through the image slices in the 2D image window to locate the approximate center of the object to be extracted. This process is repeated for the two other orthogonal views. The user can observe the 3D volume view window during this procedure to aid in determining the object center. The user then uses the mouse to specify the initial size and location of the model in the 2D image window (Fig. 6). The initial model will then be constructed and will appear embedded in the image slices in the 3D window. The user can further adjust the size and location of the model in either of the windows.

The user may specify an initial model resolution level. Typically we begin with a low resolution model and then use the mouse to globally subdivide the model. It is also useful to initially set the tension parameters α_{ij} to be significantly smaller than the rigidity parameters β_{ij}. This allows an initially coarse balloon model to stretch more easily and quickly towards the edges of the heart. Once the model reaches the edges and the model has been subdivided, β_{ij} is then increased to smooth the finer resolution model.

Once the initial model has been specified, the user may begin the model fitting (Fig. 7). Before or during the model fitting procedure the user may specify any number of pin constraints on the model. We determine by visual inspection when the fitting process is completed. The user can quickly scan the image slices in the 2D window to ascertain how well the cross sections of the model fit the object edges. A possible automatic stopping criterion might monitor the average position change of the model nodes at each iteration to assess whether the model has achieved equilibrium.

7.2 Experiments

We used the interactive system to extract and reconstruct the left-ventricular chamber from 3D CT images of a canine heart. The data set was acquired by the dynamic spatial reconstructor (DSR), a high speed volumetric X-ray CT scanner (24). Sixteen volume images representing a complete cardiac cycle were used in the experiments, with each volume image containing 118 slices of 128×128 pixels. Each slice represents an approximately 0.9 mm thick transverse cross section of the scanned anatomy, with each voxel representing a $(0.9 \text{ mm})^3$ cube of tissue.

Figure 8a shows a sagittal (y-z plane) slice of the canine heart. In a canine heart the valves may appear directly connected to the LV chamber and aorta, frustrating all attempts to fully automate the reconstruction process. Our semi-automatic approach allows a user to interact with the model as it is deforming. As mentioned previously, the user may use the mouse to apply spring forces that pull the model away from spurious edges, or to specify pins which constrain the model to interpolate fiducial features in the data. A few pins are required on one or two image slices of the canine heart data to provide an effective separation between the LV chamber and the aorta. The smoothness of the elastic surface prevents the model from straying very far in neighboring image slices.

Figure 9 shows a cross section of the balloon model in an image slice deforming to fit the edge of the ventricle. The final LV reconstruction is shown in Fig. 10. The initial model consisted of 20 triangular elements. Four global subdivisions of the model were performed during the fitting process to increase the accuracy of the reconstruction. The final model contains 5120 elements and the fitting process takes on the order of 5 minutes to complete. As the balloon model deforms in 3D, it can potentially reconstruct a globally more consistent surface than can easily be reconstructed in serial sections using deformable contours (1). It is also a potentially more robust technique—missing slices do not seriously reduce the quality of the fit—and it is

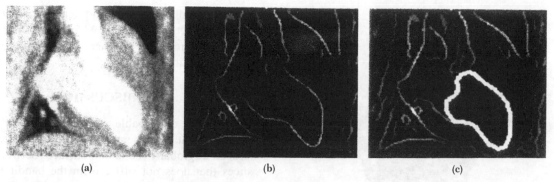

(a)   (b)   (c)

Fig. 8. Intensity and edge detected CT image slice of left ventricle. (a) Intensity image *YZ* plane slice 68. (b) Edge detected image. (c) Cross section of fitted balloon deforming to left ventricle.

far less time consuming than the traditional manual slice-editing technique.

7.3 Estimating the LV motion

We can use the balloon model to estimate the nonrigid motion of the LV over successive CT volumes in the cardiac cycle. We begin by fitting the model to the first volume in the sequence and use this fitted model as the starting point for the reconstruction of the LV in the next volume. We continue this process for all 16 volumes in the cardiac cycle. The tracking process allows the model to be "continuously" deformed by the time-varying external data forces induced by the stream of volume images. The continuous

finite element representation enables us to track the approximate motion of any point of the LV surface through the cardiac cycle (not just the nodal points).

Figure 11 shows sagittal slice 67 through the 16 successive CT volumes over one cardiac cycle. Fig. 12 shows the reconstructed LV sequence. Each fitted model contains 1280 elements and the entire fitting process, including the time required to input the 4D DSR dataset, takes only about 100 min to complete. This demonstrates the enormous potential advantage of the dynamic deformable model approach compared with the time required to manually segment the LV. Once the initial 3D model has been fitted to the first volume, relatively small deformations are needed to

(a)   (b)   (c)

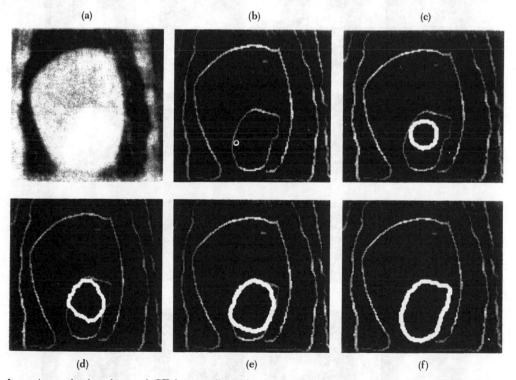

(d)   (e)   (f)

Fig. 9. Intensity and edge detected CT image slice of left ventricle. (a) Intensity image *XZ* plane slice 91. (b) Edge detected image. (c) Cross section of initial balloon model. (d–f) Cross section of balloon deforming to left ventricle.

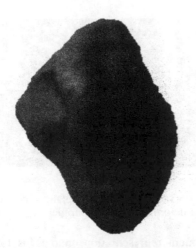

Fig. 10. Figure 10: Reconstruction of left ventricle. Model parameters: $\alpha_{ij} = 0.8$, $\beta_{ij} = 0.2$, $\kappa = 111.0$, $\kappa_1 = 110.0$, $\Delta t = 0.004$.

fit subsequent volumes; consequently very little user intervention (i.e., application of pin constraints or spring forces) is necessary. Moreover, the fitting time per volume image should decrease as images are acquired at higher rates because the interframe motion

will be smaller. This should lead to proportionally greater reductions in effort when the technique is applied to future image scanners capable of greater temporal resolution.

8 DISCUSSION

The 3D deformable model provides an efficient, semi-automatic segmentation technique which reconstructs a globally coherent surface between image slices that does not suffer from the banding artifacts often seen in surfaces reconstructed by independently contouring each serial tomographic image. The surface model approximates the data across all the slices; hence, it is much less sensitive to noise than locally interpolatory segmentation schemes (2).

An extracted surface model with the aforementioned properties provides many options for quantitative analysis of the anatomic object. In cardiology, for instance, volumetric parameters (end-diastolic and end-systolic volumes, stroke volume, and ejection ratio) are diagnostically significant, while surface curvature extrema often have anatomical significance (Fig. 13).

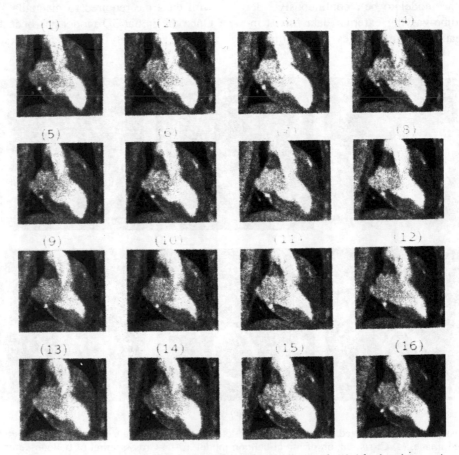

Fig. 11. Sagittal slice of successive CT volumes over one cardiac cycle (1-16) showing motion of LV.

214

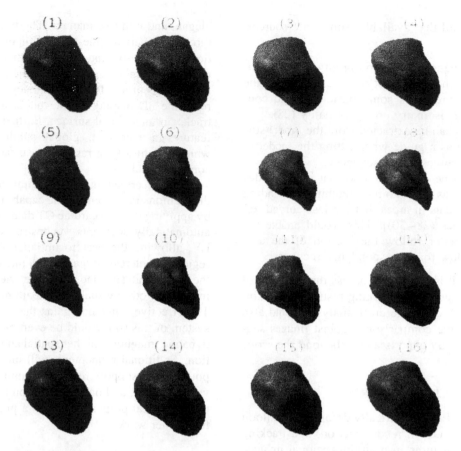

Fig. 12. Tracking of the LV motion during one cardiac cycle (1–16).

We know from differential geometry that smooth 3D surfaces are uniquely characterized (up to rigid-body transformations) by their first and second fundamental forms (25). The parametric form of our surface model (i.e., $\mathbf{x}(u, v) = [x(u, v), y(u, v), z(u, v)]^\top$) and, in particular, the nodal variables (21) of its finite element representation contain all the information needed to compute the first and second fundamental forms of the fitted model surface. The intrinsic differential characteristics of the surface, such as the unit normal and the principal curvatures, can be conveniently computed from this information, as can mean and Gaussian curvatures. Furthermore, to compute the volume of the fitted balloon we can make use of Gauss's theorem which reduces a volume calculation problem to a surface integral of the form

$$\Psi = \iint_S F(\mathbf{x}) \, d\sigma. \tag{34}$$

The balloon model is composed of M surface elements defined parametrically within an element in (25). Consequently, we can rewrite (34) as the sum of integrals over the surface elements as follows:

$$\Psi = \sum_{i=1}^{M} \iint_{S_i} F(\mathbf{x}) \, d\sigma = \iint_{S_i} F(\mathbf{x}(\xi, \eta)) \det \mathbf{J} \, d\xi \, d\eta, \tag{35}$$

where $\det \mathbf{J} = \left\| \frac{\partial \mathbf{x}}{\partial \xi} (\xi, \eta) \times \frac{\partial \mathbf{x}}{\partial \eta} (\xi, \eta) \right\|$ is the Jacobian of transformation.

By tracking a parametric surface over time, the dynamic deformable model technique permits a direct analysis of the estimated nonrigid motion. For instance, the variation in the Gaussian curvature of the fitted model over time can be used to estimate the local stretching and shrinking of the LV surface during the cardiac cycle. It should be noted, however, that for the relatively smooth LV surface, the simple tracking scheme employed in this paper estimates the tangential component of the surface velocity field much less reliably than the normal component. A more accurate estimation of the tangential component would require additional data or a priori information. For example, SPAMM images (26) depict transient magnetic tags within the heart wall whose motion can be followed over several subsequent images, providing both orthogonal components of the local velocity in the image plane (27). Our model can readily assimilate this type of information and that available from other sources. For instance,

- a priori information about nonrigidity could be included so that the model not only deforms to fit the data but also preserves some basic nonrigid constraints such as isometry or conformality (28).
- fiducial points can be extracted from the model surface and used as a guide when fitting the model to subsequent volumes in the sequence.
- the model can be generalized so that it subdivides elements in areas undergoing stretching or bending or merge elements in areas that are less curved [cf. adaptive meshes (28–30)]. This would enable the elements to better follow the motion of the data points and allow for correspondence recovery.

Obviously, it is difficult to assess the accuracy of our LV reconstruction and tracking results from a single 4D dataset. A complete error analysis would also require quantitative comparisons against images segmented manually by experts and is beyond the scope of this paper.

9 SUMMARY

We proposed a 3D elastically deformable balloon model for segmentation, reconstruction, and tracking of anatomical structures in multidimensional images. The surface of the model is composed of C^1 triangular finite elements whose nodal variables include position and first and second parametric partial derivatives of the surface. Lagrangian equations of motion make the dynamic model responsive to forces, derived from the 3D data, which deform its surface to fit the data in an elegant and intuitive manner. The fitting is carried out through numerical time-integration of the motion equations. An iterative integration method is used that exploits the parallelism of shared-memory multiprocessor architectures. This low-latency method supports real-time 3D display of the model as it extracts and tracks an anatomical surface. Furthermore, the model features a recursive, global subdivision capability which can fit a high resolution surface at low overall computational cost.

We described an experimental interactive system that demonstrates some of the capabilities of our model by applying it to 4D cardiac CT data. The system semi-automatically segments, reconstructs, and tracks the LV, allowing the user to initialize the model in the region of interest, dynamically manipulate it during the data analysis, and alter the viewpoint, shading mode, and other visualization parameters at any time. The effective efficiency gains that can accrue from a system of this sort should be even more dramatic with dynamic imaging at higher spatial and temporal resolution. Additional refinements will increase the model's potential to support reliable quantitative analysis of volume, form, and nonrigid motion for diagnostic and other medical purposes. This is a promising direction for further work.

Acknowledgments—DT is a Fellow of the Canadian Institute for Advanced Research. We thank the following people for their cooperation: The cardiac CT images were made available by Eric Hoffman of the University of Pennsylvania Medical School and were redistributed to us courtesy of Dmitry Goldgof, University of South Florida. The Monga-Deriche edge detector was provided courtesy of Nicholas Ayache and Gregoire Malandain of INRIA, Paris, France. This research was supported by the Natural Sciences and Engineering Research Council of Canada and the Information Technologies Research Center of Ontario.

REFERENCES

1. Carlbom, I.; Terzopoulos, D.; Harris, K. Computer-assisted registration, segmentation, and 3D reconstruction from images of neuronal tissue sections. IEEE Trans. Med. Imaging: 13(2):351–362; 1994.
2. Lorenson, W.E.; Cline, H.E. Marching cubes, a high resolution 3D surface construction algorithm. Comput. Graph. 21(4):163–169; 1987.
3. Sander, P.; Zucker, S. Inferring surface trace and differential structure from 3D images. IEEE Trans. Pattern Anal. Machine Intell. 12(9):833–854; 1990.
4. Sternberg, S.R. Grayscale morphology. Comput. Vision Graph. Image Process. 35:333–355; 1986.
5. Drebin, R.A.; Carpenter, L.; Hanrahan, P. Volume Rendering. Comput. Graph. 22(4):65–74; 1988.
6. Terzopoulos, D.; Witkin, A.; Kass, M. Constraints on deformable models: Recovering 3D shape and nonrigid motion. Artif. Intell. 36(1):91–123; 1988.
7. Terzopoulos, D.; Metaxas, D. Dynamic 3D models with local and global deformations: Deformable superquadrics. IEEE Trans. Pattern Anal. Machine Intell. 13(7):703–714; 1991.

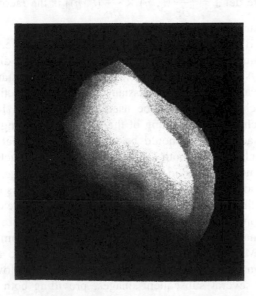

Fig. 13. End-diastolic and end-systolic surfaces of LV during cardiac cycle.

8. Pentland, A.; Horowitz, B. Recovery of nonrigid motion and structure. IEEE Trans. Pattern Anal. Machine Intell. 13(7):730–742; July 1991.

9. Cohen, L.D. On active contour models and balloons. In: CVGIP: Image understanding. vol. 53(2):211–218; March 1991.

10. Delingette, H.; Hebert, M.; Ikeuchi, K. Shape representation and image segmentation using deformable surfaces. In: Proceedings IEEE conference computer vision and pattern recognition. June 1991: 467–472.

11. Wang, Y.F.; Wang, J.F. Surface reconstruction using deformable models with interior and boundary constraints. IEEE Trans. Pattern Anal. Machine Intell. 14(5):572–579; May 1992.

12. McInerney, T. Finite element techniques for fitting deformable models to 3D data. Master's Thesis, Department of Computer Science, University of Toronto, Toronto, ON, Canada, 1992.

13. Metaxas, D.; Terzopoulos, D. Shape and nonrigid motion estimation through physics-based synthesis. IEEE Trans. Pattern Anal. Machine Intell. 15(6):580–591; 1993.

14. Terzopoulos, D. Multilevel computational processes for visual surface reconstruction. Comput. Vision, Graph., Image Process. 24:52–96; 1983.

15. Terzopoulos, D. Regularization of inverse visual problems involving discontinuities. IEEE Trans. Pattern Anal. Machine Intell. 8(4):413–424; 1986.

16. Young, A.A. Epicardial surface estimation from coronary cineangiograms. Comput. Vision Graph., Image Process. 47:11–127; 1989.

17. Young, A. Epicardial deformation from coronary cineangiograms. In: Glass, L.; Hunter, P.; McCulloch, A., eds. Theory of heart. Heidelberg: Springer-Verlag; 1991: 175–207.

18. Cohen, I.; Cohen, L.D.; Ayache, N. Introducing new deformable surfaces to segment 3D images. In: Proceedings IEEE conference computer vision and pattern recognition. June 1991: 738–739.

19. Cohen, L.D.; Cohen, I. Deformable models for 3D medical images using finite elements and balloons. In: Proceedings IEEE conference computer vision and pattern recognition. June 1992: 592–598.

20. Miller, J.V.; Breen, D.E.; Lorensen, W.E.; O'Bara, R.M.; Wozny, M.J. Geometrically deformed models. In: Computer graphics (SIGGRAPH'91). vol. 25(4). July 1991: 217–226.

21. Glass, L.; Hunter, P.; McCulloch, A., eds. Theory of heart. New York: Springer-Verlag; 1991.

22. Dhatt, G.; Touzot, G. The finite element method displayed. New York: Wiley; 1984.

23. Monga, O.; Deriche, R. 3D Edge detection using recursive filtering. In: Proceedings IEEE conference computer vision and pattern recognition. June 1989.

24. Ritman, E.L.; Robb, R.A.; Harris, L.D. Imaging physiological functions: Experience with the dynamic spatial reconstruction. New York: Praeger; 1985.

25. do Carmo, P.M. Differential geometry of curves and surfaces. Englewood Cliffs, New Jersey: Prentice Hall; 1976.

26. Axel, L.; Dougherty, L. Heart wall motion: Improved method of spatial modulation of magnetization for MR imaging. Radiology 172:349–350; 1989.

27. Young, A.; Axel, L. Non-rigid wall motion using MR tagging. In: Proceedings IEEE conference computer vision and pattern recognition. June 1992: 399–404.

28. Huang, W.C.; Goldgof, D.B. Left ventricle motion and analysis by adaptive-size physically-based models. In: SPIE Proceedings. vol. 1660-30. Feb. 1992: 299–310.

29. Huang, W.-C.; Goldgof, D.B. Adaptive-size meshes for rigid and nonrigid shape analysis and synthesis. IEEE Transactions on Pattern Analysis and Machine Intelligence. 15(6):611–616; 1993.

30. Vasilescu, M.; Terzopoulos, D. Adaptive meshes and shells: Irregular triangulation, discontinuities, and hierarchical subdivision. In: IEEE computer society conference on computer vision and pattern recognition (CVPR'92). Champaign, IL: IEEE Computer Society Press; June 1992: 829–832.

31. Singh, Ajit; von Kurowski, Lorenz; Chiu, Ming-Yee. Cardiac MRI segmentation using deformable models. In: Proceedings IEEE Conference on Computers and Cardiology. London; Sept. 1993.

About the Author—Tim McInerney is a Ph.D. candidate in the department of Computer Science at the University of Toronto, Canada. He received the M.Sc. degree in Computer Science, in 1992, and the B.A.Sc. degree in Electrical Engineering, in 1981, both from the University of Toronto. His primary research interests are surface and object modeling for medical image visualization and analysis, computer vision, and computer graphics.

About the Author—Demetri Terzopoulos received the Ph.D. degree in Artificial Intelligence from the Massachusetts Institute of Technology, Cambridge, MA, in 1984, the M.Eng. degree in Electrical Engineering, in 1980, and the B.Eng. degree with distinction in Honours Electrical Engineering, in 1978, from McGill University, Montreal, Canada.

Since 1989 he has been Associate Professor of Computer Science and Electrical and Computer Engineering at the University of Toronto and Fellow of the Canadian Institute for Advanced Research. From 1985–92 he was affiliated with Schlumberger, Inc., serving as Program Leader at the Laboratory for Computer Science, Austin, TX, and at the former Palo Alto Research Laboratory. During 1984–85 he was a Research Scientist at the MIT Artificial Intelligence Laboratory, Cambridge, MA. He has also held summer positions at the National Research Council of Canada, Ottawa, ON, (1977 & 78) and Bell-Northern Research, Montreal (1980). He has been a consultant for Digital, Ontario Hydro, Schlumberger, and Hughes.

Dr. Terzopoulos has over 120 publications in computational vision, computer graphics, biomedical image analysis, digital speech and image processing, and parallel numerical algorithms, and has been invited to speak internationally on these topics. He is the recipient of several scholarships and awards, including a Best Paper Award from the American Association for Artificial Intelligence and a Digital Media Award for Technical Excellence from the Canadian Academy of Multimedia Arts and Sciences. He serves on the editorial boards of CVGIP: Graphical Models and Image Processing and the Journal of Visualization and Computer Animation. He is a member of the Institute for Electrical and Electronics Engineers, the New York Academy of Sciences, and Sigma Xi.

Shape Modeling with Front Propagation:
A Level Set Approach

Ravikanth Malladi, James A. Sethian, and Baba C. Vemuri

Abstract — Shape modeling is an important constituent of computer vision as well as computer graphics research. Shape models aid the tasks of object representation and recognition. This paper presents a new approach to shape modeling which retains some of the attractive features of existing methods and overcomes some of their limitations. Our techniques can be applied to model arbitrarily complex shapes, which include shapes with significant protrusions, and to situations where no *a priori* assumption about the object's topology is made. A single instance of our model, when presented with an image having more than one object of interest, has the ability to split freely to represent each object. This method is based on the ideas developed by Osher and Sethian to model propagating solid/liquid interfaces with curvature-dependent speeds. The interface (front) is a closed, nonintersecting, hypersurface flowing along its gradient field with constant speed or a speed that depends on the curvature. It is moved by solving a "Hamilton-Jacobi" type equation written for a function in which the interface is a particular level set. A speed term synthesized from the image is used to stop the interface in the vicinity of object boundaries. The resulting equation of motion is solved by employing entropy-satisfying upwind finite difference schemes. We present a variety of ways of computing evolving front, including narrow bands, reinitializations, and different stopping criteria. The efficacy of the scheme is demonstrated with numerical experiments on some synthesized images and some low contrast medical images.

Index Terms — Shape modeling, shape recovery, interface motion, level sets, hyperbolic conservation laws, Hamilton-Jacobi equation, entropy condition.

I. INTRODUCTION

IN this paper, we describe a modeling technique based on a level set approach for recovering shapes of objects in two and three dimensions from various types of image data. The modeling technique may be viewed as a form of active modeling such as "snakes" [15] and deformable surfaces [34] since, the model which consists of a moving front, may be molded into any desired shape by externally applied halting criteria synthesized from the image data. The "snakes" or deformable surfaces may be viewed as Lagrangian geometric formulations

Manuscript received May 17, 1993; revised June 21, 1994.

R. Malladi's and J. Sethian's research supported in part by the Applied Mathematical Sciences Subprogram of the Office of Energy Research, US Dept. of Energy under Contract DE-AC03-76SD00098 and by the NSF ARPA under grant DMS-8919074.

B. C. Vemuri's work sponsored in part by NSF grant ECS-9210648.

R. Malladi and J. Sethian are with Lawrence Berkeley Laboratory and Department of Mathematics, University of California, Berkeley, CA 94720 USA. B. Vemuri is with the Department of Computer and Information Sciences, University of Florida, Gainesville, FL 32611 USA.

IEEECS Log Number P95015.

wherein the boundary of the model is represented in a parametric form. These parameterized boundary representations will encounter difficulties when the dynamic model embedded in a noisy data set is expanding/shrinking along its normal field [10] and sharp corners or cusps develop or pieces of the boundary intersect. By exploiting recent advances in interface techniques, our modeling technique avoids this Lagrangian geometric view and instead capitalizes on a related initial value partial differential equation. In this setting, several advantages are apparent, including the ability to evolve the model in the presence of sharp corners, cusps and changes in topology, model shapes with significant protrusions and holes in a seamless fashion, and extension to three dimensions in an extremely straightforward way.

A. Background

An important goal of computational vision is to recover the shapes of objects in 2D and 3D from various types of visual data. One way to achieve this goal is via model-based techniques. Broadly speaking, these techniques involve the use of a model whose boundary representation is matched to the image to recover the object of interest. These models can either be rigid, such as correlation-based template matching techniques, or nonrigid, as those used in dynamic model fitting techniques.

Shape recovery from raw data typically precedes its symbolic representation. Shape models are expected to aid the recovery of detailed structure from noisy data using only the weakest of the possible assumptions about the observed shape. To this end, several variational shape reconstruction methods have been proposed and there is abundant literature on the same (see [4], [27], [35], [38], [17] and references therein). Generalized spline models with continuity constraints are well suited for fulfilling the goals of shape recovery (see [6], [33]). Generalized splines are the key ingredient of the dynamic shape modeling paradigm introduced to vision literature by Kass et al [15]. Incorporating dynamics into shape modeling enables the creation of realistic animation for computer graphics applications and for tracking moving objects in computer vision. Following the advent of the dynamic shape modeling paradigm [15], [34], considerable research followed, with numerous application specific modifications to the modeling primitives, and external forces derived from data constraints [39], [18], [11], [24], [36], [37].

The final recovered shape in these schemes can depend on an initial guess which is reasonably close to the desired shape. One solution to this problem in the one-dimensional case has

Reprinted from *IEEE Trans. Pattern Analysis and Machine Intelligence*, Vol. 17, No. 2, Feb. 1995, pp. 158–175.

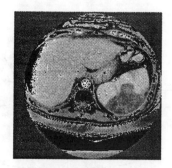 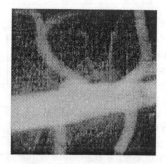 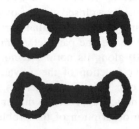

(a) CT image   (b) DSA image   (c) Shapes with holes

Fig. 1. Test bed for our topology-independent shape modeling scheme.

been presented by Amini et al [2]. They use a discrete form of dynamic programming to optimize the univariate variational problem.

The framework of energy minimization (snakes) has been used successfully in the past for extracting salient image contours such as edges and lines by Kass et al [15]. To make the final result relatively insensitive to the initial conditions, Cohen [10] suggested the use of an inflation force which makes the snake behave like an edge seeking active model. Although the inflation force prevents the curve from getting trapped by isolated spurious edges, the active contour model cannot be made to extrude through any significant protrusions that a shape may possess (see Fig. 1(b)) without resorting to cumbersome resampling techniques. In this paper, we present a technique which overcomes this problem and accurately models bifurcations and protrusions in complex shapes. Most existing shape modeling schemes require that the topology of the object be known before the shape recovery can commence. It is, however, not always possible to specify the topology of an object prior to its recovery. For example, an important concern in object tracking and motion detection applications is topological change resulting from tracking the positions of object boundaries in an image sequence through time. During their evolution, these closed contours may change connectivity and split, thereby undergoing a topological transformation. One such example is the splitting of cell boundary in a sequence of images depicting cell division. A heuristic criterion for splitting and merging of curves in 2D which is based on monitoring deformation energies of points on the elastic curve has been discussed in [26]. In the context of static problems, more recently, particle systems have been used to model surfaces of arbitrary topology [32]. Here, particles can be added and deleted dynamically to enlarge, and trim the surface respectively.

The schemes described in this paper offer a new approach to some of the above problems. To begin, the convergence to the final result is relatively independent of the shape initialization. The algorithm allows branches to sprout automatically as the front moves. The scheme described in this paper can be applied where no *a priori* assumption about the object's topology is made. A single instance of our model, when presented with an image having more than one shape of interest (see Fig. 1(c)), has the ability to split freely to represent each shape [19], [20]. We show that by using our approach, it is also pos-

sible to extract the bounding contours of shapes with holes in a seamless fashion (see Fig. 13).

Our method is inspired by ideas first introduced in Osher and Sethian [23], [29], which grew out of work in Sethian [28], to model propagating fronts with curvature-dependent speeds. Two such examples are flame propagation and crystal growth, in which the speed of the moving interface normal to itself depends on transport terms modified by the local curvature. The challenge in these problems is to devise numerical schemes for the equations of the propagating front which will accurately approximate these highly unstable physical phenomena. Osher and Sethian [23] achieve this by viewing the propagating surface as a specific level set of a higher-dimensional function. The equation of motion for this function is reminiscent of an initial value "Hamilton-Jacobi" equation with a parabolic right-hand side and is closely related to a viscous hyperbolic conservation law.

In our work, we adopt these level set techniques to the problem of shape recovery. To isolate a shape from its background, we first consider a closed, nonintersecting, initial hypersurface placed inside (or outside) it. This hypersurface is then made to flow along its gradient field with a speed $F(K)$, where K is the curvature of the hypersurface. Unknown shapes are recovered by making the front adhere to the object boundaries. This is done by synthesizing a speed term from image data which acts as a halting criterion. Finally, we note that a separate study also applying a level set approach has been performed independently by Caselles et al [7].

The outline of this paper is as follows. In Section II, we briefly explain the level set approach to front propagation problems and the accompanying numerical algorithms. In Sections III and IV, we discuss the application of this technique to shape recovery problems, and consider various speed functions and approaches to the problem, such as the effect of global speed laws, narrow band formulations, reinitialization and stopping criteria. In Section V, we present some experimental results of applying our method to some synthetic and low contrast medical images. We conclude in Section VI.

II. FRONT PROPAGATION PROBLEM

In this section we present the level set technique due to Osher and Sethian [23]. For details and an expository review, see Sethian [29].

As a starting point and motivation for the level set approach, consider a closed curve moving in the plane, that is, let $\gamma(0)$ be a smooth, closed initial curve in Euclidean plane $\Re^2$, and let $\gamma(t)$ be the one-parameter family of curves generated by moving $\gamma(0)$ along its normal vector field with speed $F(K)$, a given scalar function of the curvature K. Let $\mathbf{x}(s, t)$, be the position vector which parameterizes $\gamma(t)$ by s, $0 \le s \le S$.

One numerical approach to this problem is to take the above Lagrangian description of the problem, produce equations of motion for the position vector $\mathbf{x}(s, t)$, and then discretize the parameterization with a set of discrete marker particles lying on the moving front. These discrete markers are updated in time by approximating the spatial derivatives in the equations of motion, and advancing their positions. However, there are several problems with this approach, as discussed in Sethian [28]. First, small errors in the computed particle positions are tremendously amplified by the curvature term, and calculations are prone to instability unless an extremely small time step is employed. Second, in the absence of a smoothing curvature (viscous) term, singularities develop in the propagating front, and an entropy condition must be observed to extract the correct weak solution. Third, topological changes are difficult to manage as the evolving interface breaks and merges. And fourth, significant bookkeeping problems occur in the extension of this technique to three dimensions.

As an alternative, the central idea in the level set approach of Osher and Sethian [23] is to represent the front $\gamma(t)$ as the level set $\{\psi = 0\}$ of a function ψ. Thus, given a moving closed hypersurface $\gamma(t)$, that is, $\gamma(t = 0) : [0, \infty) \to \Re^N$, we wish to produce an Eulerian formulation for the motion of the hypersurface propagating along its normal direction with speed F, where F can be a function of various arguments, including the curvature, normal direction, etc. The main idea is to embed this propagating interface as the zero level set of a higher dimensional function ψ. Let $\psi(\mathbf{x}, t = 0)$, where $\mathbf{x} \in \Re^N$ is defined by

$$\psi(x, t = 0) = \pm d \tag{1}$$

where d is the distance from $\mathbf{x}$ to $\gamma(t = 0)$, and the plus (minus) sign is chosen if the point $\mathbf{x}$ is outside (inside) the initial hypersurface $\gamma(t=0)$. Thus, we have an initial function $\psi(\mathbf{x}, t = 0) : \Re^N \to \Re$ with the property that

$$\gamma(t = 0) = (\mathbf{x} \mid \psi(\mathbf{x}, t = 0) = 0) \tag{2}$$

As illustration, consider the example of an expanding circle. Suppose the initial front γ at $t = 0$ is a circle in the xy-plane (Fig. 2(a)). We imagine that the circle is the level set $\{\psi = 0\}$ of an initial surface $z = \psi(x, y, t = 0)$ in $\Re^3$ (see Fig. 2(b)). We can then match the one-parameter family of moving curves $\gamma(t)$ with a one-parameter family of moving surfaces in such a way that the level set $\{\psi = 0\}$ always yields the moving front (see Fig. 2(c) and Fig. 2(d)).

Our goal is to now produce an equation for the evolving function $\psi(\mathbf{x}, t)$ which contains the embedded motion of $\gamma(t)$ as the level set $\{\psi = 0\}$. Here, we follow the derivation presented

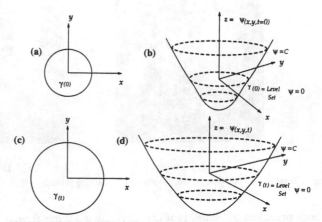

Fig. 2. Level set formulation of equations of motion – (a) and (b) show the curve γ and the surface $\psi(x, y)$ at $t = 0$, and (c) and (d) show the curve γ and the corresponding surface $\psi(x, y)$ at time t.

in [22]. Let $\mathbf{x}(t)$, $t \in [0, \infty)$ be the path of a point on the propagating front. That is, $\mathbf{x}$ $(t=0)$ is a point on the initial front $\gamma(t = 0)$, and $\mathbf{x}_t = F(\mathbf{x}(t))$ with the vector $\mathbf{x}_t$ normal to the front at $\mathbf{x}(t)$. Since the evolving function ψ is always zero on the propagating hypersurface, we must have

$$\psi(\mathbf{x}(t), t) = 0. \tag{3}$$

By the chain rule,

$$\psi_t + \sum_{i=1}^{N} \psi_{x_i} x_{i_t} = 0 \tag{4}$$

where x_i is the ith component of $\mathbf{x}$. Let

$$\left(u_1, u_2, \dots u_N\right) = \left(x_{1_t}, x_{2_t}, \dots, x_{N_t}\right).$$

Since

$$\sum_{i=1}^{N} \psi_{x_i} x_{i_t} = \left(\psi_{x_1}, \psi_{x_2}, \dots, \psi_{x_N}\right) \cdot \left(u_1, u_2, \dots, u_N\right) = F(\mathbf{x}(t))|\nabla \psi| \tag{5}$$

we then have the evolution equation for ψ, namely

$$\psi_t + F |\nabla \psi| = 0 \tag{6}$$

with a given value of $\psi(\mathbf{x}, t = 0)$. We refer to this as a Hamilton-Jacobi "type" equation because, for certain forms of the speed function F, we obtain the standard Hamilton-Jacobi equation.

There are four major advantages to this Eulerian Hamilton-Jacobi formulation. The first is that the evolving function $\psi(\mathbf{x}, t)$ always remains a function as long as F is smooth. However, the level surface $\{\psi = 0\}$, and hence the propagating hypersurface $\gamma(t)$ may change topology, break, merge, and form sharp corners as the function ψ evolves, see [23].

The second advantage of this Eulerian formulation concerns numerical approximation. Because $\psi(\mathbf{x}, t)$ remains a function as it evolves, we may use a discrete grid in the domain of $\mathbf{x}$ and substitute finite difference approximations for the spatial and temporal derivatives. For example, using a uniform mesh of spacing h, with grid nodes ij, and employing the standard notation that ψ_{ij}^n is the approximation to the solution $\psi(ih, jh, n\Delta t)$, where Δt is the time step, we might write

$$\frac{\psi_{ij}^{n+1} - \psi_{ij}^n}{\Delta t} + (F)\left(\nabla_{ij}\psi_{ij}^n\right) = 0. \tag{7}$$

Here, we have used forward differences in time, and let $\nabla_{ij}\psi_{ij}^n$ be some appropriate finite difference operator for the spatial derivative.

The correct technique for approximating the spatial derivative in the above comes from respecting the appropriate entropy condition for propagating fronts, discussed in detail in [29]. As brief motivation for these schemes, consider a periodic cosine curve propagating in its normal direction with speed $F = 1 - \varepsilon K$, where K is the curvature. This problem has been discussed extensively in [28]. For $\varepsilon > 0$, the front stays smooth for all time. For $\varepsilon = 0$, the parameterized analytic solution corresponds to a front which passes through itself and develops a swallowtail solution. In order for the propagating front to correspond to the boundary of an expanding region, we invoke the entropy condition, namely that if the boundary is viewed as a propagating flame, then *once a particle is burnt, it stays burnt*. This entropy condition yields the front which corresponds to the limiting solution as $\varepsilon \to 0$ of the smooth case.

In order to build a correct entropy-satisfying approximation to the difference operator, we exploit the technology of hyperbolic conservation laws. Following [23], we use a modification of an Engquist-Osher scheme [12]. That is, given a speed function $F(K)$, we update the front by the following scheme. First, separate $F(K)$ into a constant advection term F_0 and the remainder $F_1(K)$, that is,

$$F(K) = F_0 + F_1(K) \tag{8}$$

The advection component F_0 of the speed function is then approximated using upwind schemes, while the remainder is approximated using central differences. In one space dimension, we have

$$\phi_i^{n+1} = \phi_i^n - \Delta t \left[\left\{ \left(\max\left(D_i^-\phi, 0\right)\right)^2 + \left(\min\left(D_i^+\phi, 0\right)\right)^2 \right\}^{1/2} - F_1(K)\nabla\phi_i^n \right]. \tag{9}$$

Extension to higher dimensions are straightforward; we use the version given in [30].

The third advantage of the above formulation is that intrinsic geometric properties of the front may be easily determined from the level function ψ. For example, at any point of the front, the normal vector, is given by

$$\vec{n} = \nabla\psi \tag{10}$$

and the curvature is easily obtained from the divergence of the gradient of the unit normal vector to front, that is,

$$K = \nabla \cdot \frac{\nabla\psi}{|\nabla\psi|} = -\frac{\psi_{xx}\psi_y^2 - 2\psi_x\psi_y\psi_{xy} + \psi_{yy}\psi_x^2}{\left(\psi_x^2 + \psi_y^2\right)^{3/2}}. \tag{11}$$

Finally, the fourth advantage of the above level set approach is that there are no significant differences in following fronts in three space dimensions. By simply extending the array structures and gradients operators, propagating surfaces are easily handled.

Since its introduction in [23], the above level set approach has been used in a wide collection of problems involving moving interfaces. Some of these applications include the generation of minimal surfaces [8], singularities and geodesics in moving curves and surfaces in [9], flame propagation [25], [40], and fluid interfaces [31], [22]. Extensions of the basic technique include fast methods in [1] and extensions to triple points in [3]. The fundamental Eulerian perspective presented by this approach has since been adopted in many theoretical analyses of mean curvature flow, in particular, see [13]. In computer vision, a model for shape theory based on this work has been presented in [16].

III. SHAPE RECOVERY WITH FRONT PROPAGATION

In this section, we describe how the level set formulation for the front propagation problem discussed in the previous section can be used for shape recovery. First, note that the front represents the boundary of an evolving shape. Since the idea is to extract objects, shapes from a given image, the front should be forced to stop in the vicinity of the desired objects' boundaries. This is analogous to the force criterion used to push the active contour model towards desired shapes [15]. We define the final shape to be the configuration when all the points on the front come to a stop, thereby bringing the computation to an end.

Our goal now is to define a speed function from the image data that can be applied on the propagating front as a halting criterion. As before, we split the speed function F into two components: $F = F_A + F_G$. The term F_A, referred to as the advection term, is independent of the moving front's geometry. The front uniformly expands or contracts with speed F_A depending on its sign and is analogous to the inflation force defined in [10]. The second term F_G, is the part which depends on the geometry of the front, such as its local curvature. This (diffusion) term smoothes out the high curvature regions of the front and has the same regularizing effect on the front as the internal deformation energy term in thin-plate-membrane splines [15] (see the Fig. 9). We rewrite Equation 6 by splitting the influence of F as

$$\psi_t + F_A |\nabla \psi| + F_G |\nabla \psi| = 0. \tag{12}$$

First consider the case when the front moves with a constant speed, that is, $F_G = 0 \Rightarrow F = F_A$. Define a negative speed F_I to be

$$F_I(x, y) = \frac{-F_A}{(M_1 - M_2)} \left\{ \left| \nabla G_\sigma * I(x, y) \right| - M_2 \right\}, \tag{13}$$

where M_1 and M_2 are the maximum and minimum values of the magnitude of image gradient $|\nabla G_\sigma * I(x, y)|$, $(x, y) \in \Omega$. The expression $G_\sigma * I$ denotes the image convolved with a Gaussian smoothing filter whose characteristic width is σ. Alternately, we could use a smoothed zero-crossing image to synthesize the negative speed function. The zero-crossing image is produced by detecting zero-crossings in the function $\nabla^2 G_\sigma * I$, which is the original image convolved with a Laplacian-of-Gaussian filter whose characteristic width is σ. The value of F_I lies in the range $[-F_A, 0]$ as the value of image gradient varies between M_1 and M_2. From this argument it is clear that, if $|\nabla G_\sigma * I(x, y)|$ approaches the maximum M_1 at the object boundaries, then the front gradually attains zero speed as it gets closer to the object boundaries and eventually comes to a stop.

If $F_G \neq 0$, then it is not possible to find an additive speed term from the image that will cause the net speed of the front to approach zero in the neighborhood of a desired shape. Instead, we multiply the speed function $F = F_A + F_G$ with a quantity k_I. The term k_I, which is defined as

$$k_I(x, y) = \frac{1}{1 + |\nabla G_\sigma * I(x, y)|}, \tag{14}$$

has values that are closer to zero in regions of high image gradient and values that are closer to unity in regions with relatively constant intensity. If one desires a speed function that falls to zero faster than the reciprocal function, the following definition can be employed:

$$k_I(x, y) = e^{-|\nabla G_\sigma * I(x, y)|} \tag{15}$$

More sophisticated stopping criteria can be synthesized by using the orientation dependent "steerable" filters [14].

IV. EXTENDING THE SPEED FUNCTION

The image-based speed terms have meaning only on the boundary $\gamma(t)$, that is, on the level set $\{\psi = 0\}$. This follows from the fact that they were designed to force the propagating level set $\{\psi = 0\}$ to a complete stop in the neighborhood of an object boundary. However, the level set equation of motion is written for the function ψ defined over the entire domain. Consequently, we require that the evolution equation has a consis-

tent physical meaning for all the level sets, that is, at every point $(x, y) \in \Omega$. The speed function F_I derives its meaning not from the geometry of ψ but from the configuration of the level set $\{\psi = 0\}$ in the image plane. Thus, our goal is to construct an image-based speed function $\hat{F}_I$ that is globally defined. We call it an *extension* of F_I off the level set $\{\psi = 0\}$ because it extends the meaning of F_I to other level sets [30]. Note that the level set $\{\psi = 0\}$ lies in the image plane and therefore $\hat{F}_I$ must equal F_I on $\{\psi = 0\}$. The same argument applies to the coefficient k_I. With the extensions so defined, the equation of motion for the case $F = F_A$ is given by

$$\psi_t + (F_A + \hat{F}_I) |\nabla \psi| = 0, \tag{16}$$

and

$$\psi_t + \hat{k}_I (F_A + F_G) |\nabla \psi| = 0, \tag{17}$$

when $F = F_A + F_G$.

If the level curves are moving with a constant speed, that is, $F_G = 0$, then at any time t, a typical level set $\{\psi = C\}$, $C \in R$, is a distance C away from the level set $\{\psi = 0\}$ (see Fig. 3). Observe that the above statement is a rephrased version of *Huygen's principle* which, from a geometrical standpoint, stipulates that the position of a front propagating with unit speed at a given time t should consist of only the set of points located a distance t away from the initial front. On the other hand, for $F_G \neq 0$, the level sets will not remain a constant distance apart.

With this in mind, there are several ways to extend the speed function to the neighboring level sets.

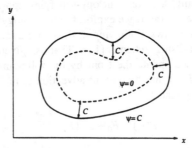

Fig. 3. Huygen's principle construction.

A. Global Extension

As a first attempt, we require that the external (image-based) speed function be such that level sets moving under this speed function cannot collide.

We can construct one such extension to the image-based speed function by (see Fig. 4) letting the value of $\hat{F}_I(\hat{k}_I)$ at a point P lying on a level set $\{\psi = C\}$ be the value of $\hat{F}_I(\hat{k}_I)$ at a point Q, such that point Q is closest to P and lies on the level set $\{\psi = 0\}$. Thus, $\hat{F}_I(\hat{k}_I)$ reduces to $F_I(k_I)$ on $\{\psi = 0\}$.

By updating the level set function on a grid, we are moving the level sets without constructing them explicitly. Therefore a straightforward algorithm consists of advancing from one time step to the next as follows:

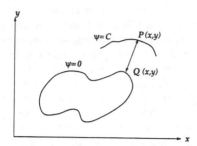

Fig. 4. Extension of image-based speed terms to other level sets.

Algorithm 1

1) At each grid point $(i\Delta x, j\Delta y)$, where Δx and Δy are step sizes in either coordinate directions, the *extension* of image-based speed term is computed. This is done in accordance with the construction described in the previous section; that is, by searching for a point q which lies on the level set $\{\psi = 0\}$, and is closest to the point $(i\Delta x, j\Delta y)$. The value of image-based speed term at the current point is simply its value at the point q.

2) With the value of extended speed term $(\hat{k}_I^n)_{i,j}$ and $\psi_{i,j}^n$, calculate $\psi_{i,j}^{n+1}$ using the upwind, finite difference schemes given in [30].

3) Construct an approximation for the level set $\{\psi = 0\}$ from $\psi_{i,j}^{n+1}$. This is required to visualize the current position of the front in the image plane. A piecewise linear approximation for the front $\gamma(t)$ is constructed as follows. Given a cell $C(i, j)$, if

$$\max(\psi_{i,j}, \psi_{i+1,j}, \psi_{i,j+1}, \psi_{i+1,j+1}) < 0$$

or

$$\min(\psi_{i,j}, \psi_{i+1,j}, \psi_{i,j+1}, \psi_{i+1,j+1}) > 0,$$

then $C(i, j) \notin \gamma(t)$ and is ignored, else, the entry and exit points where $\psi = 0$ are found by linear interpolation. This provides two nodes on $\gamma(t)$ and thus, one of the line segments which form the approximation to $\gamma(t)$. The collection of all such line segments constitutes the approximation to the level set $\{\psi = 0\}$, which is used for future evaluation of the image-based speed term in the update equation.

4) Replace n by $n + 1$ and return to step 1.

B. Global Extension with Reinitialization

The above construction can create a discontinuous velocity extension away from the zero level set, since the distance function is not differentiable. One solution to this is to reinitialization the level set function every fixed number of time steps to keep the level sets evenly spaced around the front. A straightforward way to do this is to recompute the distance from each point of the grid to the zero level set. However, this is an $O(N^3)$ operation, if we assume that there are N points in each coordinate direction, plus approximately $O(N)$ points on the interfaces.

An alternative to this reconstruction is provided by [31], based on an idea of Morel. The idea is simply to iterate on the level set function at a given time according to the following equation:

$$\psi_{k+1} = \psi_k + S(\psi)(1 - |\nabla \psi|). \tag{18}$$

In the limit as $k \to \infty$, this convergences to the distance function, with some error in relocating the original zero level set. For details, see [5].

The most expensive step in either of these algorithms is the computation of the *extension* for image-based speed term. This is because at each grid point, we must search for the closest point lying on the level set $\{\psi = 0\}$. Moreover, if $F_G = 0$, then the stability requirement for the explicit method for solving our level set equation is $\Delta t = O(\Delta x)$. For the full Equation (12), the stability requirement is $\Delta t = O(\Delta x^2)$. This could potentially force a very small time step for fine grids. These two effects, individually and compounded, make the computation exceedingly slow. In the case of reinitializing using the above iteration formula, additional labor is involved.

C. Narrow-Band Extension with Reinitialization

As a efficient alternative, we observe that the front can be moved by updating the level set function at a small set of points in the neighborhood of the zero set instead of updating it at all the points on the grid. In Fig. 5 the bold curve depicts the level set $\{\psi = 0\}$ and the shaded region around it is the narrow band. The narrow band is bounded on either side by two curves which are a distance δ apart, that is, the two curves are the level sets $\{\psi = \pm \delta/2\}$. The value of δ determines the number of grid points that fall within the narrow band. Since, during a given time step the value of ψ_{ij} is not updated at points lying outside the narrow band, the level sets $\{|\psi| > \delta/2\}$ remain stationary. The zero set which lies inside moves until it collides with the boundary of the narrow band. Which boundary the front collides with depends on whether it is moving inward or outward; either way, it cannot move past the narrow band. A complete discussion of the narrow band techniques for interface propagation may be found in [1].

As a consequence of our update strategy, the front can be moved through a maximum distance of $\delta/2$, either inward or outward, at which point we must rebuild an appropriate (a new) narrow band. We reinitialize the ψ function by treating the current zero set configuration, that is, $\{\psi = 0\}$, as the initial curve $\gamma(0)$. Chopp [8] observed that the reinitialization step can be made cheaper by treating the interior and exterior mesh points as sign holders. Note that the reinitialization procedure must account for the case when $\{\psi = 0\}$ changes topology. This procedure will restore the meaning of ψ function by cor-

223

recting the inaccuracies introduced as a result of our update algorithm. Once a new ψ function is defined on the grid, we can create a new narrow band around the zero set, and go through another set of, say l, iterations in time to move the front ahead

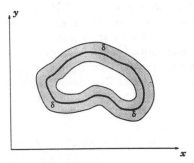

Fig. 5. A narrow band of width δ around the level set $\{\psi = 0\}$.

by a distance equal to $\delta/2$. The value of l is set to the number of time steps required to move the front by a distance roughly equal to $\delta/2$. This choice depends on some experimentation. Thus, a faster algorithm for shape recovery consists of the following steps:

Algorithm 2

1) Set the iteration number $m = 0$ and go to step 2.
2) At each grid point (i, j) lying inside the narrow band, compute the *extension* $\hat{k}_I$ of image-based speed term.
3) With the above value of extended speed term $\left(\hat{k}_I^m\right)_{i,j}$ and $\psi_{i,j}^m$, calculate $\psi_{i,j}^{m+1}$ using the upwind, finite difference scheme given in [30].
4) Construct a polygonal approximation for the level set $\{\psi = 0\}$ from $\psi_{i,j}^{m+1}$. A contour tracing procedure is used to obtain a polygonal approximation. Given a cell (i, j) which contains $\gamma(t)$, this procedure traces the contour by scanning the neighboring cells in order to find the next cell which contains $\gamma(t)$. Once such a cell is found, the process is repeated until the contour closes on itself. The set of nodes visited during this tracing process constitutes the polygonal approximation to $\gamma(t)$. In general, to collect all the closed contours, the above tracing procedure is started at a new, as yet unvisited, cell which contains the level set $\{\psi = 0\}$. A polygonal approximation is required in step 2 for the evaluation of image-based speed term and more importantly, in step 6 for reinitializing the ψ function.
5) Increment m by one. If the value of m equals l, go to step 6, else, go to step 2.
6) Compute the value of signed distance function ψ by treating the polygonal approximation of $\{\psi = 0\}$ as the initial contour $\gamma(0)$. As mentioned earlier, a more general method of reinitialization is required when $\{\psi = 0\}$ changes topology. Go to step 1.

In this approach, since we only update ψ at points lying in the narrow band, the issue of specifying boundary conditions for points lying on the edge of the band becomes pertinent. With our relatively simple speed motion, the free-end boundary condition is adequate, however, in more complex applications such as crystal growth, and flame propagation, accurate specification of boundary conditions is necessary [1].

We now show that this new faster approach provides a correct approximation to the propagating front problem. In Fig. 6, we show the result of applying narrow-band algorithm to a star shaped front propagating with speed $F = -K$, where K is the curvature as in Equation (11). The calculation was done on a unit box with 64 points in either direction, and a time step of $\Delta t = 0.00003$ was employed. The width of the narrow band has been set to $\delta = 0.075$, and the ψ function was recomputed once every ($l =$) 40 time steps. In Fig. 6(a), we show the initial curve along with the level sets $\{|\psi| < 0.2\}$. After 40 narrow-band updates (Fig. 6(b)), only the level sets $\{|\psi| < 0.0375\}$ move and the rest remain stationary. We note the inconsistency between the level sets lying on either side of the narrow band, making the reinitialization step necessary in order to restore the meaning of the ψ function. Following the reinitialization step, another 40 update steps are applied (Fig. 6(c)), which "diffuses" the high curvature regions of the front even further. In subsequent figures, the results of repeatedly applying the same strategy are shown. Finally, in Fig. 6(f), the peaks and troughs on the front get completely diffused, and it attains a smooth circular configuration after four reinitialization steps and a total of 200 time steps.

D. Straightforward Narrow-Band Extension

The narrow-band approach, in addition to being computationally efficient, allows us to return to the original construction of the speed function extension and replace it with a more mathematically appealing version. Since the narrow-band mechanism periodically "recalibrates" the front, we can in fact simply move each level set with the speed determined by the image gradient as given in Equations (14) and (15). In other words, for points inside the narrow band, the external speed values are picked directly from their corresponding image locations. Thus, we can ignore the previous extension velocity and provide a purely geometric one based on the local image gradient. Although this may cause many other level sets to temporarily stop, the narrow-band reinitialization resets them all around the zero level set. This will ensure that the zero level set is drawn close to the object boundary as well as retain other desirable properties of the level set approach, such as topological merge and split. Also, since the extension computation does not involve any search, the time complexity of this approach is identical to that of a basic narrow-band front propagation algorithm. We currently use this computationally efficient algorithm and suggest it for others interested in this work.

V. SHAPE RECOVERY RESULTS

In this section we present several shape recovery results that were obtained by applying the narrow-band level set algorithm to image data. Given an image, our method requires the user to

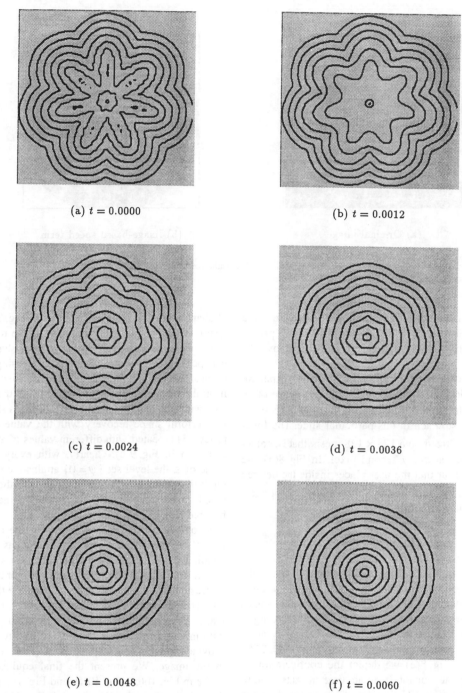

(a) $t = 0.0000$

(b) $t = 0.0012$

(c) $t = 0.0024$

(d) $t = 0.0036$

(e) $t = 0.0048$

(f) $t = 0.0060$

Fig. 6. Narrow-band algorithm applied to a star-shaped front propagating with speed $F = -K$. Calculations were done with a 64×64 grid with a time step $\Delta t = 0.00003$. Ψ was recomputed after every 40 time iterations.

provide an initial contour $\gamma(0)$. The initial contour can be placed anywhere in the image plane. However, it must be placed inside a desired shape or enclose all the constituent shapes. Our front seeks the object boundaries by either propagating inward or outward in the normal direction. This choice is made at the time of initialization. Note that after the specification of initial shape of $\gamma(0)$, our algorithm does not require any further user interaction. On the other hand, the user may interact with the model by varying the smoothness control pa-

rameter ε until a desired amount of smoothness is achieved in a given shape.

The initial value of the function ψ that is, $\psi(\mathbf{x}, 0)$ is computed from $\gamma(0)$. We first discretize the level set function ψ on the image plane and denote $\psi_{i,j}$ as the value of ψ at a grid point $(i\Delta x, j\Delta y)$, where Δx and Δy are step sizes in either coordinate directions. We define the distance from a point (i, j) to the initial curve to be the shortest distance from (i, j) to $\gamma(0)$. The magnitude of $\psi_{i, j}$ is set to this value. We use the plus sign if

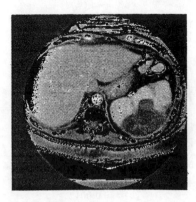
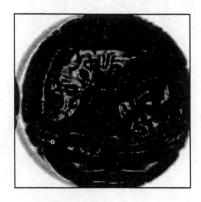

(a) Original image   (b) Image-based speed term

Fig. 7. Image-based speed term $k_I(x, y) = \dfrac{1}{1+\left|\nabla G_\sigma * I(x,y)\right|}$, with $\sigma = 3.25$, synthesized from the CT image.

is outside $\gamma(0)$ and minus sign if (i, j) is inside. Once the value of $\psi_{i,j}$ is computed at time $t = 0$ by following the above procedure, we use algorithms from the previous section to move the front.

We now present our shape recovery results in 2D. First, we consider a 256×256 CT (computed tomography) image of an abdominal section shown in Fig. 7(a), with the goal of recovering the shape of the stomach in this particular slice. The function ψ has been discretized on a 128×128 mesh, that is, calculations are performed at every second pixel. In Fig. 8(a), we show the closed contour that the user places inside the desired shape at time $t = 0$. The function ψ is then made to propagate in the normal direction with speed

$$F = \hat{k}_I(-1.0 - 0.025K).$$

We employed the narrow-band update algorithm to move the front with a time step size set to $\Delta t = 0.0005$, and the ψ function was recomputed after every 50 time steps. Fig. 7(b) shows the image-based speed term which is synthesized according to Equation (14). Note that in Fig. 7(b), $k_I(x, y)$ values lying in the interval $[0..1]$ have been mapped into the interval $[0..255]$. In Fig. 8(b) through Fig. 8(e) we depict the configuration of the level set $\{\psi = 0\}$ at four intermediate time instants. The final result is achieved after 575 time iterations and is shown in Fig. 8(f). We emphasize that our method does not require that the initial contour be placed close to the object boundary. In addition, observe how the front overshoots all the isolated spurious edges present inside the shape (see Fig. 7(b)) and settles in the neighborhood of edges which correspond to the true shape. This feature is a consequence of εK component in the speed which diffuses regions of high curvature on the front and forces it to attain a smooth shape.

As mentioned in Section III, smoothness of the front can be controlled by choosing an appropriate curvature component in the speed function $F = 1 - \varepsilon K$. The objective of our next experiment is to demonstrate smoothness control in the context of shape recovery. In Fig. 9(a) through Fig. 9(c), we show the results of applying our narrow-band shape recovery algorithm to an image consisting of three synthetic shapes. Initialization was performed by drawing a curve enclosing each one of the three shapes. We compute the signed distance function $\psi(x, y)$ from these curves. The level sets of ψ are then made to propagate with speed $F = k_I(1.0 - \varepsilon K)$. First, as shown in Fig. 9(a), we perform shape recovery with the value of $\varepsilon = 0.05$. The process is repeated with different values of ε; 0.25 in Fig. 9(b) and 0.75 in Fig. 9(c). Clearly, with every increment in the value of ε, the level set $\{\psi = 0\}$ attains a configuration that is relatively smoother. This is analogous to the smoothness provided by the second order term in the internal energy of a thin flexible rod [15].

In our third experiment we recover the complicated structure of an arterial tree. The real image has been obtained by clipping a portion of a digital subtraction angiogram. This is an example of a shape with extended branches or significant protrusions. In this experiment we compare the performance of our scheme with the active contour model. First, an attempt is made to reconstruct the arterial structure using a snake model with inflation forces [10]. In Fig. 10(a) through Fig. 10(i), we show a sequence of pictures depicting the snake configuration in the image. We present the final equilibrium state of the snake in Fig. 10(c), Fig. 10(f), and Fig. 10(i) corresponding to three distinct initializations, each better than the preceding one - in terms of the closeness to the desired final shape. In all three cases the active contour model, even after 1000 time iterations, barely recovers the main stem of the artery and completely fails to account for the branches. Due to the existence of multiple local minima in the (nonconvex) energy functional which the numerical procedure explicitly minimizes, the final result depends on the initial guess. Observe how, in the third case, despite a good initialization (Fig. 10(g)), the snake snaps back into a relatively bumpless configuration in Fig. 10(h). This is due to the snake's arc-length length (elasticity) and curvature (rigidity) minimizing property. Snakes prefer regular shapes because shapes with protrusions have very high defor

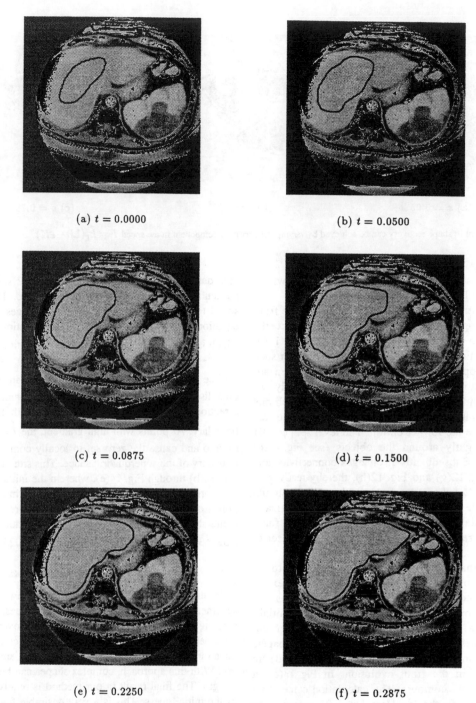

(a) $t = 0.0000$

(b) $t = 0.0500$

(c) $t = 0.0875$

(d) $t = 0.1500$

(e) $t = 0.2250$

(f) $t = 0.2875$

Fig. 8. Recovery of the stomach shape from a CT image of an abdominal section. Narrow-band computation was done on a 128×128 grid – the front was made to propagate with speed $F = \hat{k}_I(\text{-1.0 - 0.025 } K)$ and the time step Δt was set to 0.0005. ψ was recomputed once every 50 time steps.

mation energies. Note that it is important to maintain a bal-ance between the image-based force and the inflation force. Therefore, we cannot increase the latter arbitrarily. One pos-sible way to account for significant protrusions in a shape is via an adaptive resampling of the first order "balloon-snake" model. This however is a cumbersome solution to the problem. Now, we apply our level set algorithm to reconstruct the same shape. After the initialization in Fig. 11(a), the front is made to

propagate in the normal direction. We employ the narrow-band algorithm with a band width of $\delta = 0.045$ to move the front. It can be seen that in subsequent frames the front evolves into the branches and finally in Fig. 11(h) it completely reconstructs the complex tree structure. Thus, a single instance of our shape model sprouts branches and recovers all the connected compo-nents of a given shape. Calculations were carried out on a 128×128 grid and a time step $\Delta t = 0.00025$ was used. The

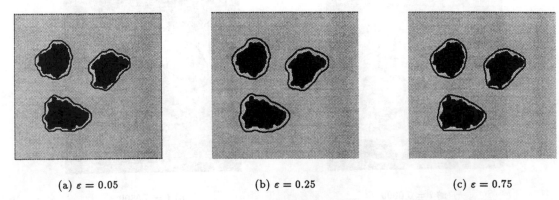

| (a) $\varepsilon = 0.05$ | (b) $\varepsilon = 0.25$ | (c) $\varepsilon = 0.75$ |

Fig. 9. Smoothness control in shape recovery can be achieved by varying the curvature component in the speed $F = \hat{k}_I(1.0 - \varepsilon K)$.

plots of $\psi(\mathbf{x}, t = 0)$ and $\psi(\mathbf{x}, t = 0.375)$ are shown in Fig. 11(b) and Fig. 11(i), respectively.

In the next experiment, we depict a situation when the front undergoes a topological transformation to reconstruct the constituent shapes in an image. The image shown in Fig. 12(a) consists of three distinct shapes. Initial curve is placed in such a way that it envelopes all the objects. The front is then advanced in the direction of the negative normal. Alternately, we could perform the initialization by placing a curve in each one of the individual shapes and propagating them in the normal direction. We choose the former option. The level set $\{\psi = 0\}$ first wraps itself tightly around the objects (see Fig. 12(d) through Fig. 12(f)). Subsequently it changes connectivity and splits twice - in Fig. 12(g) and Fig. 12(h), thereby recovering three shapes. Fig. 12(i) shows the final result. Again it should be noted that a single instance of our shape model dynamically splits into three instances to represent each object. The function ψ was discretized on a 64×64 grid and Δt was set to 0.00025.

Next, we show that our approach can also be used to recover shapes with holes. The shapes in the Fig. 13 are examples of shapes with holes. The outer and inner boundaries of a given shape are recovered without requiring separate initializations. In Fig. 13(a), we show the initial contour which encloses both the shapes. This contour is then made to propagate inward with a constant speed. Fig. 13(b) through Fig. 13(d) are intermediate stages in the front evolution. In Fig. 13(e), it splits into two separate contours. The calculation comes to a halt when, in Fig. 13(f), the level set $\{\psi = 0\}$ recovers the outer boundaries of two disconnected shapes. In the second stage of our computation, we treat the zero set configuration in Fig. 13(f) as an initial state, and propagate the front inward by momentarily relaxing the image-based speed term. This causes the zero set to move into the shapes as shown in Fig. 13(g), and recover the holes, thereby achieving a complete shape recovery (see 13(h)). The calculations for this experiment were done on a 128×128 grid, and the time step Δt was set to 0.00025.

In our last experiment, we recover the shape of a flat superquadric using the level set front propagation scheme in 3D. Vol-

ume data for this experiment consists of 32 slices each with a particular cross section of the superquadric. The image-based speed term k_I is computed from these images according to an equation in 3D which is analogous to Equation (14). A sphere, which is the level surface $\{\psi = 0\}$ of a function $\psi(x, y, z) = x^2 + y^2 + z^2 - 0.01$, forms our initialization (see Fig. 14(a)). This initial surface is moved with speed $F = \hat{k}_I$ by updating the value of ψ on a discrete 3D grid. The initial surface expands smoothly in all directions until a portion of it collides with the superquadric boundary. At points with high gradient, the $\hat{k}_I$ values are close to zero and cause the zero set to locally come to stop near the boundary of the superquadric shape. This situation is depicted in Fig. 14(b) through Fig. 14(e), wherein the initial spherical shape transforms into a flat superquadric. Finally, in Fig. 14(f), all the points on our shape model are stopped, thereby recovering the entire shape of the flat superquadric. Calculations were done on a $32 \times 32 \times 32$ grid with a time step $\Delta t = 0.0025$.

VI. CONCLUDING REMARKS

In this paper we have presented a new shape modeling scheme. Our approach retains some of the desirable features of existing methods for shape modeling and overcomes some of their deficiencies. We adopt the level set techniques first introduced in Osher and Sethian [23] to the problem of shape recovery. With this approach, complex shapes can be recovered from images. The final result in our method is relatively independent of the initial guess. This is a very desirable feature to have, especially in applications such as automatic shape recovery from image data. Moreover, our scheme makes no *a priori* assumption about the object's topology. Other salient features of our shape modeling scheme include its ability to split and merge freely without any additional bookkeeping during the evolutionary process, and its easy extensibility to higher dimensions. We believe that this shape modeling algorithm will have numerous applications in the areas of computer vision and computer graphics. For an extension of this work to a level set based shape description and recognition scheme, the reader is referred to Malladi and Sethian [21].

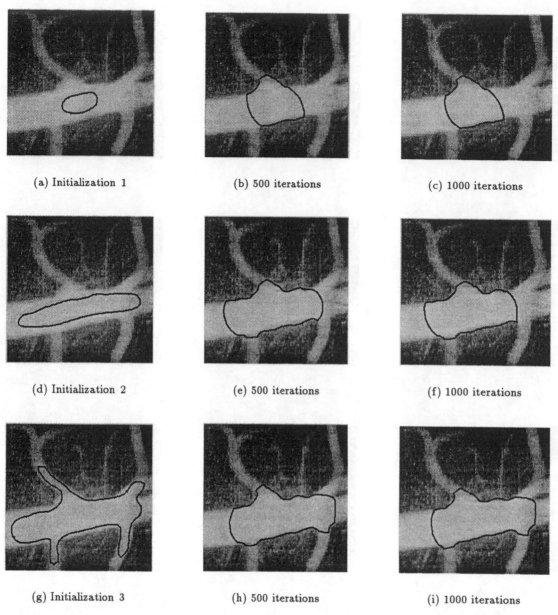

(a) Initialization 1   (b) 500 iterations   (c) 1000 iterations

(d) Initialization 2   (e) 500 iterations   (f) 1000 iterations

(g) Initialization 3   (h) 500 iterations   (i) 1000 iterations

Fig. 10. An unsuccessful attempt to reconstruct a complex shape with significant protrusions using an active contour model. Three different results are shown in parts (c), (f), and (i) corresponding to three distinct initializations in parts (a), (d), and (g), respectively. The following parameter values were employed in this experiment: γ (damping) = 1.0, Δt = 0.50, w_1 (elasticity) = 0.035, w_2 (rigidity) = 0.015, coefficient of inflation force = 0.50, and coefficient of image force = 2.50.

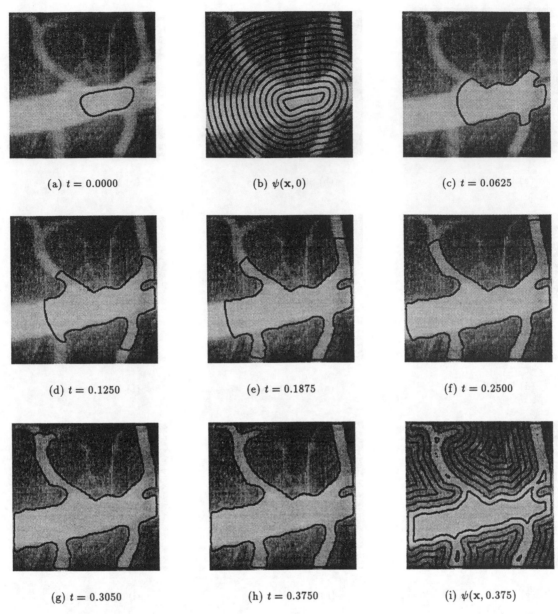

(a) $t = 0.0000$ (b) $\psi(\mathbf{x}, 0)$ (c) $t = 0.0625$

(d) $t = 0.1250$ (e) $t = 0.1875$ (f) $t = 0.2500$

(g) $t = 0.3050$ (h) $t = 0.3750$ (i) $\psi(\mathbf{x}, 0.375)$

Fig. 11. Reconstruction of a shape with significant protrusions: an arterial tree structure. Computation was done on a 128×128 grid with a time step $\Delta t = 0.00025$. The narrow-band algorithm was used with a band width of $\delta = 0.045$.

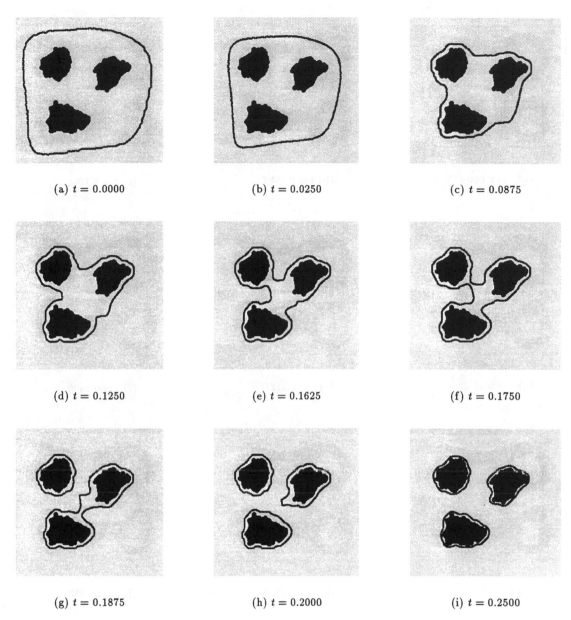

(a) $t = 0.0000$ (b) $t = 0.0250$ (c) $t = 0.0875$

(d) $t = 0.1250$ (e) $t = 0.1625$ (f) $t = 0.1750$

(g) $t = 0.1875$ (h) $t = 0.2000$ (i) $t = 0.2500$

Fig. 12. Topological split: A single instance of the shape model splits into three instances to reconstruct the individual shapes. Computation was done on a 64×64 mesh with a time step $\Delta t = 0.00025$.

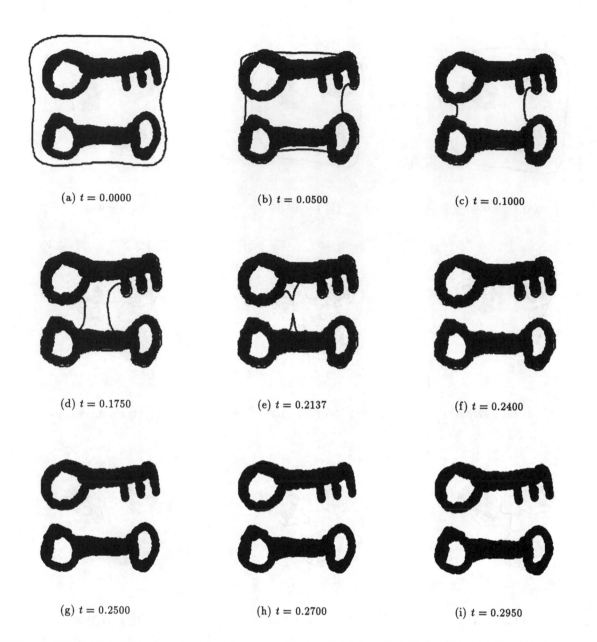

(a) $t = 0.0000$ (b) $t = 0.0500$ (c) $t = 0.1000$

(d) $t = 0.1750$ (e) $t = 0.2137$ (f) $t = 0.2400$

(g) $t = 0.2500$ (h) $t = 0.2700$ (i) $t = 0.2950$

Fig. 13. Shapes with holes: A two-stage scheme is used to arrive at a complete shape description of both simple shapes and shapes with holes. Computation was performed on 128×128 grid and the time step Δt was set to 0.00025.

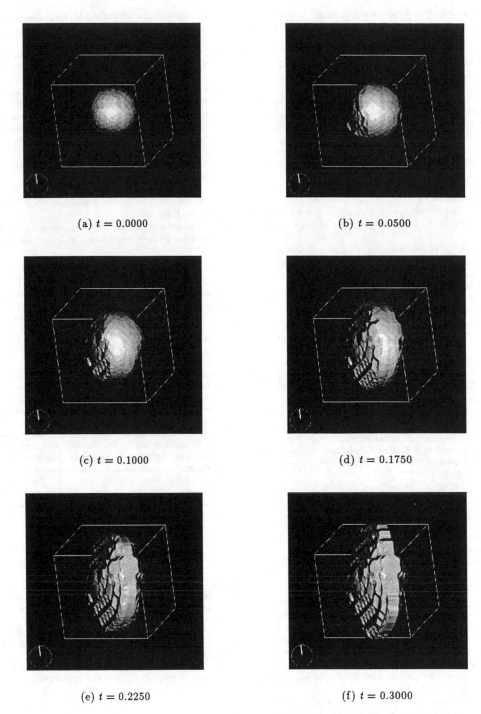

(a) $t = 0.0000$

(b) $t = 0.0500$

(c) $t = 0.1000$

(d) $t = 0.1750$

(e) $t = 0.2250$

(f) $t = 0.3000$

Fig. 14. Shape recovery in 3D: a flat superquadric shape. Calculations were done on a $32 \times 32 \times 32$ grid with a time step $\Delta t = 0.0025$.

REFERENCES

[1] D. Adalsteinsson and J. A. Sethian, "A fast level set method for propagating interfaces," submitted for publication, *J. of Computational Physics*, 1994.

[2] A. A. Amini, T. E. Weymouth, and R. C. Jain, "Using dynamic programming for solving variational problems in vision," *IEEE Trans. on Pattern Analysis and Machine Intelligence*, vol. 12, No. 9, pp. 855–867, 1990.

[3] J. Bence, B. Merriman, and S. Osher, "Motion of multiple triple junctions: A level set approach," to appear in *J. of Computational Physics*, 1994.

[4] R. M. Bolle and B. C. Vemuri, "On three-dimensional surface reconstruction methods," *IEEE Trans. on Pattern Analysis and Machine Intelligence*, vol. PAMI 13, No. 1, pp. 1–13, 1991.

[5] A. Bourlioux and J. A. Sethian, "Projection methods coupled to level set interface methods," to be submitted, *J. of Computational Physics*, 1994.

[6] A. Blake and A. Zisserman, *Visual Reconstruction*, MIT Press, Cambridge, MA.

[7] V. Caselles, F. Catte, T. Coll, and F. Dibos, "A geometric model for active contours in image processing," Internal report no. 9210, CEREMADE, Université de Paris-Dauphine, France.

[10] L. D. Cohen, "On active contour models and balloons," *Computer Vision, Graphics, and Image Processing*, vol. 53, No. 2, pp. 211–218, March 1991.

[11] H. Delingette, M. Hebert, and K. Ikeuchi, "Shape representation and image segmentation using deformable models," in *Proc. of IEEE Conf. on Computer Vision and Pattern Recognition*, pp. 467–472, Maui, Hawaii, June 1991.

[12] B. Engquist and S. Osher, "Stable and entropy satisfying approximations for transonic flow calculations," *Math. Comp.*, vol. 34, 45, 1980.

[13] L. C. Evans and J. Spruck, "Motion of level sets by mean curvature. I," *J. of Differential Geometry*, vol. 33, pp. 635–681, 1991.

[14] W. T. Freeman and E. H. Adelson, "Steerable filters for early vision, image analysis, and wavelet decomposition," *Proc. of ICCV*, pp. 406–415, Osaka, Japan, 1990.

[15] M. Kass, A. Witkin, and D. Terzopoulos, "Snakes: Active contour models," *Int'l. J. of Computer Vision*, pp. 321–331, 1988.

[16] B. B. Kimia, A. R. Tannenbaum, and S. W. Zucker, "Toward a computational theory of shape: An overview," in *Proc. of ECCV*, Antibes, France, 1990.

[17] D. Lee and T. Pavlidis, "One-dimensional regularization with discontinuities," *IEEE Trans. on Pattern Analysis and Machine Intelligence*, vol. 10, pp. 822–829, 1986.

[18] R. Malladi, "Deformable models: Canonical parameters for surface representation and multiple view integration," Master's thesis, Dept. of CIS, Univ. of Florida, Gainesville, FL, May 1991.

[19] R. Malladi, "A topology-independent shape modeling scheme," Doctoral dissertation, Dept. of CIS, Univ. of Florida, Gainesville, FL, December 1993.

[20] R. Malladi, J. A. Sethian, and B. C. Vemuri, "Evolutionary fronts for topology-independent shape modeling and recovery," in *Proc. of Third European Conf. on Computer Vision*, LNCS vol. 800, pp. 3–13, Stockholm, Sweden, May 1994.

[21] R. Malladi and J. A. Sethian, "A unified framework for shape segmentation, representation, and recognition," Report LBL-36069, Lawrence Berkeley Laboratory, Univ. of California, Berkeley, Aug. 1994.

[22] W. Mulder, S. Osher, and J. A. Sethian, "Computing interface motion in compressible gas dynamics," *J. of Computational Physics*, vol. 100, no. 2, pp. 209–228, 1992.

[23] S. Osher and J. A. Sethian, "Fronts propagating with curvature dependent speed: Algorithms based on Hamilton-Jacobi formulation," *J. of Computational Physics*, vol. 79, pp. 12–49, 1988.

[24] A. Pentland and S. Sclaroff, "Closed-form solutions for physically based shape modeling and recognition," *IEEE Trans. on Pattern Analysis and Machine Intelligence*, vol. 13, No. 7, July 1991.

[25] C. Rhee, L. Talbot, and J. A. Sethian, "Dynamical behavior of a premixed turbulent open V-Flame," submitted for publication, *J. of Fluid Mech.*, 1994.

[26] R. Samadani, "Changes in connectivity in active contour models," *Proc. of the Workshop on Visual Motion*, pp. 337–343, Irvine, CA, March 1989.

[27] L. L. Schumaker, "Fitting surfaces to scattered data," in *Approximation Theory II*, G. G. Lorentz, C. K. Chui, and L. L. Schumaker, (eds.). New York: Academic Press, 1976, pp. 203–267.

[28] J. A. Sethian, "Curvature and the evolution of fronts," *Comm. in Math. Physics*, vol. 101, pp. 487–499, 1985.

[29] J. A. Sethian, "Numerical algorithms for propagating interfaces: Hamilton-Jacobi equations and conservation laws," *J. of Differential Geometry*, vol. 31, pp. 131–161, 1990.

[30] J. A. Sethian and J. Strain, "Crystal growth and dendritic solidification," *J. of Computational Physics*, vol. 98, pp. 231–253, 1992.

[31] M. Sussman, P. Smereka, and S. Osher, "A level set approach for computing solutions to incompressible two-phase flow," UCLA CAM Report 93-18, 1993.

[32] R. Szeliski and D. Tonnesen, "Surface modeling with oriented particle systems," *Computer Graphics SIGGRAPH*, vol. 26, No. 2, pp. 185–194, July 1992.

[33] D. Terzopoulos, "Regularization of inverse visual problems involving discontinuities," *IEEE Trans. on Pattern Analysis and Machine Intelligence*, vol. 8, no. 2, pp. 413–424, 1986.

[34] D. Terzopoulos, A. Witkin, and M. Kass, "Constraints on deformable models: Recovering 3D shape and nonrigid motion," *Artificial Intelligence*, vol. 36, pp. 91–123, 1988.

[35] D. Terzopoulos, "The computation of visible surface representations," *IEEE Trans. on Pattern Analysis and Machine Intelligence*, vol. 4, no. 10, pp. 417–438, 1988.

[36] B. C. Vemuri and R. Malladi, "Surface griding with intrinsic parameters," *Pattern Recognition Letters*, vol. 13, No. 11, pp. 805–812, Nov. 1992.

[37] B. C. Vemuri and R. Malladi, "Constructing intrinsic parameters with active models for invariant surface reconstruction," *IEEE Trans. on Pattern Analysis and Machine Intelligence*, vol. 15, No. 7, pp. 668–681, July 1993.

[38] B. C. Vemuri, A. Mitiche, and J. K. Aggarwal, "Curvature-based representation of objects from range data," *Int'l. J. of Image and Vision Computing*, 4, pp. 107–114, 1986.

[39] Y. F. Wang and J. F. Wang, "Surface reconstruction using deformable models with interior and boundary constraints," in *Proc. of ICCV*, pp. 300–303, Osaka, Japan, 1990.

[40] J. Zhu and J. A. Sethian, "Projection methods coupled to level set interface techniques," *J. of Computational Physics*, vol. 102(1), pp. 128–138, 1992.

Ravikanth Malladi received his B.Eng. degree with honors in electrical engineering and an M.Sc. degree in physics from Birla Institute of Technology and Science, India, in 1988. He subsequently received the MS degree in 1991 and the PhD degree in 1993; both in computer vision from the University of Florida, Gainesville, Florida, USA. He is currently working at the Lawrence Berkeley Laboratory, University of California, Berkeley, California, USA.

In the summer of 1985 he worked at the National Geophysical Research Institute, India. During the spring of 1988, he held a research assistant position with the semiconductor physics group at the Central Electrical and Electronics Research Institute, India. From summer 1990, till fall 1993, he was a graduate research assistant at the University of Florida, and was affiliated with the Center for Computer Vision and Visualization.

His research interests are focused on computational vision, shape modeling and recognition, computer graphics, and medical image interpretation.

Dr. Malladi was awarded the NSF Postdoctoral Fellowship in Computational Science and Engineering in June 1994, and his work received best peer reviews at the Third European Conference on Computer Vision, Stockholm, Sweden, in May 1994.

James A. Sethian is professor of mathematics at the University of California, Berkeley, California, USA, and senior scientist in the physics division at the Lawrence Berkeley Laboratory. Before coming to Berkeley, he was at the Courant Institute of Mathematics.

He received a PhD in mathematics from the University of California, Berkeley, and has been a recipient of the Presidential Young Investigator Award and a Sloan Foundation Fellowship.

His research interests include computational physics, parallel processing, image processing, and material science.

Baba C. Vemuri received the PhD degree in electrical and computer engineering from the University of Texas at Austin in 1987, and joined the Department of Computer and Information Sciences at the University of Florida, Gainesville, where he is currently an associate professor of computer and information sciences and electrical engineering.

In the summer of 1988 and 1992, Prof. Vemuri was a visiting Faculty Member at the IBM Thomas J. Watson Research Center, Yorktown Heights, NY, associated with the Exploratory Computer Vision Group there. During the academic year 1989–1990, he was a Visiting Research Scientist with the German Aerospace Research Institute, DLR Oberpfaffenhofen, Germany. His research interests include computational vision, modeling for vision and

234

graphics, medical imaging, and applied mathematics. In the past several years, his research has focused primarily on efficient algorithms for 3D shape modeling and recovery from image data. He has published numerous refereed journal and conference articles in the field of computer vision and its applications.

Dr. Vemuri received the NSF Research Initiation and the Whitaker Foundation Awards in 1988 and 1994, respectively. He was a recipient of the first prize for best international paper in Computer Vision from the Norwegian branch of the IAPR in 1992. He subsequently received the best review scores for his co-authored paper in ECCV '94. Dr. Vemuri served as a guest editor for the April 1992 special issue on Range Image Understanding of the Journal of Image and Vision Computing. He also served as a program committee member for the IEEE Conference on CVPR in 1993, and was the chairman of the SPIE-sponsored conferences on Geometric Methods in Computer Vision in 1991 and 1993, respectively.

Dr. Vemuri is a member of the IEEE Computer and Signal Processing Societies,, ACM SIGGRAH and the SIAM.

Multiresolution Stochastic Hybrid Shape Models with Fractal Priors

B. C VEMURI and A. RADISAVLJEVIC
University of Florida, Gainesville

3D shape modeling has received enormous attention in computer graphics and computer vision over the past decade. Several shape modeling techniques have been proposed in literature, some are local (distributed parameter) while others are global (lumped parameter) in terms of the parameters required to describe the shape. Hybrid models that combine both ends of this parameter spectrum have been in vogue only recently. However, they do not allow a smooth transition between the two extremes of this parameter spectrum.

We introduce a *new shape-modeling scheme* that can *transform smoothly from local to global* models or vice versa. The modeling scheme utilizes a hybrid primitive called the deformable superquadric *constructed in an orthonormal wavelet basis*. The multiresolution wavelet basis provides the power to continuously transform from local to global shape deformations and thereby allow for a continuum of shape models—from those with local to those with global shape descriptive power—to be created. The multiresolution wavelet basis allows us to generate fractal surfaces of arbitrary order that can be useful in describing natural detail.

We embed these multiresolution shape models in a probabilistic framework and use them for recovery of anatomical structures in the human brain from MRI data. A salient feature of our modeling scheme is that it can naturally allow for the incorporation of prior statistics of a rich variety of shapes. This stems from the fact that, unlike other modeling schemes, in our modeling, we require relatively few parameters to describe a large class of shapes.

Categories and Subject Descriptors: G.1.8 [**Mathematics of Computing**]: Partial Differential Equations—*finite element methods;* G.3 [**Mathematics of Computing**]: Probability and Statistics—*statistical computing;* I.2.10 [**Artificial Intelligence**]: Vision and Scene Understanding—*modeling and recovery of physical attributes; shape;* I.3.5 [**Computer Graphics**]: Computational Geometry and Object Modeling—*curve, surface, solid, and object representations; hierarchy and geometric transformations; physically based modeling; splines;* I.3.7 [**Computer Graphics**]: Three-Dimensional Graphics and Realism—*fractals;* I.3.8 [**Computer Graphics**]: Applications

General Terms: Algorithms

Additional Key Words and Phrases: Bayesian estimation, deformable surfaces, fractal surfaces, multiresolution representation, orthonormal wavelet basis, stiffness matrix, superquadrics, surface fitting

This work was supported in part by the University of Florida Brain Institute.
Authors' addresses: B. C. Vemuri, Department of Computer and Information Sciences, University of Florida, Gainesville, FL 32611; email: vemuri@scuba.cis.ufl.edu; A. Radisavljevic, Department of Electrical Engineering, University of Florida, Gainesville, FL 32611.

1. INTRODUCTION

Shape modeling is an important and integral part of computer graphics as well as computer vision. In computer graphics, modeling shapes is an important ingredient of shape synthesis, while in computer vision it is needed for shape reconstruction and shape recognition from sensed data. Many shape-modeling schemes have been proposed in the graphics as well as vision literature. In this article, we will be concerned with shape modeling with a view toward facilitation of shape recovery from 3D data for computer vision/medical imaging applications. In computer vision, the motivation for modeling shapes has been driven primarily by either shape reconstruction or shape recognition tasks. Shape reconstruction from sensed data requires a broad geometric coverage. The models must recover detailed structure from noisy data using only the weakest of the possible assumptions about the observed shapes. Generalized spline models with continuity constraints are well suited for fulfilling the goals of shape reconstruction [Blake and Zisserman 1987; Terzopoulos 1986a; Vemuri et al. 1986]. Generalized splines are the key ingredient of the dynamic shape-modeling paradigm introduced by Terzopoulos et al. [1987; 1988]. Incorporating dynamics into shape modeling with generalized splines allows realistic animation for computer graphics applications and also for tracking moving objects in computer vision applications. With the advent of the dynamic shape-modeling paradigm, there was a flurry of research activity in this area, with numerous application-motivated modifications to the modeling primitives and the external forces derived from data. Additionally, methods were also presented toward improving the numerical stability by using finite-element discretization [Celinker and Gossard 1991; Cohen and Cohen 1992; Delingette et al. 1991; Vemuri and Malladi 1991; 1993; Wang and Wang 1990]. However, the distributed nature of these models—each point of the spline surface potentially contributes three spatial degrees of freedom—makes them unsuitable for shape recognition tasks. Shape recognition—a high-level vision task—requires that the shape models be characterized by a small set of parameters. Lumped parameter models are thus better suited for such tasks. Some examples of lumped parameter models include generalized cylinders [Binford 1971], superquadrics [Bajscy and Solina 1987; Barr 1981; Pentland 1986], and the parametrically deformable models [Staib and Duncan 1991; Yuille et al. 1989].

Recently, a hybrid modeling scheme, dubbed "deformable superquadrics," was introduced by Terzopoulos and Metaxas [1991]. These models have the advantage of combining the descriptive power of lumped and distributed parameter models and thus, simultaneously satisfying the requirements of shape reconstruction and shape recognition. However, these hybrid models do not exhibit a smooth transition in the number of parameters required for their description. For example, the two extremes of the spectrum are occupied by lumped models at one end and distributed models at the other. The former requiring few parameters, and the later requiring a large number of parameters for their description. Also, the lumped parameter models allow only for global deformations while the distributed parameter models allow for local deformations. The modeling scheme described in Terzopoulos and Metaxas [1991] involves a superposition of the lumped and distributed parameters to completely characterize the plethora of shapes occupying the spectrum. Although, these hybrid models can be used to generate both local and global shape deformations, they *do not depict a smooth transition between these types of deformations*. Additionally, there is *no smooth transition in the number of parameters* that can capture descriptions of the range of generated shapes.

In this article we introduce a new multiresolution hybrid modeling scheme [Vemuri and Radisavljevic 1993] that uses an orthonormal wavelet basis [Daubechies 1988; Mallat 1989]. Our hybrid models have the unique property of being able to smoothly scale up or down the range (from local to global) of possible deformations and the number of parameters required to characterize them. These properties are inherited by virtue of the multiresolution wavelet representation. Depending on the application, one may choose a set of wavelet coefficients at a particular coarse level from the multiresolution representation of the hybrid model and augment the global (lumped) parameters of the model. This augmented set of "global" (lumped) parameters defines a larger class of shapes than those characterized by purely lumped parameters. We will use this enhanced class of shapes characterized by a few global parameters as prior information in our probabilistic shape recovery algorithm. In Section 5, we describe a supervised learning method that may be used in selecting an appropriate level in the multiresolution representation for choosing the set of wavelet coefficients in the aforementioned augmentation process. Tweaking these coarse-level wavelet coefficients will produce global deformations that are *very different* from those produced by tweaking the global (lumped) parameters of the model (see the bottom four shapes in Figure 6). The number of nodes per level in the multiresolution algorithm used in our work is a power of 2, but the number of coefficients chosen in the augmentation process need not be a power of two, thus, giving the power to smoothly/"continuously" scale up or down the range of possible deformations.

A question that arises in the context of constructing hybrid models in a multiresolution wavelet basis is: *can we achieve the same results via standard finite-element subdivision techniques?* The answer is no. First, *single-level* subdivisions of the elements will not achieve the same results as a *multiresolution wavelet* representation, since there is more to a wavelet transform than subsampling or up-sampling operations (used to achieve projection from one subspace to another in the multiresolution spaces), specifically, the high-pass and low-pass filtering operations (see Section 2.2). Also, the single-level finite-element subdivision cannot lead to a smooth transition from local to global deformations since there is no scope for descending/ascending through the space of deformations. This however may be achieved via the use of a hierarchical-basis finite-element scheme. What then are the advantages of a wavelet basis in this context? There are several advantages, and some of them are (a) the number of coefficients used in a wavelet representation is the same as that in the original nodal representation of the function i.e., no additional nodes are added in creating the hierarchical wavelet-based description of a function; this leads to a compact representation technique; (b) the wavelet transform is a perfectly invertible transform, and therefore, there is no loss of information in this representation; (c) the model stiffness matrix in the wavelet basis is nearly diagonal, which leads to a very fast numerical solution to the model-fitting problem; (d) the wavelet-based representation allows us to synthesize fractal surfaces of arbitrary order without having to resort to blending approximations. These are but a few of the list of advantages of the wavelet-based representation.

One of the reasons for the nonequivalence of the hierarchical-basis finite-element representation, i.e., the multilevel splitting of the finite-element spaces as in Yeserentant [1986] and the multiresolution wavelet-based representation, is using a hierarchical basis for the finite-element spaces improves the condition number (over the one obtained with the usual nodal bases) of the model stiffness matrix. Whereas, a multiresolution orthonormal wavelet basis does not change the condition number of the stiffness matrix, since the wavelet transform is performed via a similarity transformation (a transformation that leaves the Eigen values, and hence the condition number unchanged). Even if we use an orthogonal basis in the hierarchical finite-element method, it would still not be equivalent to the multiresolution wavelet representation because not all orthogonal bases are wavelets. Finally, unlike in the construction of a wavelet basis representation, there is no high-pass filtering operation in the construction of a hierarchical-basis finite-element representation.

Unlike the windowed Fourier transform, where the analyzing sinusoid function (kernel) exists on an interval of fixed length, the analyzing wavelet's ("mother wavelet") time support reduces with increasing frequency. Wavelet analysis therefore works best for functions where low-frequency components are stationary over longer time intervals while high-frequency components are stationary over shorter time intervals. Most of the images/signals encountered in practice actually exhibit these characteristics, which accounts for the increasing popularity of wavelet analysis. For our purposes of modeling the deformable superquadrics, the choice of wavelet basis not only facilitates a hierarchical representation of the hybrid model surface, but also *provides good visual appearance due to this natural trade-off between time and frequency resolutions.* Thus, the multiresolution hybrid models can be used to synthesize a variety of shapes that look natural in the context of interactive sculpting. We present some examples of these shapes in Section 2.

Earlier work reported in Pentland [1992] on the use of wavelets in the context of shape modeling was limited to computational issues in surface-fitting applications. He used wavelets basis to approximate the Eigen vectors of the stiffness matrix assembled in the finite-element solution to the surface reconstruction problem using the thin-plate-membrane splines. The main goal of his work was to speed up the solution to the surface reconstruction problem by a change of basis, from regular nodal basis to the natural basis represented by the Eigen vectors of the stiffness matrix. Wavelet basis was used as an approximation to the natural basis, i.e., the Eigen vectors of the stiffness matrix. In the wavelet basis, the stiffness matrix is approximately diagonal, and this approximate diagonalization leads to savings in storage space as well as computation time for the solution.

Sclaroff and Pentland [1991] report techniques for generalizing implicit function representation of shapes by use of modal deformations and displacement maps. The displacement map function is defined by using a bilinear interpolation between point samples and is stored as an image array. When smoother interpolation is desired, they propose to employ a spline or pyramid-based multiresolution method [Burt and Adelson 1983]. Wavelets or quadrature mirror filter pyramids are used for data compression, leading to savings in storage of the displacement maps. Also, the modal deformations are assumed to be the free vibration modes of the object which simplifies the simulation of the dynamics of the object. The multiresolution pyramid method discussed in Burt and Adelson [1983] and *proposed for use* by Sclaroff and Pentland has several limitations compared to a wavelet-based multiresolution representation as pointed out by Mallat [1989]. Note that the wavelet-based pyramid is used in their work only for the data compression purposes. The implications of this wavelet-based representation on improving the expressive power of the modeling scheme are however left unexplored.

In our research, the *key focus* is on development of a *general shape-modeling scheme* which when embedded in a probabilistic framework can be utilized for easily incorporating a *larger class* of shapes as prior information. The reason for being able to incorporate a larger class of shapes as priors in shape extraction applications is due to the enhanced class of shapes that we can now characterize (in our modeling scheme) using a small set of global parameters. Another salient feature of our modeling scheme is that it allows for smooth transitions in the spectrum of model deformations and parameters. Additionally, we also emphasize on the efficient computation of the model-fitting process to the data. Specifically, we give a closed-form expression for the stiffness matrix computation in the wavelet basis (see Section 4.2) and employ a multiresolution relaxation process in solving the model-fitting problem.

Thin-plate-membrane splines were also used for a very different purpose by Szeliski and Terzopoulos [1989], namely, generation of constrained fractals which are useful in representing natural images. They derive the fractal characteristics of the membrane and thin-plate splines and show that the membrane splines give rise to fractals of $\beta = 2$ while the thin-plate splines yield fractals of $\beta = 4$. A fractal of in-between β (order) was approximated by using a blend of the membrane and thin-plate models. The *modeling scheme we introduce allows us to generate fractals of in-between order without having to resort to approximations with a blend of the plate membrane models.* We achieve this by modulating the frequency characteristics of the wavelet basis with a rational function (which is a reciprocal polynomial) of appropriate order. To synthesize fractal surfaces, we convert the energies into probability distributions using ideas from statistical mechanics [Geman and Geman 1984] and employ a multiresolution stochastic relaxation algorithm. We will present some examples of the synthesized fractal surfaces in a subsequent section.

Like any deformable surfaces, our multiresolution hybrid models can also be interactively manipulated to mold into desired shapes via the use of externally applied forces. In this article, external forces will be derived from volumetric medical image data (MRI brain scans), and the model will be forced into desired anatomical shapes in the MRI data of a human brain. The shape recovery from data is achieved in two stages, namely, a learning phase and an operation phase. The shape recovery process involves the use of prior information about the anatomical shape of interest in the MRI brain scan. This prior information is obtained via a *supervised learning procedure* wherein statistics on the augmented global parameters of the multiresolution hybrid model are collected. In doing so, the model is subject to external-image-based forces and also forces derived from the interactive placement of data points by an expert (neuroanatomist) on the boundary of the anatomical shape of interest. The expert anatomist has the freedom to *interactively manipulate* the model until a "satisfactory" fit to the data is obtained. The learning of a specific shape is carried out over a fairly large data set, and statistics for the augmented global parameters of the hybrid model are collected. This information is utilized in the initialization of the model during the operational phase of the shape recovery. We give a recursive algorithm for collecting the statistics on the augmented global parameters of the model in Section 5.

The rest of the article is organized as follows. In Section 2 we briefly describe the geometry of the modeling scheme and the multiresolution basis for expressing the geometry, followed by a new way to augment the global shape of the deformable superquadric primitive for achieving a smooth transition from global to local shape descriptions. Section 3 contains discussion on how to embed our models in a probabilistic framework and the derivation of the model mechanics. In Section 4 we derive the internal energy of the prior model in a wavelet basis and present the fractal characteristics of this prior model with the aid of synthesized fractal surfaces. Section 5 contains a description of the unsupervised learning technique that we use for incorporating specific a priori knowledge into our modeling framework and implementation results on model fitting to MRI data, followed by conclusions in Section 6.

2. MULTIRESOLUTION GEOMETRY OF THE MODELING SCHEME

In this section, we will briefly describe the geometry and the construction of a multiresolution wavelet basis for the modeling scheme. For a detailed description of the deformable superquadric geometry, we refer the reader to Terzopoulos and Metaxas [1991]. To dramatically increase the library of shapes that can be characterized by a small set of global parameters, and to achieve a smooth transition from global to local shape descriptions, we will present a *new* technique that will augment the global parameters of the deformable superquadric.

2.1 Geometry of the Deformable Superquadrics

The deformable superquadrics are closed surfaces in space whose intrinsic coordinates $\mathbf{u} = (u, v)$ are defined on a domain Ω. The positions of points on the model in an inertial frame of reference are given by a vector-valued function $\mathbf{x}(\mathbf{u}) = (x_1(\mathbf{u}), x_2(\mathbf{u}), x_3(\mathbf{u}))^T$. In a model-centered coordinate frame, the position vector $\mathbf{x}$ becomes

$$\mathbf{x} = \mathbf{c} + \mathbf{R}\mathbf{p} \tag{1}$$

where $\mathbf{c}$ is the location of the center of the model, and the rotation matrix $\mathbf{R}$ specifies the orientation of the model-centered coordinate frame. Hence, $\mathbf{p}(\mathbf{u})$ denotes the canonical positions of points on the model relative to the model frame. We express $\mathbf{p}$ as the sum of a reference shape $\mathbf{s}(\mathbf{u})$ and a displacement $\mathbf{d}(\mathbf{u})$, namely, $\mathbf{p} = \mathbf{s} + \mathbf{d}$ (see Figure 1). For the parameterized reference shape $\mathbf{s}(\mathbf{u})$, we use the superquadric with a bending deformation (as in Bajscy and Solina [1987]), due to its attractive global shape characterization. The reference shape $\mathbf{s}$ is given by

$$\mathbf{s} = \mathscr{B}(\tilde{\mathbf{s}}) \tag{2}$$

where $\mathscr{B}$ is a bending deformation, a function of two parameters: the radius of curvature k and angle of the bending plane α (see Bajscy and Solina for details). The parametric equation of a superquadric $\tilde{\mathbf{s}}$ is given by

$$\mathbf{s} = a \begin{pmatrix} a_1 C_u^{\epsilon_1} C_v^{\epsilon_2} \\ a_2 C_u^{\epsilon_1} S_v^{\epsilon_2} \\ a_3 S_u^{\epsilon_1} \end{pmatrix} \tag{3}$$

where, $-\pi/2 \le u \le \pi/2 - \pi \le v \le \pi$, and $S_w^{\epsilon} = sgn(sin\ w)|sin\ w|^{\epsilon}$ and $C_w^{\epsilon} = sgn(cos\ w)|cos\ w|^{\epsilon}$. Here, $0 \le a_1, a_2, a_3 \le 1$ are aspect ratio parameters; $\epsilon_1, \epsilon_2 \ge 0$ are "squareness" parameters, and $a \ge 0$ is a scale parameter. This defines the geometry of our underlying reference shape, namely, the superquadric. We collect all these shape parameters along with the two bending parameters into a vector $\mathbf{q}_s$. We will denote $\mathbf{c}$ by the vector $\mathbf{q}_c$ and use $\mathbf{q}_\theta$ to denote the vector of rotational coordinates of the model in a quaternion representation (see Terzopoulos and Metaxas [1991]).

An important aspect of our superquadric reference shape which differs from previous definitions in the work of Terzopoulos and Metaxas and Bajscy and Solina is that we have constructed a *uniform tessalation* of the superquadric. Superquadric shapes exhibit anomalous behavior when the squareness parameters ϵ_1, ϵ_2 depart from unity, causing grid lines to become unevenly spaced leading to distortion of the deformational properties of the superimposed membrane surface and inefficient use of computational resources. Additionally, numerical instabilities may be caused in the computation of derivatives due to the large grid spacing. A uniform tessalation of the superquadric can be used to overcome these problems. To achieve the uniform tessalation, we first construct uniformly spaced grid lines in the parameter direction u and apply the same technique to achieve uniform spacing along the parameter direction v. Thus, we seek a function of the parameter u (same reasoning applies to the parameter v) which when substituted into the

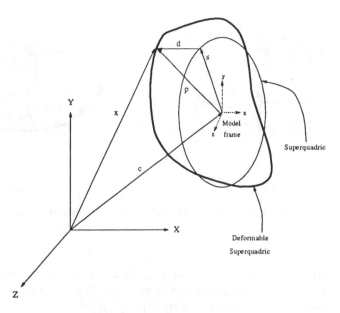

Fig. 1. Deformable superquadric geometry (adopted from Terzopoulos and Metaxas [1991]).

equation of the superquadric, i.e., Eq. 3, would yield a constant differential arc length increment for a constant differential increment in u. For a horizontal elliptical contour, we have

$$ds = \sqrt{(x')^2 + (y')^2}\, du. \tag{4}$$

Setting $ds/du = constant = (circumference/2\pi)$ and using $(x = a_1 cos^\epsilon (f(u)), y = a_2 sin^\epsilon (f(u)), z = 0)$ results in an ordinary differential equation for $f(u)$

$$\frac{df}{du} = K\frac{|tan(f)|}{\epsilon\sqrt{a_1^2|tan(f)|^4|cos(f)|^{2\epsilon} + a_2^2|sin(f)|^{2\epsilon}}} \tag{5}$$

$$f(0) = 0 \text{ as the initial condition} \tag{6}$$

where K is a constant. This ordinary differential equation can be solved numerically. In Figure 2, a superquadric with its natural *nonuniform* tessalation is shown side by side to the same superquadric *uniformly* tessalated using the method described above. Very fast retessalation of the superquadric can be achieved using the Runge-Kutta method [Dahlquist and Björk 1974]. Specifically, we use an order-three Runge-Kutta method. The retessalation needs to be done whenever the parameters of the superquadric are subject to large (greater than a preselected threshold) changes.

In the following sections, we show that the displacement vector function $\mathbf{d} = \Phi S\mathbf{q}_d$ is completely determined by a set of wavelet coefficients collected

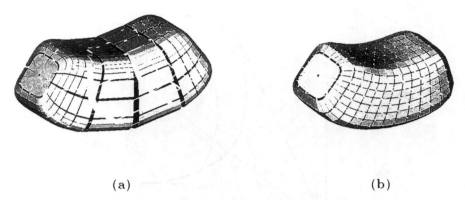

(a)   (b)

Fig. 2. Tesselations of a superquadric, (a) nonuniform (b) uniform.

into the vector $\mathbf{q}_d$, with S corresponding to the discrete wavelet transform and Φ containing nodal interpolation functions. Thus, the state of the model is fully expressed by the vector $\mathbf{q} = [\mathbf{q}_c^T, \mathbf{q}_\theta^T, \mathbf{q}_s^T, \mathbf{q}_d^T]^T$.

2.2 Multiresolution Analysis and Wavelet Bases

Multiresolution analysis has been quite popular in signal-processing and computer vision research for the past decade. It has been used quite extensively for speeding up computations in solutions to problems in computational vision [Terzopoulos 1986b] and in computer graphics for generating stochastic fractals [Szeliski and Terzopoulos 1989]. With the advent of the *wavelet transform* (WT), multiresolution analysis of functions has become more attractive due to the fact that wavelet decomposition of a function into different frequency components allows for studying each component at a resolution matched to its scale. In the following, we will very briefly describe the construction of a wavelet-based multiresolution approximation in 1D and its extension to a 2D function, specifically the membrane displacement function $\mathbf{d}(u, v)$.

2.2.1 *Detail Function from Multiresolution Approximations.* A multiresolution approximation of a scalar-valued function $d(u) \in L^2(\Re)$ at a resolution j is obtained by projecting $d(u)$ into a vector subspace $V_j \subset L^2(\Re)$ where integer (k) translates $\phi_{jk}(u) = \sqrt{2^{-j}}\,\phi(2^{-j}u - k)$ of a dilated scaling function $\phi(u)$ form the orthonormal basis of V_j. The approximation $\hat{d}^j(u)$ is expressed as

$$\hat{d}^j(u) = \sum_k \alpha_{jk}\,\phi_{jk}(u) \tag{7}$$

where the set of coefficients $\alpha_{jk} = \langle d(u), \phi_{jk} \rangle$ for all integer k corresponds to the discrete characterization of this approximation.

An important property of multiresolution approximations is that all the necessary information to compute the function at a smaller resolution $j + 1$ is contained in the function at resolution j. In other words the subspaces V_j satisfy the containment hierarchy,

$$\ldots V_3 \subset V_2 \subset V_1 \subset V_0. \tag{8}$$

The scaling function ϕ has the effect of a low-pass filter with the cutoff frequency decreasing proportionally to 2^{-j} (see Figure 3(a)). The key idea of the wavelet basis is to span the *difference spaces* W_{j+1} between the two approximations V_j and V_{j+1} such that $W_{j+1} \perp V_{j+1}$. A wavelet decomposition therefore consists of splitting the function at resolution j into the *detail function* in W_{j+1} and the next lower $(j + 1)$ resolution approximation in V_{j+1}. This leads directly to a scale wise, orthogonal decomposition of $L^2(\mathfrak{R})$. To represent the function $d(u)$ of a finite resolution we can assume $d(u) \in V_0$, where V_0 is given by

$$\ldots W_3 \oplus W_2 \oplus W_1 = V_0 \tag{9}$$

with $\oplus$ denoting the direct sum operator. The *hierarchical* orthonormal basis for $d(u)$ is given by a family of dilations and translations of a wavelet function $\psi(u)$: $\psi_{jk}(u) = \sqrt{2^{-j}}\,\psi(2^{-j}u - k)$. Thus $d(u)$ can be written in this basis as

$$d(u) = \sum_{j,\,k} \delta_{jk}\,\psi_{jk}(u) \tag{10}$$

where the discrete wavelet coefficients are computed as $\delta_{jk} = \langle d(u), \psi_{jk} \rangle$.

As in the case of the multiresolution approximation, wherein a low-pass filtering interpretation was given to the scaling function, a filtering interpretation can also be given to the WT. At each scale j the WT corresponds to a logarithmically spaced band-pass filter (see Figure 3(b)). Our work in this article is primarily based on this filter bank interpretation of the WT as discussed in Rioul and Vetterli [1991].

2.2.2 *Extension to 2D and Fast Implementation.* Extension to 2D of the multiresolution approximation using wavelet basis can be easily achieved using separable wavelets obtained from the products of one-dimensional wavelets and scaling functions [Mallat 1989]. For the multiresolution approximation of the membrane $\mathbf{d}(u, v)$ we use the tensor products of ϕ and ψ given by (see Mallat [1989]):

$$\left\{ \begin{array}{ll} \psi_{jkl}^{LH}(u, v) & = \phi(u)_{jk}\psi(v)_{jl} \\ \psi_{jkl}^{HL}(u, v) & = \psi(u)_{jk}\phi(v)_{jl} \\ \psi_{jkl}^{HH}(u, v) & = \psi(u)_{jk}\psi(v)_{jl} \end{array} \right\}_{(j,k,l)\in\mathcal{Z}} \tag{11}$$

Note that, since the displacement $\mathbf{d}$ is a vector-valued function, we have to repeat the tensor product approximations shown above for each component of the displacement vector. The superscript $H(L)$ represents high (low)-pass

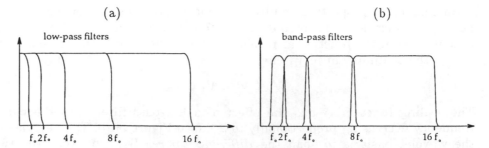

(a)   low-pass filters   (b)   band-pass filters

f_o $2f_o$ $4f_o$ $8f_o$ $16f_o$ f_o $2f_o$ $4f_o$ $8f_o$ $16f_o$

Fig. 3. Division of the frequency domain for (a) multiresolution and (b) wavelet representation.

filtering in each of the directions u and v in the parameter domain Ω, and the indices k and l represent the integer shifts (as in the 1D case) in u and v directions respectively. We collect the coefficients of the inner product of the basis and the function $\mathbf{d}(u, v)$, i.e., δ_{jkl}^{LH}, δ_{jkl}^{HL}, and δ_{jkl}^{HH} into a vector q_d as illustrated in Figure 4. This displacement vector $\mathbf{q}_d$ contains a complete hierarchical description of the membrane surface. Note that $\mathbf{q}_d$ *has the same number of elements as the original nodal discretization at $j = 0$.* For our WT implementation we adopted the specific $\phi(u)$ and $\psi(u)$ functions as given by Mallat [1989], which are based on the cubic spline interpolants. If we denote the original nodal discretization at resolution $j = 0$ by a vector $\boldsymbol{\alpha}_0$, then we have,

$$
\left.
\begin{aligned}
\boldsymbol{\alpha}_0 &= S\mathbf{q}_d \quad \text{Reconstruction} \\
\mathbf{q}_d &= S^T\boldsymbol{\alpha}_0 \quad \text{Decomposition} \\
\mathbf{d}(u, v) &= \Phi(u, v)\boldsymbol{\alpha}_0 \quad \text{Interpolation}
\end{aligned}
\right\}
\tag{12}
$$

where Φ represents a vector of interpolation functions (as in the 1D case; see Eq. 7), and multiplication by the *orthogonal* matrix S corresponds to performing the WT. A fast implementation of the WT is achieved using Quadrature Mirror Filters (QMFs). A self-explanatory block diagram of the filter-bank interpretation of the QMF is presented in Figure 5 (see Mallat [1989] for details). Figure 5 shows an efficient way to implement the WT, with a computational cost of $O(N)$ (where N is the number of grid nodes).

Finally, vector $\mathbf{q}_d$ is expressed in an orthonormal wavelet basis. Along with other parameters of the model it is subjected to the iterative minimization process, as discussed subsequently.

2.3 From Global to Local Shapes with Wavelet Coefficients

In Figure 4, we explicitly depict the hierarchical decomposition of the displacement vector $\mathbf{q}_d$ in an orthonormal wavelet basis. The coefficients δ_j toward the upper left corner are fewer than those toward the bottom right corner, i.e., the corresponding grid nodes are spaced farther apart, and the

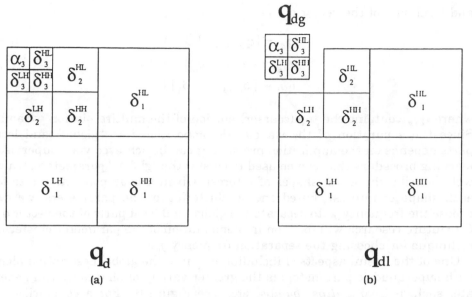

Fig. 4. (a) Organization of the displacement vector $\mathbf{q_d}$, (b) separation of the "global" and "local" parts of $\mathbf{q_d}$.

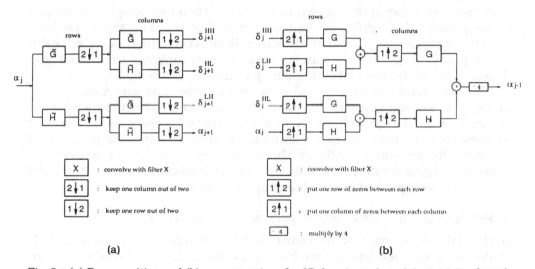

Fig. 5. (a) Decomposition and (b) reconstruction of a 2D function, adopted from Mallat [1989].

basis functions are coarser. Few parameters needed in the description and ability to depict the global shape give the low-frequency components of the wavelet representation a "semiglobal" character. Depending on the application, we can draw the boundary at an appropriate j_0 to separate the global

247

and local part of the vector $\mathbf{q}_d$, i.e.,

$$
\left.\begin{aligned}
\mathbf{q}_d &= [\mathbf{q}_{dg}, \mathbf{q}_{dl}] \\
\mathbf{q}_{dg} &= [\delta_n, \ldots, \delta_{j_0}] \\
\mathbf{q}_{dl} &= [\delta_{j_0-1}, \ldots, \delta_1]
\end{aligned}\right\} \tag{13}
$$

where $\mathbf{q}_{dg}$ contains the top (coarser) portion of the multiresolution pyramid. Since the separation of the wavelet decomposition into "global" and local parts depends on the application problem, it can be achieved via a supervised learning procedure that can be used to cluster the "global" parameters, which well describe the mean shapes of interest. Given a good population size for each shape of interest, based on the clustering of the parameters, we can choose the frequency j_0 to separate the global and local parts of the vector $\mathbf{q}_d$. Our future research will focus on implementation of the parameter-clustering technique for choosing the separation frequency j_0.

One of the useful aspects of including $\mathbf{q}_{dg}$ into the global description along with superquadric parameters is the greater variety of shapes we can generate, such as *coarse dips, bumps*, etc. (see Figure 6). For a comparison of possible global deformations generated via tweaking of superquadric parameters and the coarse-level wavelet coefficients of the displacement function, we illustrate the deformed shapes adjacent to one another. Figure 6(a) depicts the original reference shape; global deformation resulting from tweaking a superquadric parameter is shown in (b). The bottom four shapes (c) through (f) are generated via global deformations caused by tweaking the coarse-level wavelet coefficients. Note that tweaking these coarse-level wavelet coefficients produces global deformations that are *very different* from those produced by tweaking the global (lumped) parameters of the model.

When we build our prior model with mean values and covariances on $\mathbf{q}_s$ and $\mathbf{q}_{dg}$, the model assumes this enhanced shape as its new rest state, and it deforms away from this shape under the influence of sensed data. The need for incorporating more specific information such as this into the prior model is especially present in difficult shape recovery problems encountered in medical imaging applications, e.g., recovery of anatomical shapes from MR images. We will present two such examples in this article.

3. PROBABILISTIC FRAMEWORK AND MODEL MECHANICS

In the last section, we described our multiresolution deformable superquadric model in a wavelet basis. This basis provides a computationally efficient solution to the model-fitting problem and also provides us a way to enhance the library of shapes that can be described using a few global parameters. In this section, we will present a way to incorporate specific prior knowledge about the shape to be recovered from the data and then derive the mechanics of our modeling scheme.

We cast the model-fitting process in a probabilistic framework [Szeliski 1988] and incorporate prior distributions on the vector of geometric parameters that are being estimated. The combination of prior and sensor models

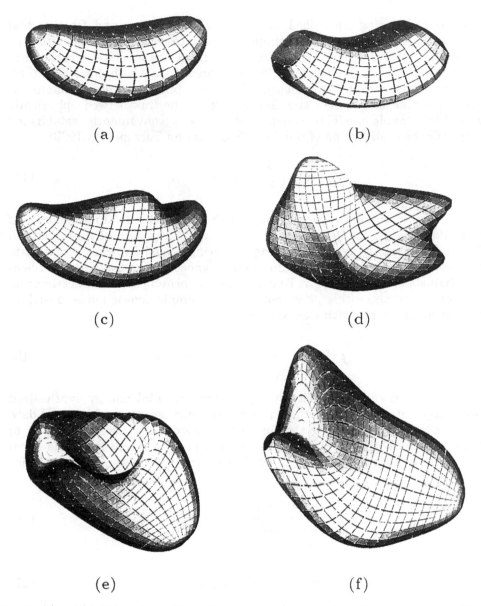

(a)

(b)

(c)

(d)

(e)

(f)

Fig. 6. (a) and (b) Global shape deformations generated via tweaking global parameters of the superquadric model; (c), (d), (e), and (f) global deformations generated by tweaking of coarse-scale wavelet coefficients.

results in a Bayesian model, since the posterior distribution of the parameters we are trying to estimate conditioned on the data can be computed using Baye's rule. In this article, we use the multiresolution physically based shape models described in earlier sections as the prior models. We collect the statistics on the global parameters of the model via a training process (*supervised learning*) described in a subsequent section, and for the local parameters we convert the continuous strain energy—which governs the deformation of the model away from its natural shape—into a probability distribution over expected shapes. This is achieved via a technique of statistical mechanics—conversion of energies into probabilities using Boltzmann, or Gibbs, distribution [Geman and Geman 1984]. The link between physically based (deformable models) models and priors is conveniently established using a Gibbs distribution of the form [Szeliski and Terzopoulos 1989]:

$$p(\mathbf{q}) = \frac{1}{Z_p} exp\left(-E_p(\mathbf{q})\right), \tag{14}$$

where $E_p(\mathbf{q})$ is the discretized version of the internal smoothness energy of the model, and Z_p (called the *partition function*) is a normalizing constant. What was originally an elastic energy restoring a model toward a rest state now becomes a probability distribution over expected shapes, with lower-energy shapes being more likely. To complete the formulation of the estimation problem, we combine this prior model with a simple sensor model based on linear measurements with Gaussian noise

$$p(\mathbf{D}/\mathbf{q}) = \frac{1}{Z_D} exp(-E_D(\mathbf{D}, \mathbf{q})), \tag{15}$$

where $E_D(\mathbf{D}, \mathbf{q})$ can be either an edge-based potential energy synthesized from image data or the potential energy in the springs attached from 3D data points to the surface of the deformable superquadric constraining it to conform to the observed data. Combining the prior and sensor models (from Eqs. 14 and 15 respectively) using Baye's rule, we obtain the posterior distribution

$$p(\mathbf{q}/\mathbf{D}) = \frac{p(\mathbf{D}/\mathbf{q})p(\mathbf{q})}{p(\mathbf{D})} = \frac{1}{Z} exp(-E(\mathbf{q})), \tag{16}$$

where

$$E(\mathbf{q}) = E_p(\mathbf{q}) + E_D(\mathbf{D}, \mathbf{q}). \tag{17}$$

Computing the *Maximum a Posteriori* (MAP) estimate, i.e., the value of $\mathbf{q}$ that maximizes the conditional probability $p(\mathbf{q}/\mathbf{D})$, provides the same result as finding the minimum energy configuration of the physically based model [Wahaba 1990]. However, the advantage of the probabilistic framework is that it allows for explicitly incorporating prior model and sensor model characteristics in addition to providing an uncertainty in the estimates.

The internal strain energy E_p of the model in our case is given by a quadratic form, $E_p = 1/2[(\mathbf{q} - \bar{\mathbf{q}})^T K_p(\mathbf{q} - \bar{\mathbf{q}})]$, where $\bar{\mathbf{q}}$ is the rest state of the model, and the matrix K_p corresponds to the stiffness of deformation. We will discuss the internal energy E_p further in a subsequent section. The two types of sensor model energies for $E_D(\mathbf{D}, \mathbf{q})$ discussed earlier are expressed as

$$
E_D(\mathbf{D}, \mathbf{q}) = \begin{cases} \frac{1}{2} \sum_i \beta(\mathbf{D}_i - \mathbf{x}(\mathbf{q}, \mathbf{u}_i))^2 & \text{spring energy} \\ \\ \int_\Omega \beta |P(\mathbf{x}(\mathbf{q}, \mathbf{u}))| & \text{image potential.} \end{cases} \tag{18}
$$

In the above equations $\mathbf{u}_i$ determines the closest point $\mathbf{x}$ to the given measured point $\mathbf{D}_i$. We adjust the locations of these grid coordinates as the shape of the model evolves (see Terzopoulos and Metaxas [1991] and Vemuri and Skofteland [1992] for more on migrating point of influence). The magnitude of parameter β is related to the uncertainty of sensor measurements. $P(\mathbf{x}(\mathbf{q}, \mathbf{u}))$ denotes an edge-based potential derived from the MR image data. Maximization of the a posteriori amounts to minimizing the total energy $E = E_p + E_D$ for which we employ a gradient descent method that amounts to iteratively solving,

$$
\mathbf{q}^{k+1} = \mathbf{q}^k - \Lambda \frac{\partial E(\mathbf{q})}{\partial \mathbf{q}} \tag{19}
$$

where Λ is a diagonal matrix containing step sizes and consequently effecting the speed of convergence. For the derivative of the energy on the right-hand side in the above equation, we use the chain rule to get $\partial E / \partial \mathbf{q} = (\partial E / \partial \mathbf{x})(\partial \mathbf{x} / \partial \mathbf{q})$ where the contribution of each parameter group—using the notation in Terzopoulos and Metaxas— is

$$
\frac{\partial \mathbf{x}}{\partial \mathbf{q}} = \left[\frac{\partial \mathbf{c}}{\partial \mathbf{q}_c}, \frac{\partial (\mathbf{R}\mathbf{p})}{\partial \mathbf{q}_\theta}, \frac{\mathbf{R} \partial_S}{\partial \mathbf{q}_s}, \frac{\mathbf{R} \partial (\Phi \mathbf{S} \mathbf{q}_d)}{\partial \mathbf{q}_d} \right] \tag{20}
$$

$$
= [\mathbf{I} \quad \mathbf{B} \quad \mathbf{RJ} \quad \Phi \mathbf{S}] \tag{21}
$$

$$
= \mathbf{L} \tag{22}
$$

Partial derivatives of the prior model and data energies defined above can be now written as

$$
\frac{\partial E_p}{\partial \mathbf{q}} = K_p(\mathbf{q} - \bar{\mathbf{q}}) \tag{23}
$$

and

$$
\frac{\partial E_D}{\partial \mathbf{q}} = \mathbf{f_q} = \begin{cases} -\sum_i \beta(\mathbf{D}_i - \mathbf{x}(\mathbf{q}, \mathbf{u}_i))\mathbf{L} & \text{spring energy} \\ \\ \int_\Omega \beta \nabla |P(\mathbf{x}(\mathbf{q}, \mathbf{u}))|\mathbf{L} & \text{image potential.} \end{cases} \tag{24}
$$

By substituting Eqs. 23 and 24 into the equation for gradient descent (19), we obtain an expression for iterative updating of the state vector $\mathbf{q}$

$$
\mathbf{q}^{(k+1)} = \mathbf{q}^{(k)} + \Lambda \left(\mathbf{f}_q^{(k)} - K(\mathbf{q}^{(k)} - \bar{\mathbf{q}}) \right). \tag{25}
$$

251

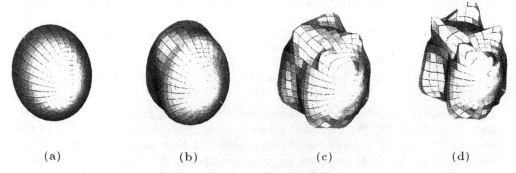

Fig. 7. Evolution of a deformable superquadric, (a) initialization; (b), (c), and (d) configurations of the model after 10, 20, 40, iterations, respectively.

Close similarity of this evolution equation to the one derived in Terzopoulos and Metaxas [1991] reveals that Eq. (25) can be modified slightly and effectively used to generate motion sequences corresponding to first-order dynamics $C\dot{\mathbf{q}} + K(\mathbf{q} - \bar{\mathbf{q}}) = \mathbf{f}_q$ (see Figure 7). The damping matrix C determines the velocity-dependent dissipation of the kinetic energy which governs the exponentially decaying motion of the model toward the equilibrium state. For simplicity, the equations can be decoupled by assuming the C matrix to be diagonal and constant over time. In addition to producing the statistically most likely state $\hat{\mathbf{q}}$, the Bayesian framework provides the uncertainty in the estimate via the associated covariance matrices.

While the above iterative equation will eventually converge to the correct estimate, in practice it may be unacceptably slow. To accelerate convergence we use coarse-to-fine search on a multiresolution pyramid corresponding to the wavelet basis. The problem is first solved on a coarser mesh; then this solution serves as a starting point for the next finer mesh. Figure 8 shows the evolution of the model at three successive resolutions. This was achieved by incorporating wavelet coefficients of increasingly finer levels in Eq. (25). Besides improving computational efficiency, this framework leads to significant smoothing of the energy potential at coarser resolutions, which consequently reduces the problem of entrapment in local minima.

4. PRIOR MODEL IN WAVELET BASIS

In the previous section we describe a probabilistic framework for embedding our model. We now derive the explicit form of the internal energy of the model in the wavelet basis. This energy is then converted to a Gibbsian probability distribution using the technique discussed earlier.

4.1 Internal Energy of the Prior Model

In addition to generic smoothness assumptions, a prior model should incorporate the information about the possible shapes that an observed object can

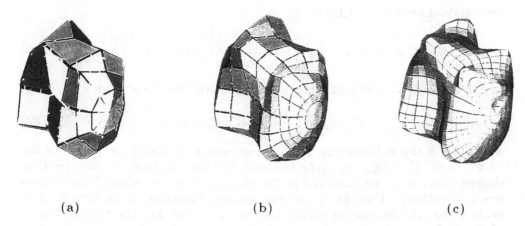

(a)   (b)   (c)

Fig. 8.   Coarse to fine model fitting; from (a) through (c) resolution of the membrane increases.

assume. This can be very important in applications involving recovery of known natural shapes from "unfriendly" (low contrast and noisy) images. We express the probability of a given configuration $\mathbf{q}$ through a Gibbs distribution (see Section 3), which assigns a low probability to configurations with large energy E_i and vice versa. The configuration with $E_i = 0$ represents the *rest state* of the model. The internal energy of the membrane spline (which augments the reference superquadric shape $\mathbf{s}$ of the model), in the continuous form, is given by (see Terzopoulos and Metaxas [1991]):

$$E_i = \int w_0 \mathbf{d}^2 + w_1 \left(\left(\frac{\partial \mathbf{d}}{\partial u} \right)^2 + \left(\frac{\partial \mathbf{d}}{\partial v} \right)^2 \right) d\mathbf{u}, \qquad (26)$$

where the functions $\omega_0(\mathbf{u})$ and $\omega_1(\mathbf{u})$ control the local magnitude and variation of the deformation respectively. In this article, we will assume these functions to be known scalar parameters.

With no additional prior information about the shapes being modeled, the underlying global shape of the model, namely, the superquadric, can be interpreted as the mean value or the rest state of the membrane surface—expressed by the displacement function $\mathbf{d}$. If we rewrite the deformation energy in terms of vector $\mathbf{p} = \mathbf{s} + \mathbf{d}$ we have an equivalent expression to (26),

$$E_i = \int w_0 (\mathbf{p} - \mathbf{s})^2 + w_1 \left(\left(\frac{\partial (\mathbf{p} - \mathbf{s})}{\partial u} \right)^2 + \left(\frac{\partial (\mathbf{p} - \mathbf{s})}{\partial v} \right)^2 \right) d\mathbf{u}, \qquad (27)$$

where the role of the global (reference) shape $\mathbf{s}$ as the rest state becomes apparent. We extend our underlying global shape $\mathbf{s}$ with a low-resolution mean displacement function $\overline{\mathbf{d}} = \hat{\mathbf{d}}^{j_0}$ corresponding to parameters $\mathbf{q_{dg}}$ as defined in Eq. (13) and shown in Figure 4. This is done by altering the

253

deformation energy Eq. (26) to

$$E_i = \int w_0(\mathbf{d} - \overline{\mathbf{d}})^2 + w_1\left(\left(\frac{\partial(\mathbf{d} - \overline{\mathbf{d}})}{\partial u}\right)^2 + \left(\frac{\partial(\mathbf{d} - \overline{\mathbf{d}})}{\partial v}\right)^2\right) d\mathbf{u}. \qquad (28)$$

The discrete version of this internal strain energy can be written as

$$E_i = \frac{1}{2}(\mathbf{q}_d - \overline{\mathbf{q}}_d)^T K_d(\mathbf{q}_d - \overline{\mathbf{q}}_d), \qquad (29)$$

where K_d is the stiffness matrix that determines the elastic properties of the model, and $\overline{\mathbf{q}}_d^T = [\overline{\mathbf{q}}_{dg}, 0, \ldots, 0]$ incorporates the statistics of the possible shapes that can be encountered in the shape recovery problem. These statistics are gathered through a training process described in Section 5. It is evident that the number of parameters in $\overline{\mathbf{q}}_{dg}$ is low, i.e., the representation of the model remains compact and thus making the training process feasible. We include other global shape parameters of the model in our prior statistics by extending the above energy as follows

$$E_i = \frac{1}{2}(\mathbf{q}_{\tilde{s}} - \overline{\mathbf{q}}_{\tilde{s}})^T C_{\tilde{s}}^{-1}(\mathbf{q}_{\tilde{s}} - \overline{\mathbf{q}}_{\tilde{s}})$$

$$+ \frac{1}{2}(\mathbf{q}_b - \overline{\mathbf{q}}_b)^T C_b^{-1}(\mathbf{q}_b - \overline{\mathbf{q}}_b)$$

$$+ \frac{1}{2}(\mathbf{q}_d - \overline{\mathbf{q}}_d)^T K_d(\mathbf{q}_d - \overline{\mathbf{q}}_d) \qquad (30)$$

where $\tilde{s}$ denotes the superquadric shape without the bending, while C represent the covariance matrices which are accumulated in the iterative training phase. In Section 4.2, we give the derivation for the stiffness matrix K in the wavelet basis and comment on its structure.

4.2 The Stiffness Matrix in Wavelet Basis

The stiffness matrix for the membrane operator is a very large, sparse, and banded matrix in the ordinary nodal basis. By expressing this in an orthonormal wavelet basis, we can achieve near diagonalization of this matrix. We will shown how the filter bank interpretation of WT (see Figure 3) relates directly to the diagonal entries of the stiffness matrix K. This approach in turn gives us a straightforward and *inexpensive* way to compute K.

The standard way to obtain stiffness matrix in wavelet basis is essentially a similarity transformation. By combining Eqs. (12), (28), and (29), and for simplicity depicting the 1D case, we get

$$K_d^0 = w_0 S^T\left(\int \Phi\Phi^T \, du\right)S \qquad (31)$$

$$K_d^1 = w_1 S^T\left(\int \left(\frac{\partial \Phi}{\partial u} \frac{\partial \Phi^T}{\partial u}\right) du\right)S \qquad (32)$$

$$K = K_d^0 + K_d^1. \qquad (33)$$

Here K_d^0 controls the local magnitude and K_d^1 the local variation of the (membrane) displacement function. Due to orthogonality of the interpolation functions in Φ and orthogonality of S, Eq. (31) simplifies to $K_d^0 = w_0 I$. However, the part K_d^1 of the stiffness matrix in Eq. (33) needs to be computed by a similarity transformation $K_d^1 = S^T \hat{K}_d^1 S$, where $\hat{K}_d^1$ represents the membrane stiffness matrix in nodal basis (see Pentland [1992]). The drawback of computing K_d^1 using this similarity transformation is the large computational cost incurred ($O(N^3)$, where N is the number of nodal variables), which can be avoided by using the property that differential operators in wavelet basis remain sparse (see Alpert [1992]) and have strong diagonal dominance (see Pentland [1992]). This allows us to compute the diagonal elements of the stiffness matrix directly by taking inner products of the corresponding finite-element basis function (an $O(N)$ computational cost)

$$(K_d^1)_{jk} = w_1 \int_{-\infty}^{\infty} |j\omega|^2 |\Psi_{jk}(\omega)|^2 \, d\omega, \tag{34}$$

which is done in frequency domain by employing Parseval's theorem [Bracewell 1978]. Extension to the 2D case is straightforward and achieved by using the tensor product of the basis functions. The factor $j\omega$ in (34) results from the Fourier transform of the first derivatives representing the membrane regularizer. Note that both K_d^0 and K_d^1 have diagonal structure and that only the relative magnitude of their diagonal entries determines the smoothing effects of each matrix. The filter bank interpretation of WT (Figure 3) explains how coefficients corresponding to lower resolutions j contribute less energy than those corresponding to higher resolutions. Figure 9 illustrates two aspects of the modeling: (a) the membrane displacement function which has a spectral density characterized by ω^{-2} and is a *fractal* process of $\beta = 2$ can be used to modulate the ideal bandpass characteristics of the wavelet basis for creating the appropriate stiffness matrix. Additionally, one can synthesize fractals of arbitrary order (β) by using a function $\omega^{-\beta}$ to modulate the bandpass characteristic of the wavelet basis for creation of the appropriate stiffness matrix; (b) the concept of increasing energy contributions with increasing resolution via a 1D example. For instance, if we assume an ideal bandpass characteristic for $\Psi_j(\omega)$ between ω_j and $2\omega_j$ we would have the following relationship between elements of K^1 at j and $(j + 1)$ resolutions.

$$(K_d^1)_{jk} = w_1 \int_{\omega_j}^{2\omega_j} |j\omega|^2 \, d\omega = 8(K_d^1)_{j+1)k}. \tag{35}$$

Therefore, for the membrane regularizer, we notice that the energy at a resolution j is eight times that at the next lower resolution ($j + 1$).

For a verification of the above discussed scaling behavior, we computed the diagonal entries of the K_d^1 matrix for a (32×32) grid of nodes using a similarity transformation technique discussed earlier. Figure 10 depicts the diagonal entries as an elevation map, where the elevation corresponds to the magnitude of the entries. The entries are organized as in a standard repre-

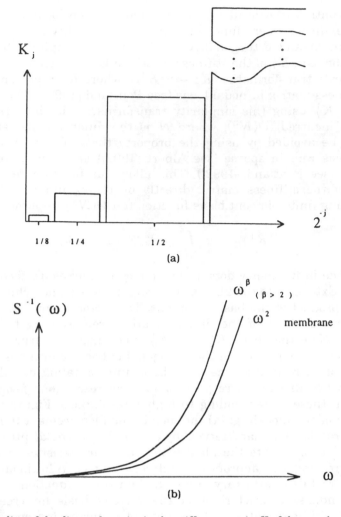

Fig. 9. (a) Scaling of the diagonal entries in the stiffness matrix K of the membrane model with spectral density, ω^{-2}, and an arbitrary density $\omega^{-\beta}$; (b) increasing energy with increasing resolution.

sentation of images in wavelet basis (see Figure 4 for the standard organization).

4.3 Prior Model of General Fractal Degree

Splines and stochastic fractals are complementary techniques for modeling free-form shapes [Szeliski and Terzopoulos 1989]. Splines are well suited for modeling smooth man-made objects and are easily controlled. Fractals on the other hand are well suited for modeling irregular shapes and are difficult to constrain. There is abundant literature on fractal generation algorithms, and we refer the reader to Barnsley [1988], Fournier et al. [1982], and Voss [1985]. However, these algorithms do not describe techniques to constrain

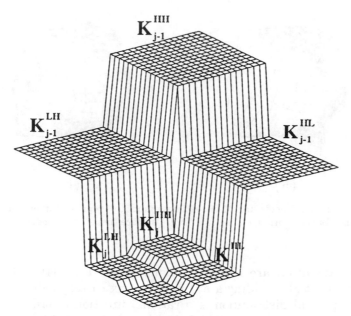

Fig. 10. Diagonal entries of K as an elevation map, for a (32×32) grid computed via a similarity transformation.

fractals. Szeliski and Terzopoulos describe a novel technique for constraining fractals by establishing a formal connection between splines and fractals using Fourier analysis of energy-minimizing splines.

Our prior model corresponding to the membrane spline is a Markov random field with a Gibbsian distribution. Its spectrum can be determined using Fourier analysis techniques [Szeliski and Terzopoulos 1989]. In their work on constrained fractals Szeliski and Terzopoulos show how prior models corresponding to a membrane and thin-plate regularizers possess a spectral density proportional to ω^{-2} and ω^{-4} respectively, which are fractal, i.e., they are self-affine over scale. These spectra characterize special cases of fractals of general form possessing a density given by

$$S(\omega) \propto \frac{1}{\omega^{\beta}}. \tag{36}$$

The spectral density of a stochastic fractal obeys the inverse power law in Eq. (36) and characterizes a fractal Brownian function with $2H = \beta - E$, whose fractal dimension is $D = E + 1 - H$ [Voss 1985]. Here, E denotes the dimension of the Euclidean space.

In Szeliski and Terzopoulos [1989] fractals of an in-between β, namely, $2 \leq \beta \leq 4$ were approximated by blending the membrane and thin-plate terms. *In contrast*, our multiresolution wavelet-based modeling scheme discussed earlier allows us to construct fractals of any β directly by utilizing the natural scale space characteristics of wavelet basis. Elements of K governing

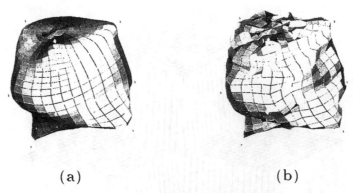

(a)   (b)

Fig. 11. Model-fitting result (a) MAP estimate and (b) representative sample from the a posteriori distribution, corresponding to a fractal surface (membrane model).

the prior distribution are computed using either Eq. (34) or (35) with ω^2 replaced by ω^β, thus yielding a stiffness matrix corresponding to a regularizer whose spectral distribution is a rational function of order β. A random sample from the corresponding Gibbsian distribution of this prior model will be a fractal surface of order β.

Figure 11 shows a surface-fitting result to 3D point data set with (a) MAP estimate and (b) representative sample from the Gibbs distribution $p(\mathbf{q}|\mathbf{D})$ depicting the underlying fractal prior. For the purpose of visually comparing surfaces of various fractal orders β, we choose to normalize the cumulative energy contributed by stiffness matrix K. Normalization was achieved by setting the Frobenious norm of K to be constant for various β. As a result, the only factor governing the behavior of fractal surfaces in Figures 12 is the relative distribution of energy along the frequency axis according to curve $\omega^{-\beta}$. As expected, a higher value of β emphasizes low-frequency content and deemphasizes higher frequencies. These surfaces were obtained by taking a representative sample from the associated Gibbsian distributions that describe the surface probabilistically. The explicit evaluation of the Gibbs distribution is very difficult due to the large computational requirements (summation over all possible states) in evaluating the partition function $\mathbf{Z}$. As in Szeliski and Terzopoulos [1989] this difficult computation can be circumvented by generating random samples from the Gibbs distribution using a simple technique called the Gibbs Sampler [Geman and Geman 1984]. In the Gibbs Sampler technique, at each iteration, a new random state is selected from the Gibbs distribution associated with the local energy function of the variable being updated. The convergence of this updating scheme to a random sample from the overall distribution is guaranteed. However, the rate of convergence may be very slow. We employ the multiresolution wavelet-based pyramid to accelerate the convergence by using the results at a coarse level as the starting point of the relaxation for a finer level.

The implementation of the coarse-to-fine relaxation in a wavelet basis is quite different from that discussed by Szeliski and Terzopoulos [1989].

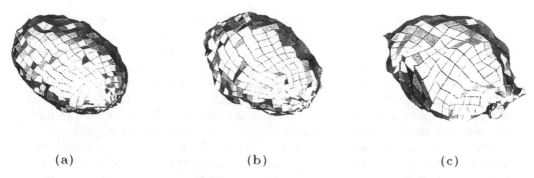

(a)   (b)   (c)

Fig. 12. Fractal surfaces of varying order β; (a), (b), and (c)—$\beta = 1.5,:2.0, 2.5$, respectively.

Specifically, after transformation of the nodal basis to the wavelet basis, the solution is obtained at a coarse resolution; to this solution, we add fine detail (detail function) and then recompute the new solution and so on. White noise is added to the surface at each iteration in a given level. The retransformation to nodal basis is done only after the entire solution is obtained at the finest level in the wavelet basis. Strictly speaking, if the model stiffness is perfectly diagonal, then the multiresolution solution can be obtained directly in one step. In our model, the stiffness matrix (inverse covariance) is for all practical purposes diagonal, and therefore, neglecting the near-zero off-diagonal terms, the white noise was added to the final solution surface to produce a representative sample (fractal surface) from the corresponding Gibbs distribution.

Fractal surfaces are very useful for modeling natural detail. In our application of medical imaging, our goal is to create realistic shape models of the anatomical structures found in the human body, specifically the brain. Future experiments will focus on achieving this goal.

5. SUPERVISED LEARNING AND MODEL-FITTING RESULTS

From an application point of view, our goal is *to apply the new multiresolution shape-modeling scheme* described in previous sections for recovering the 3D shape of cortical and subcortical structures such as the gyrus and hippocampus, from brain MRI data. The shapes will be accurately quantified by a parameter vector that can be used in computing shape measures such as volume. Volumetric analysis of structures contributes to understanding of various neurological disorders such as dyslexia, specific language impairment, etc. [Leonard et al. 1992]. Nontrivial shapes, low-contrast images, and high noise levels in this application domain prompted us to take advantage of our statistical modeling scheme by incorporating object-specific information into our prior model. To facilitate construction of such specialized prior models we divide the shape recovery process into a training phase and an operational phase. In the training phase human supervision via interaction and manipulation is needed to provide good training samples, while in the operational phase the model-fitting process becomes fully autonomous and relies heavily on statistics accumulated in the prior model.

Shape recovery from poor-quality data can be formidable. Any approach that does not make use of prior knowledge of the shape of interest is doomed to fail due to the underconstrained nature of the problem. Imperfect data can be augmented with a priori information that a model of the structure of interest provides. For example, when dealing with specific anatomical shapes, one can use models of these shapes to guide the recovery algorithms. In the earlier sections, we have described a new modeling scheme that captures global as well as semiglobal shape using a *small set of parameters*. This key attractive feature of the modeling scheme makes it conducive to perform statistical data collection on global model parameters which are then used (in combination with the Gibbsian probability distribution of the local part of the model) as prior information in the model-fitting process.

As discussed in Section 3, Bayesian modeling requires knowledge of the a priori probability $p(\mathbf{q})$ of the model $\mathbf{q}$ and the probability of $\mathbf{q}$ conditioned on the sensed data, i.e., $p(\mathbf{q}|\mathbf{D})$. Unfortunately, in surface-modeling applications we rarely if ever have this kind of complete knowledge about the probabilistic structure of the problem. Typically, we have a number of representative samples of what we want to model. In an approach known as *Bayesian learning* [Duda and Hart 1973], these samples are used to estimate the unknown probabilities which in turn are used as if they were the true values. It is important to distinguish between *supervised learning* and *unsupervised learning*. The distinction being, in supervised learning we know the class (label) of each sample in advance, whereas in unsupervised learning the natural clustering of samples is used to define the classes. In our work, prior knowledge about the object shapes that are to be recovered from the MRI data is collected via a supervised learning technique. A training sequence of several iterations provides samples of correctly reconstructed shapes for specific classes of objects—in our experiments a *gyrus* and the *hippocampus* from the human brain. Parameter sets $\mathbf{q}(i)$ corresponding to these shapes represent the training sequence for the global part $(\mathbf{q}_s + \mathbf{q}_{dg})$ of our prior model (see Figure 13). With each iteration i we improve estimates of the mean vector $\overline{\mathbf{q}}$ and covariance matrix C through a simple equation for accumulating measurements as indicated in the Figure 13. Since we update only the statistics of the global parameters of the model, the local deformations remain constrained only by smoothness assumptions captured in the stiffness matrix K (refer to Eq. (30)). Therefore, most of the flexibility of the locally deformable surface remains unchanged. We recommend human visual supervision of the model fitting in the training stage to assure that only good model-fitting results enter the statistics of the prior model. An extension to multiclass case is straightforward and can be achieved by defining multiple prior distributions $p_j(\mathbf{q})$ for each class j.

This method clearly demonstrates the useful aspect of global models which offer a compact description of the overall features of the object. Deformable superquadrics with the global shape extended by some offset deformation (as presented in previous sections) allow a much wider range of shapes to be

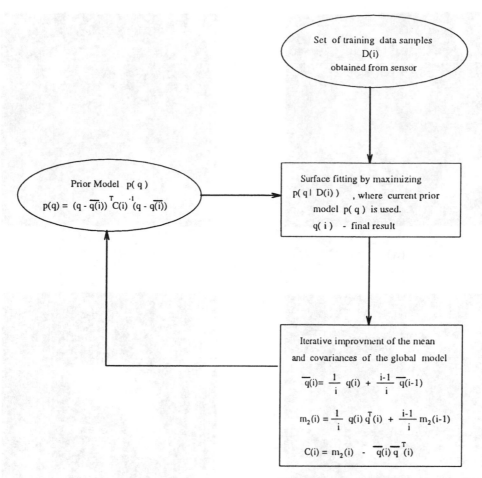

Fig. 13. Supervised learning to incorporate information into the prior model.

representable in the prior model, all at the expense of few additional parameters. This makes our model very attractive for shape recognition as well as shape reconstruction tasks.

We now present two examples depicting the model-fitting process to a gyrus and a hippocampus shape, given MRI data of a human brain. The data set consisted of 64 slices, with each slice of 1.25mm thickness. Figure 14 illustrates our results for a **gyrus**. From left to right and top to bottom, the displayed images are : (a) a sagittal section of the brain showing a region of interest (containing a gyrus) indicated in a box, (b) a slice of the initialized 3D shape model superimposed on the corresponding slice from the original data, (c) superimposition of a slice from the final recovered shape on a corresponding slice from the original data, and (d) the 3D recovered shape. The initialization shown here has incorporated statistical information (mean and variance) of the gyrus from a small sample data set. The initialized model was subject to externally applied forces synthesized from a 3D edge-based

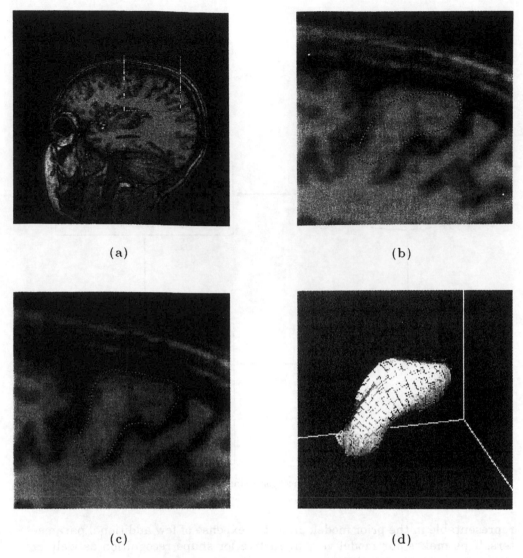

(a)

(b)

(c)

(d)

Fig. 14. 3D shape recovery results for a gyrus.

potential obtained by computing edges in 3D using the recursive filtering discussed by Monga and Deriche [1989]. Figure 15 depicts the reconstruction results for a *hippocampus*, arranged left to right, top to bottom in sequence. Figure 15(a) is a slice of the raw MRI data showing the region of interest (ROI); (b) is a slice from the 3D model initialization superimposed on the ROI; (c) depicts a slice from the model initialization superimposed on the edge-based potential field computed using the recursive-filtering method in Monga and Deriche; (d) is a slice from the recovered 3D shape superimposed on the ROI; and (e) depicts the recovered 3D shape of the hippocampus.

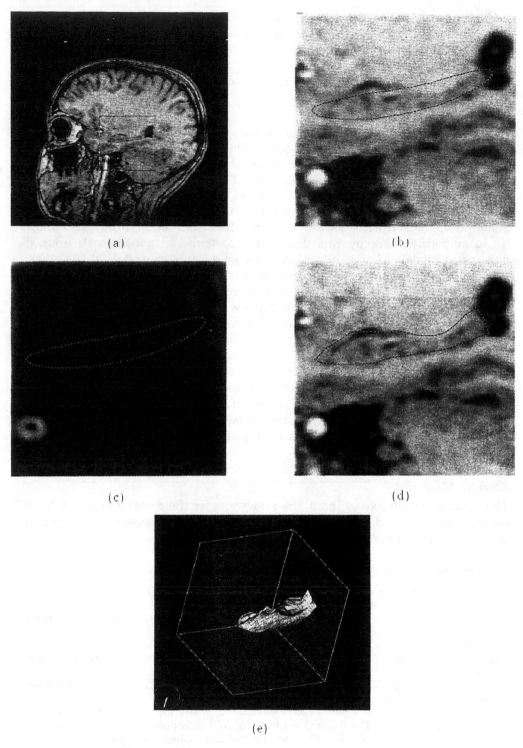

Fig. 15.   3D shape recovery results for a hippocampus.

Further experimentation with our modeling scheme is currently under way, and we expect to better our results by using (a) larger data sets for collecting the statistics, (b) better 3D edge-finding methods, and (c) adaptive clustering for automatically choosing the cut-off frequency j_0 in separating the global and local parameters of the model.

6. CONCLUSION

In this article, we introduced a *new shape-modeling scheme* that can *transform smoothly from local* to *global* models or vice versa. The modeling scheme utilizes a hybrid primitive called the deformable superquadric *constructed in an orthonormal wavelet basis*. These bases provide the power to continuously transform from local to global shape deformations and thereby allow for a continuum of shape models—from those with local to those with global shape descriptive power—to be created. Additionally, they also allow us to smoothly scale up and down the spectrum of models with lumped parameter models at one end and distributed parameter models at the other. The multiresolution wavelet basis allows us to generate fractal surfaces of arbitrary order, which can be useful in describing natural detail.

When embedded in a probabilistic framework, our modeling scheme allows us to incorporate more detailed prior information than when using lumped parameter models, while keeping the number of parameters required to describe the shape low. The same level of detail may also be incorporated by using some existing modeling techniques [Staib and Duncan 1991; Terzopoulos and Metaxas 1991] but, at the expense of increasing the number of parameters tremendously. From a computational point of view, our modeling scheme is very *attractive* for segmentation purposes since multiresolution relaxation is a natural by-product of implementing the gradient relaxation method in the wavelet basis.

ACKNOWLEDGMENTS

The authors would like to thank the reviewers, for their useful and insightful comments, and Mr. S. H. Lai, for the fruitful technical discussions and help in preparing the figures in LATEX.

REFERENCES

ALPERT, B. K. 1992. Wavelets and other bases for fast numerical linear algebra. In *Wavelets—A Tutorial in Theory and Applications*, C. K. Chui, Ed., Academic Press, New York, 181–216.

BAJSCY, R. AND SOLINA, R. 1987. Three-dimensional object representation revisited. In *IEEE First Conference on Computer Vision*. IEEE, New York, 231–240.

BARNSLEY, M. 1988. *Fractals Everywhere*. Academic Press, New York.

BARR, A. H. 1981. Superquadrics and angle-preserving transformations. *IEEE Comput. Graph. Appl. 18*, 1 (Jan.), 21–30.

BINFORD, T. O. 1971. Visual perception by computer. In the *IEEE Systems and Control Conference*. IEEE, New York.

BLAKE, A. AND ZISSERMAN, A. 1987. *Visual Reconstruction*, MIT Press, Cambridge, Mass.

BRACEWELL, R. N. 1978. *The Fourier Transform and Its Applications*. McGraw-Hill, New York.

BURT, P. J. AND ADELSON, E. H. 1983. A multiresolution spline with application to image mosaics. *ACM Trans. Graph. 2*, 4, 217–236.

CELINKER, G. AND GOSSARD, D. 1991. Deformable curve and surface finite-elements for free-form shape design. *Comput. Graph. 25*, 4, 257–266.

COHEN, L. D. AND COHEN, I. 1992. Deformable models for 3D medical images using finite elements and balloons. In the *IEEE Conference on Computer Vision and Pattern Recognition*. IEEE, New York.

DAHLQUIST, G. AND BJÖRCK, A. 1974. *Numerical Methods.* Prentice-Hall, Englewood Cliffs, N.J.

DAUBECHIES, I.. 1988. Orthonormal bases of compactly supported wavelets. *Commun. Pure Appl. Math. 41*, 909–996.

DELINGETTE, H., HEBERT, M., AND IKEUCHI, K. 1991. Shape representation and image segmentation using deformable surfaces. In the *IEEE Conference on Computer Vision and Pattern Recognition*. IEEE, New York, 467–472.

DUDA, R. O. AND HART, P. E. 1973. *Pattern Classification and Scene Analysis.* Wiley, New York.

FOURNIER, A., FUSSEL, D., AND CARPENTER, L. 1982. Computer rendering of stochastic models. *Commun. ACM. 25*, 6, 371–384.

GEMAN, S. AND GEMAN, D. 1984. Stochastic relaxation, Gibbs distribution, and Bayesian restoration of images. *IEEE Trans. Patt. Anal. Mach. Intell. 6*, 6, 721–724.

LEONARD, C. M., WILLIAMS, C. A., NICHOLLS, R. D., AND AGEE, O. F. 1992. Angelman and Prader-Willi syndrome: A magnetic resonance imaging study of differences in cerebral structure. *Am. J. Med. Genet. 46*, 26–33.

MALLAT, S. G. 1989. A theory of multi-resolution signal decomposition: The wavelet representation. *IEEE Trans. Patt. Anal. Mach. Intell. 11*, 7, 674–693.

MONGA, A. AND DERICHE, R. 1989. 3D edge detection using recursive filtering: Application to scanner images. In *Proceedings of the IEEE Conference on Computer Vision and Pattern Recognition*. IEEE, New York, 28–35.

PENTLAND, A. P. 1992. Fast solutions to physical equilibrium and interpolation problems. In *Visual Computer*. Vol. 8. Springer-Verlag, New York, 303–314.

PENTLAND, A. P. 1986. Parts: Structured descriptions of shape. In *Proceedings of AAAI*. AAAI, Menlo Park, Calif., 695–701.

RIOUL, O. AND VETTERLI, M. 1991. Wavelets and signal processing. *IEEE SP Mag. 8* (Oct.) 14–38.

SCLAROFF, S. AND PENTLAND, A. 1991. Generalized implicit functions for computer graphics. *Comput. Graph. 25*, 4, 247–250.

STAIB, L. H. AND DUNCAN, J. S. 1991. Boundary finding with parametrically deformable contour models. *IEEE Trans. Patt. Anal. Mach. Intell. 14*, 11, 1061–1075.

SZELISKI, R. 1988. Bayesian modeling of uncertainty in low-level vision. Ph.D. thesis, Carnegie Mellon Univ., Pittsburgh, Pa.

SZELISKI, R. AND TERZOPOULOS, D. 1989. Constrained fractals. *Comput. Graph. 23*, 1, 51–60.

TERZOPOULOS, D. 1986a. Regularization of inverse visual problems involving discontinuities. *IEEE Trans. Patt. Anal. Mach. Intell. PAMI-8*, 413–424.

TERZOPOULOS, D. 1986b. Image analysis using multigrid relaxation methods. *IEEE Trans. Patt. Anal. Mach. Intell. PAMI-8*, 2, 129–139.

TERZOPOULOS, D. AND METAXAS, D. 1991. Dynamic 3D models with local and global deformations: Deformable superquadrics. *IEEE Trans. Patt. Anal. Mach. Intell. 13*, 7, 703–714.

TERZOPOULOS, D., WITKIN, A., AND KASS, M. 1988. Constraints on deformable models: Recovering 3D shape and nonrigid motion. *Artif. Intell. 36*, 91–123.

TERZOPOULOS, D., PLATT, J., BARR, A., AND FLEISCHER, K. 1987. Elastically deformable models. *Comput. Graph. 21*, 4, 205–214.

VEMURI, B. C. AND MALLADI, R. 1993. Constructing intrinsic parameters with active models for invariant surface reconstruction. *IEEE Trans. Patt. Anal. Mach. Intell. 15*, 7 (July), 668–681.

VEMURI, B. C. AND MALLADI, R. 1991. Deformable models: Canonical parameters for invariant surface representation and multiple-view integration. In *Proceedings of the IEEE Conference on Computer Vision and Pattern Recognition*. IEEE, New York.

VEMURI, B. C. AND RADISAVLJEVIC, A. 1993. From global to local, a continuum of shape models with fractal priors. In *Proceedings of the IEEE Conference on Computer Vision and Pattern Recognition (CVPR)*. IEEE, New York, 307–313.

VEMURI, B. C. AND SKOFTELAND, G. 1992. Invariant surface and motion estimation from sparse range data. *J. Math. Imaging and Vis. 1*, 1 (Mar.), 48–62.

VEMURI, B. C., MITICHE, A., AND AGGARWAL, J. K. 1986. Curvature-based representation of objects from range data. *Image Vis. Comput. 4*, 2 (May), 107–114.

VOSS, R. F. 1985. Random fractal forgeries. In *Fundamental Algorithms for Computer Graphics*, R. A. Earnshaw, Ed. Springer-Verlag, Berlin.

WAHABA, G. 1990. *Spline Models for Observational Data*. CBMS-NSF Regional Conference Series in Applied Mathematics, SIAM, Philadelphia, Pa.

WANG, Y. F. AND WANG, J. F. 1990. Surface reconstruction using deformable models with interior and boundary constraints. In *Proceedings of the IEEE Conference on Computer Vision*. IEEE, New York, 300–303.

YESERENTANT, H. 1986. On the multi-level splitting of finite element spaces. *Numerische Mathematik 49*, 379–412.

YUILLE, A. L., COHEN, D., AND HALLINAN, P. W. 1989. Feature extraction from faces using deformable templates. In the *IEEE Conference on Computer Vision*. IEEE, New York, 104–109.

EXTENDED BIBLIOGRAPHY

BARSKY, B. A. 1981. The Beta-spline: A local representation based on shape parameters and fundamental geometric measures. Ph.D. thesis, Univ. of Utah, Salt Lake City, Utah.

BESL, P. J. AND JAIN, R. 1985. Three-dimensional object recognition. *ACM Comput. Surv. 17*, 1, 75–145.

BOULT, T. E. AND KENDER, J. R. 1986. Visual surface reconstruction using sparse depth data. In *Proceedings of the IEEE Conference on Computer Vision and Pattern Recognition*. IEEE, New York, 68–76.

BOLLE, R. M. AND VEMURI, B. C. 1991. On surface reconstruction methods. *IEEE Trans. Patt. Anal. Mach. Intell. 13*, 1, 1–13.

HOPPE, H., DEROSE, T., DUCHAMP, T., MCDONALD, J., AND STUETZLE, W. 1992. Surface reconstruction for unorganized points. *Comput. Graph. 26*, 2 (July), 71–78.

MALLAT, S. G. AND HWANG, W. L. 1992. Singularity detection and processing with wavelets. *IEEE Trans. Inf. Theor. 38*, 2, 617–643.

MAYBECK, P. S. 1982. *Stochastic Models, Estimation, and Control*. Vol. 1, Academic Press, New York.

MILLER, J. V., BREEN, D. E., LORENSEN, W. E., O'BARA, R. M., AND WOZNY, M. J. 1991. Geometrically deformed models: A method for extracting closed geometric models from volume data. *Comput. Graph. 25*, 4, 217–226.

MURAKI, S. 1991. Volumetric description of range data using the Blobby Model. *Comput. Graph. 25*, 4, 227–235.

REQUICHA, A. A. G. 1980. Representations of rigid solid objects. *ACM Comput. Surv. 12*, 4 (Dec.), 437–464.

SZELISKI, R. AND TONNESEN, D. 1992. Surface modeling with oriented particle systems. *Comput. Graph. 26*, 2 (July), 185–194.

Received April 1993, Revised December 1993; accepted September 1993

SECTION III

Motion Analysis and Tracking

An Overview of Motion Analysis and Tracking Issues in Medical Image Analysis

Ajit Singh
Siemens Medical Systems
Iselin, New Jersey

Dmitry B. Goldgof
Department of Computer Science and Engineering
University of South Florida, Tampa, Florida

Demetri Terzopoulos
Department of Computer Science
University of Toronto, Toronto, Ontario

This section of the book deals with applications of deformable models to the problems of motion analysis and tracking. Motion analysis has been an important research area in computer vision applications for the past two decades. However, until recently most of the work was done with the assumption that all the objects involved have constant shapes throughout the time sequence. The rigidity assumption fails in numerous motion analysis situations, since many real-world objects are nonrigid. That is especially true for many biomedical applications.

The nonrigid motion analysis problem is difficult because it implies varying shape. A nonrigid object cannot be represented by a fixed set of parameters unless certain restrictions are placed on the object's behavior. Thus, we cannot have a general algorithm for determining motion parameters as we can for rigid motion. Consequently, we need a classification for nonrigid motion that can guide the choice of applicable approaches. Nonrigid objects can be separated into different types such as articulated objects, elastic objects, and fluids. Different methods for motion analysis may be suitable for each type. Narrowing the scope of nonrigid analysis problem to a particular type allows one to define specific "nonrigidity assumptions" which may be incorporated as computational constraints within nonrigid motion analysis algorithms. These "nonrigidity" constraints can be classified two ways: (1) general versus specific, and (2) local versus global.

The first classification refers to the amount of a priori knowledge that is incorporated into the motion analysis algorithm. General constraints will, for example, specify that the object of interest is elastic and that some degree of smoothness is maintained (both in space and time). Specific constraints, on the other hand, can go as far as to include known material properties into the motion analysis algorithm.

The second classification refers to the degree to which global shape models are utilized. It is important to realize that the questions of motion analysis and shape modeling become inseparable when we consider nonrigid motion. Local modeling schemes concentrate on local shape representations, which include differential geometric methods and physics-based finite-element techniques. Global modeling schemes include various parameterized models (which are often suitable for both rigid and nonrigid objects) such as spherical harmonics, global polynomial models, hyperquadrics, and so forth.

Deformable models are flexible enough to implement both general and specific constraint (depending on the amount of a priori information available). They are usually considered as local models. However, they can be combined with global modeling techniques. The past decade has brought both advances in theory needed to approach the problem of nonrigid motion analysis and advances in the state of the art of image acquisition technology providing two- and three-dimensional, time-varying, high-resolution data. This section of the book deals with these advances.

Chapter 19 gives a brief review of the recent work in nonrigid motion analysis. It starts with a classification of various approaches used in nonrigid motion analysis based on the assumptions made by each approach. It also presents the survey of the state of the art in nonrigid motion research with the goal of providing a guideline for matching existing approaches to a given application. In that, it presents various approaches and not only those using deformable models.

The following chapters deal with several specific approaches based on the idea of deformable models. Most of the applications are in the areas of cardiac imaging, possibly the most obvious application involving nonrigid motion, and, arguably, the technology area that enjoyed the fastest technological advances (both in 3D CT and cardiac MR). They deal with both 2D and 3D data with the goal of tracking cardiac boundary and reconstruction of local strain parameters.

Chapter 20 deals with multiresolution matching. Chapters 21 and 22 deal with 2D motion analysis. Specifically, Chapter 21 considers the problem of tracking 2D boundaries of the cardiac ultrasound images. It combines the idea of a deformable 2D model with analysis of the curvature of the boundary lines, and does pointwise tracking of the boundary of the mitral valve. Chapter 22 concentrates on MR SPAMM—a modality catching up very quickly among radiologists and cardiologists. It utilizes the snake model to track tagged grid lines and maintain correspondence between grid line intersections. Chapter 23 deals with 3D point correspondence recovery. Chapters 24 through 26 are devoted to cardiac motion understanding in 3D, using CT DSR, MR, and MR SPAMM modalities, respectively. Finally, Chapters 27 through 29 address several general issues pertaining to physically based analysis of non-rigid deformation. They use CT DSR images of the left ventricle, MR images of the head and the heart, and ultrasound images of the mitral valve to illustrate the issues.

Nonrigid Motion Analysis

Chandra Kambhamettu
Department of Computer and Information Sciences
University of Delaware
Newark, Delaware 19716

Dmitry B. Goldgof
Department of Computer Science and Engineering
University of South Florida
Tampa, Florida

Demetri Terzopoulos
Department of Computer Science
University of Toronto
Toronto, Canada

Thomas S. Huang
Department of Electrical and Computer Engineering
University of Illinois at Urbana-Champaign
Champaign, Illinois

1. Introduction

Motion analysis has been an important research area in computer vision for the past two decades. The motion analysis problem was defined traditionally as the problem of finding the motion of an object based on 2D or 3D images of it acquired at two or more time instances. The so-called structure from motion problem has an additional goal, which is to obtain the geometrical structure as well as the motion parameters from a sequence of projections. A large body of work has been done in this area because of its importance in dynamic scene understanding [1, 2], essentially under the assumption that all the objects involved have constant shapes throughout the time sequence. The rigidity assumption fails in numerous motion analysis situations as many real-world objects are nonrigid. For example, trees sway, a piece of paper bends, cloth wrinkles, and the living human body is in continuous nonrigid motion.

In recent years, a growing trend toward research in nonrigid motion analysis has become apparent. A significant impetus for this work derives from potential applications in areas such as medical imaging and model-based image compression. Numerous applications exist in the biomedical area, such as the study of heart and lung motion, blood flow, and analysis of tumor growth. One of the goals in cardiac imaging, for instance, is to analyze nonrigid motion and estimate the deformation characteristics of the heart. In this application, computed tomography (CT) or magnetic resonance imaging (MRI) scanners collect 3D density data of the heart at a series of time instants during the cardiac cycle. An analysis of the range of motion parameters can help screen patients and decide on the extent of cardiac injury. Another example is model-based image compression in high-speed teleconferencing. Once the motion parameters or point correspondences of a facial movement can be estimated, they can be encoded and transmitted. This reduces the information bandwidth significantly when compared to the traditional statistical approaches.

There are many more applications of nonrigid motion analysis. They include the study of lip motion for lip reading, human face recognition for security applications, material deformations for visual inspection of structures (such as dams, bridges, and crystal-growth inspection), and the tracking of cloud formations for weather prediction. Machine vision for robotics applications will also need to handle nonrigid shapes: articulated and bendable parts are found in industrial settings. Nonrigid objects are also clearly unavoidable for a robot operating in natural environments. Additionally, virtual reality applications require methods for the construction and simulation of both rigid and nonrigid object models.

The nonrigid motion analysis problem is difficult because nonrigid motion implies varying shape and possibly varying topological structure. A nonrigid object cannot be represented by a fixed set of parameters unless certain restrictions are placed on the object's behavior. Thus, we cannot have a general algorithm for determining motion parameters as we can have for rigid motion. Consequently, we need a classification for nonrigid motion that can guide the choice of applicable approaches. Nonrigid objects can be separated into different types such as articulated objects, elastic objects, and fluids. Different methods for motion analysis may be suitable for each type. Narrowing the scope of nonrigid analysis problem to a particular type allows one to define specific "nonrigidity assumptions" that may be incorporated as computational constraints within nonrigid motion analysis algorithms.

The past 5–10 years have seen significant progress in the analysis of nonrigid motion. In this chapter, we classify the different approaches in nonrigid motion analysis and indicate the assumptions and conditions that they utilize. Our goal in surveying the state of the art in nonrigid motion research is not to attempt an exhaustive review of the literature, but to provide some guidance in deciding the approaches most suitable to particular applications.

It is important to realize that the questions of motion analysis and shape modeling become inseparable when we consider nonrigid motion. Our review therefore includes some of the relevant work on shape modeling. The modeling perspective suggests one possible classification of nonrigid shape and motion research. Nonrigid shape models may be categorized into two main groups: local models and global models. Local modeling schemes concentrate on local shape representations, which include differential geometric methods and physics-based finite-element techniques. Global modeling schemes include various parameterized models (which are often suitable for both rigid and nonrigid objects) such as spherical harmonics, global polynomial models, hyperquadrics, and so on. The local/global classification is not the only one possible, and, in fact, recent research has yielded shape models with both global and local characteristics.

A coarse classification of nonrigid motion was first proposed by Huang [3]. He suggested three broad groups of objects: articulated, elastic, and fluid objects. We will follow this broad classification and supplement it with the curvature-based classification of elastic nonrigid motion suggested by Goldgof, Lee, and Huang [4]. This will yield

what we believe to be a natural classification ranging from near rigid objects to highly nonrigid objects. Our survey concentrates on the analysis of 3D objects at the expense of work related to 2D curve deformations and fluid motion.

Section 2 presents an overview of our nonrigid motion classification. Sections 3 and 4 survey the literature associated with each motion class. Section 5 discusses local and global shape models for nonrigid objects. Section 6 concludes the chapter with a summary.

2. Classification of Nonrigid Motion

This section proposes a classification of nonrigid motion. Figure 1 is a chart depicting the classification of nonrigid motion analysis algorithms, together with some of the references. A much larger set of references is mentioned in the text throughout this chapter and in the reference section. The motion of objects can generally be classified according to the degree of nonrigidity. We will consider primarily the motion of 3D objects, especially of their surfaces.

Rigid motion preserves the 3D distances between any two points in an object. The object does not stretch or bend; hence both mean curvature and Gaussian curvature on the surface of the object remains invariant.

Articulated motion is piecewise rigid motion. It involves motion of rigid parts connected by nonrigid joints. Examples are animal skeletons and robot manipulators. Clearly, the rigidity constraint is more relaxed in this case.

Quasi-rigid motion restricts the deformation to be small. A general nonrigid motion is quasi-rigid when viewed in a sufficiently short time interval, say between image frames when the sampling rate is high enough.

Isometric motion is nonrigid motion that preserves lengths along the surface as well as angles between curves on the surface.

Homothetic motion is a uniform expansion or contraction of a surface.

Conformal motion is nonrigid motion that preserves angles between curves on the surface, but not lengths of the curves.

Elastic motion is a nonrigid motion whose only constraint is some degree of continuity or smoothness. This kind of solid object motion is the most difficult to analyze.

Fluid motion is general nonrigid motion that need not be continuous. It may involve topological variations and turbulent deformation.

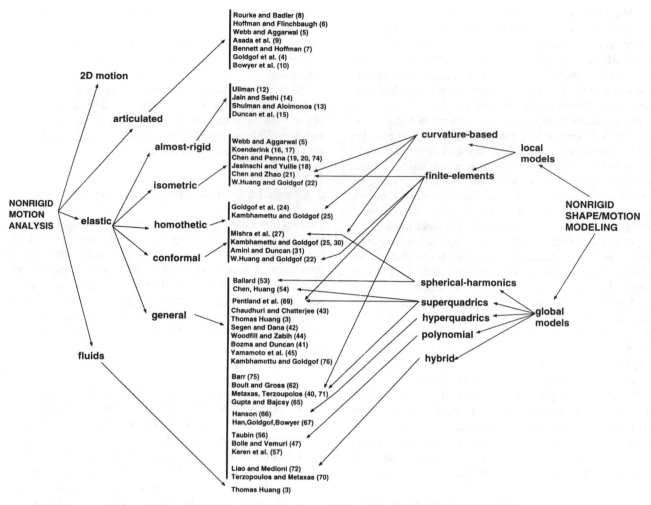

Figure 1. Classification of nonrigid motion analysis algorithms.

3. Restricted Classes of Nonrigid Motion

3.1 Articulated Motion

Articulated motion is piecewise rigid motion. It involves motion of rigid parts connected by nonrigid joints. Examples are animal skeletons and robot manipulatros. Clearly, the rigidity constraint is more relaxed in this case. An *articulated* object is a very restricted type of nonrigid object that is composed of rigid parts with connections between them that may allow defined ranges of movement. Arms, legs, scissors, and pliers are some simple examples of articulated objects. The relevance of articulated motion in robot movement is one of the reasons for its importance in motion analysis.

An object can be categorized as articulated by observing its behavior over some time period and comparing the image sequences with all the valid shapes that can be generated by an articulated model in the database. Another reliable approach is to consider all the image sequences of an object and integrate them depending on the articulation degrees of freedom at each point. Extensive research has been done in the modeling, recognition, and analysis of articulated motion. Webb and Aggarwal [5] considered the *fixed-axis assumption*; that is, that all movements consist of translations and rotations about an axis that is fixed in direction for short periods of time. Hoffman and Flinchbaugh [6] and Bennet and Hoffman [7] discuss the movement of linked rigid rods in one plane, and points in motion rotating about a fixed axis. O'Rourke and Badler [8] and Asada, Yachida, and Tsoji [9] also consider restricted motion of articulated objects. Goldgof, Lee, and Huang [4] use surface curvature to segment an articulated object into its rigid parts. The computation of aspect graphs for 3D articulated object recognition is proposed by Sallam and Bowyer [10]. The representation of articulated objects for purposes of machine vision is considered by Bruno, et al. [11]. Additionally, authors suggest function-based models which allow the generic recognition of all objects that are the members of the modeled category. For more details, see Chapter 2 of this book.

On the whole, there has been significant development in the research of articulated motion when compared to other kinds of nonrigid motion analysis. This is because once we break up the articulated body into its rigid parts, we can apply rigid motion analysis. We will now proceed to different approaches in nonrigid motion analysis, in increasing degrees of nonrigidity.

3.2 Quasi-Rigid Motion

Quasi-rigid motion restrics the degree of deformation. A general non-rigid motion is quasirigid when viewed in a sufficiently short time interval, say, between image frames when the sampling rate is sufficiently high.

Initial work in nonrigid motion was premised on the fact that a real-world object cannot change shape instantaneously due to inertia. When a translating, rotating, and deforming object is imaged at high temporal sampling rates, the nonrigid motion that occurs between image frames will be small.

Ullman [12] proposed an incremental rigidity scheme to recover the shape of an object from its motion, based on the human perception of nonrigid transformations. The scheme has an internal model of the viewed object, which it modifies at each instant by the minimal nonrigid change which suffices to account for the observed transformation; that is, at each instant the estimated 3D structure of the viewed object is updated over that of the previous model. It integrates information from an extended viewing period to improve the approximation of the current 3D structure. However, the success of the scheme depends on the reliability of its initial model of the 3D structure, as well as the availability of point correspondences between 2D frames, which itself is a hard task in nonrigid motion. On similar lines, Shulman and Aloimonous [13] used a regularization approach to find the smoothest motion consistent with image data and the known object structure. The assumption was that the parameters characterizing the motion are approximately constant in any sufficiently small region of the image.

The problem of point correspondences in nonrigid motion is addressed by Jain and Sethi [14]. They presented a method of establishing correspondences of nonrigid objects in a sequence of image frames using a motion smoothness constraint. Using path coherence, they formulate an optimization problem that assumes that the object cannot change its shape instantaneously. Their approach involves hypothesizing the 2D trajectories of points (that is, projections of 3D trajectories) to be smooth over an extended space-time region. Thus, they choose maximally smooth trajectories from the set of all possible trajectories. This automatically solves the correspondence problem. However, this approach is computationally intensive (complexity depends on the number of frames) and relies on the smoothness of the 2D motions. A similar approach for measuring the point trajectories on deformable objects from image sequences is addressed by Duncan [15]. They model the boundary of the object as a deformable contour and then track the local segments of the contour through the temporal sequence. Small motion is assumed between tokens from frame to frame to hypothesize the candidate match points. The motion estimation is done by matching the local segments between pairs of contours by minimizing the deformation between the segments using a measure of bending energy. They have used this approach for tracking left ventricle (LV) endocardial motion.

3.3 Isometric Motion

Isometric motion is defined as a motion that preserves lengths along the surface as well as angles between curves on the surface. It can be described as a motion that preserves Gaussian but not mean curvature. A well-known example is a bending deformation: a piece of paper or metal plate bending from a planar configuration into a cylindrical shape (Figure 2). Isometric motion severely limits the nonrigidity, since for many curved objects, such as spheres, no isometry is possible.

There have been several approaches to estimating isometric motion from 2D image sequences. It is important to note that all of them assume known point correspondences between images.

Koenderink considered the shape from motion assuming bending deformation in [16]. Koenderink and Doorn [17] proposed a method for solving shape from motion under bending deformations, using polyhedral approximations of a smooth surface. Polyhedral approximation results in a piecewise rigid surface, unless there is sufficient spatial resolution. The authors concentrate on obtaining partial solutions of 3D shape and motion up to a relief transformation using the projected positions of points and their temporal derivatives.

In contrast, Jasinschi and Yuille [18] triangulate the surface approximation. They use Regge calculus to approximate a general surface by a net of triangles, and allow bending at the common edges of these triangles to accommodate flexing motion. Again, a jointed triangulation may be suitable only for articulated motion unless the spatial resolution is sufficiently high. The authors have modified Ullman's incremental rigidity scheme to estimate depth information at the vertices of triangles, assuming correspondences between vertices of triangles. They initially consider the object to be a flat structure and update the model between time frames by assuming a minimal nonrigidity (quasi-rigidity) occurring between time frames. The minimal change is enforced by a cost function, thus yielding a series of estimated depth values that converge toward the correct result.

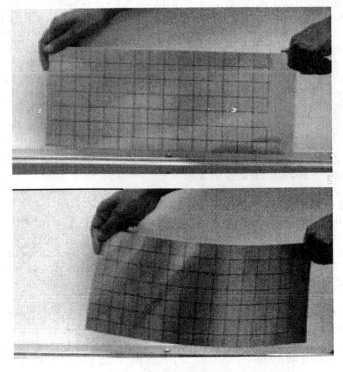

Figure 2. Bending of a metal.

Chen and Penna [19, 20] apply differential geometry to nonrigid motion analysis. They relax the rigidity constraint but consider mostly isometric motion. Their approach is to approximate the transformation using Taylor expansion. They first consider a general elastic motion, and present three approaches for motion recovery. These are: (1) an infinitesimal approach, (2) a global approach, and (3) a hybrid of the former two approaches. The infinitesimal approach is based on the local surface geometry of the object. The authors first recover the image transformation between two images using point correspondences and a least-squares approach. The Jacobian of the image transformation is coupled with the Jacobian of the orthographic or planar perspective projection to recover the Jacobian (that is, linear approximation) of the generalized motion. A closed-form solution is only possible in the case of isometric motion in this approach. The global approach is concerned with determining the generalized motion completely from point correspondences. They illustrate this approach by using projective geometry under affine transformations. The hybrid approach is based on the spherical perspective model, which is a reasonable model for human perception. Chen and Zhao [21] further developed this work and presented an analysis of the geometric structure of moving, nonrigid point patterns and their orthographically projected images. The authors provide ways to represent and encode an image sequence of moving, nonrigid objects in terms of the initial frame and the motion parameters. They consider only a class of nonrigid motions: constant affin emotions in 3D space. They utilize a "localization principle" to reduce nonrigid motion into a collection of affine motions.

Huang and Goldgof [22, 23] allow the inclusion of an isometric motion assumption in adaptive-size physically based models. They have demonstrated the result of using the isometric constraint in an adaptive-size finite-element model of the bending surface.

3.4 Homothetic Motion

Homothetic motion involves uniform expansion or contraction of a surface; that is, the stretching (amount of expansion or contraction) is equal at every point of the surface. Isometric motion is a special case of homothetic motion with the stretching parameter equal to 1 at all points on the surface. Examples of homothetic motion include a balloon being expanded or contracted, or a sphere as its radius increases or decreases (Figure 3).

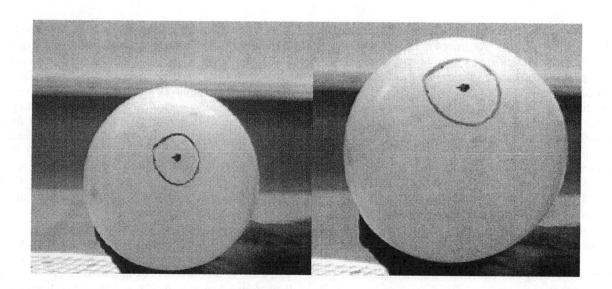

Figure 3. Expansion of a balloon.

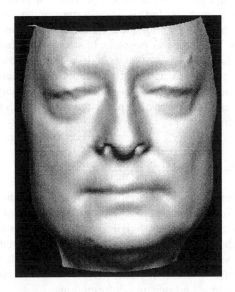

Figure 4. Rendered facial data–Frame 1.

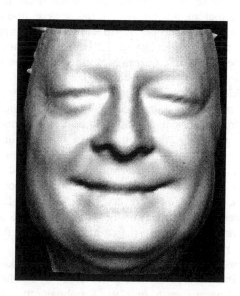

Figure 5. Rendered facial data—Frame 2.

Goldgof, Lee, and Huang [4] consider the use of mean and Gaussian curvatures for motion classification, and deal with both articulated and homothetic motion. Stretching of the surface during motion is the additional motion parameter. They extract the stretching of the surface undergoing homothetic transformation (constant at all points), and also detect the parts of the surface where homothetic motion is violated. The same authors have also applied the above algorithm to cineangiographic left ventricular data [24] to recover stretching parameters of the heart wall. Extending this approach, Kambhamettu and Goldgof [25] proposed a curvature-based approach toward point correspondence and stretching recovery of conformal motion, with homothetic motion as a special case. The idea here is that by hypothesizing point correspondences, one can detect the correct correspondence through minimizing the deviation from the assumed homothetic motion.

3.5 Conformal Motion

Conformal motion is defined as a motion that preserves angles between curves on the surface, but not lengths. It is shown [26] that a necessary and sufficient condition for the motion to be conformal is that the ratios of the coefficients of the first fundamental form remain constant (t^2). The infinitesimal lengths are stretched by a factor of t at the given point. The parameter t can vary at different points on the surface; however, at each point the stretching is the same in all directions. Thus, recovering t will give us information on the amount of stretching at each point. *Mercator's chart* and *stereographic projection* are some of the many conformal deformations of a sphere into a plane. Stereographic projection is the most general conformal representation of the sphere upon the plane possessing the property that circles on the sphere correspond to circles in the plane. Homothetic motion is a restricted class of conformal motion where the parameter t is the same for all points on the surface.

Mishra, Goldgof, and Huang, and Mishra et al. [27, 28] first presented an algorithm for local stretching recovery from Gaussian curvature, based on polynomial (linear and quadratic) approximations of the stretching function under conformal motion. Their expression for linear stretching in conformal motion requires at least three point correspondences. A feature of this algorithm is that it does not require a preservation of the coordinate system between any two frames of data. They have applied this algorithm to estimate the stretching of the left ventricular wall in the data obtained by coronary angiography. An extension of this approach that incorporates knowledge of the line correspondences is described by Mishra, Goldgof, and Kambhamettu in [29]. Kambhamettu and Goldgof

[30] proposed another extension and developed algorithms for point correspondence recovery in nonrigid motion under local conformal motion with constant (homothetic), linear, and polynomial stretching. They first hypothesize possible point correspondences, and they form an error function for each hypothesis that represents the deviation from conformal motion. The error function is then minimized for estimating point correspondences and stretching. The advantage of this approach is that the coordinate system can be different for each frame. The authors have applied the algorithm to volumetric CT data of the left ventricle to derive stretching and point correspondences between frames.

Figure 6 shows three frames of left-ventricle data (represented by the surface below the cutting plane). One can observe different elastic motions between each frame. There are 16 time frames of this data over one heart cycle. Each frame consists of $128 \times 128 \times 118$ binary voxels containing previously extracted surface information. This data was acquired by Dr. Eric Hoffman's group, now at the University of Iowa.

A similar approach was used by Amini and Duncan [31]. However, they use an additional bending model along with the stretching model for tracking point correspondences of the LV in motion. They consider the physical model of the LV as a thinplate, and then they track the motion involved by minimizing the bending and deviation from conformal stretching. Principal directions before and after the motion are used for setting up the coordinate system.

4. General Nonrigid Motion

Many researchers are working on the problem of general nonrigid motion analysis. In this domain, motion has few restrictions other than topological invariance. General nonrigid motion analysis is possible in situations where we have specialized models that encode a priori knowledge about the intended application (model-based methods). More general approaches to nonrigid motion analysis, however, can make use of generic constraints such as motion smoothness.

4.1 Elastic Motion

Elastic motion is nonrigid motion whose only constraint is some degree of continuity or smoothness. Examples are the motion of elastic materials such as rubber, viscoelastic materials such as modeling clay, and plastic materials. This kind of solid-object motion is the most difficult to analyze. Elastic motion includes rigid motions plus stretching, bending, and twisting deformations.

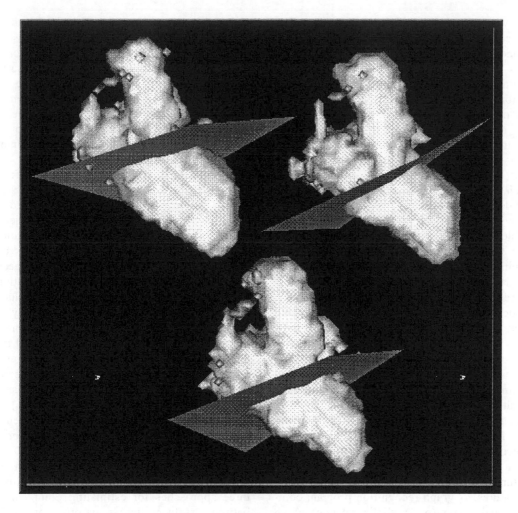

Figure 6. Frames of left ventricle.

Terzopoulos, Witkin, and Kass [32] introduced a general physics-based approach to the estimation of elastic motion. Their work makes use of *deformable models.* These models are dynamic primitives made of a simulated elastic material. The material, represented mathematically in terms of generalized splines [33], provides intrinsic smoothness constraints that permit the recovery of continuous nonrigid motions. Like real-world objects, deformable models will move in response to applied forces according to the principles of Lagrangian mechanics. In this dynamic approach, external force fields serve to couple the deformable models to imaged objects. These fields are derived from potential functions that are computed from input images. As the deformable model achieves equilibrium in its external force field, it reconstructs the shape of the imaged object. When presented with image sequences of objects in nonrigid motion, deformable models are capable of estimating and tracking the motion.

The physics-based approach is also applicable to planar nonrigid motion. A simplified deformable curve model popularly known as a *snake* [34], has been used by Terzopoulos and Waters [35] to track nonrigidly moving eyebrows, lips, and other facial features of an expressive face for the purposes of expression estimation and resynthesis.

The most common implementations of deformable models make use of finite-difference methods (as does the model in [32]) and finite-element methods. McInerney and Terzopoulos develop a "balloon" model that makes use of a quintic triangular finite element whose nodal variables include the time-varying positions and partial derivatives of the deformable surface up to the second order [36]. They apply their balloon model to the reconstruction and tracking of the LV in dynamic CT data.

Recursive nonrigid motion estimators have recently been developed which employ the deformable model equations of motion as system models within a nonlinear Kalman estimation framework [37–40]. The system model synthesizes nonrigid motions in response to generalized forces arising from the inconsistency between the incoming observations and the estimated model state. The observation forces also account formally for instantaneous uncertainties and incomplete information. A Riccati procedure updates a covariance matrix that transforms the forces in accordance with the system dynamics and the prior observation history. The transformed forces induce changes in the translational, rotational, and deformational state variables of the system model in order to reduce inconsistency, thus deriving robust nonrigid motion estimates from time-varying visual data.

Bozma and Duncan [41] chose a deformable model-based approach, where reliable models are required for recognition of deformable objects. They have described a segmentation system for model-based recognition of multiple deformable objects in which the modules are integrated using a game-theoretic approach. The segmentation is accomplished using an extended model-based recognition that is a combination of deformable object matching and relational matching. The deformable (flexible) model is defined as a set of independent deformable objects coupled together by loose (inequality) constraints. The matching is decomposed into individual tasks to form N-functional modules in the vision system. The authors arrive at a correspondence between the vision system and an N-player game and then use a game-theoretic approach to solve for multiple coexisting modules.

Another model-based approach is proposed by Segen and Dana [42]. The authors have implemented a symbolic method for recognition of deformable shapes, which is distributed in a network of general-purpose processors. Structural features were used to get a symbolic relation among local features. A graph recognition program compares the generated graph (or symbolic relation) of an object with graph models stored in a model library to select the best match. The graph model is a layered graph with a probability distribution over labels attached to each vertex. The criterion for recognition is the minimal representation complexity for a given object. Hence it tries to find the least possible graph description for an object by relating it to one of the graph models in the library.

As we observed in the earlier work on nonrigid motion, most of the approaches need point correspondences. This problem is relaxed to subset correspondences by Chaudhuri and Chatterjee [43]. They have proposed the estimation of translation, rotation, and the deformation parameters for a nonrigid object using subset correspondences. Explicit point-to-point correspondence is not required in this approach. Subsets are created by grouping points lying on a single surface. Thus, the correspondence problem is simplified to identifying the same surface (say, a planar patch) at two different time frames. This approach needs at least six subset correspondences to determine the motion parameters.

An algorithm for real-time tracking of nonrigid objects is presented by Woodfill and Zabih [44]. It requires that the object's approximate initial location is available, and the object can be distinguished from the background by motion or stereo. They use a massively parallel bottom-up approach to track and segment the object specified along the temporal sequence. The main restriction however is that the object's shape and position should not change too drastically. So, given a pair of images together with the position of an object in the first image, their algorithm computes the position of the object in the second image. This implies determining the 2D motion of the object.

Yamamoto et al. [45] presented an approach that can estimate the deformable motion parameters by solving a system of linear equations that are obtained by substituting a linear transformation of nonrigid objects expressed by the Jacobian matrix into a set of motion constraints. They use a general-motion model that is composed of connected links, forming a grid. The displacement of any point can be expressed by a linear combination of the link deformations. The motion constraints include the depth constraint during motion, and the intensity constraint of the image. The input data considered is from a video rate range camera, which provides a registered range and intensity image sequences. The prime advantage of this approach is that point correspondences are not necessary in order to determine the nonrigid motion parameters.

Kambhamettu and Goldgof [46, 76] proposed a method for estimating point correspondences between surfaces under small deformation using normal and curvature information. They estimate the displacement function using a first-order approximation, and then derive the motion parameters. The authors have designed three approaches for estimating point correspondences between surfaces under deformation. All three approaches can be used with and without a priori knowledge of point correspondences. The first approach involves using the changes in discriminants during small deformation. The second approach involves using changes in unit normal direction to estimate the point correspondences. The third approach uses the changes in Gaussian curvature, along with the changes in unit normal direction to estimate point correspondences.

Huang [3] chose an application-motivated approach to general nonrigid motion analysis. As we mentioned previously, he proposed a classification of nonrigid motion into articulated objects, elastic objects, and fluids. The research of his group includes modeling and analysis of heart wall motion, human face/head motion analysis and synthesis in model-based image compression, and studying the evolution of coherent structures in fluid motion. They use spherical harmonics for the modeling and analysis of heart wall motion, based on the biplane cineangiograms and CT and MRI data of the human heart. Face/head motion analysis is studied with applications toward visual communication such as teleconferencing. The surface of the face/head is approximated by triangular patches, and the facial motion is interpreted as motion at the vertices of these triangles. Figures 4 and 5 represent rendered images of two different facial expressions, which are being used for face/head motion analysis. The surface points of the face were obtained in a cylindrical fashion. The data consist of 512 slices, where each slice has 512 points distributed radially around a central axis. This data was acquired using the Cyberware range scanner.

4.2 Fluid Motion

Fluid motion is the most general type of nonrigid motion. It includes the motion of liquid and gaseous objects. These motions, which need not be continuous, can exhibit highly variable topological structure as well as nonsmooth behavior such as turbulence. Compared to the other classes of motion, relatively little work has been done on fluid motion analysis.

Huang [3] and his group have been investigating the fluid motion analysis problem in order to develop automated analysis and visualization techniques for fluid flow. These techniques have applications in the acquisition of flow data, interpretation of complicated fluid motions, and the active control of flows and flow systems. The ultimate goal of this research is to study the similarities and differences among these problems and more traditional motion analysis problems, as well as to develop concepts, methodologies, and techniques applicable to various types of nonrigid motion.

5. Shape Models for Nonrigid Objects

Shape modeling for nonrigid motion analysis is attracting increasing attention. Powerful shape models are needed to efficiently represent deformable objects and track their nonrigid motions. Globally parameterized primitives such as superquadrics and hyperquadrics have emerged as useful representations of shape. These primitives allow solids and surfaces to be constructed and easily modified using only a few parameters. Globally parameterized models are useful for object recognition using model libraries. Another useful class of shape models is the free-form mesh and spline models whose definition involves many local parameters. These models are useful for local shape control and for representing shape details as the number of parameters is increased. Recently, hybrid models have been proposed that combine the features of globally and locally parameterized representations. Dynamic, physics-based versions of certain models in all three model classes have been proposed and more are currently under development. For a survey of shape-modeling methods for surface representation, see Bolle and Vemuri [47].

5.1 Local Models

Significant work in computer vision has gone into the development of reconstruction algorithms based on local shape models using generalized splines [33, 48]. Dynamic generalizations of these local models were surveyed in Section 4.1 [32, 36].

Terzopoulos and Vasilescu [49] developed adaptive meshes that can nonuniformly sample and reconstruct intensity and range data. Adaptive meshes are discrete dynamic models, which are assembled by interconnecting nodal masses with adjustable nonlinear springs. The nodes are mobile and can move over the surface. The springs can automatically adjust their stiffness based on the locally sampled information about depth, gradient, and/or curvature, in order to concentrate nodes near rapid shape variations. Hence the position of the nodes, and the stiffness of the springs connecting them, automatically change depending on the surface (or image) properties.

Along similar lines, Huang and Goldgof [50, 22] presented a new approach to sampling and surface reconstruction that uses dynamic models. They have introduced adaptive-size meshes that will automatically update the size of the meshes (number of nodes) as the distance between the nodes changes. They have implemented algorithms for sampling of the intensity data, surface reconstruction of the range data, and surface reconstruction of the 3D computed-tomography left-ventricle data. These models can also incorporate isometric and conformal constraints.

Recent work in this area includes that of Huang and Goldgof [51], who use a non-linear finite element method (FEM) to describe the object behavior. They exploit a priori information about the object's material properties and force information, and then model the object surface using nonlinear FEM. This method allows for material nonlinearity (that is, non-Hookean materials with nonlinear stress-strain relationships) and large displacement during motion. The correct point correspondences can be obtained using image information and knowledge of material properties.

5.2 Global Models

Spherical harmonics are popular in designing global models. The spherical harmonic model [52] is a parametric representation of the closed surface that can be described by a radial function $r(\theta, \phi)$. The model, similar in concept to the Fourier descriptor, decomposes the function $r(\theta, \phi)$ into many orthogonal basis functions. The disadvantage in such a model is that its basis function is global, just like the sine and cosine functions in Fourier descriptor. Schudy and Ballard used time-varying spherical harmonics for heart-volumetric representation [53]. Recently, Chen and Huang [54] used superquadrics as modeling primitives for deformation analysis of 3D data. They have developed a recursive algorithm for estimating global motion and object shape, which incorporates a priori knowledge of the object information into the estimation and object shape irrespective of the biased distribution of 3D points. Matheny and Goldgof [55] extended spherical harmonics to surface harmonics that are defined on domains other than the sphere and to 4D spherical harmonics. These harmonics enable the representation of shapes that cannot be represented as a global function in spherical coordinates, but can be represented in other coordinate systems. Nonrigid shapes are hence represented as functions of space and time either by including time-dependence as a separate factor or by using 4D spherical harmonics.

Quadric surfaces are the simplest models for curved shapes. They were used for position and orientation estimation, object recognition, and range data segmentation in the early 80s [47]. The disadvantage of using quadric surfaces is that the objects are described by many quadric patches. Taubin [56] and Keren, Cooper, and Subrahmonia [57] have been studying higher degree polynomials. They proposed the bounded shape polynomials for recovery and recognition. They use fourth-degree-bounded polynomials as their primitives (since the third degree polynomials are unbounded) and report very strong descriptive power. A significant advantage of shape polynomials is that they have algebraic invariants and, thus, become very useful for recognition purposes. However, higher degree polynomials also give rise to certain disadvantages, since such polynomials involve ambiguity in representation, recovery, and recognition. Subrahmonia, Cooper, and Keren used a Bayesian method to cope with such a nonuniqueness problem [58].

In the past five years, superquadrics have become the focus of several computer vision researchers. Different from shape polynomials, superquadrics extend the quadric models by allowing the exponents to be real values. Superquadrics have a small number of parameters but are flexible and powerful for describing the parts of natural objects. With the same compact equation, superquadrics can generate a continuum of forms: spheres, cuboids with rounded corners, cubes, or diamond shapes. Such shapes are difficult to model with traditional constructive solid geometry systems. Pentland's [59] *Supersketch* modeling system uses superquadrics as the basic shape primitive. The system also includes deformations to define more complex shapes.

Pentland [60] originally suggested analytically solving for all independent parameters in the superquadric parametric equation. The input might be 2D contours and shading. His second approach [61] is a combination of part model recovery and segmentation based on exhaustive search through the entire superquadric parameter space (at 84,000 locations) to find the best initial values. Input is 3D points from range images.

Boult and Gross [62] used a gradient descent minimization method for the superquadrics recovery, but had problems with convergence of cylindrically shaped objects. Solina and Bajcsy [63] used a modified error-of-fit function and obtained better results. Gross and Boult [64] also discussed several different error-of-fit functions and compared their effect on the shape recovery. Gupta and Bajcsy [65] presented an integrated framework for segmenting dense range data of complex 3D scenes into constituent parts using bi-quadrics and superquadrics.

Although powerful in describing shapes, superquadrics still have some drawbacks. They are intrinsically symmetric along x, y, and z axes and their geometric bounds are just simple Cartesian cubes. In 1988, Hanson [66] extended superquadrics, proposing hyperquadrics for computer graphics applications. Hyperquadrics may be composed of any number of terms, their geometric bounds are arbitrary convex polyhedra, and the modeled shapes are not necessarily symmetric. Other properties of hyperquadric model include compactness, semilocal control, hierarchical structure, and intuitive meaning, which are all advantageous for shape representation. Han, Goldgof, and Bowyer [67] presented a fitting method that uses the hyperquadric model for the recovery of complex shapes from range data.

Pentland and Horowitz [68] presented an approach to the recovery of nonrigid motion based on a 20-node, hexahedral isoparametric, elastic finite element. The element applies a parameterized global deformation to an enclosed geometric model such as a sphere, cube, or superquadric. Their algorithm applies approximate modal analysis to decouple the degrees of freedom of the element into rigid and nonrigid vibration modes. They modeled and simulated the physics of elastic motion to estimate object shape and velocity. In [69] they obtain estimates of both object shape and velocity from contour data. Shape estimates are integrated over time by using an extended Kalman filter, resulting in a stable estimate of both 3D shape and 3D velocity.

5.3 Hybrid Models

Terzopoulos and Metaxas [70] present a physically based approach to fitting complex 3D shapes using a new class of dynamic models that can deform both locally and globally. They formulate deformable superquadrics that incorporate the global shape parameters of a conventional superellipsoid with the local degrees of freedom of a spline. In [71], they present an approach for recursively estimating 3D object shape and general nonrigid motion, which makes use of these physically based dynamic models. The models provide global deformation parameters that represent the salient shape features of natural parts, and local deformation parameters that capture shape details. They formulate constraints that allow them to construct multibody models with deformable parts. Using these models as dynamic system models, they derive a shape and nonrigid motion estimator that takes the form of an extended Kalman filter.

Liao and Medioni [72] present representation of range

data using deformable models. They have used B-spline surface patches to model the given data using an initial approximation of the surface as a simple surface, such as a cylinder or a plane. This initial surface is deformed using internal and external forces. The deformation takes place in each iteration, as the control vertices are moved around under the influence of features of the surface data. The internal and external energies are defined according to the surface derivatives, and the distance function between control vertices and the data points.

6. Summary

Nonrigid motion is ubiquitous since there is no such thing as a perfectly rigid object in the real world. In this chapter we reviewed a large body of work on nonrigid motion analysis. The reason for the recent wave of interest in nonrigid motion is twofold: First, recent research has uncovered several promising new approaches to nonrigid motion analysis. Second, a wealth of potential applications has become apparent, including human face/head recognition for teleconferencing, gesture recognition for virtual reality, model construction of nonrigid objects, lip reading, material deformation and soil pressure studies, tracking of cloud formations for weather prediction, crystal growth observation, and fluid-flow analysis. There are also numerous biomedical applications, such as left-ventricle motion analysis, lung motion studies, and tumor growth, among others.

Nonrigid motion analysis is a burgeoning research area and the available body of research has begun to make inroads into only a few of the many difficult problems. There are numerous open theoretical issues in motion tracking from 3D data or from projections, analysis of objects undergoing large deformation, and analysis of unrestricted viscoelastic and fluid motion. For nonrigid objects, the issues of motion representation and shape representation are much more closely related than for rigid objects. Only a few researchers have considered the problems of representing nonrigid objects more complex than articulated objects. Most of this work describes "single-part" nonrigid objects. It is clear that multiple-part representations are more suitable for many nonrigid objects. Often, each part is itself a nonrigid object. Consider, for example, the human body with its numerous deformable parts, a reclining office chair with soft cushions, child swings formed by two ropes and a rubber seat, and quasi-articulated objects such as beads on a rope or a metal mesh woven out of bendable wires. Representation issues become critically important as we go beyond motion tracking and motion analysis to problems of nonrigid object recognition. New ideas for efficient representation, storage, and indexing of nonrigid shapes are needed to make automated nonrigid object recognition a practical reality.

References

[1] J.W. Roach and J.K. Aggarwal, "Determining the Movement of Objects from a Sequence of Images," *IEEE Trans. Pattern Analysis and Machine Intelligence*, Vol. 2, No. 6, 1980, pp. 554–562.

[2] T.S. Huang, "Motion Analysis," *Encyclopedia of Artificial Intelligence*, Vol. 1, 1986, pp. 620–632.

[3] T.S. Huang, "Modeling, Analysis, and Visualization of Nonrigid Object Motion," *Proc. 10th ICPR*, IEEE Computer Society Press, Los Alamitos, Calif., 1990, pp. 361–364.

[4] D.B. Goldgof, H. Lee, and T.S. Huang, "Motion Analysis of Nonrigid Surfaces," *Proc. IEEE Computer Society Conf. Computer Vision and Pattern Recognition,* IEEE Computer Society Press, Los Alamitos, Calif., 1988, pp. 375–380.

[5] J.A. Webb and J.K. Aggarwal, "Structure from Motion of Rigid and Jointed Objects," *Artificial Intelligence*, Vol. 19, No. 1, 1983, pp. 107–130.

[6] D.D. Hoffman and B.E. Flinchbaugh, "The Interpretation of Biological Motion," *Biological Cybernetics*, 1982, pp. 195–204.

[7] B.M. Bennett and D.D. Hoffman, "The Computation of Structure from Fixed Axis Motion: Non Rigid Structures," *Biological Cybernetics*, 1985, pp. 293–300.

[8] J. O'Rourke and N. Badler, "Model-Based Image Analysis of Human Motion Using Constraint Propagation," *IEEE Trans. Pattern Analysis and Machine Intelligence*, Vol. 2, 1980, pp. 522–536.

[9] M. Asada, M. Yachida, and S. Tsuji, "Understanding of 3D Motion in Block World," *Pattern Recognition*, Vol. 17, No. 1, 1984, pp. 57–84.

[10] M. Sallam and K. Bowyer, "Generalizing the Aspect Graph Concept to Include Articulated Assemblies," *Pattern Recognition Letters*, Vol. 12, Mar. 1991, pp. 171–176.

[11] B. Bruno, et al., "Modeling of Articulated Objects for Machine Perception," *Proc. 5th Florida AI Research Symp.*, 1992, pp. 247–251.

[12] S. Ullman, "Maximizing Rigidity: The Incremental Recovery of 3D Structure from Rigid and Nonrigid Motion," *Perception*, Vol. 13, 1984 , pp. 255–274.

[13] D. Shulman and J.Y. Aloimonos, "Nonrigid Motion Interpretation: A Regularized Approach," *Proc. Royal Society of London B233*, 1988, pp. 217–234.

[14] R. Jain and T.K. Sethi, "Establishing Correspondence of Non-Rigid Objects Using Smoothness of Motion," *Proc. Workshop Computer Vision: Representation and Control*, 1984, pp. 83–87.

[15] J. Duncan, et al., "Measurement of Non-Rigid Motion Using Contour Shape Descriptors," *Proc. Computer Vision and Pattern Recognition*, IEEE Computer Society Press, Los Alamitos, Calif., 1991, pp. 318–324.

[16] J.J Koenderink, "Shape from Motion and Bending Deformation in AI," *J. Optical Society of America*, 1984, pp. 1265–1266.

[17] J.J. Koenderink and A.J. van Doom, "Depth and Shape from Different Perspective in the Presence of Bending Deformations," *J. Optical Society of America*, Vol. 3, No. 2, Feb. 1986.

[18] R. Jasinschi and A. Yuille, "Nonrigid Motion and Regge Calculus," *J. Optical Society of America*, 1989, pp. 1088–1095.

[19] S.S. Chen, "Structure-from-Motion without the Rigidity Assumption," *Proc. 3rd Workshop Computer Vision: Representation and Control,* 1985, pp. 105–112.

[20] S.S. Chen and M. Penna, "Motion Analysis of Deformable Objects," *Advances in Computer Vision and Image Processing*, T.S. Huang, ed., JAI Press, Cambridge, Mass., 1988.

[21] S.-S. Chen and A.-G. Zhao, "Image Representation of Moving Nonrigid Objects," *J. Visual Communication and Image Representation*, Academic Press, New York, N.Y., 1991.

[22] W.-C. Huang and D.B. Goldgof, "Adaptive-Size Physically-Based Models for Non-Rigid Motion Analysis," *Proc. IEEE Conf. Computer Vision and Pattern Recognition*, IEEE Computer Society Press, Los Alamitos, Calif., 1992, pp. 833–835.

[23] W.-C. Huang and D.B. Goldgof, "Adaptive-Size Meshes for Rigid and Nonrigid Shape Analysis and Synthesis," *IEEE Trans. Pattern Analysis and Machine Intelligence*, Vol. 15, No. 3, Mar. 1993.

[24] D.B. Goldgof, H. Lee, and T.S. Huang, "Parameter Estimation of the Heart Motion from Angiography Data," *SPIE/SPSE Symp. Electronic Imaging, Conf. Biomedical Image Processing*, Vol. 1245, No. 15, Feb. 1990, pp. 171–181.

[25] C. Kambhamettu and D.B Goldgof, "Towards Finding Point Correspondences in Non-Rigid Motion," *Proc. 7th Scandinavian Conf. Image Analysis*, 1991, pp. 1126–1133.

[26] W.C. Graustein, *Differential Geometry*, Macmillan, New York, N.Y., 1935.

[27] S.K. Mishra, D.B. Goldgof, and T.S. Huang, "Non-Rigid Motion Analysis and Epicardial Deformation Estimation from Angiography Data," *Proc. IEEE Conf. Computer Vision and Pattern Recognition,* IEEE Computer Society Press, Los Alamitos, Calif., 1991, pp. 331–336.

[28] S.K. Mishra, et al., "Curvature-Based Non-Rigid Motion Analysis from 3D Point Correspondences," *Int'l J. Imaging Systems and Technology*, 1993.

[29] S.K. Mishra, et al., "Estimating Non-Rigid Motion from Point and Line Correspondences," *Pattern Recognition Letters*, 1993.

[30] C. Kambhamettu and D.B. Goldgof, "Point Correspondence Recovery in Nonrigid Motion," *Proc. IEEE Conf. Computer Vision and Pattern Recognition*, IEEE Computer Society Press, Los Alamitos, Calif., 1992, pp. 222–227.

[31] A.A. Amini and J.S. Duncan, "Pointwise Tracking of Left-Ventricular Motion in 3D," *Proc. IEEE Workshop on Visual Motion*, IEEE Computer Society Press, Los Alamitos, Calif., 1991, pp. 294–299.

[32] D. Terzopoulos, A. Witkin, and M. Kass, "Constraints on Deformable Models: Recovering 3D Shape and Nonrigid Motion," *Artificial Intelligence*, Vol. 36, No. 1, 1988, pp. 91–193.

[33] D. Terzopoulos, "Regularization of Inverse Visual Problems Involving Discontinuities," *IEEE Trans. Pattern Analysis and Machine Intelligence*, Vol. 8, No. 4, 1986, pp. 413–424.

[341] M. Kass, A. Witkin, and D. Terzopoulos, "Snakes: Active Contour Models," *Int'l J. Computer Vision*, Vol. 1, No. 4, 1988, pp. 321–331.

[35] D. Terzopoulos and K. Waters, "Analysis and Synthesis of Facial Image Sequences using Physical and Anatomical Models," *IEEE Trans. Pattern Analysis and Machine Intelligence*, Vol. 15, July 1993. Also in *Proc. 3rd Int'l Conf. Computer Vision (ICCV'90)*, IEEE Computer Society Press, Los Alamitos, Calif., 1990, pp. 727–732.

[36] T. McInerney and D. Terzopoulos, "A Finite Element Model for 3D Shape Reconstruction and Nonrigid Motion Tracking," *Proc. 4th Int'l Conf. Computer Vision (ICCV'98)*, IEEE Computer Society Press, Los Alamitos, Calif., 1993.

[37] R. Szeliski and D. Terzopoulos, "Physically-Based and Probabilistic Modeling for Computer Vision," *Proc. SPIE 1070, Geometric Methods in Computer Vision*, Soc. Photo-Optical Instrumentation Engineers, 1991, pp. 140-152.

[38] D. Terzopoulos and R. Szeliski, "Tracking with Kalman Snakes," in *Active Vision*, A. Blake and A. Yuille, eds., MIT Press, Cambridge, Mass., 1992, pp. 3–20.

[39] D. Terzopoulos and D. Metaxas, "Tracking Nonrigid 3D Objects," in *Active Vision*, A. Blake and A. Yuille, eds., MIT Press, Cambridge, Mass., 1992, pp. 75–89.

[40] D. Metaxas and D. Terzopoulos, "Shape and Nonrigid Motion Estimation through Physics-Based Synthesis, *IEEE Trans. Pattern Analysis and Machine Intelligence*, Vol. 15, Sept. 1993. Also in *Proc. IEEE Computer Vision and Pattern Recognition Conf. (CVPR'91)*, IEEE Computer Society Press, Los Alamitos, Calif., 1991, pp. 337–343.

[41] H.I. Bozma and J.S. Duncan, "Model-Based Recognition of Multiple Deformable Objects Using a Game-Theoretic Framework," *Proc. 12th Int'l Conf. IPMI'91*, 1991, pp. 358–372.

[42] J. Segen and K. Dana, "Parallel Symbolic Recognition of Deformable Shapes," in *From Pixels to Features II*, H. Burkhardt, Y. Neuvo, and J.C. Simon, eds., Elsevier Science Publishers B.V., North-Holland, 1991.

[43] S. Chaudhuri and S. Chatterjee, "Estimation of Motion Parameters for a Deformable Object from Range Data," *Proc. IEEE Conf. Computer Vision and Pattern Recognition*, IEEE Computer Society Press, Los Alamitos, Calif., 1989, pp. 991–295.

[44] J. Woodfill and R. Zabih, "An Algorithm for Real-Time Tracking of Non-Rigid Objects," *AAAI-91, Proc. 9th Nat'l*

Conf. Artificial Intelligence, Vision, and Sensor Interpretation, Vol. 2, Morgan Kaufman, San Francisco, Calif., 1991, pp. 718–723.

[45] M. Yamamoto, et al., "Direct Estimation of Range Flow on Deformable Shape from a Video Rate Range Cameras," *IEEE Trans. Pattern Analysis and Machine Intelligence*, Vol., 15, No. 1, 1993, pp. 82–89.

[46] C. Kambhamettu and D.B. Goldgof, "Estimating Point Correspondences in Small Deformations," TR. 93-01, Dept. Computer Science and Engineering, Univ. of South Florida, 1993.

[47] R.M. Bolle and B.C. Vemuri, "On Three-Dimensional Surface Reconstruction Methods," *IEEE Trans. Pattern Analysis and Machine Intelligence*, Vol. 13, No. 1, 1991, pp. 1–13.

[48] D. Terzopoulos, The Computation of Visible-Surface Representations," *IEEE Trans. Pattern Analysis and Machine Intelligence*, Vol. 10, No. 4, 1988, pp. 417-438.

[49] D. Terzopoulos and A. Vasilescu, "Sampling and Reconstruction with Adaptive Meshes," *Proc. IEEE Conf. Computer Vision and Pattern Recognition,* IEEE Computer Society Press, Los Alamitos, Calif., 1991, pp. 70–75.

[50] W.-C. Huang and D.B. Goldgof, "Sampling and Surface Reconstruction with Adaptive-Size Meshes," *Proc. SPIE Applications of Artificial Intelligence X: Machine Vision and Robotics*, Vol. 1708, 1992, pp. 760–770.

[51] W.-C. Huang and D.B. Goldgof, "Qualitative Vision Using Non-Linear Finite Element Modeling," *SPIE/SPSE Symposium on Electronic Imaging, Conf. Geometric Methods in Computer Vision*, 1993.

[52] D.H. Ballard and C.M. Brown, *Computer Vision*, Prentice-Hall, Englewood Cliffs, N.J., 1982, pp. 271–274.

[53] R.B. Shudy and D.H. Ballard, "Towards an Anatomical Model of Heart Motion as Seen in 4-D Cardiac Ultrasound Data," *Proc. 6th Conf. Computer Applications in Radiology and Computer-Aided Analysis of Radiological Images*, Springer Verlag, Berlin, 1979.

[54] C.-W. Chen and T.S. Huang, "Nonrigid Object Motion and Deformation Estimation from Three-Dimensional Data," *Int'l J. Imaging Systems and Technology*, 1990, pp. 385–394.

[55] A. Matheny, "The Use of Three- and Four-Dimensional Surface Harmonics for Rigid and Non-Rigid Shape Recovery and Representation," Masters Thesis, Dept. Computer Science and Engineering, Univ. of South Florida, Apr. 1993.

[56] G. Taubin, "Estimation of Planar Curves, Surfaces, and Nonplanar Curves Defined by Implicit Equations with Applications to Edge and Range Image Segmentation," *IEEE Trans. Pattern Analysis and Machine Intelligence*, Vol. 13, No. 11, Nov. 1991.

[57] D. Keren, D. Cooper, and J. Subrahmonia, "Describing Complicated Objects by Implicit Polynomials," TR lems-102, Division of Eng., Brown University, Feb. 1992.

[58] J. Subrahmonia, D.B. Cooper, and D. Keren, "Practical Reliable Bayesian Recognition of 2D and 3D Objects Using Implicit Polynomials and Algebraic Invariants," TR lems-107, Division of Eng., Brown University, 1992.

[59] A. Pentland, "Towards an Ideal CAD Systems," *Proc. SPIE Conf. Machine Vision and Man-Machine Interface*, SPIE, Jan. 1986.

[60] A. Pentland, "Perceptual Organization and the Representation of Natural Form," *AI*, Vol. 28, No. 3, pp. 3-331, 1986.

[61] A. Pentland, "Recognition by Parts," *Proc. 1st Int'l Conf. Computer Vision*, IEEE Computer Society Press, Los Alamitos, Calif., 1987, pp. 612–620.

[62] T.E. Boult and A.D. Gross, "Recovery of Superquadrics from 3-D Information," *Proc. Spatial Reasoning and Multi-Sensor Fusion Workshop*, 1987, pp. 128–137.

[63] F. Solina and R. Bajcsy, "Recovery of Parametric Models from Range Images: The Case for Superquadrics with Global Deformations," *IEEE Trans. Pattern Analysis and Machine Intelligence*, Vol. 12, No. 2, Feb. 1990, pp. 131–147.

[64] A.D. Gross and T.E. Boult, "Error of Fit Measurements for Recovering Parametric Solids," *Proc. 2nd Int'l Conf. Computer Vision*, IEEE Computer Society Press, Los Alamitos, Calif., 1988, pp. 690–694.

[65] A. Gupta and R. Bajcsy, "An Integrated Approach for Surface and Volumetric Segmentation of Range Images Using Biquadrics and Superquadrics," *SPIE Proc. Applications of AI X: Machine Vision and Robotics*, Vol. 1708, 1992, pp. 210–227.

[66] A.J. Hanson, "Hyperquadrics: Smoothly Deformable Shapes with Convex Polyhedral Bounds," *Computer Vision, Graphics, and Image Processing*, Vol. 44, 1988, pp. 191–210.

[67] S. Han, D.B. Goldgof, and K.W. Bowyer, "Using Hyperquadrics for Shape Recovery from Range Data," *Proc. 4th Int'l Conf. Computer Vision*, IEEE Computer Society Press, Los Alamitos, Calif., 1993, pp. 492–496.

[68] B. Horowitz and A. Pentland, "Recovery of Non-Rigid Motion and Structure," *Proc. IEEE Conf. on Computers*, IEEE Computer Society Press, Los Alamitos, Calif., 1991, pp. 288–293.

[69] A. Pentland, B. Horowitz, and S. Sclaroff, "Non-Rigid Motion and Structure from Contour," *Proc. IEEE Workshop on Visual Motion*, IEEE Computer Society Press, Los Alamitos, Calif., 1991, pp. 288–293.

[70] D. Terzopoulos and D. Metaxas, "Dynamic 3D Models with Local and Global Deformations: Deformable Superquadrics," *IEEE Trans. Pattern Analysis and Machine Intelligence*, Vol. 13, July 1991, pp. 703–714.

[71] D. Metaxas and D. Terzopoulos, "Recursive Estimation of Shape and Nonrigid Motion," *Proc. IEEE Workshop on Visual Motion*, IEEE Computer Society Press, Los Alamitos, Calif., 1991, pp. 306–311.

[72] C.-W. Liao and G. Medioni, "Representation of Range Data with B-Spline Surface Patches," *Proc. 11th IAPR Int'l*

Conf. Pattern Recognition, IEEE Computer Society Press, Los Alamitos, Calif., 1992, pp. 745–748.

[73] A. Matheny and D.G. Goldgof, "The Use of Three- and Four-Dimensional Surface Harmonics for Rigid and Nonrigid Shape Recovery and Representation," Tech. Report TR 93-04, Department of Computer Science and Eng., Univ. of South Florida.

[74] S.S. Chen and M. Penna, "Shape and Motion of Nonrigid Bodies*," Computer Vision, Graphics, and Image Processing,* Vol. 36, 1986, pp. 175–207.

[75] A.H. Barr, "Superquadrics and Angle Preserving Transformations," *IEEE Computer Graphics and Applications,* Vol. 1, 1981, pp. 11–23.

[76] C. Kambhamettu, D.B. Goldgof, and M. He, "Determination of Motion Parameters and Estimation of Point Correspondeces in Small Nonrigid Deformations," *Proc. IEEE Conf. Computer Vision and Pattern Recognition,* IEEE Computer Society Press, Los Alamitos, Calif., 1994, pp. 943–946.

Multiresolution Elastic Matching*

Ruzena Bajcsy

*Department of Computer and Information Sciences, University, of Pennsylvania,
Philadelphia, Pennsylvania 19104-6389*

AND

Stane Kovačič

Fakulteta za elektrotehniko, E. Kardelj University, Ljubljana, Yugoslavia

Received November 5, 1987; accepted October 7, 1988

Matching of locally variant data to an explicit 3-dimensional pictorial model is developed for X-ray computed tomography scans of the human brain, where the model is a voxel representation of an anatomical human brain atlas. The matching process is 3-dimensional without any preference given to the slicing plane. After global alignment the brain atlas is deformed like a piece of rubber, without tearing or folding. Deformation proceeds step-by-step in a coarse-to-fine strategy, increasing the local similarity and global coherence. The assumption underlying this approach is that all normal brains, at least at a certain level of representation, have the same topological structure, but may differ in shape details. Results show that we can account for these differences. © 1989 Academic Press, Inc.

1. INTRODUCTION AND MOTIVATION

Matching is a process in which two existing representations are put into correspondence [1]. Given a stored model and some input data from sensors, the purpose of matching is to interpret the input in terms of the model. This paper describes an approach to matching an explicit 3-dimensional pictorial model to locally variant data. The representations of the model and the data are similar, thus matching is used in its familiar sense. First the model and the input data are globally aligned or registered. After global alignment the model is deformed like a piece of rubber, without tearing or folding. Deformation proceeds step-by-step in a coarse-to-fine strategy, increasing the local similarity and global coherence.

Elastic matching mimics a manual registration process. Assume that we have two objects, one of them made from an elastic material, the other serving as a reference. By applying external forces we can change the shape of the elastic object so that it matches the reference. Manual matching proceeds step-by-step, correcting larger disparities first and making improvements afterwards. The process stops when a satisfactory match and an equilibrium state between the applied forces and the forces resisting deformation are achieved.

Applications of this approach are in medicine, geography, and in recognition of 3D shapes in general. In this paper we concentrate on a medical application. The input data are X-ray computed tomography scans of the brain. The model is a voxel

*Acknowledgment: This work was in part supported by NSF grant DCR-8410771, Air Force grant AFOSR F49620-85-K-0018, Army/DAAG-29-84-K-0061, NSF-CER/DCR82-19196 Ao2, DARPA/ONR NIH grant NS-10939-11 as part of Cerebrovascular Research Center, NIH 1-RO1-NS-23636-01, NSF INT85-14199, NSF DMC85-17315, ARPA N0014-85-K-0807, NATO grant No. 0224/85. By DEC Corp., IBM Corp. and LORD Corp., and IREX.

representation of an anatomical human brain atlas. A CT scanner captures 3-dimensional information slice-by-slice, with each slice representing a cross section through a human body. By stacking several parallel slices on top of each other a truly 3-dimensional image can be obtained. The developed matching process is 3-dimensional without giving preference to the slicing plane. This is important, since the slicing plane can vary from patient to patient. The matching results are, however, visualized as 2-dimensional cross sections through the tissue, as is usually done by physicians. The assumption underlying elastic matching approach is that all normal brains, at least at a certain level of representation, have the same topological structure, but may differ in shape details. The results show that we can account for these differences.

This paper is organized in the following way: the rest of this section gives a brief overview of the previous and related work, Section 2 is about matching in general, and Section 3 describes the implementation and shows some results of matching CT images and brain models. Section 4 consists of conclusions and directions for our future work.

1.1. *Background and Related Work*

The idea for using deformations in matching goes back to Widrow [2], who deformed prototypical patterns to match the real data. Similar motivations led Fischler and Elschlager [3] to a more elaborate technique, with a physical analog consisting of a templates-and-springs model. An iterative cooperative method for matching dot patterns and grey-valued images was proposed by Burr [4]. A model based object matching through elastic deformation formulated as a minimization problem of the cost function, $cost = cost(deformation) - cost(similarity)$, was originated by Broit [5]. Based on this theory the elastic matching was implemented on reduced resolution CT images [6], later on partial CT images of original resolution [7], and finally attempting to combine them [8]. Broit's elastic model and a similar derivation of forces is used in this paper, extending it to an (incremental) multistage deformation using a coarse-to-fine strategy. We do not try to explain deformations biologically. The measurement of biological shape and shape change can be found in [9, 10].

Recently, modeling of objects as deformable elastic bodies has gained more attention in computer graphics and computer vision. Terzopoulos *et al.* proposed energy constraints on deformable models for recovering shape and non-rigid body motion through elastic deformation [11] and for computer graphics animation [12]. Kass *et al.* [13] investigated active models for solving computer vision problems using the energy minimization framework with forces and deformations as basic tools. Matching signals through scale–space balancing the similarity between the signals with the smoothness of deformation has been described by Witkin *et al.* [14]. Dengler [15] developed a dynamic pyramid for solving the correspondence problem in moving image sequences, where the physical model of the elastic membrane is combined with a multilevel technique. Recovery of parametric models and global deformations for shape recognition have been reported by Bajcsy and Solina [16]. Multilevel (multigrid) techniques by themselves are an exciting, rapidly growing field. They were introduced in numerical analysis by Fedorenko and Bakhvalov and later promoted by Brandt, (see historical remarks in [17]). For multiresolution techniques in computer vision and image processing good references are [18, 19].

The basic matching process can be formulated in the following way: given two sets of data, the model M and the pattern P, use some essential information from the model and the pattern to find a mapping T which, under certain constraints, gives the best possible match in terms of predefined similarity measure S. The mapping T usually consists of registration, which is always global, and matching, which can be local or global, depending on the information used.

This formulation applies regardless of the diversity of the matching problems and possible solutions to them. As we proceed, the nature of the problem becomes important, since we have to define:

—what to match, i.e., what are the features to be used in matching;

—what are the constraints we have to consider;

—how to match, i.e., the matching process for achieving a consistent match;

—how to evaluate the match, i.e., define the similarity measure.

We are interested in matching 3D objects, located in space, which may change position and shape as a result of the physical processes acting on them. What we want for such 3D objects is:

—to account for global misalignment;

—to deal with small and local shape changes and possibly model them;

—to use only reliable matching information and propagate it in a consistent way;

—to account for boundary and homogeneous region interactions;

—to achieve scale independence.

The propagation of information and boundary-region interaction are properties of the elastic matching process, which will be described later in the paper. Elastic matching can also efficiently deal with small and local shape changes, but fails if global misalignment is too large. Hence, before elastic matching can take place, some global (or rigid) alignment, such as the one described in the Appendix is necessary.

Small or local change as well as difference are relative terms. When we say small or local we refer to the overall object size and interpret those terms with respect to the resolution used. What is local for one resolution can be global for the other. Equivalently, depending on the resolution used, the objects may be similar or different. Since no sufficient single resolution exists, and because we do not want to make an a priori assumption about how much the objects may differ, a multiresolution technique is combined with elastic matching.

2.1. Global Matching

Global matching or registration involves translation, rotation and scaling of the whole object. In this step we approximate each object by an ellipsoid-like scatter of particles uniformly distributed in space. The translational difference between objects is eliminated by aligning the centers of mass. For rotation and scaling correction we use the method of principal axes, often used for solving similar problems [20, 21]. First the covariance matrices for both objects are computed and then an attempt is made to equalize the matrices through rotation and scaling. The procedure is described in the Appendix.

2.2. *Elastic Matching*

When the relative positions of particles in a continuous body are altered, we say that the body is strained and the change in the relative position of points is a deformation [22]. A nondeformable, or rigid body, is only an abstraction of the real world for which the distance between every pair of its particles remains invariant throughout the history of the body. All material bodies are to some extent deformable. Deformations maybe local or global, small or large, elastic or plastic. The elastic matching considered in this paper models small local elastic deformations. Such an elastic matching model was introduced and developed by Broit [5].

When the external forces are applied, the object is deformed until an equilibrium state between the external forces and internal forces resisting the deformation is achieved. The equilibrium state for an isotropic homogeneous body is described by the partial differential equations which are associated with the name of Navier [22] and serve as the constraint equations in the elastic matching [5]:

$$\mu \nabla^2 u_i + (\lambda + \mu)\frac{\partial \theta}{\partial x_i} + F_i = 0 \qquad (i = 1, 2, 3), \tag{1}$$

where θ is cubical dilation,

$$\theta = \frac{\partial u_1}{\partial x_1} + \frac{\partial u_2}{\partial x_2} + \frac{\partial u_3}{\partial x_3}. \tag{2}$$

$x = (x_1, x_2, x_3)^T$ refers to the coordinate system before deformation and $F = (F_1, F_2, F_3)^T$ are the external forces distributed everywhere in the body. Elastic constants μ and λ define the elastic properties of the body and $u = (u_1, u_2, u_3)^T$ are the displacements we want to find. The forces and displacements can be set to zero at the boundary, which is the frame of the image, or they can be derived by global matching. For given displacements and forces at the boundary, the displacements everywhere else are completely determined by the external forces and elastic constants. Thus, matching through elastic deformations turns into the problem of deriving forces and selecting elastic properties leading to consistent displacements.

2.2.1. *Elastic Properties*

The results of matching depend on the elastic properties of the object, i.e., on selection of the *Lame's* elastic constants μ and λ. The most we can do is to model the goodness of fit. We set λ to zero and use the remaining parameter μ for balancing the internal and external forces. For large elastic constants (in comparison to the forces), the object becomes more rigid, the effects of forces are attenuated, and the disparities between the objects are underestimated. For small elastic constants the solution is mostly controlled by forces. Moreover, noise effects show up and false matches are more likely to occur. The consequences are very unrealistic deformations, since the smoothness constraint is weak. Thus, deforming the object step-by-step, using moderately large elastic constants, should be safer. The physical meaning of *Lame's* elastic coefficients is better understood in terms of Young's modulus E and Poisson ratio σ [22]:

$$E = \mu(3\lambda + 2\mu)/(\lambda + \mu), \qquad \sigma = \lambda/2(\lambda + \mu). \tag{3}$$

σ is the ratio between lateral shrink and longitudinal stretch. E relates tension of the object and its stretch in the same direction. In real world objects σ is around $1/3$. For a highly incompressible body, like rubber, σ is $1/2$ and λ approaches ∞. In our elastic matching model, λ, as well as σ, is zero, so that a tensile stress produces only a stretch without a lateral shrink.

2.2.2. *External Forces*

Perhaps the most important part of the elastic matching model is where and how the external forces are applied in order to obtain consistent deformation. The solution strongly depends on the forces and with the appropriate force modeling we can guide the solution locally as well as globally. There are many different ways to derive forces [13], such as using information from the input data, from external knowledge (i.e., interactively or from a knowledge base) or from some other processes.

In the matching process the task of the forces is to bring similar regions in both objects into correspondence. What we need then is the local similarity measure between the region at some particular position $x = (x_1, x_2, x_3)^T$ in one object and corresponding regions in the other object at position $x + u, u = (u_1, u_2, u_3)^T$. Let us denote the similarity function at some particular position x with $S(u)$. The best possible local match is expected for the displacement vector u which maximizes S. Provided the similarity function has a maximum, we can apply a force proportional to the gradient vector of the similarity function $S(u)$, causing the similarity to increase. Assuming that the function $S(u)$ has continuous second derivatives, it is possible to approximate it in a small neighborhood by using the first three terms of the Taylor series expansion,

$$S(u + \delta u) = S(u) + \delta u^T g(u) + \tfrac{1}{2}\delta u^T H(u)\delta u. \tag{4}$$

The necessary and sufficient condition for the function to have an (unconstrained local) maximum at u^m is that gradient vector $g(u^m) = 0$ and that the Hessian matrix $H(u^m)$ is negative definite [23]. For the quadratic function Eq. (4) holds exactly since the higher order derivatives are zero. All functions with continuous second derivatives behave quadratically over a sufficiently small region, and as long as the deformations needed are small we can use the quadratic approximation of $S(u)$,

$$S(u) = \tfrac{1}{2}u^T A u + b^T u + c. \tag{5}$$

The explicit expression for the applied force, which can be substituted in (1), then becomes

$$F(u) = g(u) = Au + b, \tag{6}$$

289

or when written out in full notation,

$$F_i = 2a_{i1}u_1 + 2a_{i2}u_2 + 2a_{i3}u_3 + b_i \qquad (i = 1, 2, 3). \tag{7}$$

Those forces will be applied in regions for which the local similarity function exhibits a substantial maximum. All other regions are not used for matching since they lack reliable matching information and as such should behave in the matching process as constrained by the elastic matcher. What remains to be described is the local similarity measure.

2.2.3. Local Similarity Measure

The derivation of the local similarity function $S(u)$ resembles the template matching process. For a small set of displacements u the similarity between some particular small region $f(x)$ in one object and the corresponding regions $g(x + u)$ in the other object is calculated using the normalized correlation $C(f, g)$, $S(u) = C(f(x), g(x + u))$. To be more selective we decompose f and g into components and take those components which are relevant for matching. Let us take some complete system of orthonormal functions h_i defined over domain D. Any piecewise continuous function f defined over domain D can then be described by its projections F_i on the h_i:

$$f = \sum_{i=0}^{\infty} F_i h_i, \qquad \text{where } F_i = (f, h_i) = \int_D f(x) h_i(x) \, dx, \tag{8}$$

and $(f, g) = \int_D f(x) g(x) \, dx$ is by definition the scalar product between functions f and g. In this case the normalized cross correlation of the two functions f and g can be computed from their projections,

$$C(f, g) = \frac{(f, g)}{(f, f)^{1/2} (g, g)^{1/2}} = \frac{\displaystyle\sum_{i=0}^{\infty} F_i G_i}{\left[\displaystyle\sum_{i=0}^{\infty} F_i^2\right]^{1/2} \left[\displaystyle\sum_{i=0}^{\infty} G_i^2\right]^{1/2}}. \tag{9}$$

The complete orthonormal system of functions $\psi_n(t)$ of one variable, which are orthogonal with respect to the weighting function $w(t) = e^{-t^2}$ can be derived from Hermite polynomials H_n [24],

$$\psi_n(t) = H_n(t) \frac{1}{\sqrt{2^n n! \sqrt{\pi}}} e^{-t^2/2} \qquad (n = 0, 1, 2, \ldots), \tag{10}$$

where

$$H^n = (-1)^n e^{t^2} \frac{d^n e^{-t^2}}{dt^n} \qquad (-\infty < t < +\infty). \tag{11}$$

For instance, the first three Hermite polynomials are $H_0 = 1$, $H_1 = 2t$, and $H_2 =$

$4t^2 - 2$. Functions of three variables $h_i(x) = h_i(x_1, x_2, x_3)$ can be constructed by multiplication,

$$h_0(x_1, x_2, x_3) = \psi_0(x_1)\psi_0(x_2)\psi_0(x_3), \tag{12a}$$

$$h_1(x_1, x_2, x_3) = \psi_1(x_1)\psi_0(x_2)\psi_0(x_3), \tag{12b}$$

$$h_2(x_1, x_2, x_3) = \psi_0(x_1)\psi_1(x_2)\psi_0(x_3), \tag{12c}$$

$$h_3(x_1, x_2, x_3) = \psi_0(x_1)\psi_0(x_2)\psi_1(x_3), \tag{12d}$$

$$\vdots$$

The exponential weighting function gives progressively less importance to more distant points. Indeed, the first component F_0 can be interpreted as a Gaussian weighted grey-value average, the next three components correspond to the Gaussian weighted gradient operator (compare [25]). These are the only components used in matching, since we want the matching to be based on edges which are in turn detected at different resolutions. The similarity function needs to be estimated only for a small neighborhood. In the multiresolution approach at any particular level we attempt to correct only relatively small disparities, which can be smoothed out fast. Larger disparities should be corrected at coarser levels, and smaller disparities at finer levels—they should not be "seen" at that level.

2.2.4. *Multiresolution Elastic Matching Process*

Multiresolution elastic matching was inspired by the contributions to multilevel (multigrid) techniques in numerical mathematics [26], computational vision [27, 28], and multiresolution picture processing [29]. Broadly speaking, multiresolution techniques are a systematic way for structuring local information into global and allowing local and global processes to interact and are associated with various schemes for propagating information, vertically (interlevel communication) and horizontally (intralevel communication), see [19, 30]. The major motivation for using a multiresolution technique, in combination with incremental deformations, is to alleviate the following deficiencies of the one-resolution model:

— the fact that matching is based on local information only,
— the limitation that deformations should be small,
— the computational complexity.

To detect larger differences we cannot simply extend the similarity measure to a larger area since then the similarity function does not have a unique maximum and false matches are very likely to occur. Also, it is difficult and computationally more expensive to apply large deformations and achieve good accuracy at the same time. In multiresolution a coarse level match is obtained first, which is later improved on finer resolution levels. Some limitations for small deformations remain even when the multiresolution technique is applied. As the object undergoes deformations its appearance can change substantially and the similarity functions should be computed from the already deformed object (compare [5, 14]). Thus, the multiresolution approach compensates for local information, while the incremental deformations compensate for large deformations.

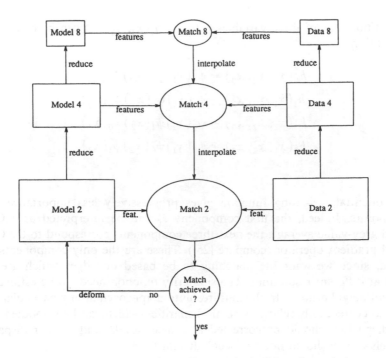

FIG. 1. A multiresolution deformation scheme. Features obtained from the resolution pyramid for the model M and the data D are entered into elastic matcher. Matching starts on a coarse resolution level. The interpolated solution from coarser level is entered as the first approximation to the next finer level. The finest level solution is used to incrementally deform the model until a satisfactory match is achieved.

Figure 1 shows one of the possible multiresolution incremental deformation schemes. Each deformation cycle consists of image reduction, feature extraction, and matching the model with the data by deforming the model. Three reduced resolution images are generated from each of the original 3D images. Each image in sequence is derived from the previous one by a low-pass filtering followed by resampling by a factor of two. From these images, features (projections) are extracted to be passed on to the elastic matcher. Elastic matching is first performed on the coarsest resolution level. The resulting displacements are entered after linear interpolation as initial displacements to the middle resolution level where elastic matching is performed again. The same procedure is repeated on the finest resolution level. The finest level displacements field is used to deform the model. The model is incrementally deformed until a satisfactory match is achieved. Appropriate stopping criteria, such as residual global mismatch $\int |u(x)|\, dx$, are readily available.

3. IMPLEMENTATION AND EXPERIMENTS

Code for elastic matching is written completely in the C Language, and can be installed on an HP 9000 Series 300 or a similar workstation running UNIX. Input to the elastic matching system consists of CT scans of the human brain. The model is a voxel representation of the anatomical brain atlas. The steps involved in the matching process are CT scan preprocessing, preparing the brain atlas for matching,

matching the brain atlas with the CT brain, and overlaying the brain atlas over the CT brain after matching.

3.1. *Preprocessing CT Scans*

We used CT scans of normal subjects obtained from a GE8800 scanner, located at the Hospital of the University of Pennsylvania. Each patient was represented by 22 to 24 slices. Slices were 5 mm apart with a pixel size in the perpendicular slice direction of 0.64×0.64 mm. Pixel grey values varied between 0 and 4095. Pixels representing brain had grey values somewhere between 900 and 1200. The steps involved in preprocessing CT scans are:

—optional low-pass filtering of CT slices before resampling;

—resampling of CT slices from original (0.64×0.64 mm) pixel size to the atlas brain pixel size (1.098×1.098 mm);

—interpolating by linear interpolation additional slices between original slices, which were 5 mm apart to get cubically shaped voxels of size ($1.098 \times 1.098 \times 1.098$ mm);

—selecting an 8-bit grey value window in the original 12-bit range, usually somewhere between 900 and 1200;

—removing the skull to isolate the brain in CT scans;

—optional removal of large calcifications (white spots) if present.

This sequence of steps gives us a 3D image of the patient's brain which is used later in the matching process. The brain isolation, or skull removal, is slice oriented, yet it accounts for 3D connectivity. The isolation proceeds slice-by-slice, starting with the upper-most slice, where the brain area can be easily isolated. The processing of each slice consists of shrinking the brain area, filling in the shrunken brain area, and expanding back the filled brain area to compensate for shrinking. The purpose of shrinking the brain area is to prevent filling algorithm of leaking out of the skull. To start filling, the brain area in the upper (previously) processed slice is used as a "seed". The grey values of pixels representing the brain are not altered in this process. Figure 2 shows the results of that process. Seed-filling technique is used also for removing larger calcifications.

3.2. *The Brain Atlas*

The purpose of the brain atlas is to represent a 3-dimensional model of a healthy human brain. Such an atlas can provide a wealth of information, since geometrical, topological anatomical, metabolic, or any other information, as well as relations among them, can be associated with it.

The anatomy brain atlas formerly used in this work was created in 1976 by Robert Livingston at the University of California, San Diego. A normal human brain was sectioned at narrow intervals (1.098 mm) and the slices were photographed and aligned in the slicing direction. The contours of 45 anatomic structures in the photographs were manually traced and stored on computer tape.

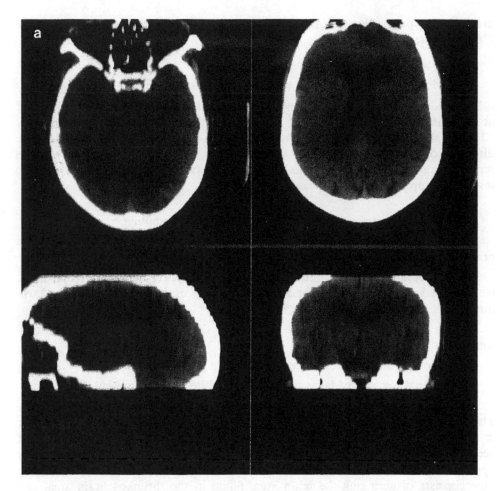

FIG. 2. (a) CT scan before isolating brain. Two horizontal, one sagittal, and one coronal sections are shown. (b) CT scan after isolating brain. Two horizontal, one sagittal, and one coronal sections are shown.

From the atlas any subset of brain structures can be selected. Currently, a more complete new atlas is under development. Having two atlases is also of special value for the development of the matching process. Later in the paper some illustrative matching results between the atlases will be shown.

In our matching process the brain atlas should have the same representational form as the data obtained from the scanners. To obtain a volumetric representation of the brain atlas, the structures delineated by contour lines were "colored" uniformly, using some appropriate grey values. To get cubically shaped voxels, the slicing distance of 1.098 mm was chosen as the voxel size. Figure 3 shows three slices each from horizontal, sagittal, and coronal views, respectively. Only ventricles, brainstem, cerebellum, caudate nucleus, putamen, thalamus, and globus pallidus were the structures chosen from the original brain atlas. Deformations resulting from matching will be ultimately applied on this atlas.

b

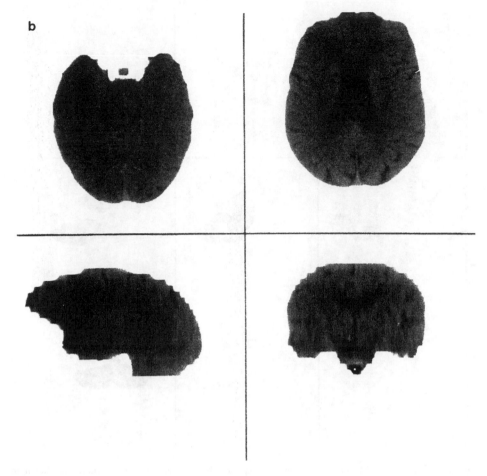

FIG. 2.—*Continued*.

3.3. *Global Matching Example*

After preprocessing of the brain atlas and CT data, global matching (as described in the Appendix) is performed first. Results obtained by a global match of one of the CT brains with the atlas brain are tabulated (see Table 1). Quantities show the number of overlapping and non-overlapping voxels in the atlas brain and in the CT brain. Usually, global matching results in roughly 80% overlap. The most unreliable part of the transformation is rotation. When rotation does not give us a better overlap (or overlap is almost the same), then rotation is not performed.

Figure 4 shows the brain atlas superimposed on the CT brains after global alignment. Three different CT brains were used in this experiment. Unfortunately, the top-most and/or the bottom-most slices in CT scans are often missing, causing problems in global alignment as well as in elastic matching. To compensate for missing slices the superfluous atlas slices were removed.

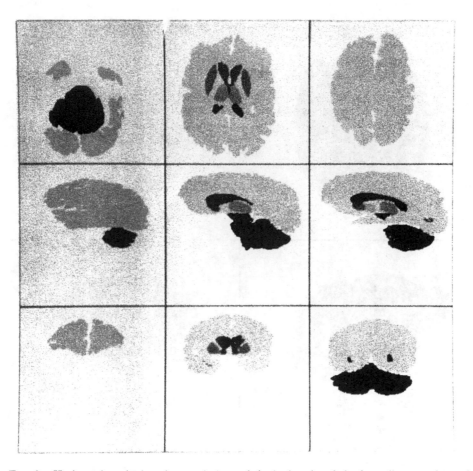

FIG. 3. Horizontal, sagittal, and coronal views of the brain atlas. Only three slices are shown for each view.

3.4. *Elastic Matching Implementation*

3.4.1. *The Features*

In order to perform elastic matching we need reliable information on both the brain atlas and the CT brain. From the brain atlas any subset of well-delineated structures can be used to measure similarity with the CT brain anatomy. Unfortunately, edges of only a very limited number of structures can be detected in the CT brain. So far two matching structures have been used, the outer edge of the brain atlas was matched to the outer edge of the CT brain, and brain atlas ventricles were matched to the CT brain ventricles. Other anatomical structures in the brain atlas are deformed as a side-effect of ventricle and outer edge matching because deformations propagate through the elastic matching process. For matching purposes the atlas brain ventricles and the rest of the brain were colored using an average grey value of the corresponding regions in the real CT brain.

296

TABLE 1

Global Matching Example

	No. of voxels	%
Overlap of CT brain and atlas brain	671158	82.2
Non-overlapped part of atlas brain	74060	9.1
Non-overlapped part of CT brain	70938	8.7
Atlas brain total	745218	
CT brain total	742096	

From the original 3D images three reduced resolution images are generated for the brain atlas as well as for the CT brain. The next coarser image in sequence is derived from the previous one using a $3 \times 3 \times 3$ weighted averaging followed by resampling by a factor of two, resulting in eight times less data. Projections are computed for the three reduced resolution images for each other voxel. A Gaussian-like weighting function in Eq. (10) gives progressively less importance to more

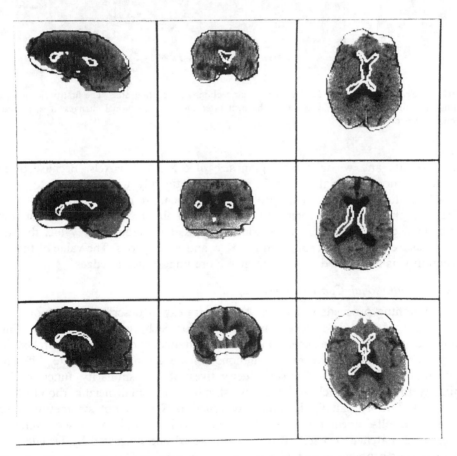

FIG. 4. The brain atlas and the CT brains superimposed after global matching. Each row shows a different CT brain. The brain atlas is represented by contour lines. Shown from left to right are, one section each of sagittal, coronal, and horizontal views.

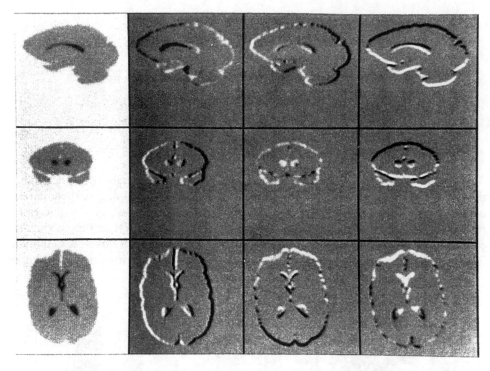

FIG. 5. Features computed for some particular sections of the brain atlas. The first projection (left column) measures the average grey value, the next three measure directional changes in *x*, *y*, and *z* direction, respectively.

distant points and we take the region size of 5 × 5 × 5 voxels. Because of the enormous amount of data it would be computationally too expensive to match original resolution images, hence projections for them are not computed.

Figure 5 shows features computed for one of the fine resolution images for some particular sections. The first projection measures the average grey value, the next three measure directional changes in the *x*, *y*, and *z* directions. The value of the first projection was attenuated in order to give more importance to edges.

3.4.2. *Computational Considerations*

The matching proceeds in a coarse-to-fine strategy as described in Section 2.2.4. The system of Eq. (1) is solved numerically for each resolution level by finite difference approximation using Jacobi's simultaneous displacements relaxation sweeps. Coefficients in the force equations (7) are estimated by finite difference approximation to first and second derivatives of the similarity function. The similarity function at each grid point is estimated in a small neighborhood of size 3 × 3 × 3. Unfortunately, the similarity function $S(u)$ is not symmetric, which introduces a self-deformation effect. Thus, deformations would be present even if an object were matched to itself. This was also noted and corrected by Dengler [15]. We solve that problem in a similar way.

From time to time we expect the similarity function to obtain a minimum. Such situations should be detected and corrected because they would cause convergence problems. When this happens, we set positive eigenvalues of Hessian matrix to a small negative value, making it negative definite.

Most of the computation time in each iteration is spent for computing and recomputing the similarity function. Only the similarity function, not the projections, is recomputed. Recomputation is necessary as long as changes in displacements from iteration to iteration demand it. This happens in the first few iterations. The last iterations take much less computation time and, rather than checking for a stopping condition, the number of iterations is fixed to an empirically derived value of 16. The initial displacements at the coarsest level are set to zero. The solution, i.e., displacements obtained at a coarser level, is entered after a tri-linear interpolation as the first approximation to the next finer level. Corrections computed at each level of resolution are roughly in the range between -1 and $+1$ and can be smoothed out quickly. The grid ratio of $1:2$ is about optimal [31] and the time needed for one iteration on the finer level is comparable to the time spent to obtain the solution on the coarser level. Matching on the original resolution images is not performed. Deformations for them are linearly interpolated in the same way as done whenever a process goes from lower to finer resolution images. The multiresolution approach accelerates and improves the matching substantially, although the accepted scheme is a simple one and does not take full advantage of multigrid techniques [26].

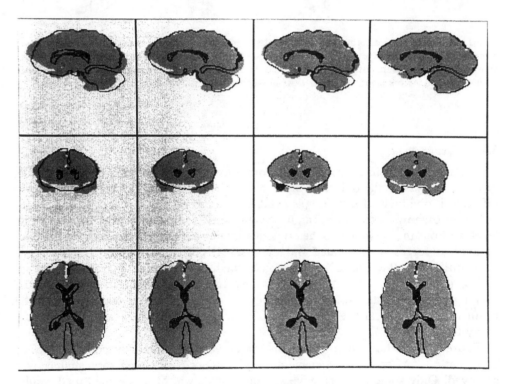

FIG. 6. Matching between two brain atlases using different elastic constants. The deformed atlas is represented by contour lines. The first column shows globally aligned brains, the next three columns show deformation results using elastic constants of eight, four, and one units, respectively. From the top down: one section each of sagittal, coronal, and horizontal views are shown.

299

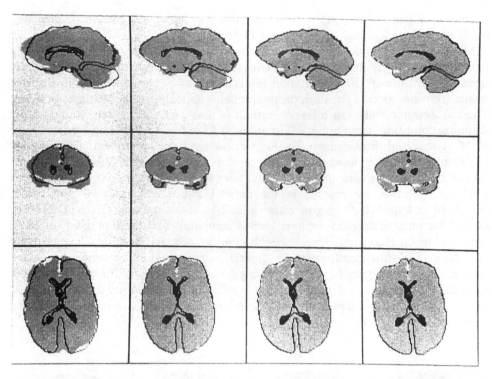

FIG. 7. Incremental deformations with the elastic constant set to two units. The deformed atlas is represented by contour lines. The first column shows globally aligned brains, the next three columns show deformation results after first, second, and third deformations. From the top down: one section each of sagittal, coronal, and horizontal views are shown.

3.4.3. *Experiments*

Matching results in terms of elastic constants are demonstrated for match of the new brain atlas to the old brain atlas. Note that atlases in fact correspond to two different individuals, thus testing is valid. CT preprocessing however, is not needed.

Figure 6 shows some representative sections as computed at the finer resolution level, without interpolation to the original size. For a large elastic constant the effect of applied forces is attenuated and the residual difference between the objects is substantial. As the elastic constant gets smaller, matching in regions with no ambiguity is improved. In atlas-to-atlas matching the noise is not problematic, although some questionable deformations are seen. However, when matching the brain atlas to the real CT data, noise is unavoidable and false matches are more likely to occur.

Figure 7 shows how one of the brain atlases was deformed at successive stages of deformation. After three incremental deformations a satisfactory match was achieved. Only some representative sections are shown. More detailed final results are shown in Fig. 8.

Figure 9 shows the results obtained in matching the brain atlas to three different CT brains. The scanning position and shape of the individual CT brains, as well as

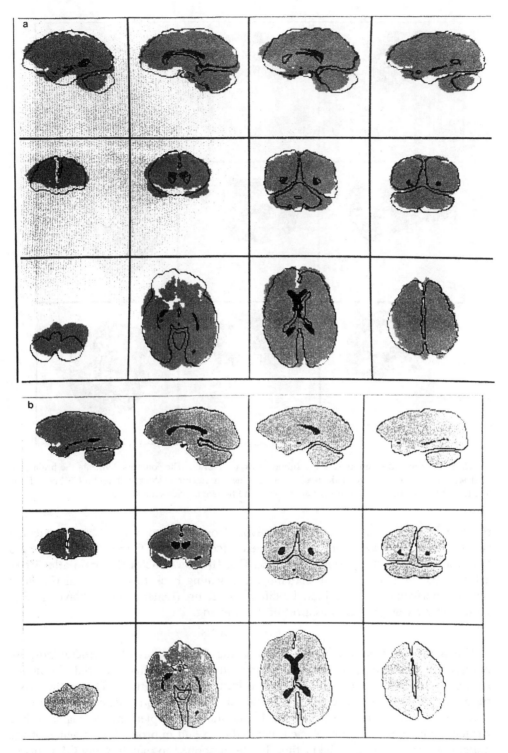

FIG. 8. (a) The two brain atlases superimposed after global alignment: one of them is represented by contour lines, the other by the shaded region. Shown are sagittal, coronal, and horizontal planes, respectively. Only four sections are shown for each view. (b) The two brain atlases superimposed after elastic matching; the deformed atlas is represented by contour lines.

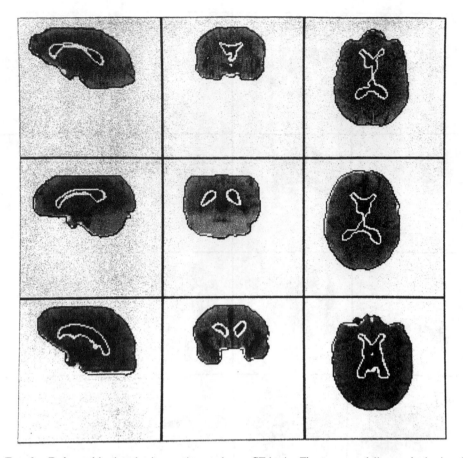

FIG. 9. Deformed brain atlas is superimposed over CT brain. The contours delineate the brain atlas ventricles and the outer edge of the brain after deformation. Each row shows a different CT brain. From left to right: one section each of sagittal, coronal, and horizontal views are shown.

the size of brain ventricles differ noticeably from brain to brain. Elastic matching substantially improves shape correspondence (compare Fig. 9 and 4). Superimposed over the corresponding original CT slice, Fig. 10 shows one of the brain atlas slices after global matching, elastic matching, and scaling back to the original CT pixel size was performed. An additional anatomic structure (thalamus) is displayed in Fig. 10 to show its deformation as a result of matching.

4. CONCLUSIONS

The main contribution of this paper is the development of a general purpose method for matching 3D pictorial information with an explicit pictorial 3D model. It can also serve as a tool for measuring local shape variations. The method uses rigid transformation to account for global misalignment and elastic deformation to account for local shape differences. In addition, it implements a coarse-to-fine strategy, which allows more efficient computation and improves convergence of the matching process. So far, the method has been applied to match X-ray CT scans to the anatomical brain atlas. Matching is performed in three dimensions, rather than on a slice-by-slice basis. In the described experiments we investigated the influence

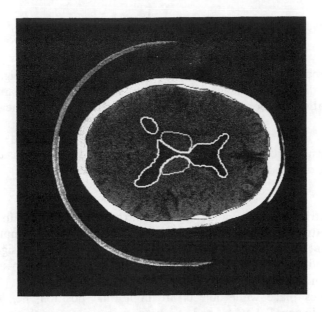

FIG. 10. A brain atlas slice is superimposed over the corresponding original CT slice, after global matching, elastic matching, and scaling up to the original CT pixel size was performed. An additional anatomic structure (thalamus) is displayed to show its deformation as a result of matching.

of the elastic constraints on the matching process. In the future we anticipate that more anatomical structures with different elastic properties will be used in matching and hence elastic constants will be selected locally. We believe that this method can contribute to a more objective interpretation as well as to a quantitative analysis of the anatomical information in CT images. Evaluation of the method is in progress.

We also want to investigate different multiresolution incremental deformation schemes and their convergence behavior, study elastic properties in terms of the regularization theory, make computational improvements by using more advanced multigrid techniques, and integrate global alignment into the cooperative multiresolution process.

APPENDIX: GLOBAL MATCHING

Let us approximate each of two given objects by an ellipsoid-like scatter of particles uniformly distributed in space. The translational difference between the tow objects is eliminated by aligning the centers of mass. For rotational correction the objects are rotated around the center of mass $(\bar{x}_1, \bar{x}_2, \bar{x}_3)$. For that purpose the covariance matrix C is computed:

$$C = [c_{ij}] \qquad (i, j = 1, 2, 3), \qquad (A.1)$$

where

$$c_{ij} = c_{ji} = \frac{1}{N} \sum_{n=1}^{N} (x_{i_n} - \bar{x}_i)(x_{j_n} - \bar{x}_j),$$

and N is the number of particles, i.e., voxels. The covariance matrix C is symmetric and can always be diagonalized by and orthogonal similarity transformation:

$$\Lambda = Q^{-1}CQ = Q^{T}CQ. \qquad (A.2)$$

The transformation matrix Q consists of the orthonormal set of eigenvectors of C. Matrix Λ is diagonal, containing eigenvalues λ_i of C on the main diagonal. An arbitrary rotation of coordinate axes transforms matrix C into a new matrix D:

$$D = RCR^{T}. \qquad (A.3)$$

Of our concern are rotations for which the transformed matrix D is diagonal. Thus, the transpose of Q is the rotation matrix we are interested in:

$$R = Q^{T}. \qquad (A.4)$$

However, matrix Q is not unique due to arbitrary signs and positions of eigenvectors in the matrix. To make matrix Q unique, two additional assumptions are made. First, diagonal elements of the matrix Q should have positive signs in order to prevent reflection. Next, the eigenvectors are positioned in such a way that the object rotation is minimal.

Scaling takes place while objects are in normal position, i.e., the covariance matrices are diagonal. Let Λ_1 and Λ_2 be such matrices for the two objects after rotations R_1 and R_2, respectively. Then scaling a matrix K having k_1, k_2, k_3 in the main diagonal follows from relation (A.5):

$$\lambda_{i_1} = k_i^2 \lambda_{i_2}. \qquad (A.5)$$

We need to change the position of one of the objects, while the position of the other remains unaltered. In this case the overall transformation matrix M for rotation and scaling correction becomes:

$$M = R_1^{-1}KR_2 = R_1^{T}KR_2. \qquad (A.6)$$

Matrix K is the scaling matrix defined before, and rotation matrices R_1 and R_2 are associated with the first and the second object, respectively. To apply the transformation, we usually compute the inverse of matrix M and perform a tri-linear interpolation in the original object position.

Since alignment is based on purely global geometric information which does not (up to some extent) depend on the resolution used, the same matching result can be obtained at a very coarse resolution with substantially less computation. Thus, it can serve as a top level in the multiresolution elastic matching approach.

ACKNOWLEDGMENTS

The authors thank Robert Dann and John Hoford for their active participation in the project. We thank Eleanor Kassab for providing us with CT scans from the Radiology Research Section of the University of Pennsylvania and to Martin Reivich for encouragements and interest in our work. We are grateful to Franc Solina for discussions and generous help.

REFERENCES

1. D. H. Ballard and C. M. Brown, *Computer Vision*, Prentice–Hall, Englewood Cliffs, NJ, 1982.
2. B. Widrow, The rubber mask technique, Part I, *Pattern Recognit.* **5**, No. 3, 1973, 175–211.
3. M. Fischler and R. Elschlager, The representation and matching of pictorial structures, *IEEE Trans. Comput.* **22**, No. 1, 1973, 67–92.

4. D. J. Burr, A dynamic model for image registration, *Comput. Graphics Image Process.* **15**, 1981, 102–112.

5. C. Broit, *Optimal Registration of Deformed Images*, Doctoral dissertation, University of Pennsylvania, Philadelphia, August 1981.

6. R. Bajcsy, R. Lieberson, and M. Reivich, A computerized system for the elastic matching of deformed radiographic images to idealized atlas images, *J. Comput. Assisted Tomography* **5**, 1983, 618–625.

7. S. Schwartz and R. Bajcsy, Three-dimensional elastic matching of ventricles, in *Computer Graphics '85*, the conference of the National Computer Graphics Association, 1985.

8. R. Bajcsy and S. Kovacic, *Toward an Individualized Brain Atlas Elastic Matching*, Technical Report MS-CIS-86-71 GRASP LAB 76, Dept. of Computer and Information Science, University of Pennsylvania, Philadelphia, 1986.

9. F. Bookstein, *The Measurement of Biological Shape and Shape Change*, Lecture Notes in Biomathematics, Vol. 24, Springer-Verlag, New York, 1978.

10. F. Bookstein, B. Chernoff, R. Elder, J. Humphries, G. Smith, and R. Strauss, *Morphometrics in Evolutionary Biology*, The Academy of Natural Sciences, Philadelphia, 1985.

11. D. Terzopoulos, A. Witkin, and M. Kass, Energy constraints on deformable models: Recovering shape and non-rigid motion, in *Proceedings, AAAI 87, Vol. 2*, July 1987, pp. 755–760.

12. D. Terzopoulos, J. Platt, A. Barr, and K. Fleischer, Elastically deformable models, in *Proceedings, SIGGRAPH '87, July 1987*.

13. M. Kass, A. Witkin, and D. Terzopoulos, Snakes: Active contour models, *Int. J. Comput. Vision*, **1**, No. 4, 1988, 321–331.

14. A. Witkin, D. Terzopoulos, and M. Kass, Signal matching through scale space, *Int. J. Comput. Vision*, **1** No. 2, 1987, 133–144.

15. J. Dengler, Local motion estimation with the dynamic pyramid, in *Eighth Int. Conference on Pattern Recognition, Paris*, 1986, 1289–1292.

16. R. Bajcsy and F. Solina, Three-dimensional shape representation revisited, in *Proceedings, First International Conference on Computer Vision, London, England*, June 1987, 231–240.

17. K. Stuben and U. Trottenberg, Multigrid methods: Fundamental algorithms, model problem analysis and applications, in *Multigrid Methods*, Lecture Notes in Mathematics Vol. 960, Springer-Verlag, New York/Berlin, 1982.

18. D. Terzopoulos, Image analysis using multigrid relaxation methods, *IEEE Trans. Pattern Anal. Mach. Intell.*, **PAMI-8**, No. 2, 1986, 129–139.

19. A. Rosenfeld (Ed.), *Multiresolution Image Processing and Analysis*, Springer Series in Information Sciences, Vol. 12, Springer-Verlag, New York/Berlin, 1984.

20. B. K. P. Horn, *Robot Vision*, MIT, Cambridge, MA, 1986.

21. A. Rosenfeld and A. Kak, *Digital Picture Processing*, Academic Press, New York, 1982.

22. I. S. Sokolnikoff, *Mathematical Theory of Elasticity*, McGraw–Hill, New York, 1956.

23. L. E. Scales, *Introduction to Non-Linear Optimization*, Springer-Verlag, New York, 1985.

24. R. Courant and D. Hilbert, *Methods of Mathematical Physics*, Interscience, New York, 1966.

25. R. Hartley, A Gaussian-weighted multiresolution edge detector, *Comput. Vision Graphics, Image Process.*, **30**, No. 1, 1985, 70–83.

26. A. Brandt, Multi-level adaptive techniques for boundary-value problems, *Math. Comput.*, **31**, No. 138, 1977, 333–390.

27. D. Terzopoulos, Multilevel computational processes for visual surface reconstruction, *Comput. Vision Graphics Image Process.*, **24**, No. 1, 1983, 52–96.

28. D. Terzopoulos, *Multiresolution Computation of Visible-Surface Representations*, Doctoral dissertation, MIT, January 1984.

29. P. Burt and T. Adelson, The Laplacian pyramid as a compact image code, *IEEE Trans. Commun.*, **31**, No. 4, 1983, 532–540.

30 W. Hackbusch and U. Trottenberg (Ed.), *Multigrid Methods*, Lecture Notes in Mathematics, Vol. 960, Springer-Verlag, New York, 1982.

31. A. Brandt, Multilevel approaches to large scale problems, survey lecture at *ICM-86, Berkeley, August* 1986.

Tracking Points on Deformable Objects Using Curvature Information*

Isaac COHEN, Nicholas AYACHE, Patrick SULGER

INRIA, Rocquencourt
B.P. 105, 78153 Le Chesnay CEDEX, France.
Email isaac@bora.inria.fr, na@bora.inria.fr.

Abstract

The objective of this paper is to present a significant improvement to the approach of Duncan et al. [1, 8] to analyze the deformations of curves in sequences of 2D images. This approach is based on the paradigm that high curvature points usually possess an anatomical meaning, and are therefore good landmarks to guide the matching process, especially in the absence of a reliable physical or deformable geometric model of the observed structures.

As Duncan's team, we therefore propose a method based on the minimisation of an energy which tends to preserve the matching of high curvature points, while ensuring a smooth field of displacement vectors everywhere.

The innovation of our work stems from the explicit description of the mapping between the curves to be matched, which ensures that the resulting displacement vectors actually map points belonging to the two curves, which was not the case in Duncan's approach.

We have actually implemented the method in 2-D and we present the results of the tracking of a heart structure in a sequence of ultrasound images.

1 Introduction

Non-rigid motion of deformable shapes is becoming an increasingly important topic in computer vision, especially for medical image analysis. Within this topic, we concentrate on the problem of tracking deformable objects through a time sequence of images.

The objective of our work is to improve the approach of Duncan et al. [1, 8] to analyze the deformations of curves in sequences of 2D images. This approach is based on the paradigm that high curvature points usually possess an anatomical meaning, and are therefore good landmarks to guide the matching process. This is the case for instance when deforming patients skulls (see for instance [7, 9]), or when matching patient faces taken at different ages, when matching multipatients faces, or when analyzing images of a beating heart. In these cases, many lines of extremal curvatures (or ridges) are stable features which can be reliably tracked between the images (on a face they will correspond to the nose, chin and eyebrows ridges for instance, on a skull to the orbital, sphenoid, falx, and temporal ridges, on a heart ventricle to the papillary muscle etc...).

As Duncan's team, we therefore propose a method based on the minimisation of an energy which tends to preserve the matching of high curvature points, while ensuring a smooth field of displacement vectors everywhere.

The innovation of our work stems from the explicit description of the mapping between the curves to be matched, which ensures that the resulting displacement vectors actually

---

* This work was partially supported by Digital Equipment Corporation.

306

map points belonging to the two curves, which was not the case in Duncan's approach. Moreover, the energy minimization is obtained through the mathematical framework of Finite Element analysis, which provides a rigorous and efficient numerical solution. This formulation can be easily generalized in 3-D to analyze the deformations of surfaces.

Our approach is particularly attractive in the absence of a reliable physical or deformable geometric model of the observed structures, which is often the case when studying medical images. When such a model is available, other approaches would involve a parametrization of the observed shapes [14], a modal analysis of the displacement field [12], or a parametrization of a subset of deformations [3, 15]. In fact we believe that our approach can always be used when some sparse geometric features provide reliable landmarks, either as a preprocessing to provide an initial solution to the other approaches, or as a post-processing to provide a final smoothing which preserves the matching of reliable landmarks.

2 Modelling the Problem

Let C_P and C_Q be two boundaries of the image sequence, the contour C_Q is obtained by a non rigid (or elastic) transformation of the contour C_P. The curves C_P and C_Q are parameterized by $P(s)$ and $Q(s')$ respectively.

The problem is to determine for each point P on C_P a corresponding point Q on C_Q. For doing this, we must define a similarity measure which will compare locally the neighborhoods of P and Q.

As explained in the introduction, we assume that points of high curvature correspond to stable salient regions, and are therefore good landmarks to guide the matching of the curves. Moreover, we can assume as a first order approximation, that the curvature itself remains invariant in these regions. Therefore, we can introduce an energy measure in these regions of the form:

$$E_{curve} = \frac{1}{2} \int_{\delta S} \left(K_Q(s') - K_P(s) \right)^2 ds \qquad (1)$$

where K_P and K_Q denote the curvatures and s, s' parameterize the curves C_P and C_Q respectively. In fact, as shown by [8, 13], this is proportional to the energy of deformation of an isotropic elastic planar curve.

We also wish the displacement field to vary smoothly around the curve, in particular to insure a correspondence for points lying between two salient regions. Consequently we consider the following functional (similar to the one used by Hildreth to smooth a vector flow field along a contour [11]) :

$$E = E_{curve} + R \, E_{regular} \qquad (2)$$

where

$$E_{regular} = \int_{C_P} \left\| \frac{\partial (Q(s') - P(s))}{\partial s} \right\|^2 ds$$

measures the variation of the displacement vector **PQ** along the curve C_P, and the $\|.\|$ denotes the norm associated to the euclidean scalar product $\langle .,. \rangle$ in the space $\mathbb{R}^2$.

The regularization parameter $R(s)$ depends on the shape of the curve C_P. Typically, R is inversely proportional to the curvature at P, to give a larger weight to E_{curve} in salient regions and conversely to $E_{regular}$ to points inbetween. This is done continuously without annihiling totally the weight of any of these two energies (see [4]) .

3 Mathematical Formulation of the Problem

Given two curves C_P and C_Q parameterized by $s \in [0, 1]$ and $s' \in [0, \alpha]$ (where α is the length of the curve C_Q), we have to determine a function $f : [0, 1] \to [0, \alpha]$; $s \to s'$ satisfying

$$f(0) = 0 \quad \text{and} \quad f(1) = \alpha \tag{3}$$

and

$$f = ArgMin(E(f)) \tag{4}$$

where

$$E(f) = \int_{C_P} (K_Q(f(s)) - K_P(s))^2 \, ds + R \int_{C_P} \left\| \frac{\partial(Q(f(s)) - P(s))}{\partial s} \right\|^2 ds \tag{5}$$

The condition (3) means that the displacement vector is known for one point of the curve. In the model above defined we assumed that:

- the boundaries have already been extracted,
- the curvatures K are known on the pair of contours (see [9]).

These necessary data are obtained by preprocessing the image sequence (see for more details [4]).

The characterization of a function f satisfying $f = ArgMin(E(f))$ and the condition (3) is performed by a variational method. This method characterizes a local minimum f of the functional $E(f)$ as the solution of the Euler-Lagrange equation $\nabla E(f) = 0$, leading to the solution of the partial differential equation:

$$\begin{cases} f'' \|Q'(f)\|^2 + K_P \langle N_P, Q'(f) \rangle + \frac{1}{R} [K_P - K_Q(f)] K'_Q(f) = 0 \\ + \text{ Boundary conditions (i.e. condition 3).} \end{cases} \tag{6}$$

where Q is a parametrization of the curve C_Q, $Q'(f)$ the tangent vector of C_Q, K'_Q the derivative of the curvature of the curve C_Q and N_P is the normal vector to the curve C_P.

The term $\int_{C_P} (K_Q(f(s)) - K_P(s))^2 \, ds$ measures the difference between the curvature of the two curves. This induces a non convexity of the functional E. Consequently, solving the partial differential equation (6) will give us a local minimum of E. To overcome this problem we will assume that we have an initial estimation f_0 which is a good approximation of the real solution (the definition of the initial estimation f_0 will be explained later). This initial estimation defines a starting point for the search of a local minimum of the functional E. To take into account this initial estimation we consider the associated evolution equation:

$$\begin{cases} \frac{\partial f(s)}{\partial t} + f''(s) \|Q'(f(s))\|^2 + K_P(s) \langle N_P(s), Q'(f(s)) \rangle + \frac{1}{R} [K_P(s) - K_Q(f(s))] K'_Q(f(s)) = 0 \\ f(0, s) = f_0(s) \text{ Initial estimation.} \end{cases} \tag{7}$$

Equation (7) can also be seen as a gradient descent algorithm toward a minimum of the energy E, it is solved by a finite element method and leads to the solution of a sparse linear system (see for more details [4]).

3.1 Determining the Initial Estimation f_0

The definition of the initial estimation f_0 has an effect upon the convergence of the algorithm. Consequently a good estimation of the solution f will lead to a fast convergence. The definition of f_0 is based on the work of Duncan *et al* [8]. The method is as follows:

Let $s_i \in [0, 1]$, $i = 1 \ldots n$ be a subdivision of the interval $[0, 1]$. For every point $P_i = (X(s_i), Y(s_i))$ of the curve C_P we search for a point $Q_i = (X(s'_i), Y(s'_i))$ on the curve C_Q, and the function f_0 is then defined by $f_0(s_i) = s'_i$.

For doing so we have to define a pair of points P_0, Q_0 which correspond to each other. But, first of all, let us describe the search method. In the following, we identify a point and its arc length (*i.e.* the point s_i denotes the point P_i of the curve C_P such that $P(s_i) = P_i$, where P is the parametrization of the curve C_P).

For each point s_i of C_P we associate a set of candidates S_i on the curve C_Q. The set S_i defines the search area. This set is defined by the point s' which is the nearest distance point to s_i belonging to the curve C_Q, along with $(N_{search} - 1)/2$ points of the curve C_Q on each side of s' (where N_{search} is a given integer defining the length of the search area).

Among these candidates, we choose the point which minimizes the deformation energy (1).

In some situations this method fails, and the obtained estimation f_0 is meaningless, leading to a bad solution. Figure 1 shows an example where the method described in [8] fails. This is due to the bad computation of the search area S_i.

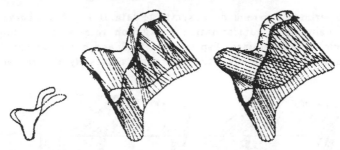

Fig. 1. This example shows the problem that can occur in the computation of the initial estimate based only on the search in a given area. The initial estimation of the displacement field and the obtained solution.

To compute more accurately this set, we have added a criterion based on the arc length. Consequently, the set defining the search area S_i is defined by the point s' which is the nearest distance point to s_i belonging to the curve C_Q such that $s'_i \approx s_i/\alpha$, along with $(N_{search} - 1)/2$ points of the curve C_Q on each side of s'_i. Figure 2 illustrates the use of this new definition of the set S_i for the same curves given in Fig. 1. This example shows the ability to handle more general situations with this new definition of the search area S_i.

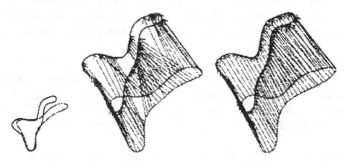

Fig. 2. In the same case of the previous example, the computation of the initial estimate based on the local search and the curvilinear abscissa, gives a good estimation f_0, which leads to an accurate computation of the displacement function.

As noted above, the search area S_i can be defined only if we have already chosen a point P_0 and its corresponding point Q_0. The most salient features in a temporal sequence undergo small deformations at each time step, thus a good method for choosing the point P_0 is to take the most distinctive point so that the search for the corresponding point becomes a trivial task. Consequently the point P_0 is chosen among the points of C_P with maximal curvature. In many cases this method provides a unique point P_0. Once we have chosen the point P_0, the point Q_0 is found by the local search described above.

4 Experimental Results

The method was tested on a set of synthetic and real image sequences. The results are given by specifying at each discretization point P_i $i = 1\ldots N$ of the curve C_P the displacement vector $\mathbf{u_i} = \mathbf{P_i Q_i}$. At each point P_i the arrow represents the displacement vector $\mathbf{u_i}$.

The first experiments were made on synthetic data. In Fig. 3, the curve C_Q (a square) is obtained by a similarity transformation (translation, rotation and scaling) of the curve C_P (a rectangle). The obtained displacement field and a plot of the function f are given. We can note that the algorithm computes accurately the displacements of the

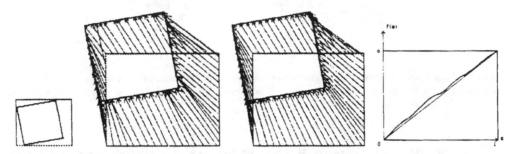

Fig. 3. The rectangle (in grey) is deformed by a similarity (translation, rotation and scaling) to obtain the black square. In this figure we represent the initial estimation of the displacement vector of the curves, the obtained displacement field and the plotting of the solution f.

four corners. This result was expected since the curves C_P and C_Q have salient features which help the algorithm to compute accurately the displacement vector $\mathbf{u_i}$. Figure 4 give an example of the tracking of each point on an ellipse deformed by a similarity. In this case, the points of high curvature are matched together although the curvature varies smoothly.

As described in section (3.1) the computation of the initial estimation is crucial. In the following experimentation we have tried to define the maximal error that can be done on the estimation of f_0 without disturbing the final result. In Fig. 5 we have added a gaussian noise ($\sigma = 0.05$) to a solution f obtained by solving (7). This noisy function was taken as an initial estimation for Eq. 7. After a few iterations the solution f is recovered (5).

It appears that if $|f - f_0| \leq 4h$ (where h is the space discretization step), starting with f_0 the iterative scheme 7 will converge toward the solution f. The inequality $|f - f_0| \leq 4h$ means that for each point P on the curve C_P the corresponding point Q can be determined with an error of 4 points over the grid of the curve Q.

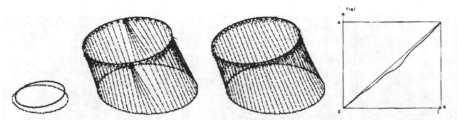

Fig. 4. Another synthetic example, in this case the curvature along the curves C_P and C_Q varies smoothly. This often produces as a consequence in the computation of the initial estimation f_0 that several points of the curve C_P (in grey) match the same point of C_Q (in black). We remark that, for the optimal solution obtained by the algorithm, each point of the black curve matches a single point of the grey curve, and that, maximum curvature points are matched together.

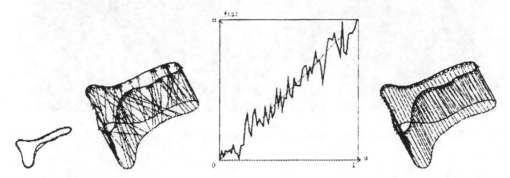

Fig. 5. In this example we have corrupted an obtained solution with a gaussian noise ($\sigma = 0.05$) and considered this corrupted solution as an initial estimate f_0. The initial displacement field, the initial estimate f_0 and the obtained solution are shown in this figure.

The tracking of the moving boundaries of the valve of the left ventricle on an ultrasound image helps to diagnose some heart diseases. The segmentation of the moving boundaries over the whole sequence was done by the snake model [6, 2, 10]. In Fig 6 a global tracking of a part of the image sequence is showed[2]. This set of curves are processed (as described in [4]) to obtain the curvatures and the normal vector of the curves. The Fig. 7 shows a temporal tracking of some points of the valve in this image sequence. The results are presented by pairs of successive contours. One can visualize that the results meet perfectly the objectives of preserving the matching of high curvature points while insuring a smooth displacement field.

---

[2] Courtesy of I. Herlin [10]

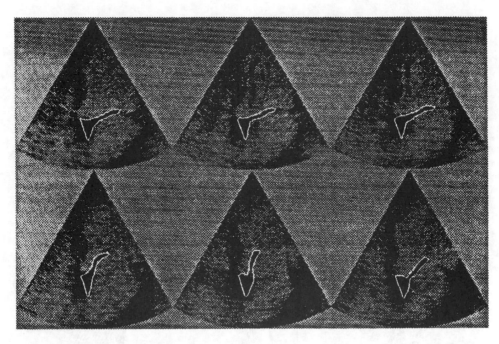

Fig. 6. Temporal tracking of the mitral valve, obtained by the snake model [10], for images 1 to 6.

5 3-D Generalization

In this section we give a 3-D generalization of the algorithm described in the previous sections. In 3-D imaging we must track points on located surfaces, since the objects boundaries are surfaces (as in [1]). In [16] the authors have shown on a set of experimental data, that the extrema of the larger principal curvature often correspond to significant intrinsic (i.e. invariant by the group of rigid transformation) features which might characterize the surface structure, even in the presence of small anatomic deformations.

Let S_P and S_Q be two surfaces parameterized by $P(s,r)$ and $Q(s',r')$, and let κ_P denote the larger value of the principal curvature of the surface S_P at point P.

Thus the matching of two surfaces, leads to the following problem:
find a function

$$f : \ \mathbb{R}^2 \rightarrow \mathbb{R}^2; \quad (s,r) \mapsto (s',r')$$

which minimizes the functional:

$$E(f) = \int_{S_P} \left(\kappa_Q(f(s,r)) - \kappa_P(s,r)\right)^2 ds\,dr$$

$$+ R_s \int_{S_P} \left\| \frac{\partial(Q(f(s,r)) - P(s,r))}{\partial s} \right\|^2 ds\,dr + R_r \int_{S_P} \left\| \frac{\partial(Q(f(s,r)) - P(s,r))}{\partial r} \right\|^2 ds\,dr$$

where $\|.\|$ denotes the euclidean norm in $\mathbb{R}^3$. Its resolution by a finite element method can be done as in [5], and the results should be compared to those obtained by [1]. This generalization has not been implemented yet.

312

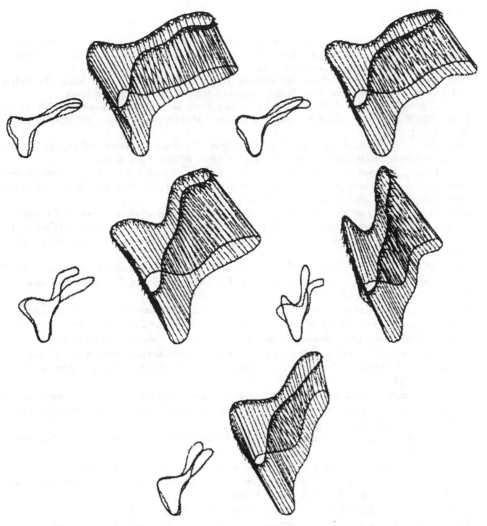

Fig. 7. Applying the point - tracking algorithm to the successive pairs of contours of Fig. 6 (from left to right and top to bottom).

6 Conclusion

We presented a significant improvement to Duncan's team approach to track the motion of deformable 2D shapes, based on the tracking of high curvature points while preserving the smoothness of the displacement field. This approach is an alternative to the other approaches of the literature, when no physical or geometric model is available, and can also be used as a complementary approach otherwise.

The results on a real sequence of time varying anatomical structure of the beating heart perfectly met the defined objectives [2]. Future work will include the experimentation of the 3-D generalization.

References

1. A. Amini, R. Owen, L. Staib, P. Anandan, and J. Duncan. *non-rigid motion models for tracking the left ventricular wall.* Lecture notes in computer science: Information processing in medical images. 1991. Springer-Verlag.

2. Nicholas Ayache, Isaac Cohen, and Isabelle Herlin. Medical image tracking. In *Active Vision*, Andrew Blake and Alan Yuille, chapter 20. MIT Press, 1992. In press.

3. Fred L. Bookstein. Principal warps: Thin-plate splines and the decomposition of deformations. *IEEE Transactions on Pattern Analysis and Machine Intelligence*, PAMI-11(6):567–585, June 1989.

4. Isaac Cohen, Nicholas Ayache, and Patrick Sulger. Tracking points on deformable objects using curvature information. Technical Report 1595, INRIA, March 1992.

5. Isaac Cohen, Laurent D. Cohen, and Nicholas Ayache. Using deformable surfaces to segment 3-D images and infer differential structures. *Computer Vision, Graphics, and Image Processing: Image Understanding*, 1992. In press.

6. Laurent D. Cohen and Isaac Cohen. A finite element method applied to new active contour models and 3-D reconstruction from cross sections. In *Proc. Third International Conference on Computer Vision*, pages 587–591. IEEE Computer Society Conference, December 1990. Osaka, Japan.

7. Court B. Cutting. Applications of computer graphics to the evaluation and treatment of major craniofacial malformation. In Jayaram K.Udupa and Gabor T. Herman, editors, *3-D Imaging in Medicine*. CRC Press, 1989.

8. J.S. Duncan, R.L. Owen, L.H. Staib, and P. Anandan. Measurement of non-rigid motion using contour shape descriptors. In *Proc. Computer Vision and Pattern Recognition*, pages 318–324. IEEE Computer Society Conference, June 1991. Lahaina, Maui, Hawaii.

9. A. Guéziec and N. Ayache. Smoothing and matching of 3D-space curves. In *Proceedings of the Second European Conference on Computer Vision 1992*, Santa Margherita Ligure, Italy, May 1992.

10. I.L. Herlin and N. Ayache. Features extraction and analysis methods for sequences of ultrasound images. In *Proceedings of the Second European Conference on Computer Vision 1992*, Santa Margherita Ligure, Italy, May 1992.

11. Ellen Catherine Hildreth. *The Measurement of Visual Motion*. The MIT Press, Cambridge, Massachusetts, 1984.

12. Bradley Horowitz and Alex Pentland. Recovery of non-rigid motion and structures. In *Proc. Computer Vision and Pattern Recognition*, pages 325–330. IEEE Computer Society Conference, June 1991. Lahaina, Maui, Hawaii.

13. L.D. Landau and E.M. Lifshitz. *Theory of elasticity*. Pergamon Press, Oxford, 1986.

14. Dimitri Metaxas and Demetri Terzopoulos. Constrained deformable superquadrics and nonrigid motion tracking. In *Proc. Computer Vision and Pattern Recognition*, pages 337–343. IEEE Computer Society Conference, June 1991. Lahaina, Maui, Hawaii.

15. Sanjoy K. Mishra, Dmitry B. Goldgof, and Thomas S. Huang. Motion analysis and epicardial deformation estimation from angiography data. In *Proc. Computer Vision and Pattern Recognition*, pages 331–336. IEEE Computer Society Conference, June 1991. Lahaina, Maui, Hawaii.

16. O. Monga, N. Ayache, and P. Sander. From voxel to curvature. In *Proc. Computer Vision and Pattern Recognition*, pages 644–649. IEEE Computer Society Conference, June 1991. Lahaina, Maui, Hawaii.

Automatic Tracking of SPAMM Grid and the Estimation of Deformation Parameters from Cardiac MR Images

Senthil Kumar and Dmitry Goldgof, *Member, IEEE*

Abstract—In this paper, we present a new approach for the automatic tracking of SPAMM (Spatial Modulation of Magnetization) grid in cardiac MR images and consequent estimation of deformation parameters. The tracking is utilized to extract grid points from MR images and to establish correspondences between grid points in images taken at consecutive frames. These correspondences are used with a thin plate spline model to establish a mapping from one image to the next. This mapping is then used for motion and deformation estimation. Spatio-temporal tracking of SPAMM grid is achieved by using snakes—active contour models with an associated energy functional. We present a minimizing strategy which is suitable for tracking the SPAMM grid. By continuously minimizing their energy functionals, the snakes lock on to and follow the in-slice motion and deformation of the SPAMM grid. The proposed algorithm was tested with excellent results on 123 images (three data sets each a multiple slice 2D, 16 phase Cine study, three data sets each a multiple slice 2D, 13 phase Cine study and three data sets each a multiple slice 2D, 12 phase Cine study).

I. Introduction

A COMMON APPROACH to motion and deformation estimation is to identify feature points from images taken at two different times and then to establish the correspondence between these feature points. Feature points are usually extracted by some low level image processing algorithm such as corner detection and then, correspondences are established between features obtained at different time instances. In this paper, we provide a method for tracking the spatio-temporal motion and deformation of SPAMM grid in MR images [3]. This tracking can viewed as a mechanism for extracting feature points in MR images and establishing correspondences between them. With this new method, once the features are detected, point correspondences are automatically known. No explicit step is necessary for the matching of corresponding points.

MR Imaging with Spatial Modulation of Magnetization (SPAMM) [2]–[4] is a technique in which regions of the heart wall are tagged so that their motion can be followed in subsequent images. The tagging is done by producing localized

Manuscript received November 25, 1992; revised August 31, 1993. This work was supported in part by SUN and BRSG grant from USF, in part by a grant from Siemens, and in part by the grant from the Whitaker Foundation. The associate editor responsible for coordinating the review of this paper and recommending its publication was E. M. Haacke.

The authors are with the Center for Engineering and Medical Image Analysis (CEMIA), Department of Computer Science and Engineering, University of South Florida, Tampa FL 33620.

IEEE Log Number 9215319D.

regions of altered magnetization. The generation of magnetic saturation in a thin sheet perpendicular to the imaging plane will result in the appearance of a dark band (corresponding to the intersection of the saturated sheet with the imaging plane) in subsequent images acquired in times on the order of or less than the longitudinal relaxation time, $T1$. This altered magnetization is a property of the tissue and will move with it. Therefore, any motion of the tissue will be reflected in a corresponding displacement of the dark band in the images.

The use of SPAMM can simultaneously produce parallel families of such tagging bands. Two sequential applications of SPAMM in orthogonal orientations produce a tagging grid. This grid has a set of parallel lines in one direction and another set of parallel lines in the perpendicular direction. The grid lines are typically two pixels wide with a interline spacing of five pixels (Fig. 2). As the grid undergoes motion and deformation from one time frame to next, the intersection points of these lines can be used as markers for establishing point correspondences. In MR images obtained with the SPAMM technique, the magnetically tagged points can function as noninvasive fiducial markers, and their motion can be quantitatively analyzed like the motion of invasively implanted markers [10], [17], [16], [21]. Further, the drawbacks of the invasive techniques, namely, the mechanical alteration of the cardiac motion due to the implanted markers and the practical limitations to the number of markers that can be implanted, are absent in the SPAMM technique.

Once point correspondences are established, the motion and deformation parameters can be estimated by total least squares estimation [8]. For example, for every set of four point correspondences, we can use the total least squares technique to determine the deformation parameters for the region enclosed by those four points. But, since SPAMM technique provides a somewhat sparse set of intersection points and since the region enclosed by any set of four points is fairly large, the deformation estimates based on these intersection points alone may not be precise enough. Therefore, we first compute a mapping from one image to the next using the intersection points. This mapping is achieved using a thin plate spline model [6] as an interpolant. With this mapping we can take an arbitrary point in one image and find its corresponding point in the next image. Such correspondences are then used to estimate the deformation parameters of arbitrarily small region.

Reprinted from *IEEE Trans. Medical Imaging,* Vol. 13, No. 1, Mar. 1994, pp. 122–132.

Point correspondences can be obtained from the SPAMM data by tracking the spatio-temporal movement of the grid from one time frame to the next. Axel et al. [4] have analyzed the regional heart wall motion by manually tracking these intersection points. According to them, "Two dimensional analysis of a typical subject as mentioned above [in their paper] takes a few hours. Most of this time involves the interactive measurement of grid intersection locations; the actual calculation of the motion variables can be performed quickly." The need for a fast automated tracking technique is rather obvious. Edge detection and edge tracking from one time frame to the next is not very suitable for the SPAMM data due to the inherent poor localization properties of edge detectors. For example, while the grid lines are two pixels wide, Canny's edge detector [7] gives two edges separated by a distance of one pixel. Further, matching the corresponding points is by no means easy.

Prince and McVeigh [18] have proposed an algorithm for tracking the SPAMM grid using optical flow. In standard optical flow (SOF) technique, the time derivative of brightness of the material point under consideration is assumed to be zero. But in SPAMM-MR data, the SPAMM grid fades away with time. Prince and McVeigh develop a new equation called the *variable brightness optical flow (VBOF) equation* which takes into account the variation in intensity of the SPAMM grid with time. The VBOF equation is very similar to the SOF equation except that it has an additional term that describes the time rate of change of intensity. This equation is then solved using the regularization approach of Horn and Schunck [11]. Solving this equation requires estimates of the time derivative of brightness and these estimates are obtained from the MR imaging equation [20], which describes the time variation of the intensity of the image of a material point in terms of the longitudinal relaxation time T_1, the transverse relaxation time T_2 and the spin density D_0. Consequently, this approach requires that the MR parameters over the entire field of view be accurately known or measured. This is one drawback of this approach. Another drawback, as discussed in [18], is that the positional estimates given by VBOF are dependent on the previous estimates and hence the performance degrades with each new image.

Another approach to tracking the grid is given by McVeigh and Zerhouni [15]. In this approach, to track a single grid line, the user first zooms in on the desired region and places certain seed points on the grid line with the help of a mouse. A third-order polynomial is then fit through these points. After this, at each point of the polynomial curve, a search for the exact center of the grid line is conducted in a direction perpendicular to the curve. This is done as follows. The grid line's profile was found to fit very well with a Gaussian curve model. Therefore, seven points are sampled along the perpendicular line and fit to the Gaussian model of the profile. The mean of the Gaussian gives the center of the grid line. This procedure is repeated at all points along the polynomial. The centers computed are used as new seeds and the whole procedure is repeated until convergence. This technique requires user interaction and is certainly time consuming. In this paper we propose a new method which requires only minimal user interaction and minimal *a priori* knowledge of the MR data.

In our approach, we follow the spatio-temporal motion of the SPAMM grid by using active contours which are commonly known as snakes. Some preliminary results were presented in [13]. We give a brief overview of snakes in Section II. In Section III, we discuss energy measures for snakes that are suitable for MR SPAMM data and we also discuss our minimization algorithm. In Section IV, we compute a mapping from one image to the next using the thin-plate spline model. Section V discusses the estimation of deformation parameters and Section VI discusses the accuracy of the tracking algorithm and the thin-plate spline interpolant. Section VII provides some conclusions.

II. SNAKES

A snake [12] is an energy-minimizing spline guided by external forces and influenced by image forces that pull it towards features such as lines and edges. Snakes are active contour models which lock on to nearby edges localizing them accurately. Kass, Witkin, and Terzopoulos [12] define an energy functional for the contour and determine the minimum energy contour using variational calculus. Williams and Shah [23] provide a fast greedy algorithm for finding the minimum energy contour. They define the energy of the snake as

$$\mathbf{E} = \int (\alpha(s)E_{\text{cont}}(s) + \beta(s)E_{\text{curv}}(s) + \gamma(s)E_{\text{img}}(s))ds \quad (1)$$

Here s denotes the arc-length along the snake, the energy term E_{cont} denotes a first-order continuity constraint and is given by

$$E_{\text{cont}} = \left| \overline{d} - \|\mathbf{v}_i - \mathbf{v}_{i-1}\| \right| \quad (2)$$

where $\mathbf{v}_i$ denotes the coordinates of the ith snaxel[1], $\|\mathbf{v}_i - \mathbf{v}_{i-1}\|$ denotes the distance between $\mathbf{v}_i$ and $\mathbf{v}_{i+1}$ and $\overline{d}$ denotes the average distance between neighbors. Minimizing this term forces the snaxels to be uniformly spaced. The second term E_{curv} is the curvature energy and is defined as

$$E_{\text{curv}} = \left\| \frac{\mathbf{u}_{i+1}}{\|\mathbf{u}_{i+1}\|} - \frac{\mathbf{u}_i}{\|\mathbf{u}_i\|} \right\|^2 \quad (3)$$

Here $\mathbf{u}_i = \mathbf{v}_i - \mathbf{v}_{i-1}$ and $\frac{\mathbf{u}_i}{\|\mathbf{u}_i\|}$ is a discreet approximation unit tangent at $\mathbf{u}_{i-1}$.

The third term E_{img} is the image energy and is set equal to the negative of either gradient magnitude or intensity. Minimizing this term would cause the snake to seek points of maximum gradient or maximum intensity respectively. All the three energy terms must be scaled to lie in the same range.

In Williams and Shah [23], a greedy iterative algorithm is presented in which each snaxel is moved to a new point in its neighborhood whose energy is a minimum relative to other points in the neighborhood. The algorithm terminates when the number of points moved becomes less than a preset threshold.

The above algorithm is not readily applicable to MR SPAMM data and has to be modified to suit the MR SPAMM data. We provide suitable energy measures and discuss a minimization algorithm in the next section.

---

[1] Following [14], we will refer to the snake points as snaxels.

316

III. Energy Measures and Minimization

The parallel and perpendicular lines that make up the SPAMM grid are typically two pixels wide. If we use a snake of pixel width one to track a grid line, the snake may choose either of these two pixels leading to a zig-zag snake. This problem is avoided by using thick snakes.

A thick snake has a width of two pixels. Each line of the grid is tracked by a thick snake which consists of a sequence of pairs of pixels. Each pair lies along the width of the grid line. The pixels forming a pair move together, always maintaining their relative positions. An initial approximate position for the snakes is obtained by template matching. Minimization of the energy of each snake makes the snake to lock on to the grid lines and move with them. The new energy measures for the thick snake are given below.

A. Image Energy

The image energy term is modified so that the snakes track the grid lines faithfully. Specifically, for the current pair of snaxels, E_{img} is defined as the product of the image intensities at the two snaxels. Minimizing this term would cause the snakes to seek pairs of adjacent pixels with minimum intensity. Since the grid is the darkest object in the MR SPAMM image, this would make the snakes to seek the lines of the grid. Also, since the search is always done for pairs of pixels of minimum intensity, the tracking is relatively immune to noise.

The continuity and curvature terms are modified as given below and are computed for the upper element of each pair.

B. Continuity and Curvature Energies

The purpose of the continuity term is to provide a uniform spacing between the snaxels and the purpose of the curvature term is to provide a smooth contour for the snake. For the curvature term we use the same formulation as given in [23]. Since the thick snake consists of two parallel rows of snaxels, we can use either of these rows in the computation of curvature and continuity energies. Therefore, in what follows, we will talk about only one of these rows.

It is worth mentioning that the curvature measure as given by (3) performs better than the one given by Kass *et. al.* [12]. The curvature measure given in [12] is

$$E_{curv} = \|\mathbf{v}_{i-1} - 2\mathbf{v}_i + \mathbf{v}_{i+1}\|^2 \qquad (4)$$

The basic definition of curvature is $\kappa = |\frac{d\tau}{ds}|$ where τ is the unit tangent and s is the arc length. Equation (3) approximates κ as the difference of two unit tangents whereas (4) approximates κ as the difference of two tangents. Therefore, (3) is a better approximation of κ when the distance between the snaxels is not unity.

The continuity measure as given by (2) guarantees that $snaxel_i$ does not get too close to or too far away from $snaxel_{i-1}$. While this measure is suitable for the original algorithm of Kass et. al. [12] where the energy is integrated over the length of the snake, it is not appropriate for the greedy algorithm. This is due to the local nature of the greedy algorithm and the fact that this energy measure does not concern itself with the distance between $snaxel_i$ and $snaxel_{i+1}$.

$Snaxel_i$ can move anywhere on a circle of radius $\bar{d}$ centered about $snaxel_{i-1}$ without changing the continuity energy. In fact it can move to the other side of $snaxel_{i-1}$ changing the ordering of the snaxels from $snaxel_{i-1} \rightarrow snaxel_i \rightarrow snaxel_{i+1}$ to $snaxel_i \rightarrow snaxel_{i-1} \rightarrow snaxel_{i+1}$. $Snaxel_{i+1}$, in trying to minimize its energy, will move close to the other two snaxels and this will cause a pile up of snaxels in a way some what similar to that in the original algorithm by Kass et. al. [12, 1]. So, for the continuity measure, we bring in another term which takes into account the distance between $snaxel_i$ and $snaxel_{i+1}$. We define the continuity energy to be

$$E_{cont} = \left|\bar{d} - \|\mathbf{v}_i - \mathbf{v}_{i-1}\|\right| + \left|\bar{d} - \|\mathbf{v}_{i+1} - \mathbf{v}_i\|\right| \qquad (5)$$

The next subsection discusses a method for minimizing the snake's energy.

C. Minimization of Snake's Energy

We follow an algorithm which is similar to the one presented in Williams and Shah [23]. We first find an initial approximate position for the snakes by template matching. We assume that the orientation of the grid lines and the spacing between them is known. To find the location of a grid line, we place a line template on the image and slide it over a distance equal to the spacing between the grid lines. The position that gives the least image energy corresponds to a grid line. Successive grid lines can be found by sliding the template further. The perpendicular set of grid lines can be found similarly. The minimum energy positions of the template are used as the initial positions for the snakes. Then, for each thick snake, we move from one snaxel-pair to the next. For each snaxel-pair, we search a small neighborhood and move the snaxel-pair to a new location that will yield a smaller energy for the snake. For each snake, the above procedure is repeated until the number of snaxels moved becomes less than a preset threshold or until a fixed number of iterations. In this subsection we will discuss the choice of the neighborhood and the choice of the coefficients $\alpha(s)$, $\beta(s)$ and $\gamma(s)$ (see (1)).

The choice of the coefficients α, β and γ is a difficult one. If we need to track the low-intensity grid lines, we need a high γ. But, a high γ will make the snaxels sensitive to even minor intensity variations. Since the image intensity along the grid lines is not a constant, a high sensitivity to intensity will cause snaxel-pairs to pile up on a pair of points that have the lowest energy in the neighborhood. To avoid this we must increase the other two coefficients, but how much to increase them is a difficult issue. If we increase α and β too much the snakes will not move from their initial position because any bending will increase the energy. To avoid this dilemma, we allow the snaxel-pairs to move only in a direction perpendicular to the length of the snake. In other words, the search for minimum energy is conducted only along a line through the current pair that is perpendicular to the length of the snake.

The first few iterations for each snake are performed with only the image energy—the coefficients α and β are set to zero. This will make the snake lie on the grid line in all places except those where a perpendicular grid line intersects the current grid line. The snaxels at these intersections may

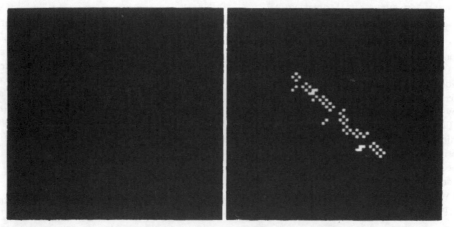

Fig. 1. Snake with image energy only: (a) Original image with one snake; (b) Magnified image.

wander along the perpendicular grid line, if this line has a lower intensity. The final contour a snake takes when it is governed by only image energy is shown in Fig. 1. Fig. 1(a) shows the original image with one snake. Fig. 1(b) shows a magnified view of the region around the snake. Note that the snake has correctly identified the grid line everywhere except at intersections. We need a way to prevent this wandering of snaxels at intersections. We do this in two steps. First, we increase the curvature and continuity coefficients for snaxels lying at points of high curvature. Second, at the regions of intersections we neutralize small variations in intensity of the grid pixels. In other words, if two grid pixels at the regions of intersections differ in intensity by a small value then their intensities are set to the same value.

It is possible to divide the set of all image pixels into two sets: grid pixels, those that lie on the SPAMM grid and background pixels, those that do not lie on the SPAMM grid. This division can be done by clustering the intensity values. We consider all the pixels in the area of interest and cluster the intensity values into two clusters using K-means clustering [9]. The cluster corresponding to the lower intensity values will contain approximately all the grid pixels. Clustering can be done locally over the region of interest or globally over the entire image. For the typical intensity distribution of SPAMM images, the difference between local and global clustering is negligible.

Having found an approximate set of grid pixels, we proceed as follows. For each snake, we perform several iterations with the curvature and continuity coefficients set to zero. Then, we look for points of high curvature. We give nonzero values for the curvature and continuity coefficients of the snaxels at these locations. Also, all the grid pixels that lie in a small neighborhood about these snaxels are set to the same value and minimization is continued. The algorithm is terminated either when the number of points moved is less than a threshold or when the number of iterations reaches a preset maximum value. We found that on an average, after about eight to 10 iterations less than 8% of the snaxels change their position and it is a good time to terminate the algorithm. The algorithm is given in the next subsection.

D. The Algorithm

The minimization algorithm is as follows.

1. For the first frame, find an initial approximate position of the grid by template matching.
2. Track each line of the grid by a separate snake.
3. For each snake do

    iteration ← 1.

    For all snaxels s, set $\alpha[s] = \beta[s] = 0;\ \gamma[s] = 1;$

    Repeat

        for each snaxel s do

            if (iteration $\geq$ 3) and (curvature[s] $\geq$ HIGH){

                $\alpha[s] = \beta[s] = 1;$

                Set all the grid pixels in a small neighborhood to the same value;

            }

            Move the snaxel to a new position in the neighborhood where the energy is a local minimum;

        iteration++;

    Until *points_moved < threshold*;

4. End of algorithm.

When the algorithm terminates, the entire set of snakes will be lying on the grid. We now have the location of each point of the grid and we can compute the intersection points. Since each snake is two pixels wide, the intersection point of two orthogonal snakes is computed as the intersection point of the two inter-pixel curves that pass through the center of each snake. Using the final contours of the snakes of one image as the starting point for the next image, we can track the entire spatio-temporal motion of the grid.

Fig. 2 shows the first time slice of the MRI SPAMM data. It can be seen that the snakes have correctly localized the grid lines. Figs. 3–5 correspond to time slices 2–4. Note that as time passes, the grid lines in the intraventricular chambers get washed away by blood flow and become invisible. In such regions, the snakes maintain straight contours due to their internal energies. The grid intersection points in these regions do not correspond to cardiac muscle tissue and should not be

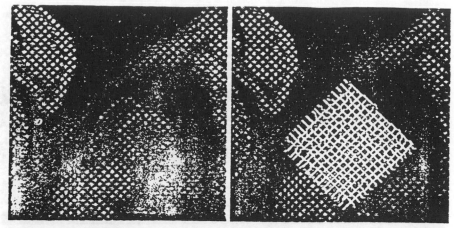

Fig. 2. Time slice 1: (a) Original image; (b) Image with snakes.

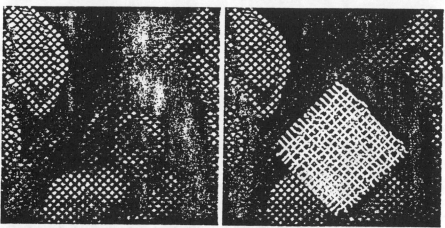

Fig. 3. Time slice 2: (a) Original image; (b) Image with snakes.

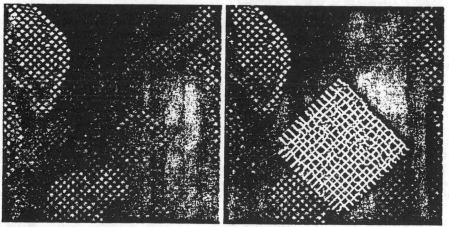

Fig. 4. Time slice 3: (a) Original Image. (b) Image with snakes

included in the strain computations. Intersection points within the myocardium must be identified and only these points must be used.

An automated technique for the identification of grid intersection points within the myocardium can be devised by using a new MR imaging technique (suggested to us by the scientists at Siemens). This technique gives two MR cardiac images for each slice and each phase. One of them is the SPAMM image (contains the tagging grid) and the other is a "normal" image (does not contain the tagging grid). The ventricular boundaries can be determined in the normal image by using, for example, an algorithm devised by Singh et al. [19]. Since

319

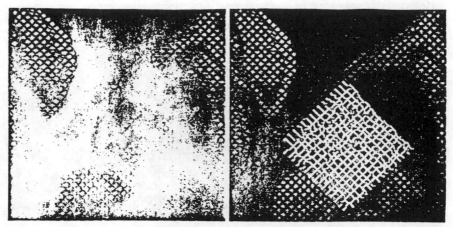

Fig. 5.   Time slice 4: (a) Original image; (b) Image with snakes.

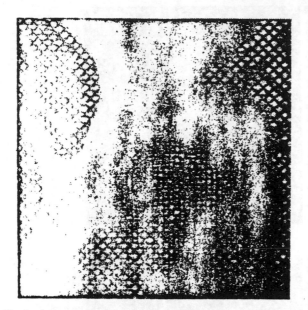

Fig. 6.   Intersection points superimposed on original image.

the normal and the SPAMM image are taken from the same phase, the positions of the ventricular boundaries are identical in both images. Having extracted the ventricular boundaries, the grid intersection points that lie within the myocardium can be identified and used in the strain computations. We are continuing our research in this direction. In this paper, however, we have used all the intersection points in the computation of the thin plate spline interpolant to be discussed in the next section.

Fig. 6 shows the computed intersection points superimposed on the original image (time slice 1). The ability of the snakes to track the grid intersections accurately is evident.

IV. A Thin Plate Spline Interpolant

We can use the intersection points extracted from multiple frames for the estimation of deformation parameters. Note that since the snakes and the snaxels are ordered, we already know the correspondence between the intersection points extracted from multiple frames—no explicit matching is necessary. However, the number of intersection points depends on the resolution of the grid and is somewhat small. In deformation estimation one typically takes three or more pairs of points and estimates the deformation parameters for the region enclosed by these points. Since the intersection points are fairly far apart, we need to find points that are closer together in one time frame and their correspondences in the next time frame. For this we compute a mapping from one time frame to the next. This mapping is defined everywhere in the plane of the picture and for any point in the first image, we can compute the corresponding point in the next image. This is the subject of the this section.

Bookstein [6] has proposed an algebraic approach to the description of deformations specified by a finite number of point correspondences. He gives a mapping function from one image to the next based on a finite number of correspondences. This mapping is based on a thin plate spline model and can be viewed as minimizing a certain bending energy. Bookstein has used this mapping to analyze the Apert Syndrome. This mapping is described below.

Let $(x_1, y_1), (x_2, y_2), \ldots, (x_n, y_n)$ be n feature points in one image and let (x_i', y_i') be the point homologous to (x_i, y_i) in the next image. Define

$$U(r) = r^2 \log(r^2) \qquad (6)$$

Let r_{ij} be the distance between points i and j. Define the matrices

$$K = \begin{pmatrix} 0 & U(r_{12}) & \ldots & U(r_{1n}) \\ U(r_{21}) & 0 & \ldots & U(r_{2n}) \\ \ldots & \ldots & \ldots & \ldots \\ U(r_{n1}) & U(r_{n2}) & \ldots & 0 \end{pmatrix} \quad n \times n \qquad (7)$$

$$P = \begin{pmatrix} 1 & x_1 & y_1 \\ 1 & x_2 & y_2 \\ \ldots & \ldots & \ldots \\ 1 & x_n & y_n \end{pmatrix} \quad 3 \times n \qquad (8)$$

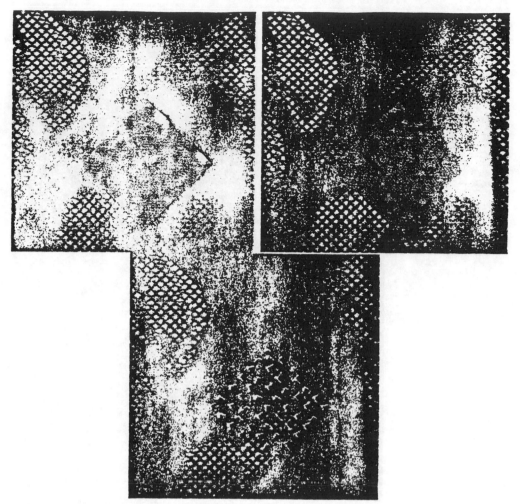

Fig. 7. Principal strains for motion from time slice 1 to time slice 2.

$$L = \begin{pmatrix} K & P \\ K^T & \emptyset \end{pmatrix} \quad (n+3) \times (n+3) \qquad (9)$$

where $\emptyset$ is a 3×3 matrix of zeros.

Let $V = (v_1, v_2, \ldots, v_n)$ be any n-vector. Write $Z = (V \mid 0\ 0\ 0)^T$. Z is a column vector of length $n+3$. Define the vector $W = (w_1, w_2, \ldots, w_n)$ and the coefficients a_1, a_x, a_y by the equation

$$L^{-1}Z = (W \mid a_1\ a_x\ a_y)^T \qquad (10)$$

Define $f(x, y)$ for all x and y as

$$f(x, y) = a_1 + a_x x + a_y y + \sum_{i=1}^{n} w_i U(|P_i - (x, y)|) \qquad (11)$$

Let $f_x(x, y)$ and $f_y(x, y)$ be the functions obtained when we substitute the vectors $(x_1', x_2', \ldots, x_n')$ and $(y_1', y_2', \ldots, y_n')$, respectively, for V. Then $f_x(x, y)$ and $f_y(x, y)$ give the desired mapping from one image to the next. A point (x, y) in the first image gets mapped onto the point $(f_x(x, y), f_y(x, y))$ in the next image. These two functions are the thin-plate spline mappings proposed by Bookstein [6].

In our implementation, we typically have 15 snakes tracking one set of parallel lines and another 15 snakes tracking the perpendicular set of lines. The intersection of these two snake groups gives $15 \cdot 15 = 225$ intersection points per time frame. We use 225 points from one image with the corresponding 225 points from the next image to determine the thin-plate spline mapping from the first image to the second. The matrix $\mathbf{K}$ is of size 225×225 and the matrix $\mathbf{L}$ that is to be inverted is of size 228×228. Once the mapping is constructed, we can take any three or more arbitrarily close points in the one image and find their homologs in the next. These correspondences can then be used for the deformation estimation.

V. Estimation of Generalized Motion Parameters

We compute the deformation tensor at each pixel by surrounding it with an equilateral triangle centered about that pixel. The corners of the triangle are chosen to lie at a distance of 0.5 pixels from its center. We then use the thin plate spline mapping to compute the positions of these corners in the next image. This gives us the positions of three points before and after motion. The deformation tensor is estimated as follows.

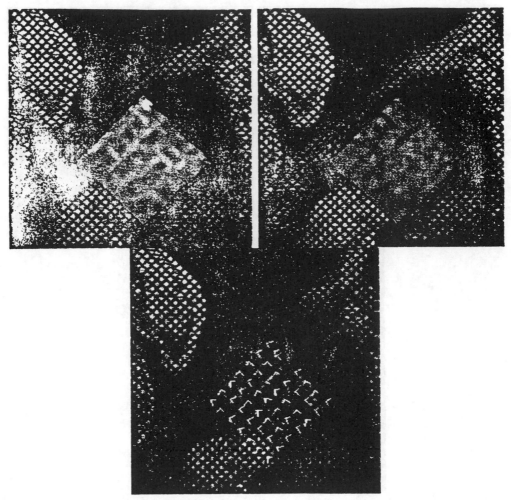

Fig. 8. Principal strains for motion from time slice 2 to time slice 3.

Let $p_i = [x_i \ y_i \ z_i]$ be the row vector representing the coordinates of the ith point and q_i be the coordinate vector of the same point after deformation. Then p_i and q_i are related by

$$q_i = p_i K + t + \eta_i \tag{12}$$

where the 3 by 3 matrix K represents both the rotation and deformation, t the translation and η_i the measurement noise. Assuming an object centered coordinate frame, we can express the above equation as $q_i = p_i K + \eta_i$.

Let $n \geq 3$ be the number of data points available. Then, assuming that K is the same at these points, the above equation can be expressed in matrix form as follows.

$$Q = PK + \eta \tag{13}$$

where Q, P and η are n by 3 matrices. Then K can be found either by least squares estimation or by total least squares estimation [8]. Note the assumption that K is the same at these n points. For this to be true, the n points must be close together and this explains the need for an interpolant.

When the deformation can be represented as an affine transformation, K can be expressed as $K = RD$ [24], [22],

TABLE I
MEAN ERROR IN PIXELS BETWEEN THE MANUALLY
EXTRACTED POINTS AND THOSE FOUND BY THE ALGORITHM

Time Frame	Mean Error	Variance
1	0.275	0.201
2	0.356	0.072
3	0.215	0.061
4	0.369	0.175
5	0.292	0.261
6	0.372	0.141

where R and D denote the rotation and deformation tensors respectively. Here, R is orthonormal and D is symmetric positive definite. Therefore, $K^T K = D^T D$. But, since D is symmetric, there exists a unique decomposition of $K^T K$ in terms of $D^T D$ such that D is symmetric and positive definite. Once D is estimated, R can be estimated uniquely as KD^{-1}. The eigenvalues of D give the principal strains and the associated eigenvectors give a set of orthogonal directions in which these strains act.

Figs. 7–9 show the principal strains and the associated directions. Fig. 7 corresponds to motion from frame 1 to frame

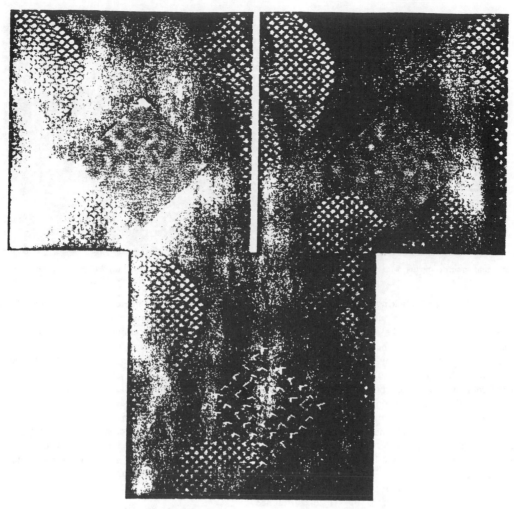

Fig. 9. Principal strains for motion from time slice 3 to time slice 4.

2, Fig. 8 corresponds to motion from frame 2 to frame 3 and Fig. 9 corresponds to motion from frame 3 to frame 4. In each figure, the left image gives the maximum strain and the right image gives the minimum strain. The bottom image shows the directions of minimum and maximum strains at selected points. At each selected point, the longer line shows the direction of maximum strain and the shorter line shows the direction of minimum strain. As we discussed at the end of Section III, one must use only those intersection points that lie within the myocardium in the strain computations. The strain parameters displayed in regions other than the myocardium do not have any relevance to cardiac analysis.

The need for the thin-plate interpolant is obvious from Fig. 10. This figure shows the maximum strains computed with and without the thin-plate interpolant. Fig. 10(a) shows the maximum strain computed with the thin plate spline interpolant. Fig. 10(b) shows the maximum strain computed without the thin plate spline interpolant. To get this estimate, we used only the intersection points and the deformation tensor was computed for every region enclosed by four neighboring

intersection points. The deformation estimate is the same for all points inside any such region. Therefore, to get a better estimate our feature points must be close to one another and hence the need for an interpolant.

VI. EXPERIMENTAL RESULTS

We used six data sets consisting a total of 87 images provided to us by Dr. Eric Hoffman, University of Iowa Medical School. The data sets shown in this paper correspond to two axial spatial positions in the same patient. Figs. 2–5 correspond to the first four time slices at the first spatial position and Figs. 7 and 8 correspond to the first two time slices at the second spatial position. We also tested our algorithm on 36 images provided by Siemens.

We now turn to a discussion on the accuracy of the tracking algorithm and that of the thin-plate spline interpolant. We also discuss the extent of user interaction required by our algorithm.

To estimate the accuracy of tracking, we manually selected the intersection points and compared them with those given by the algorithm. The manual selection was done by magnifying

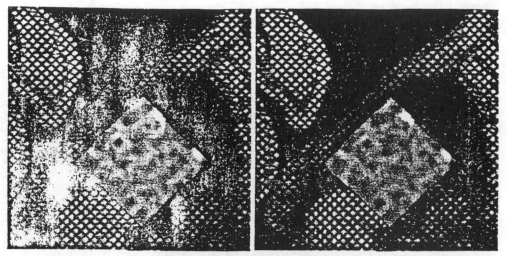

Fig. 10. Maximum strains computed with and without the thin plate spline interpolant: (a) With interpolant; (b) Without interpolant.

the image four times and clicking the intersection points with a mouse. This manual technique is tedious and becomes inaccurate as we move towards the end of the time sequence. The inaccuracy arises because of the fact that the intensity of the grid decays with time. At many intersections quite a few pixels look alike and it is difficult to pick the correct one. We compared the manually extracted points in each image with those given by the algorithm. In each image, we computed the absolute distances between the manually extracted points and those given by the algorithm. We then computed the mean of these absolute distances. The process was repeated for the next five frames. The mean error in pixels for the first six frames is shown in Table I.

To compute the distribution of error, we calculated the error vector for each intersection point as the vector difference between the manually extracted point and that given by the algorithm. The error vectors for the first time frame are shown as points in Fig. 11.

To arrive at an error estimate for the thin-plate spline mapping, we first selected 224 out of the 225 point-pairs computed by the algorithm. We used these 224 point-pairs to construct the mapping. This mapping was then used to predict the position of the 225th point. We repeated the procedure for all the 225 points, every time leaving one point out, and predicting its position using the mapping constructed from the other 224 points. The vector difference between the predicted position and the correct position was computed each time. The 225 error vectors are shown as points in Fig. 12. The mean of these error vectors has magnitude of 0.801 pixel.

We must also mention that, in any given image sequence the intensity of the grid decays with time and we soon reach a stage where the grid lines are not distinguishable from the background. In places where a grid line is not distinguishable from the background, the snake tracking that grid line is guided more by its internal energy than the image energy and hence, the snake assumes a straight contour.

The proposed tracking algorithm requires some user interaction in the initial placement of snakes. First, the user has to specify the region of interest, i.e. the position of the heart in the image. Next, for the template matching phase, the algorithm has to know the directions of the grid lines and the spacing between two grid lines. The directions can be input either by the user or can be determined by the Hough Transform [5]. To find the locations of the grid lines, we must know how far we should slide our template before looking for the position of minimum average intensity. This requires a knowledge of the interline spacing which must be supplied by the user. Thus our algorithm requires three parameters—the region of interest, the orientation of the grid and the interline spacing of the grid. We are currently developing a friendly user interface for the input of these three parameters.

VII. CONCLUSION

We have provided a reliable mechanism for establishing point correspondences in MR SPAMM images. Point correspondences are obtained by successfully tracking the SPAMM grid through consecutive time slices. The use of snakes avoids the problem of explicit matching of feature points belonging to different time frames. We also provided energy measures suitable for the SPAMM grid tracking. To get an accurate estimate of the deformation tensor, we used the intersection points to construct the thin-plate spline mapping that maps arbitrary points in one image to their homologs in the next image. This mapping allows us to compute the deformation parameters for arbitrarily small regions. This is desired because the discussion in Section V is based on the assumption that the deformation tensor is a constant in the region enclosed by the feature points. The relationship between the deformation parameters and the cardiac dynamics is under current investigation.

In all our test images, the inter-frame movement was quite small. However, it is quite probable for a set of stripes to move more than half a stripe spacing between frames, especially in higher resolution images. In other words, a stripe adjacent to the one being tracked by a particular snake might move closer

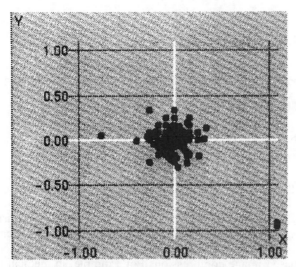

Fig. 11.   Error vectors between manually tracked points and those found by the algorithm. Distances are in pixels.

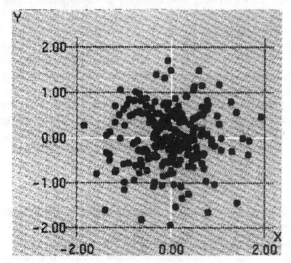

Fig. 12.   Error vectors between the actual and the predicted intersection points. Distances are in pixels.

to the snake than the correct one. The snake always seeks the closest local minimum and hence, in this case, it will choose the wrong stripe. Should this happen, some form of manual interaction is necessary to pull the snake towards the correct contour. A second limitation of our algorithm is its inability to analyze the myocardial region selectively. However, as we discussed at the end of Section III, this limitation can be easily overcome and this will be a part of our future research. Another limitation to cardiac analysis using SPAMM data is the decay of SPAMM grid with time. This is due to the imaging technique and is not a limitation of our algorithm.

The algorithm requires three parameters for the initial placement of the snakes. These parameters are readily available and can be easily input by the user. Experimentation with seven data sets consisting of multiple time frames has shown that correct tracking is achieved. The software is available through anonymous FTP at figment.csee.usf.edu (ethernet: 131.247.2.2) in the directory "/home/figment/grad1/ftp/pub/snakes".

ACKNOWLEDGMENT

We would like to thank Dr. Eric A. Hoffman, University of Iowa College of Medicine, for providing data and valuable advice.

REFERENCES

[1] A. A. Amini, Tehrani and T. E. Weymouth, "Using dynamic programming for minimizing the energy of active contours in the presence of hard constraints." in *Proc., Second Int. Conf. on Comput. Vision*, pp. 55–99. 1988.
[2] L. Axel and L. Dougherty, "Heart wall motion: Improved method of spatial modulation of magnetization for MR imaging." *Radiology*, vol. 172, pp. 349–350, 1989.
[3] L. Axel and L. Dougherty, "MR imaging of motion with spatial modulation of magnetization," *Radiology*, 171, pp. 841–845, 1989.
[4] L. Axel, R. Goncalves, and D. Bloomgarden, "Regional heart wall motion: Two-dimensional analysis and functional imaging with MR imaging." *Radiology*, 183, pp. 745–750, 1992.
[5] D. H. Ballard and C. M. Brown, *Computer Vision*. Englewood Cliffs, NJ: Prentice Hall, Inc., 1982.
[6] F. L. Bookstein, "Principal warps: Thin plate splines and the decomposition of deformations." *IEEE Trans. Pattern Anal. and Mach. Intell.*, pp. 567–585, 1989.
[7] J. Canny, "A computational approach to edge detection," *IEEE Trans. on Pattern Anal. and Mach. Intell.*, PAMI-8, no. 6, pp. 679–698, 1986.
[8] S. Chaudhuri and S. Chatterjee, "estimation of motion parameters for a deformable object from range data," in *Proc. IEEE Conf. on Comput. Vision and Pattern Recognition*, pp. 291–295, 1989.
[9] R. O. Duda and P. E. Hart, *Pattern Classification and Scene Analysis*. New York: Wiley Interscience, 1973.
[10] T. R. Fenton, J. M. Cherry, and G. A. Klassen, "Transmural myocardial deformation in the canine left ventricular wall," *Am. J. Physiol.*, vol. 253, pp. H523–H530, 1978.
[11] B. K. P. Horn and B. G. Schunck, "Determining optical flow," *Artificial Intell.*, vol. 17, pp. 185–203, 1981.
[12] M. Kass, A. Witkin, and D. Terzopoulos, "Snakes: Active contour models," *Int. J. Comput. Vision*, vol. 1, no. 4, pp. 321–331, 1988.
[13] S. Kumar and D. Goldgof, "Automatic tracking of SPAMM grid in MR images," In *Proc. IEEE Nuclear Sci. Symp. and Med. Imaging Conf.*, 1992, pp. 1319–1321.
[14] F. Leymarie, "Tracking and describing deformable objects using active contour models." MS thesis, Department of Electrical Engineering, McGill University, 1990.
[15] E. R. McVeigh and E. A. Zerhouni, "Noninvasive MR imaging." *Radiology*, vol. 180, pp. 677–683, 1991.
[16] G. D. Meier, A. Bove, and W. P. Santamore, "Contractile function in canine right ventricle." *Am. J. Physiol.*, vol. 239, pp. H794–H804, 1980.
[17] G. D. Meier, M. C. Ziskin, W. P. Santamore, and A. Bove, "Kinematics of the beating heart," *IEEE Trans. Biomed. Eng.*, vol. 27, pp. 319–329, 1980.
[18] J. L. Prince and E. R. McVeigh, "Motion estimation from tagged MR image sequences." *IEEE Trans. on Medical Imaging*, vol. 11, no. 2, pp. 238–249, 1992.
[19] A. Singh, L. Kurowski, and M. Chiu, "Cardiac MR image segmentation using deformable models." in *Proc. IS&T/SPIE's Symp. on Electron. Imaging: Sci. & Technol.; Biomed Image Processing and Biomed. Visualization* 1993, pp. 8–28.
[20] S. L. Thomas and R. L. Dixon, NMR in medicine: The instrumentation and clinical applications, *American Assoc. of Physicists, Medical Physics Monograph 14*,1986..
[21] L. K. Waldman, Y. C. Fung, and J. W. Covell, "Transmural myocardial deformation in the canine left ventricle," *Circ. Res.*, vol. 57, pp. 152–163, 1985.
[22] K. R. Walley, M. Grover, G. L. Raff, J. W. Benge, B. Hannaford, and S. A. Glantz, "Left ventricular dynamic geometry in the intact and open chest dog." *Circ. Res.*, vol. 50, no. 4, pp. 573–589, 1982.
[23] D. J. Williams and M. Shah, "A fast algorithm for active contours and curvature estimation." *CVGIP: Image Understanding*, vol. 55, no. 1, pp. 14–26, 1992.
[24] T. Y. Young and S. Gunasekaran, "A regional approach to tracking 3D motion in an image sequence," *Advances in Computer Vision and Image Processing*, T. S. Huang, Ed., pp. 63–99, 1988.

Curvature-Based Approach to Point Correspondence Recovery in Conformal Nonrigid Motion*

Chandra Kambhamettu and Dmitry B. Goldgof

Department of Computer Science and Engineering, University of South Florida, Tampa, Florida 33620

Received December 22, 1991; revised October 25, 1993

This paper describes a novel method for the estimation of point correspondences on a surface undergoing conformal nonrigid motion based on changes in its Gaussian curvature. The use of Gaussian curvature in nonrigid motion analysis is justified by its invariancy towards rigid motion and the type of surface parameterization. Input to the algorithm is the set of 3D points before and after the motion. We deal with a restricted class of nonrigid motion called conformal motion. In conformal motion, the stretching is equal in all directions, but different at different points. Small motion assumption is utilized to hypothesize all possible point correspondences. Curvature changes are then computed for each hypothesis. Finally, the error between computed curvature changes and the one predicted by the conformal motion assumption is calculated. The hypothesis with the smallest error gives point correspondences between consecutive time frames. The algorithm requires calculation of the Gaussian curvature at points on surface before and after the motion. It also requires computation of the coefficients of the first fundamental form at points on surface before the motion. Estimation of point correspondences and stretching can also be refined so as to reduce the error introduced by sampling. Simulations are performed on an ellipsoidal data to illustrate performance and accuracy of derived algorithms. Then, the proposed algorithm is applied to volumetric CT data of the left ventricle (LV) of a dog's heart. Stretching of the LV wall during its expansion and contraction phases is depicted along with the estimated point correspondences. Stretching comparisons are made between the normal and abnormal LV. ⓒ 1994 Academic Press, Inc.

1. INTRODUCTION

Motion analysis has been an important research area in computer vision for several decades. It can be defined traditionally as the process of finding the 3D motion of an object based on its 2D images taken during two or more time instances. There has been extensive research in this area due to its importance in dynamic scene understanding [31, 15, 27]. In most of the work, rigidity is assumed in estimating motion parameters. In the last few

* This work is supported by the National Science Foundation Grant IRI-90-10357 and the Whitaker Foundation Grant 2108-097-LO.

years, an increasing trend towards research in nonrigid motion analysis has become apparent due to its potential applications in such areas as medical imaging and model-based image compression. For example, in medical cardiac imaging, one of the goals is to analyze nonrigid motion and estimate corresponding motion parameters involved in the deformation of the heart. In this application, a CT or MRI scanner collects data of a person's heart during a series of frames over a cardiac cycle. Analysis can be made on the range of motion parameters in order to screen patients and decide on the extent of cardiac injury. Another potential application is model-based image compression for teleconferencing. Once the motion parameters or point correspondences of a facial movement can be recovered, they can be encoded and transmitted. This would reduce the information bandwidth significantly when compared to the traditional statistical approaches.

Research in nonrigid motion is complicated by the fact that nonrigid motion has varying structure which cannot be defined by any specific set of parameters unless there are certain restrictions in the object's behavior. *Differential geometry* is one of the tools used in the analysis of nonrigid motion. Classical differential geometry provides a complex local description of smooth surfaces. We use such surfaces descriptors and follow curvature-based approach (first proposed by Goldgof, Lee, and Huang [9]) in recovering point correspondences in nonrigid motion.

Although, 3D nonrigid motion, in general, can involve arbitrary deformation, it can be classified into certain classes depending on the nature of the deformation involved. The three major classes of nonrigid objects are: articulated objects, elastic objects, and fluids [16].

In recent years, several research groups have been working on visual analysis of articulated and elastic objects. Below we mention some of the previous work. Webb and Aggarwal [37] considered the case of *fixed axis assumption*, Bennet and Hoffman [3] discussed the movement of linked rigid rods in one plane, O'Rourke and Badler [28], and Asada, Yachida, and Tsuji [2] also considered restricted motion of articulated objects. Goldgof, Lee, and Huang [9] used surface curvature to segment an articulated object into its rigid parts and distinguish among rigid, isometric, homothetic, conformal, and general nonrigid motion. Chen and Penna [5] presented three approaches for the recovery of generalized motion: an infinitesimal approach to determine the linear approximation of the generalized motion, a global approach to completely determine generalized motion, and a hybrid of the infinitesimal approach and the global approach. However, the solutions can only be obtained under the assumption of isometry. Isometric motion severely limits the nonrigidity, since for many curved objects no isometry is possible. Webb and Aggarwal [36] studied a special case of elastic objects where the object is assumed to be locally rigid; i.e., an affine transform exists between two images under local parallel projection. Huang *et al.* [16] chose an application-motivated approach. Their research includes an initial approach to modeling and an analysis of heart wall motion, human face/head motion analysis and synthesis in model-based image compression, and studying the evolution of coherent structures in fluid motion. The ultimate goal here is to study the similarities and differences among these problems and develop the concepts, methodologies, and techniques applicable to various types of nonrigid motion. Chen and Huang [4] presented a model-based approach for nonrigid object motion and deformation analysis from 3D data. The modeling primitives used here are the superquadrics. Horowitz and Pentland [14] presented an approach for recovery of nonrigid motion based on finite element methods. They have proposed to model and simulate the physics of nonrigid motion and obtain object shape and velocity, as opposed to recovery of nonrigid structure on a patch-by-patch basis. They have also utilized a similar approach in [29] to obtain estimates of both object shape and velocity from contour data. Terzopoulos and Metaxas [34] presented a physically based approach in fitting complex 3D shapes using a new class of dynamic models that can deform both locally and globally. They formulated deformable superquadrics which incorporate the global shape parameters of a conventional superellipsoid with the local degrees of freedom of a spline. In [23], they have presented an approach for recursively estimating 3D object shape and general nonrigid motion, which makes use of physically based dynamic models. Other research work in this area include Cheng and Don [6], Ullman [35], and Shulman and Aloimonous [33]. For a detailed review on nonrigid motion analysis, see [20].

Goldgof, Lee, and Huang [9] first proposed a curvature-based approach to nonrigid motion analysis. They have chosen stretching as an additional motion parameter and have extracted the stretching of a surface which is undergoing homothetic transformation. The authors have also applied the proposed algorithm to cineangiographic data [10] to recover surface stretching parameters. Later, this approach was extended by Mishra, Goldgof, Huang, and Kambhamettu [25] in estimating nonrigid deformation of moving surface. They have presented an algorithm for local stretching recovery from Gaussian curvature based on polynomial (linear and quadratic) approximations of the stretching function. All of the above algorithms require point correspondences between time frames. Mishra, Goldgof, and Kambhamettu have further extended this approach to incorporate knowledge about the line correspondences [26]. Based on the above work, Kambhamettu and Goldgof [8, 17] first proposed the curvature-based approach to point correspondence recovery in nonrigid motion. A local homothetic motion assumption (i.e., conformal motion with constant stretching) was used in estimating point correspondences. They have extended this work to include conformal motion of surface with polynomial stretching in [18].

Amini and Duncan [1] have proposed a similar approach; however, they employed a bending and stretching model for tracking point correspondences in nonrigid motion. They considered the physical model of a surface as a thin plate, and then tracked the motion involved by minimizing the bending and deviation from conformal stretching. Principal directions before and after the motion were used for setting up the coordinate system. One main drawback with this approach is that the energy functions are sensitive to parameterization of the surface. Mean curvature and first fundamental coefficients need the same parameterization of the surface before and after the elastic motion. Principal directions may not always provide the necessary parameterization due to noise and the nonrigid motion involved. Bending energy provides regularization over the estimation of point correspondences, although conformal motion by itself includes bending (isometric) motion. A better formulation may be achieved using the invariant measures such as Gaussian curvature and the use of parameterization sensitive factors such as fundamental coefficients in only one time frame in order to estimate point correspondence. This would allow us to choose independent parameterization for different time frames.

In this paper, we present an extended version of [18], having detailed derivations and experiments on simulated and real data. It is not necessary to preserve parameterization between frames, as we use the coefficients of first fundamental form (which depends on surface parameterization) in only one time frame. Input to the algorithm is the set of 3D points before and after the motion. Our method then estimates point correspondences and stretching parameters of a surface undergoing conformal motion with constant (homothetic), linear and polynomial stretching. We also refine the point correspondences so as to allow the estimated point correspondences to fall between sampled points after the motion. The algorithm has been tested for both simulated and real data. In particular, we have applied our algorithm for endocardial left ventricular motion analysis.

2. BACKGROUND

Differential geometry is an important tool that can be used to derive properties of surfaces and eventually analyze the motion between surfaces. The geometric property of any surface can be extrinsic, which is dependent on the surface representation and its orientation in space. Thus, the extrinsic properties of a surface in space are not invariant to motion and parameterization of the surface in space. Properties of surfaces which are invariant to rigid motion and representation are called intrinsic properties. We are more interested in the study of these invariant properties of a surface. Nonrigid motion can be estimated in terms of the invariant properties, such as curvature (Gaussian curvature in 3D) and other differential geometric measurements. The material in this section is presented for completeness. More details of differential geometry can be found in various books, such as [22, 11].

2.1. First Fundamental Form

A surface in E^3 is uniquely determined by certain local invariant quantities called the fundamental forms. Let $x = x(u, v)$ be a coordinate patch on a surface. Then the differential of the mapping, $x = x(u, v)$ at (u, v) is a one-to-one linear mapping, $ds = x_u du + x_v dv$ of the vectors (du, dv) in the uv-plane onto the vectors $x_u du + x_v dv$ parallel to the tangent plane at $x(u, v)$. ds represents the image $x_u du + x_u dv$, on the tangent plane; ds is a first-order approximation to the vector $x(u + du, v + dv)$ from the point $x(u, v)$ on the patch to the neighboring point $x(u + du, v + dv)$.

Consider a curve $C : u = u(t)$, $v = v(t)$ on surface S. The differential of arc, ds of C, is given by

$$ds^2 = ds \cdot ds$$
$$= (x_u \cdot x_u)du^2 + (x_u \cdot x_v)dudv + (x_v \cdot x_v)dv^2, \quad (1)$$

where $du = u'dt$, $dv = v'dt$. The expression (1) is a homogeneous function of second degree in du, dv. It is known as the *first fundamental differential quadratic form* of S which defines the differential of arc for an arbitrary curve C on S as a linear element of S. We denote the coefficients in (1) by E, F, G. We will then have

$$ds^2 = Edu^2 + Fdudv + Gdv^2, \quad (2)$$

where

$$E = (x_u \cdot x_u), \quad F = (x_u \cdot x_v), \quad G = (x_v \cdot x_v). \quad (3)$$

The coefficients E, F, and G are called the *first funda-mental coefficients*, which are functions of u and v and vary from point to point on the coordinate patch.

The discriminant, denoted by D^2 is given as

$$D^2 = EG - F^2.$$

Consequently, $D = \sqrt{EG - F^2}$ is positive at every regular point.

Also from Eq. (2),

$$ds = \pm \sqrt{Edu^2 + Fdudv + Gdv^2},$$

where the plus or minus sign is to be taken according as $dt > 0$ or $dt < 0$. The linear element enables us to find not only the lengths of arcs, but also angles between curves. We observe that the length of arc defined in terms of the coefficients of first fundamental form is invariant to the coordinate system in space but it does depend on representation (direction of the curve) [22, 11].

2.2. Second Fundamental Form

Consider now a patch $x = x(u, v)$ on a surface. Since the components of $x_u \times x_v$ are direction components of the normal to S at $P : (u, v)$, and since $(x_u x_v \cdot x_u x_v) = D^2$, the direction cosines of normal are given by $(x_u \times x_v)/D$ or $-(x_u \times x_v)/D$, according to the sense in which the normal is directed. Thus, the unit normal is given by

$$n = \frac{x_u \times x_v}{D}.$$

The second fundamental form is then defined as

$$-dx \cdot dn = Ldu^2 + 2Mdudv + Ndv^2. \quad (4)$$

Formula (4) is a homogeneous function of second degree in du and dv with coefficients L, M, N, called the second fundamental coefficients, which are continuous functions of u and v.

Expressing dx and dn in terms of u, v, we have $dx = x_u du + x_v$ and $dn = n_u + n_v$. Hence, L, M, N can be defined as

$$L = -(x_u \cdot n_u) = (x_{uu} \cdot n) = \frac{x_{uu} x_u x_v}{D},$$

$$M = -(x_u \cdot n_v) = (x_{uv} \cdot n) = \frac{x_{uv} x_u x_v}{D}, \quad (5)$$

$$N = -(x_v \cdot n_v) = (x_{vv} \cdot n) = \frac{x_{vv} x_u x_v}{D}.$$

It can be shown that the second fundamental form is invariant in the same sense that the first fundamental form is invariant under a parameter transformation which preserves the direction of n; otherwise it changes sign.

The local surface shape is uniquely determined by the first and second fundamental forms of the surface. Gaussian and mean curvatures combine the first and second fundamental forms intrinsically and extrinsically to obtain scalar surface features that are invariant to rotations, translations, and changes in parameterization.

2.3. Gaussian Curvature

Let P be a point on a surface, and $x = x(u, v)$ is a patch containing P. Let $x = x(u(t), v(t))$ be a regular curve C of class C^2 through P. The normal curvature vector to C at P, denoted by k_n, is the vector projection of the curvature vector k of C at P onto the normal N at P, given by

$$k_n = (k \cdot N)N. \tag{6}$$

Where k_n is independent of the sense of N. It is also independent of the sense of C, since k is independent of the sense of C. The component of k_n in the direction N is called the normal curvature of C at P and is denoted by κ_n. Here the sign of κ_n depends upon the sense of N; but it is independent of the sense of C. The normal curvature at point P on a surface in the direction $dv : du$, $du^2 + dv^2 \neq 0$ is given by

$$\kappa_n = \frac{Ldu^2 + 2Mdudv + Ndv^2}{Edu^2 + 2Fdudv + Gdv^2}. \tag{7}$$

It follows that κ_n is invariant under a parametric transformation which preserves the sense of N and that κ_n changes sign under a parametric transformation which reverses the sense of N. The two perpendicular directions for which the values of κ_n take on maximum and minimum values are called the principal directions, and the corresponding normal curvatures κ_1 and κ_2 are called the principal curvatures. At an elliptic point, $\kappa_n = \text{const} \neq 0$ and all directions are called principal directions. At a planar point $\kappa_n = \text{const} = 0$ and all directions are principal directions. A point on the surface at which $\kappa_n = \text{const}$ is called an umbilical point. Figure 1 shows the principal directions for an elliptic point. The two extreme values of the normal curvature are called the principal normal curvatures [22, 11] and is given by roots of

$$(EG - F^2)\kappa^2 - (EN - 2FM + GM)\kappa + (LM - N^2) = 0.$$

We designate the product and the sum of the roots as

$$K = \kappa_1 \kappa_2 = \frac{LN - M^2}{EG - F^2} \tag{8}$$

and

$$H = \kappa_1 + \kappa_2.$$

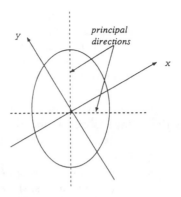

FIG. 1. Principal directions for elliptic point.

The product K is called the *total curvature,* or the *Gaussian curvature,* of the surface at P, and the sum H is called the *mean curvature* of the surface. Since the normal curvature κ_n of a curve at most changes sign with a change in orientation of the surface, the extreme values of κ_n remain extreme values and, at most, both change sign with a change in orientation (for example, maximum becomes minimum and vice versa). Hence it follows that the Gaussian curvature is an invariant property of the surface, independent of its representation. However, the mean curvature is the relative invariant of two fundamental forms.

3. 3D MOTION CLASSIFICATION

The following *classification of motion* has been suggested in [20]. We follow this classification throughout our discussion.

Rigid motion preserves the 3D distances between any two points in an object. The object does not stretch or bend; hence both mean curvature and Gaussian curvature on the surface of the object remain invariant.

Articulated motion is piecewise rigid motion. It involves motion of rigid parts connected by nonrigid joints. Examples are, animal skeletons and robot manipulators. Clearly, the rigidity constraint is more relaxed in this case.

Quasi-rigid motion restricts the deformation to be "very small." A general nonrigid motion is quasirigid when viewed in a sufficiently short time interval, say between image frames when the sampling rate is high enough. Motion analysis algorithms for this type of motion will usually minimize the nonrigidity.

Conformal motion is nonrigid motion which preserves angles between curves on the surface during motion, but not lengths. It is shown [11] that a necessary and sufficient condition for the motion to be conformal is that the ratios of the coefficients of the first fundamental form remain constant (t^2). The infinitesimal distances are stretched by a factor of t at the given point. The parameter t can vary at different points on the surface; however, at each point the stretching is the same in all directions. Thus, recovering t will give us information on the amount of stretching at each point.

Isometric motion is conformal motion which preserves lengths along the surface as well as angles between curves on the surface. Parameter t is equal to 1 at all points on the surface in this case.

Homothetic motion is conformal motion, having uniform expansion or contraction of a surface (parameter t is constant for all points). In such a motion, we can show that the Gaussian curvature at each point changes by a factor inversely proportional to t^2.

Elastic motion is a nonrigid motion whose only constraint is some degree of continuity or smoothness. This kind of solid object motion is the most difficult to analyze.

Fluid motion is a general nonrigid motion that need not be continuous. It may involve topological variations and turbulent deformations.

4. CURVATURE CHANGES AND CORRESPONDENCE RECOVERY

This section presents the solution for estimating point correspondences of a surface S which has undergone a nonrigid transformation. We assume conformal motion between the surfaces S (before motion) and $\overline{S}$ (after motion). First, we derive expressions for estimating point correspondences and stretching of a surface undergoing *homothetic motion*. Then, a similar procedure is used to derive expressions required for estimating point correspondences and stretching of a surface undergoing *conformal motion* with linear or higher-order polynomial stretching.

Our approach in estimating point correspondences involves first formulating possible hypotheses about point correspondences. Under small motion assumption, correspondence hypotheses can be formed in some small neighborhood around the point of interest. Curvature changes are computed for each hypothesis. Then, the error between computed curvature changes and the one predicted by the conformal motion assumption is computed. The hypothesis with the smallest error gives point correspondence between two consecutive time frames. This process is repeated for all points of interest (i.e., the whole surface).

Figure 2 shows all correspondence hypotheses of a point, $P(x, y, z)$, on a surface S which has undergone nonrigid motion to map onto $\overline{S}$. Here, point $P(x, y, z)$ can map onto any point within some region, $\mathfrak{R}$ (region of interest). $\mathfrak{R}$ is the region we check for the point correspon-

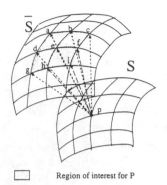

FIG. 2. Correspondences in 3D surfaces.

dences; it is defined by small motion assumption. This region could be the neighborhood of the position of point before motion, and its boundary depends on the maximum amount of motion generated. For small motion, it is defined as a small window around the position of the point.

In the estimation of point correspondences, neighborhood points are also considered for error computations; i.e., we consider local patches at each point under consideration. This provides consistency in estimation of point correspondences and stretching. The mapping of a set of neighboring points P_i onto another set $\overline{P}_i$ satisfies the curvature change equation for the nonrigid motion (presented later in this section). Figure 3 shows the neighborhood region of a point P on S which is mapped to $\overline{P}_i$ on $\overline{S}$. A least square error is thus defined for each hypothesis correspondence following the underlying motion assumption. Minimizing this error in the local neighborhood will guide us in estimating point correspondences.

It is known [11] that the mapping (motion) of S to $\overline{S}$ is conformal if the angle between two directed curves through a point P of S is equal to the angle between the two corresponding directed curves through the corresponding point $\overline{P}$ of $\overline{S}$. In addition, a necessary and sufficient condition for the motion to be conformal is the proportionality of the coefficients of the first fundamental form:

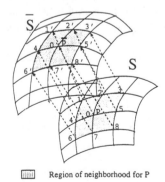

Region of neighborhood for P

FIG. 3. Region of the neighborhood.

330

$$\frac{\overline{E}}{E} = \frac{\overline{F}}{F} = \frac{\overline{G}}{G} = t^2. \tag{9}$$

In (9), (E, F, G) are the coefficients of the first fundamental form for any point on S, mapped onto a point on $\overline{S}$ having coefficients of the first fundamental form $(\overline{E}, \overline{F}, \overline{G})$.

The above theorem shows that it is characteristic of a conformal motion that the corresponding infinitesimal distances at corresponding points are proportional and that the factor of proportionality (t) depends only on the pair of corresponding points chosen, (u, v).

As discussed in the previous section, homothetic motion is a special kind of conformal motion, having constant stretching of the surface during motion. It can be described using Gaussian curvatures of the surface before and after the motion. It has been shown [9] that for a homothetic motion,

$$\frac{\overline{K}}{K} = \frac{1}{t^2} \quad \text{or} \quad K = \overline{K}t^2, \tag{10}$$

where K and $\overline{K}$ represent Gaussian curvature of the surface at a given point before and after the motion, respectively; t is the stretching undergone by the surface at that point during motion. Stretching is constant under the homothetic motion assumption for a given region.

For conformal (nonhomothetic) motion, the following expression was derived for the Gaussian curvature change [24, 25]:

$$\overline{K} = \frac{K}{t^2} + f(E, F, G, t). \tag{11}$$

The function f (see section 4.2) in the above equation represents the deviation of conformal motion from homothetic motion. Hence, if a given region on a surface has undergone conformal motion (non-homothetic), the above equation will be satisfied for some nonzero f; f is zero for homothetic motion.

Equation (11) allows us to complete surface stretching using Gaussian curvature of a point before and after the motion for a patch which has undergone conformal motion, as was done in [24, 25]. However, point correspondence is required in order to form Eq. (11) and to find stretching at any point. In our work, we hypothesize possible point correspondence and compute curvature changes for each hypothesis. The error between computed curvature changes and the one predicted by conformal motion assumption is computed. Correspondence hypothesis with the smallest error is chosen as the one indicating true point correspondence and true stretching of the surface region under consideration.

In the following sections, we derive the necessary ex-

pressions involved in estimating point correspondences under conformal motion with constant (homothetic), linear, and polynomial stretching.

4.1. Conformal Motion with Constant (Homothetic) Stretching

From Eq. (10), the least square error under homothetic motion assumption is defined as

$$ER = \sum_{i \in \eta} (K_i - t^2\overline{K}_i)^2; \tag{12}$$

η represents the region of the neighborhood chosen for any point on the surface in error calculation. Error ER can be used to measure the deviation from homothetic motion for each hypothesis correspondence; t is, however, not known in this error function. We know that the error (ER) is ideally zero for homothetic motion. Hence, we calculate t which minimizes ER. The resulting equation can be used to determine the stretching for each hypothesis correspondence. The error for each hypothesis correspondence is calculated by substituting the estimated stretching values back in (12). The hypothesis with minimum error gives the correct point correspondence and surface stretching. Strictly speaking, hypothesis with large error can be rejected and all hypotheses with very small error should be kept (see discussion on error utilization in Section 7). Let us minimize ER with respect to stretching (t):

$$\frac{dER}{dt} - \sum_{i \in \eta} 2(K_i - t^2\overline{K}_i)(2t\overline{K}_i) = 0$$
$$\Rightarrow \sum_{i \in \eta} (\overline{K}_i K_i - t^2\overline{K}_i^2)t = 0. \tag{13}$$

Solving this equation for t, which is a positive nonzero value gives

$$t - \sqrt{\sum_{i \in \eta}(\overline{K}_i K_i)/\sum_{i \in \eta}(\overline{K}_i^2)}. \tag{14}$$

The above expression (14) has to be calculated for each correspondence hypothesis to find the corresponding stretching. The error for each correspondence hypothesis can then be calculated using Eq. (12). We then choose the point from correspondence hypotheses having minimum error. Corresponding value of t is the stretching at the given point.

If a surface is expanded elastically, such that the stretching remains constant at all points, the point correspondences and the stretching factor can be estimated using the above procedure. The point correspondences and the stretching will be determined precisely if the surface follows homothetic motion assumption. The accuracy of estimation depends on the amount of deviation from homothetic motion assumption.

4.2. Conformal Motion with Linear Stretching

The above approach can be modified for a more general motion, where the stretching (t) is described by a linear function, $t(u, v)$. Consider the linear function for t,

$$t(u, v) = au + bv + c, \tag{15}$$

where (u, v) is the position of the point on the surface; (u, v) are the parameters in any given parameterization. For example, they can be the polar coordinates (θ, ϕ), or rectangular coordinates (x, y) of any given point. We have three unknowns (a, b, c) in the linear stretching function defined by Eq. (15). The necessary equations to calculate these unknowns can be obtained by minimizing the error ER. From (11) and (15),

$$ER = \sum_{i \in \eta} \left\{ \overline{K}_i - \frac{K_i}{(au + bv + c)^2} - f_{\text{linear}}(E_i, F_i, G_i, a, b, c) \right\}^2, \tag{16}$$

where ER is the least square error, or deviation from conformal motion with linear stretching. The least square error (ER) is a minimum when the motion is well approximated by conformal motion with linear stretching. Hence, we compute the partial derivatives of ER over a, b, and c in order to obtain the minimum (ideally, zero).

$(ER)_{\min}$ is determined by equating the partial derivatives $\partial ER/\partial a$, $\partial ER/\partial b$, $\partial ER/\partial b$ to zero. The correct values of a, b, and c correspond to the minimum error $(ER)_{\min}$. After solving for a, b, and c, we use them to compute the error for all correspondence hypotheses. The correspondence hypothesis with minimum error $(ER)_{\min}$ gives us point correspondence and stretching information.

We now proceed to derive the necessary equations using the above criteria. First, we state the necessary equations for conformal motion with linear stretching from [25]. The function f_{linear} in Eq. (16) is given by

$$
\begin{aligned}
&f_{\text{linear}} \\
&= \frac{\begin{array}{c} 2EG[Ga^2 + Eb^2] - EG(au + bv + c) \\ [G_u a + E_v b] + (au + bv + c)[G^2 E_u a + E^2 G_v b] \end{array}}{2(au + bv + c)^2 G^2 E^2}. \tag{17}
\end{aligned}
$$

The error function (ER) can now be minimized to obtain necessary expressions for estimating point correspondences and the stretching. Let

$$\Delta_i = \overline{K}_i - \left\{ \frac{K_i}{(au + bv + c)^2} + f_{\text{linear}}(E_i, F_i, G_i, a, b, c) \right\}$$

$$ER = \sum_{i \in \eta} \Delta_i^2. \tag{18}$$

Now, set

$$\frac{\partial ER}{\partial a} = \frac{\partial ER}{\partial b} = \frac{\partial ER}{\partial c} = 0$$

$$\frac{\partial ER}{\partial a} = \sum_{i \in \eta} 2\Delta_i \left\{ \frac{-2K_i u}{(au + bv + c)^3} + \frac{\partial}{\partial a}(f_{\text{linear}}(E_i, F_i, G_i, a, b, c)) \right\} \tag{19}$$

$$\frac{\partial ER}{\partial b} = \sum_{i \in \eta} 2\Delta_i \left\{ \frac{-2K_i v}{(au + bv + c)^3} + \frac{\partial}{\partial b}(f_{\text{linear}}(E_i, F_i, G_i, a, b, c)) \right\} \tag{20}$$

$$\frac{\partial ER}{\partial c} = \sum_{i \in \eta} 2\Delta_i \left\{ \frac{-2K_i}{(au + bv + c)^3} + \frac{\partial}{\partial c}(f_{\text{linear}}(E_i, F_i, G_i, a, b, c)) \right\}. \tag{21}$$

Thus, we have three nonlinear equations to solve for a, b, c (for complete equations see [21]). Alternative derivations of these equations using tensors is explained in [13].

A mathematica package [38] may be used which is based on Grobner basis construction for finding the numerical solution. It does not require an initial guess. Alternatively, any iterative approach may be used such as the Newton–Raphson method for the solution of a nonlinear system of equations [30]. It requires a good initial guess for fast convergence to a correct local minimum. We have used the latter method in our implementation, with the initial guess generated by the algorithm which uses homothetic motion assumption. Homothetic motion (constant stretching) algorithm is a subset of the conformal motion (with linear stretching) algorithm described above. This leads us to believe that it provides a reliable initial guess for the linear conformal algorithm to converge. This, together with "small motion assumption," helps in avoiding the "valley problem," common in most of the nonlinear minimization problems. Results from both simulation and experimental data (explained later) suggest to us that the minimization algorithm performs satisfactorily.

4.3. Conformal Motion with Polynomial Stretching

Clearly, the approach of the previous section can be extended to the quadratic (or higher order polynomial) approximation of the stretching function $t(u, v)$. In particular, let

$$t(u, v) = au^2 + bv^2 + cuv + du + ev + f. \qquad (22)$$

Substituting t from (22) in the general expression for Gaussian curvature changes (11), we obtain

$$\overline{K} = \frac{K}{(au^2 + bv^2 + cuv + du + ev + f)^2}$$
$$+ f_{quadratic}(E, F, G, a, b, c, d, e, f). \qquad (23)$$

Hence, error ER can now be defined as

$$ER = \left[\overline{K} - \frac{K}{(au^2 + bv^2 + cuv + du + ev + f)^2} \right.$$
$$\left. - f_{quadratic}(E, F, G, a, b, c, d, e, f) \right]^2. \qquad (24)$$

The above error term (ER) can be minimized by taking partial derivatives with respect to a, b, c, d, e, f and equating them to zero. We will then have six equations and six unknowns, which can be solved using nonlinear techniques as discussed in a previous section.

This can be similarly extended to the polynomial stretching of order n. However, the number of unknown terms in the stretching function increase as n increases. This means that we have to solve for more unknowns in estimating each point correspondence. This would increase the computations involved and, hence, the time taken to estimate point correspondence (it will also complicate the minimization problem). Therefore, there has to be a trade-off between the order of polynomial approximation of stretching and the computation time involved in estimating point correspondence.

4.4. Algorithm Description

The algorithm involves three basic steps: (1) curvature calculation and (for nonhomothetic conformal motion) calculation of the coefficients of the first fundamental form and their derivatives, (2) hypotheses formulation and error computation, (3) hypotheses verification and stretching estimation:

1. Gaussian curvature and coefficients of the first fundamental form and its derivatives are calculated. The algorithm for conformal motion assumption (nonhomothetic) needs both Gaussian curvature (before and after motion) and coefficients of the first fundamental form and its derivatives (before motion) at each point on the surface under consideration. However, the algorithm for homothetic motion does not require coefficients of the first fundamental form or its derivatives. Gaussian curvature and coefficients of the first fundamental form and its derivatives can be estimated from the data by invariant fitting [7] of a quadratic surface over a square window and calculating the directional derivatives of this surface.

2. The correspondence hypotheses are formulated using the window around the point under consideration. Points in this window are the candidates for point correspondence. Stretching is calculated for each point in correspondence hypotheses using (14) or (15). Error for each candidate correspondence is then computed using (12) or (16).

3. The above step provides us with the set of correspondence hypotheses, with corresponding stretching and error values. The third step involves evaluating which of these hypotheses satisfies the underlying motion assumption. This is done by choosing the hypothesis with minimum error. There may be more than one hypothesis with small (close to minimum) error, in which case we have several probable point correspondences. This may be due to the insufficient sampling of data points (see Section 6 for point correspondence refinement). In addition, the computed point correspondences are not reliable if the minimum error is large (as discussed in Section 5). Hence a threshold can be chosen for the error term. The point correspondence is estimated if the minimum error is less than this threshold. The output of this last step is the estimated point correspondences and the corresponding stretching.

The computational complexity of this algorithm depends on (1) the nature of surface fitting (quadratic in our case) to calculate differential geometric parameters, (2) the number of correspondence hypothesis, and (3) the iterations taken for solving the nonlinear equations in case of conformal (nonhomothetic) motion assumption. For a chosen order of surface fitting and a chosen window of correspondence hypotheses, the algorithm dealing with conformal (nonhomothetic) assumption solely depends on the computational complexity for solving nonlinear equations used in estimating the stretching parameter. This in turn depends on the initial guess to the algorithm and the tolerance of error, or the number of iterations permitted in the search for a global minimum.

5. SIMULATION RESULTS

Simulations are performed on a surface patch of an ellipsoid by generating a nonrigid motion. The following are the equations governing an ellipsoid in rectangular and polar coordinate systems:

$$\frac{x^2}{a^2} + \frac{y^2}{b^2} + \frac{z^2}{c^2} = 1 \qquad (25)$$

$$x = a \sin(\phi) \cos(\theta), \quad y = b \sin(\phi) \sin(\theta), \quad z = c \cos(\phi) \qquad (26)$$

Any point on the surface in a rectangular coordinate system can be represented in Monge patch form such as (x, y, $z(x, y)$). The parametric curves are orthogonal in this

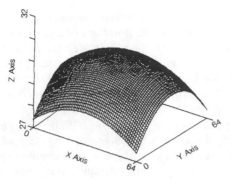

FIG. 4. Ellipsoid patch before motion.

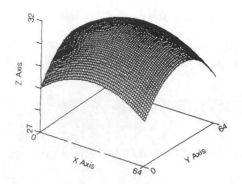

FIG. 6. Ellipsoid patch after motion.

case, as well as in the polar coordinate system (i.e., the first fundamental coefficient $F = 0$).

5.1. Homothetic Motion

We use a patch of the ellipsoid represented by (25) in the simulations. Homothetic motion can be generated by expanding the object in equal proportions in all directions. In the case of an ellipsoid, it can be achieved by increasing in equal proportions the parameters of ellipsoid, a, b, c which control its dimensions [12]. This results in expansion of the ellipsoid. Hence, the equation governing the ellipsoid after homothetic motion is given by

$$\frac{x^2}{(\delta \cdot a)^2} + \frac{y^2}{(\delta \cdot b)^2} + \frac{z^2}{(\delta \cdot c)^2} = 1, \qquad (27)$$

or in the polar coordinate system,

$$x = \delta \cdot a \sin(\phi) \cos(\theta), \quad y = \delta \cdot b \sin(\phi) \sin(\theta),$$
$$z = \delta \cdot c \cos(\phi), \qquad (28)$$

where δ controls the amount of expansion of the ellipsoid. In the simulation tests, we have generated motion on the ellipsoidal patch (65 by 65 points) by increasing a, b, c by 5% (i.e., $\delta = 1.05$). We have used both the implicit equations ((25) and (27)) and explicit equations ((26) and

(28)) in estimating point correspondence and stretching. In the case of Eqs. (26) and (28), the parameters θ and ϕ are preserved during homothetic motion. We have obtained the exact point correspondences and stretching in this simulation, when the polar coordinate system is used. Such an exact estimation is due to the fact that sampling of data points in polar coordinates corresponds one-to-one with the point correspondences. In other words, there is perfect sampling of a surface in polar coordinates such that the point correspondences will not fall between the grid points. On the other hand, the point correspondences between surfaces generated by Eqs. (25) and (27) may fall between grid points. This might introduce some error in estimating point correspondences and stretching in rectangular coordinates. Such an error can be minimized by using better sampling and by performing a refinement procedure described later. The following is the description of simulations utilizing a rectangular coordinate system.

Figures 4 and 6 show the surface patch of an ellipsoid before and after motion respectively given by Eq. (25) and (27). Following the steps of the algorithm discussed before, we compute the curvature of the surface patches before and after the motion. Curvature at each point was computed locally by considering a moving 3 by 3 window with the origin at the center of the window. Figures 5 and 7 show the calculated curvature before and after motion, respectively.

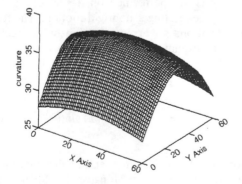

FIG. 5. Curvature before motion.

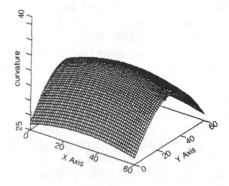

FIG. 7. Curvature after motion.

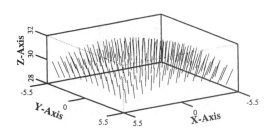

FIG. 8.   Point correspondences.

# of Sample Points	Stretching	
	True	Estimated
4225	1.05	1.053184
16900	1.05	1.049889

FIG. 10.   Sampling.

Next, we need to define the region of interest ($\Re$), or the set of correspondence hypotheses for each point on the surface. For any point, $P_{i,j}$, we consider the region of interest as a 5 by 5 window of points with $P_{i,j}$ as its center. Hence, there will be a set of 25 points as correspondence hypotheses for any $P_{i,j}$. We can now estimate the stretching and error for each correspondence hypothesis. The least of 25 errors (corresponding to each correspondence hypothesis) gives us an estimation of point correspondences and stretching.

Figure 8 shows the point correspondences obtained using the Gaussian curvature-based algorithm with the homothetic motion assumption. This figure consists of line vectors, whose initial points indicate the points on the surface patch before motion, and the final points indicate points on the surface patch after motion. It can be observed that for the points away from the origin, the vectors are more inclined. This phenomenon characterizes the expansion of an ellipsoid. The point correspondences are verified by converting the rectangular coordinates into polar coordinates and comparing them (note that polar coordinates will not change during homothetic motion). The stretching estimation obtained is shown in Fig. 9. It can be observed that the estimated stretching is constant throughout the surface patch.

The precision of estimated point correspondences and stretching can be effected due to the correspondences falling between grids. The precision can be improved by increasing the number of data points on the surface (i.e., increasing sampling points on surface). Figure 10 shows the table with the estimated stretching for two different sets of sample points of the same surface undergoing homothetic motion. It can be observed that the estimated stretching is more accurate with higher sampling. Refinement of the estimated point correspondences and stretching is explained in Section 6.

5.2.   Non-conformal Motion

Improved performance of the algorithm which uses a conformal motion assumption with linear stretching over the algorithm with the homothetic motion assumption can be illustrated by comparing the performance of these algorithms when applied to the surface undergoing nonconformal motion. This is done by testing the results of each approach on the surface patch of an ellipsoid with nonconformal expansion. This motion can be generated by increasing a, b, c nonproportionately (i.e., $a = \delta_x \cdot a$, $b = \delta_y \cdot b$, $c = \delta_z \cdot c$). In this simulation, $\delta_x = 1.02$, $\delta_y = 1.04$, and $\delta_z = 1.06$. Figure 11 shows the surface patch after motion, and Fig. 12 represents its corresponding curvature. In this simulation, the deformation along the y axis (controlled by δ_y) is greater than the deformation along the x axis (controlled by δ_x). It is expected that point correspondences should move away from the center of

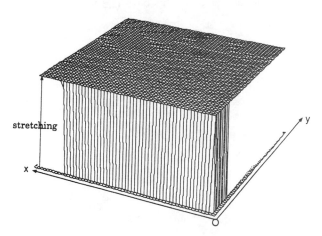

FIG. 9.   Estimated stretching.

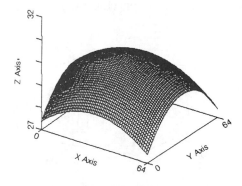

FIG. 11.   Ellipsoid patch after motion.

335

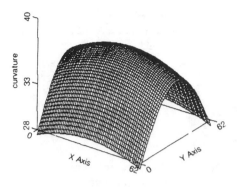

FIG. 12. Curvature after motion.

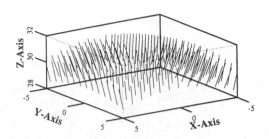

FIG. 14. Point correspondences under linear stretching.

the ellipsoid as the ellipsoid is being expanded. However, they will not be uniform as in homothetic motion.

Figure 13 represents point correspondences generated by the algorithm utilizing the homothetic motion assumption. Clearly, it fails to give correct point correspondences, as the estimated point correspondences here are directed towards the center of the patch instead of moving away. On the other hand, we note better estimation of point correspondences in the case of conformal motion with the linear stretching assumption in Fig. 14. Figure 15 represents the estimated stretching generated by the algorithm under conformal motion with the linear stretching assumption. Note the larger deformation along the y Axis which corresponds to $\delta_x < \delta_y$.

Next, we generate motion on the surface patch of the ellipsoid by pulling each point on the patch (2D mesh in our case) vertically, without changing its x and y coordinates. Figure 16 shows the surface patch after motion, and Fig. 17 represents its corresponding curvature. Here, we have known correspondences in the rectangular coordinate system, as we know that the x and y coordinates of each point are not changed during motion. Any point on the surface patch before motion will have the same x and y coordinates after the motion, enabling us to test the results of the algorithm. In this simulation, the motion on the surface is generated by pulling each point vertically, using ($\bar{z} = \delta \cdot z$). Since this motion is not conformal, we are using higher resolution (130 by 130) and a 9 by 9

window of the correspondence hypotheses around the point under consideration (we will discuss this fact again later in this section).

Figure 18 shows the point correspondences with $\delta = 1.003$. As we have discussed before, the point correspondences are known a priori since the motion is in a vertical direction. Hence we can also calculate the error in the estimated correspondence. It can be seen from Fig. 18 that the algorithm estimates correct correspondences at most of the points on the surface. Correspondence error can be defined as the absolute value of the number of steps (pixels); that the estimated correspondence is away from the correct correspondence. The minimum value of the correspondence error is zero. For the above motion, the average error in each estimated correspondence is 0.62.

The algorithm generates correct estimation of point correspondences if the motion can be well approximated by conformal motion (as in the previous simulation). As the amount of displacement in the z direction increases, the motion starts to deviate more from conformal motion, resulting in the increase of correspondence error. In the case where $\delta = 1.003$, the motion is small and thus it can be well approximated to conformal motion. However, this will not be true as the motion increases. Figure 19 shows the point correspondences with $\delta = 1.05$. The average correspondence error in this case is 3.85.

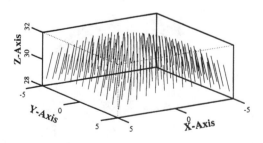

FIG. 13. Point correspondences under constant stretching.

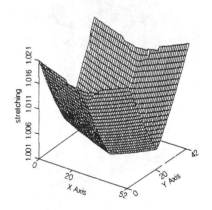

FIG. 15. Estimated stretching.

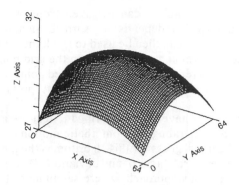

FIG. 16. Ellipsoid patch after motion.

The algorithm may also estimate more than one point correspondence, as the minimum least square error (*ER*, defined by Eq. (12) or (16)) can be associated with more than one correspondence hypothesis. In addition, several errors can be "very close" to the minimum least square error. Figure 20 shows the error distribution of the correspondence hypotheses of a point on the surface for the above simulation. We know that the correct correspondence is always the center of the correspondence hypotheses, as the motion is vertical (5 by 5 window in this case). In an ideal case, the center of the error distribution must be a minimum, in order that the algorithm can choose the correct point correspondence. However, we observe that there are more than one correspondence hypothesis close to the minimum error, as indicated in Fig. 20. Hence with real data, the smallest error may not provide good estimation of point correspondence, when there is more than one error close to the minimum. In such cases, more than one point correspondence is generated, indicating probable correspondences at each point. One way of solving such a problem is to introduce more equations to satisfy the underlying constraints. The next section deals with this problem and also alleviates the error introduced by sampling.

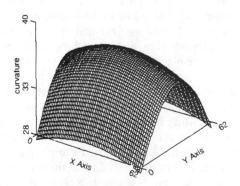

FIG. 17. Curvature after motion.

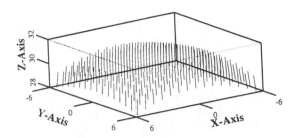

FIG. 18. Point correspondences (for $\delta = 1.003$).

6. REFINEMENT OF ESTIMATED POINT CORRESPONDENCES

The estimation of point correspondences in our approach described above involves an error due to the sampling of data points. This is because, the point correspondences can lie between sampled data points, in which case our algorithm chooses the closest true correspondence. In this section, we present an algorithm which is able to track accurate point correspondences (with a small error introduced due to the surface approximation).

Gaussian curvature of a surface $z(x, y)$ at any point (x, y) is given by

$$K = \frac{z_{xx}z_{yy} - z_{xy}^2}{(1 + z_x^2 + z_y^2)^2}. \quad (29)$$

Consider fitting a quadratic surface in the local neighborhood. The quadratic surface can be

$$z(x, y) = \gamma_1 + \gamma_2 x + \gamma_3 y + \gamma_4 xy + \gamma_5 x^2 + \gamma_6 y^2. \quad (30)$$

It may be noted that higher order approximation of the surface reduces the error in estimating the differential geometric parameters used in our algorithm. Higher sampling rate also improves the fit, thus contributing to the accurate estimation of parameters used and, eventually, in estimating point correspondences and stretching. The partial derivatives of the quadratic surface are given by

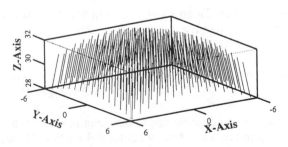

FIG. 19. Point correspondences (for $\delta = 1.05$).

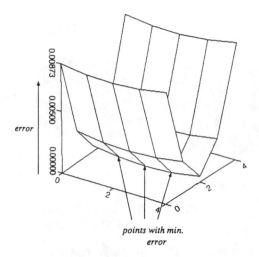

FIG. 20. Error distribution.

$$z_x = \gamma_2 + \gamma_4 y + 2\gamma_5 x, \quad z_y = \gamma_3 + \gamma_4 x + 2\gamma_6 y$$

$$z_{xx} = 2\gamma_5, \quad z_{yy} = 2\gamma_6, \quad z_{xy} = \gamma_4.$$

Using these expressions, Gaussian curvature is given by

$$K$$

$$= \frac{4\gamma_5\gamma_6 - \gamma_4^2}{(1 + (\gamma_2 + \gamma_4 y + 2\gamma_5 x)^2 + (\gamma_3 + \gamma_4 x + 2\gamma_6 y)^2)^2}. \quad (31)$$

From Mishra *et al.*, any conformal motion is of the form

$$\overline{K} = \frac{K}{t^2} + \frac{f}{t^2}; \quad (32)$$

f is a polynomial function of (u, v); f_{linear} (Eq. (17)) is discussed in Section 4.2. The error term can be defined from the above equation as

$$ER = \left[\frac{4\gamma_5\gamma_6 - \gamma_4^2}{(1 + (\gamma_2 + \gamma_4\overline{y} + 2\gamma_5\overline{x})^2 + (\gamma_3 + \gamma_4\overline{x} + 2\gamma_6\overline{y})^2)^2} \right. $$
$$\left. - \frac{K}{t^2} - \frac{f}{t^2} \right]^2. \quad (33)$$

K is a constant for any given point in the above equation. On the other hand, f, t, and points after the motion $(\overline{x}, \overline{y})$ are unknowns. ER can be rewritten as

$$ER = [(4\gamma_5\gamma_6 - \gamma_4^2)t^2 - (K + f)(1 + (\gamma_2 + \gamma_4\overline{y} + 2\gamma_5\overline{x})^2$$
$$+ (\gamma_3 + \gamma_4\overline{x} + 2\gamma_6\overline{y})^2)^2]^2. \quad (34)$$

The above equation has to be a minimum for the point correspondences to follow conformal motion. Hence we minimize ER w.r.t. the unknowns t, f, $\overline{x}$, $\overline{y}$. An initial

guess to this solution can be given from our previous algorithm (which depends on surface sampling). The above equation can then be used to track the point correspondences which may fall between the grid points. This step acts as a refinement to the estimated point correspondences and stretching generated by the previous algorithm.

Simulations have been performed to test the above approach by generating the homothetic motion on an ellipsoid. The initial guess for this algorithm is the point correspondences, stretching (t), and deviation (f), as generated by the previous approach, where sampling of the points introduced some error. It has been observed that this error, due to sampling, has been rectified to give better estimation. Using the new algorithm, the error is reduced to one-fifth the error between the initial guess (which lies on the closest grid point) and the actual point correspondence. This remaining error can be attributed to the surface fitting in calculating the differential parameters.

7. EXPERIMENTS ON REAL DATA

The algorithm has been applied to volumetric CT data of the left ventricle of a dog's heart. We have 16 time frames of two sets of data over one heart cycle. One set corresponds to the healthy heart, and the other one corresponds to the heart with abnormal condition (atrial fibrillation). Each frame consists of 128 by 128 by 118 binary voxels containing previously extracted surface information. The surface information was extracted manually and supplied to us by Dr. Eric Hoffman at the University of Iowa. The data was obtained by the Dynamic Spatial Reconstructor—a high temporal resolution, synchronous volume (three-dimensional), computed tomography scanner [32]. We have performed experiments on healthy heart data first and then compared against the atrial fibrillation case. The following experiments correspond to the healthy heart.

Figure 21 shows the volumetric data at frame 4. Only the voxels above the plane (which is the left ventricle) are considered. Figure 22 shows the volume changes of the left ventricle (LV) data used in our experiments. It can be observed that frames 1 to 7 undergo contraction and frames 7 to 16 undergo expansion in the heart cycle. Point correspondences and stretching have been estimated using the algorithm which employs the assumption of conformal motion with linear stretching in the local neighborhood. Gaussian curvature and coefficients of the first fundamental form and its derivatives are calculated by invariant fitting of a quadratic surface over a 5 by 5 square window and estimating the directional derivatives at each point on the LV surface. Fitting a quadratic surface provides a certain level of smoothing of the surface and partially reduces the noise. Region of interest ($\Re$) is defined as a 5 by 5 window around the point under

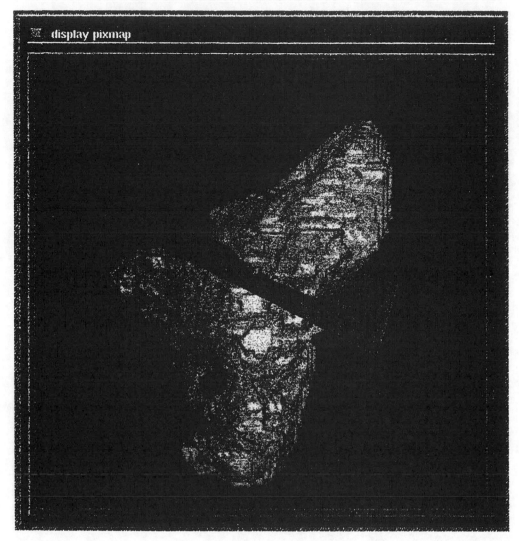

FIG. 21.   Left ventricle at frame 4.

consideration. Refinement of the estimated point correspondences have been performed (as explained in Section 6); however, there is no significant improvement; this is due to the dense sampling of the LV data set. Results on frames 4–5 and 9–10 are explained below, which are in contraction and expansion phase, respectively.

The points in the lower part of the surface shown are not on the LV; hence they are not considered in our calculations. The error can be large in the following cases: (a) where small motion assumption is not satisfied, or (b) where motion is not conformal. *ER* can hence be used as a measure of confidence in the estimated stretching and point correspondences. In addition, planar patches (zero curvature) will have a large number of hypotheses with small errors. Hence, we ignore these patches in estimating correspondences. Figure 23 shows the stretching and

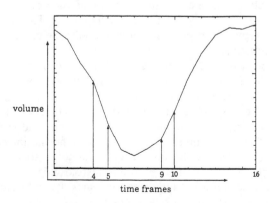

FIG. 22.   Volume changes of LV.

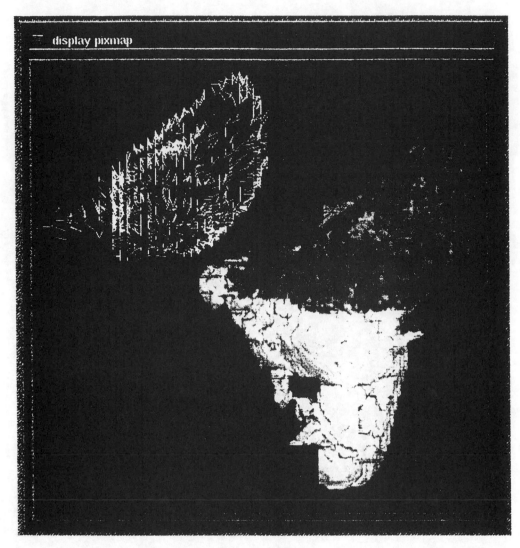

FIG. 23. Point correspondences and stretching between frames 4 and 5.

point correspondences between frames 4–5. The line vectors represent point correspondences between the frames 4 and 5. The darker region indicates contraction (close to black color), and the lighter region indicates expansion (close to white color). It can be seen that the algorithm estimates contraction at most points of the surface. At points where the point correspondences have not been determined, the average stretching in the (3 by 3) neighborhood is used to determine surface stretching. Thus, stretching for certain regions, where the algorithms has failed to estimate, due to the reasons explained above, can also be approximated. Figure 24 shows the stretching and point correspondences between frames 9 and 10. It can be observed again that the algorithm estimates expansion for most points of the LV surface. Figure 25 depicts

the error (*ER*) distribution during correspondence recovery between frames 4 and 5. The magnitude of the error increases from dark-light in increasing order. The isolated white regions represent the points having the error above the threshold.

Comparison of stretching between the healthy LV and the LV affected by atrial fibrillation has been performed to verify the results of the algorithm. According to radiologists, there is less stretching on the LV wall between end-diastole (time frame of maximum volume) and end-systole (time frame of minimum volume) in atrial fibrillation case. Figure 26 shows the curves corresponding to average stretching of frames between end-diastole and end-systole in the case of normal and diseased hearts. It can be clearly observed that the atrial fibrillation case has smaller

340

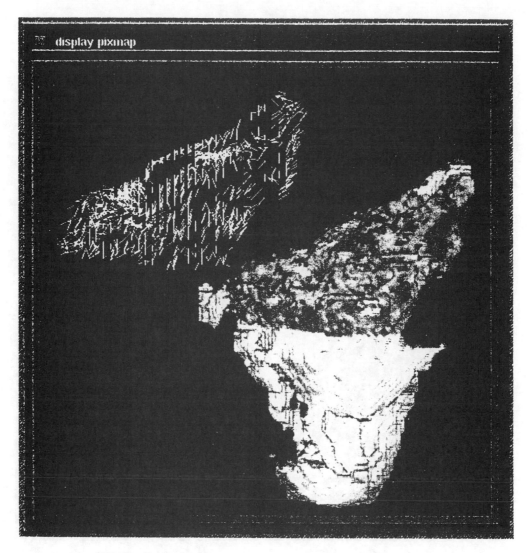

FIG. 24.   Point correspondences and stretching between frames 9 and 10.

stretching (i.e., closer to stretching = 1.0) than the normal heart. This gives an indication that conformal motion can be a reasonable approximation of the LV in motion.

8.   DISCUSSIONS

We have presented a new curvature-based method for estimating point correspondences and stretching of a surface in nonrigid motion. Our approach uses assumptions of a locally constant, linear, or polynomial surface stretching to estimate point correspondences in conformal motion.

The algorithm requires the calculation of Gaussian curvature at points on the surface at each frame. It also requires the computation of the coefficients of the first fundamental form and their derivatives at points on the surface before motion in case of conformal motion with nonhomothetic stretching. The algorithm is invariant to the surface parameterization, as it uses Gaussian curvature (invariant property of the surface) in the point correspondence estimation. Although coefficients of the first fundamental form and their derivatives depend on parameterization, that does not affect the algorithm, since these coefficients are used in only one time frame (before motion). A small motion assumption is utilized to hypothesize possible point correspondences. The least square error is framed as the difference between computed curvature changes and the one predicted by the conformal motion assumption. A hypothesis with the smallest error is estimated as the point correspondence. Refinement can also be performed on the estimated point correspondence

341

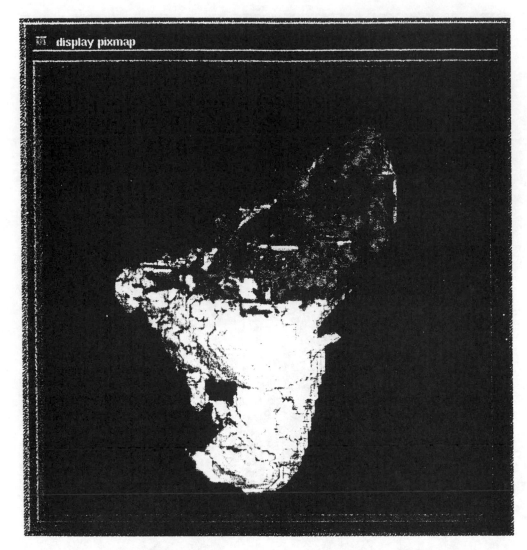

FIG. 25. Error distribution during correspondence recovery between frames 4 and 5.

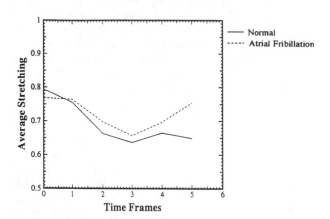

FIG. 26. Comparisons.

and stretching in order to reduce the error caused by sampling.

Simulations are performed on ellipsoidal data to illustrate the performance and the accuracy of the derived algorithms. Then, the proposed algorithm is applied to volumetric CT data of the LV for endocardial left ventricular motion analysis. Comparisons of surface stretching are made between the normal and abnormal LVs.

Future work will include both theoretical and practical aspects. First, future investigations will involve other invariance measures (in addition to curvature) that can be used in tracking point correspondences in a general nonrigid motion [19]. Second, it is also necessary to consider the problem of point tracking and the estimation of motion parameters for nonconformal motion which is less restrictive than conformal motion. Multiframe analysis of non-

342

rigid motion may also simplify the extraction of nonrigid motion parameters and help in the estimation of point correspondences. Finally, extensive testing of the proposed algorithm on numerous real data sets is warranted to determine its clinical usefulness in cardiac studies.

REFERENCES

1. A. A. Amini and J. S. Duncan, Pointwise tracking of left-ventricular motion in 3D, in *Proceedings, IEEE Workshop on Visual Motion, October 1991*, pp. 294–299.

2. M. Asada, M. Yachida, and S. Tsuji, Understanding of 3D motion in block world, *Pattern Recognit.* **17**(1), 1984, 57–84.

3. B. M. Bennet and D. D. Hoffman, The computation of structure from fixed axis motion: Nonrigid structures, *Biol. Cybernet* **51**, 1985, 293–300.

4. C. W. Chen and T. S. Huang, Nonrigid object motion and deformation estimation from three-dimensional data, *Int. J. Imaging Systems Technol.* **2**, 1990, 385–394.

5. S. S. Chen and M. Penna, *Motion Analysis of Deformable Objects*, Vol. 3, JAI Press, Greenwich, CT, 1988.

6. J. Cheng and H. Don, A structural approach to finding the point correspondences between two frames, in *Proceedings, IEEE International Conference on Robotics and Automation, April 1988*, Vol. 3, pp. 1810–1815.

7. D. B. Goldgof, T. S. Huang, and H. Lee, A curvature-based approach to terrain recognition, *IEEE Trans. Pattern Anal. Mach. Intell.* **PAMI-11**(11), 1989, 1213–1217.

8. D. B. Goldgof and C. Kambhamettu, Application of the nonrigid shape matching algorithm to volumetric cardiac images, in *SPIE/SPSE Symposium on Electronic Imaging, Conference on Biomedical Image Processing, February, 1991*, pp. 264–276.

9. D. B. Goldgof, H. Lee, and T. S. Huang, Motion analysis of nonrigid surfaces, in *Proceedings, IEEE Computer Society Conference on Computer Vision and Pattern Recognition, 1988*, pp. 375–380.

10. D. B. Goldgof, H. Lee, and T. S. Huang, Parameter estimation of the heart motion from angiography data, in *SPIE/SPSE Symposium on Electronic Imaging, Conference on Biomedical Image Processing, February 1990*, 1245(15), 171–181.

11. W. C. Graustein, *Differential Geometry*, Macmillan, New York, 1935.

12. H. W. Guggenheimer, *Differential Geometry*, McGraw–Hill, Polytechnic Institute of New York, 1977.

13. M. He, D. B. Goldgof, and C. Kambhamettu, Variation of gaussian curvature under conformal mapping and its application, *Comput. Math. Appl.* 1993, **26**(1), 63–74.

14. B. Horowitz and A. Pentland, Recovery of non-rigid motion and structure, in *Proceedings, IEEE Conf. on Computers June 1991*, pp. 288–293.

15. T. S. Huang, Motion analysis, in *Encyclopedia of Artificial Intelligence*, Vol. 1, pp. 620–632, Wiley, New York, 1986.

16. T. S. Huang, Modeling, analysis, and visualization of nonrigid object motion, in *Proceedings, of 10th ICPR, December 1990*, pp. 361–364.

17. C. Kambhamettu and D. B. Goldgof, Towards finding point correspondences in nonrigid motion, in *The 7'th Scandinavian Conference on Image Analysis, August 1991*, pp. 1126–1133.

18. C. Kambhamettu and D. B. Goldgof, Point correspondence recovery in nonrigid motion, in *Proceedings, IEEE Conference on Computer Vision and Pattern Recognition, June 1992*, pp. 222–227.

19. C. Kambhamettu, D. B. Goldgof, and M. He, On a study of invariant features in nonrigid transformations, in *Proceedings, IEEE Workshop on Qualitative Vision, June 1993*, pp. 118–127.

20. C. Kambhamettu, D. B. Goldgof, D. Terzopoulos, and T. S. Huang, Nonrigid motion analysis, in *Handbook of PRIP: Computer Vision*, Vol. II (T. Young, Ed.), Academic Press, San Diego, CA, 1994.

21. C. Kambhamettu, *Curvature-Based Approach to Point Correspondence Recovery in Nonrigid Motion*, Master's thesis, Department of Computer Science and Engineering, University of South Florida, 1991.

22. M. M. Lipschutz, *Schaum's Outline of Theory and Problems of Differential Geometry*, McGraw-Hill, New York, 1969.

23. D. Metaxas and D. Terzopoulos, Recursive estimation of shape and nonrigid motion, in *Proceedings, IEEE Workshop on Visual Motion, October 1991*.

24. S. K. Mishra, D. B. Goldgof, T. S. Huang, Non-rigid motion analysis and epicardial deformation estimation from angiography data, in *IEEE Conference on Computer Vision and Pattern Recognition, June 1991*.

25. S. K. Mishra, D. B. Goldgof, T. S. Huang, and C. Kambhamettu, Curvature-based non-rigid motion analysis from 3D point correspondences, *Int. J. Imaging Systems Technol.* **4**, 1993, 214–225.

26. S. K. Mishra, D. B. Goldgof, and C. Kambhamettu, Estimating nonrigid motion from point and line correspondences, *Pattern Recognit. Lett.*, in press.

27. A. N. Netravali, T. S. Huang, A. S. Krishnakumar, and R. J. Holt, Algebraic methods in 3-D motion estimation from two-view point correspondences, *Int. J. Imaging Systems Technol.* **1**, 1989, 78–99.

28. J. O'Rourke and N. Badler, Model-based image analysis of human motion using constraint propagation, *IEEE Trans. Pattern Anal. Mach. Intell.* **PAMI-2**, 1980, 522–536.

29. A. Pentland, B. Horowitz, and S. Sclaroff, Non-rigid motion and structure from contour, in *Proceedings, IEEE Workshop on Visual Motion, October 1991*, pp. 288–293.

30. W. H. Press, B. P. Flannery, S. A. Teukolsky, and W. T. Vetterling, *Numerical recipes in C: The Art of Scientific Programming*, Cambridge Univ. Press, Cambridge, UK, 1988.

31. J. W. Roach and J. K. Aggarwal, Determining the movement of objects from a sequence of images, *IEEE Trans. Pattern Anal. Mach. Intell.* **PAMI-2**(6), 1980, 554–562.

32. R. A. Robb, E. A. Hoffman, L. J. Sinak, L. D. Harris, and E. L. Ritman, High-speed three-dimensional X-ray computed tomography: The dynamic spatial reconstructor, *Proc. IEEE* **71**(3), 1983, 308–320.

33. D. Shulman and J. T. Aloimonos, Nonrigid motion interpretation: A regularized approach, *Proc. R. Soc. London B* **233**, 1988, 217–234.

34. D. Terzopoulos and D. Metaxas, Dynamic 3D models with local and global deformations: Deformable superquadrics, *IEEE Trans. Pattern Anal. Mach. Intell.* **13**, 1991, 703–714.

35. S. Ullman, Maximizing rigidity, MIT AI Memo 721, 1983.

36. J. A. Webb and J. K. Aggarwal, Shape and correspondence, *Comput. Vision Graphics Image Process.* **21**, 1983, 145–160.

37. J. A. Webb and J. K. Aggarwal, Structure from motion of rigid and jointed objects, *Artif. Intell.* **19**(1), 1983, 107–130.

38. S. Wolfram, *Mathematica: A System for Doing Mathematics by Computer*, Addison-Wesley, Reading, MA, 1988.

Pointwise Tracking of Left-Ventricular Motion in 3D

Amir A. Amini and James S. Duncan
Departments of Diagnostic Radiology and Electrical Engineering
Yale University
New Haven, Connecticut 06510

Abstract

The problem of motion-tracking of the left-ventricular wall from 4D image data is addressed. We first discuss the forms of 4D data available to us, namely cine-X-Ray CT, and gated and cine Magnetic-Resonance Image data. We then discuss the approach that is utilized for tracking the movement of the endocardium. Based on these ideas, an algorithm is developed, and experimental results are presented.

1 Introduction

Non-invasive techniques for measuring the dynamic behavior of the left ventricle (LV) can be an invaluable tool in the diagnosis of heart disease. The results gained from quantifying this motion can yield insight into the general health of the heart and provide clues regarding specific events affecting cardiac performance. The motion of the LV chamber has been of major interest to the medical community since the left ventricle is the chamber responsible for pumping out oxygenated blood to the body. To assess functionality of the LV, knowledge of regional motion of the endocardial surface will be of substantial value.

From the standpoint of computer vision, measuring the LV motion is a challenging problem mainly because the motion is non-rigid. Rigid motion, as opposed to non-rigid motion, is better-understood, and a number of techniques dealing with it have been proposed [1]. Motion of non-rigid objects, on the other hand, is more complicated. This is because the *structure* of the object no longer remains the same, and deforms with time [11]. Previous work in the measurement of cardiac motion has dealt with data from two-dimensional image sequences. Several methods have been devised attempting to extract motion information based on such data (see [8] for an overview). The alternate route to cardiac motion analysis has been to artificially create distinct features that are visible in images. One method is to surgically implant markers on the LV wall [14]. These techniques usually require manual registration of the markers ([4] is an example) and in the past have often been restricted to finding motion of the epicardium which clinically is felt to be not as useful of a measure as the endocardial motion. A new, non-invasive technique that offers a different approach for tracking of points is Magnetic Resonance (MR) tagging [15]. This approach, based on MR imaging principles, creates a magnetization grid tagging

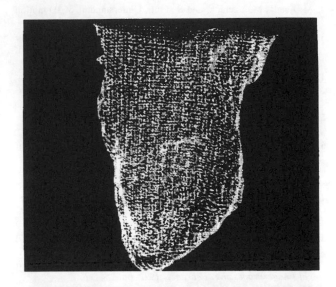

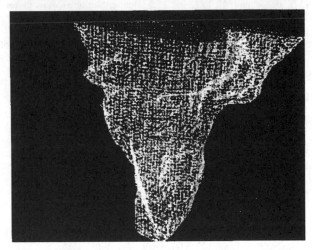

Figure 1: Triangular tesselation of the left-ventricle at diastole, and systole of DSR data.

Reprinted from *Proc. IEEE Workshop Visual Motion,* 1991, pp. 294–300.

344

the underlying tissue, and uses the grid in following the tissue over a 2D image sequence. Since the magnetic tags decay over time, however, MR-tagging has limited ability in tracking points over the entire cardiac cycle. Furthermore, one needs to locate the tagged points that fall on the LV wall, and movement in the z direction is difficult to follow.

2 Cardiac Image Data

In comparison to 2D image-sequence analysis, 3D image-sequence analysis has not received a great deal of attention. Primarily, this has been due to the lack of available 4D (3-space and time) imaging methods. However, these methods are becoming increasingly available. There are four major methods: Echochardiography, 4D Cine Computed-Tomography (CT), gated Single-Photon Emission Computed Tomography (SPECT), and Magnetic Resonance Imaging (MRI) [6]. Among these methods, MRI is most likely to provide the highest resolution and blood/heart wall contrast. Cine-CT data are comparable to MR in this respect and in addition, Cine-CT data can be acquired extremely fast.

The basis for MRI is spatial encoding of the nuclear magnetic resonance signal. Both gated spin-echo and gradient-echo cine MR are popular acquisition techniques. To acquire images from a single phase of the cardiac cycle and to improve the resolution, MR images are obtained by synchronizing to the electrocardiographic (ECG) signal where the acquisition is triggered by the ECG R-wave. To get volumetric data, the 2D slices which are obtained from different time instants in the R-R phase of the cardiac cycle are stacked to achieve "averaged" three-dimensional image frames of the heart. Another MR methodology for imaging the heart is the gradient-echo cine technique. In gradient echo, after all the data is collected, data sets representative of each cardiac phase are generated retrospectively. This results in faster acquisitions at the expense of more noise. In addition to MR, we are utilizing data from cine-CT. For this purpose, we have acquired *Dynamic Spatial Reconstructor* (DSR) data from the Mayo clinic. DSR is the only machine of its kind for acquiring real-time 4D data. To get an idea about the speed of acquisition, in the time (5 seconds) that an average CT scanner produces one cross section image of the body, the DSR can generate 75,000 cross sections. IMATRON, a commercial manufacturer, builds cine-CT machines which can quickly acquire several image slice sequences. Figure 1 shows surface triangulations of manually traced DSR contour data at diastole and systole. The complete data set contains 18 3D image volumes, each having roughly 90 slices. Employing 3D information greatly enhances the accuracy of various motion measures, and has clear advantages over 2D analysis.

3 LV Motion Models

Our approach to non-rigid motion computation can be summarized in determining the local bending and stretch-

ing of the LV surface. There is an important theorem in differential geometry which assures us that finding these quantities is equivalent to determination of the 3D-surface in a lapsed time (fundamental theorem of curves and surfaces) [12]. This is important to recognize, since bending and stretching will be unique to the pair of geometric entities.

3.1 Differential Geometry

In this section, we review relevant concepts from differential geometry [3,5,9,12] which will be used in the formulation of non-rigid motion computation. Computing non-rigid motion will include measurement of bending and stretching deformation of shape based on differential geometry. Our notation will follow that of Do Carmo [5].

Differential geometry is the branch of mathematics that deals with local description of smooth curves and surfaces. Here, we will concern ourselves only with differential geometry of surfaces. We will refer to a surface S in some parametrized neighborhood as $\mathbf{x}(u,v)$; i.e., we will assume that there exists an open neighborhood $U \in \Re^2$ such that $\mathbf{x} : U \rightarrow \Re^3$. Let $\beta : [a,b] \rightarrow U$ be a differentiable path and let us ask the question: what is the arc length of the curve $\mathbf{x}(\beta(t))$ on the surface S? The stretching of a surface is clearly related to change of length of such a curve on the surface as a function of time. Consider the tangent plane $T_p(S)$ of S at point p, and consider any two vectors w_1 and w_2 on T_p. The quadratic form associated with the inner product $< w_1, w_2 >$ is

$$I_p(w) = < w, w > = |w|^2 \tag{1}$$

which is referred to as the first fundamental form of the surface and measures length of vectors on $T_p(S)$. Since the length of the curve $\alpha(t) = \mathbf{x}(\beta(t))$ is $\int_a^b |\alpha'(t)| dt$, applying the chain rule of differential calculus to $\mathbf{x}(\beta(t))$ with $\beta(t) = (u(t), v(t))$,

$$
\begin{aligned}
|\alpha'(t)| &= (\alpha'(t) \cdot \alpha'(t))^{1/2} \\
&= [\mathbf{x}_u \cdot \mathbf{x}_u (u')^2 + 2\mathbf{x}_u \cdot \mathbf{x}_v (u'v') + \\
&\quad \mathbf{x}_v \cdot \mathbf{x}_v (v')^2]^{1/2}
\end{aligned}
\tag{2}
$$

where the subscript in each case denotes differentiation with respect to the variable of interest. Letting $E = \mathbf{x}_u \cdot \mathbf{x}_u$, $F = \mathbf{x}_u \cdot \mathbf{x}_v$, $G = \mathbf{x}_v \cdot \mathbf{x}_v$, the length of a curve on the surface can be described by the E, F, G functions directly from the parameter space U. In addition to length, one can show that area on the surface, also, may be calculated with knowledge of the same functions in the parameter space. It should be clear that stretching properties of the surface are related to the *coefficients of the first fundamental form*, E, F, and G.

Curvature properties of the surface S on the other hand are related to how the normal to the surface varies. Consider the normal to the surface defined as the mapping from S to the unit sphere ($x^2 + y^2 + z^2 = 1$) as

$$N_p = \frac{\mathbf{x}_u \times \mathbf{x}_v}{|\mathbf{x}_u \times \mathbf{x}_v|} \tag{3}$$

for a point p in S. This is the familiar Gauss map. Now, consider the restriction of the Gauss map to the curve $\alpha(t)$ with $\alpha(0) = p$. Then with $N(t) = N(\alpha(t))$, $N'(0) = dN_p(\alpha'(0))$ is a vector in the tangent plane at p (one can show that the tangent plane at p and the tangent plane at N_p on the Gauss map are parallel and thus the two can be treated as being the same here). dN_p measures how N pulls away from N_p in a neighborhood of p. In the case of curves, this measure is given by a number, the curvature. In the case of surfaces, this measure is characterized by dN_p, a linear map which is self-adjoint, that is,

$$< dN_p(w_1), w_2 > = < w_1, dN_p(w_2) > \tag{4}$$

for all $w_1, w_2 \in T_p(S)$. Specifically, for a vector $v \in T_p(S)$, a quadratic form

$$II_p(v) = - < dN_p(v), v > \tag{5}$$

can be associated with dN_p since (4) is bilinear and symmetric. II_p is called the second fundamental form of the surface at p. A related concept is that of the normal curvature of a curve on the surface. Consider the intersection of a plane with the surface such that the plane contains the point p, and the normal to the surface at p. The curvature of the curve found as a result of the intersection of the plane with S is called the normal curvature, κ_n, of the surface at p in the direction of the tangent vector to the curve and takes on the value of the second fundamental form at p (in this case $|v| = 1$ in equation (5). In general, $\kappa_n = II_p(v)/I_p(v)$.) The maximum and minimum of the normal curvature (found by rotating the said intersecting plane about N_p) are κ_1 and κ_2, which are known as the principal curvatures. There are directions associated with these quantities namely, the principal directions (directions of maximal and minimal change of the normal vector), which may be found by diagonalizing the matrix of dN_p.

To calculate II_p, the methods discussed above are not easily adaptable. Instead, consider the curve $\alpha(t)$ on the surface. Since $\alpha' = \mathbf{x}_u u' + \mathbf{x}_v v'$ and $dN(\alpha') = N'(u(t), v(t)) = N_u u' + N_v v'$,

$$\begin{aligned} II_p(\alpha') &= - < dN(\alpha'), \alpha' > \\ &= - < N_u u' + N_v v', \mathbf{x}_u u' + \mathbf{x}_v v' > \\ &= e(u')^2 + 2fu'v' + g(v')^2 \end{aligned} \tag{6}$$

where $e = - < N_u, \mathbf{x}_u > = < N, \mathbf{x}_{uu} >$, $f = - < N_v, \mathbf{x}_u > = < N, \mathbf{x}_{uv} > = - < N_u, \mathbf{x}_v >$ and $g = - < N_v, \mathbf{x}_v > = < N, \mathbf{x}_{vv} >$.

Since a local basis for the tangent plane is $\{\mathbf{x}_u, \mathbf{x}_v\}$, we can express N_u and N_v as linear combinations of these two basis elements in the following way [5]:

$$\begin{bmatrix} N_u \\ N_v \end{bmatrix} = \begin{bmatrix} E & F \\ F & G \end{bmatrix}^{-1} \begin{bmatrix} e & f \\ f & g \end{bmatrix} \begin{bmatrix} \mathbf{x}_u \\ \mathbf{x}_v \end{bmatrix} \tag{7}$$

The change of coordinate matrix above is known as the Weingarten mapping, which we refer to by $\mathbf{W}$, and is the matrix of dN_p expressed in tangent plane coordinates.

The Gaussian curvature function K of a surface is defined in terms of both the principal curvatures and in *Gauss*'s notation by

$$K(u, v) = \kappa_1 \kappa_2 = det(\mathbf{W}) = \frac{eg - f^2}{EG - F^2} \tag{8}$$

Note that the second equality follows because diagonalizing a matrix leaves its determinant unchanged. The same will be true of the trace of the matrix when computing the mean curvature. The mean curvature of the surface is defined as

$$H(u, v) = \frac{\kappa_1 + \kappa_2}{2} = \frac{1}{2} tr(\mathbf{W}) = \frac{Eg + Ge - 2Ff}{2(EG - F^2)} \tag{9}$$

Our approach to measurement of non-rigid shape change of the LV draws from the concepts described in this section.

3.2 A Bending and Stretching Model for the LV

Our formulation is based on a bending and stretching model. The physical model of the LV used is a thin-plate constrained to stretch in a predetermined way as will be shown later. The potential energy of an ideal-thin-flexible flat plate of elastic material which is a measure of the strain energy of the deformation is given in [7]:

$$\begin{aligned} \epsilon_{be}(u, v) &= \frac{\kappa_1^2 + \kappa_2^2}{2} \\ &= 2H^2(u, v) - K(u, v) \end{aligned} \tag{10}$$

The measure is invariant to 3D rotation and translation. The energy required to bend a curved plate to a new deformed state (assuming known matches between (u, v) and $\bar{u}, \bar{v})$ is:

$$\begin{aligned} \epsilon_{be}(u, v, \bar{u}, \bar{v}) = \{ \sqrt{2H^2(u, v) - K(u, v)} - \\ \sqrt{2\bar{H}^2(\bar{u}, \bar{v}) - \bar{K}(\bar{u}, \bar{v})} \}^2 \end{aligned} \tag{11}$$

Mean and Gaussian curvature of surface at time t_0 are given with no bars. The same quantities at $t_0 + \Delta t$ are specified with bars.

A number of motion types can be described in terms of the first and second fundamental form coefficients. Rigid motion, which is the motion of an object without any bending or stretching and involving only translation and rotation, renders the (H, K) quantities unaltered. Isometric motion is a more general motion type and can be stated as a motion that preserves distances along the surface. It can be shown that under isometric motion K remains the same while H changes. An example of this type of motion occurs when for example rolling a piece of paper into the shape of a cylinder or a cone. Clearly, this is non-rigid, and bending occurs, but note that no stretching of the surface takes place and thus distances remain unaltered. Conformal motion is more general and has the important property that it preserves angles between curves, but is not required to preserve distances between points. As a result of angle preservation under conformal motion, it can be shown that if a motion has the property that the stretching factor is uniform around a point, the motion necessarily is conformal

[9]. When the stretching is constrained further such that it is not only the same around a point but is the same for all points around the surface, homothetic motion results. An example of homothetic motion occurs for example when a balloon is inflated. Of interest also, might be a motion that preserves corresponding areas. If it is known that such a motion takes place, and also conformality holds, it can be shown that the result is equivalent to an isometry.

There are important results in differential geometry that may be brought to bear which characterize mappings between surfaces. The following general result may be stated. If there exists $\eta(u, v) > 0$ such that

$$\frac{E}{\bar{E}} = \frac{F}{\bar{F}} = \frac{G}{\bar{G}} = \eta(u, v) \quad (12)$$

the object's motion is conformal. Again, no bars specify values of quantities at time t_0, and bars specify the same quantities at the same position on the surface at $t_0 + \Delta t$. η which may vary around the surface is called the stretching factor. If in (12), $\eta(u, v)$ is a constant, homothetic motion occurs, and yet if the constant is identity, isometric motion takes place. Possible models based on the isometric and homothetic assumptions imply invariant and proportional Gaussian curvatures (*Theorema Egregium* of Gauss [5] states the invariance property of the Gaussian curvature under isometries). Instead, let us consider the more general conformal motion. As examples of important conformal maps between surfaces, Mercator, and stereographic projections of the unit sphere on to the plane may be mentioned. Also, in complex analysis, any analytic function satisfying the Cauchy-Riemann equations is a conformal map of $\Re^2$ into itself. In general, "exact" conformal maps are angle-preserving maps. The objective function given below favors matching points that are close to the conformal model:

$$\epsilon_{st}(u, v, \bar{u}, \bar{v}) = (\frac{E}{\bar{E}} - \frac{F}{\bar{F}})^2 + (\frac{F}{\bar{F}} - \frac{G}{\bar{G}})^2 + (\frac{E}{\bar{E}} - \frac{G}{\bar{G}})^2 \quad (13)$$

Note that parametrizations of S and $\bar{S}$ have a subtle role in (13). A natural choice for local surface parametrization of a patch centered at p is to have coordinate axes along the principal directions of S on $T_p(S)$. This can be set up for most surface points. Our model for the "approximate" conformal stretching involves this choice of a local coordinate system. As can be seen, the stretching model as formulated favors the same value for η at each point on the surface. However, since this is the sum of three quadratic error measures, the uniformity of errors is not enforced. In order to force this uniformity in error calculations, we have also used the minimax procedure which as the name implies, minimizes the maximum of the three error terms. In statistical terms, minimax is a more *robust* error norm than sum of quadratic errors. We note that Goldgof and Huang [10] have used an H-K map for classifying motion into rigid and non-rigid components, ultimately aimed at obtaining the epicardial motion of the LV. Also, Mishra, Goldgof, and Huang [13] have proposed a method for recovering a conformal stretching function, linear in coordinates of parameterization, assuming knowledge of three point correspondences and involving the solution to a system of three

fourth order equations with the stretching function and its derivatives as the unknowns. This approach yields an interesting, but computationally expensive solution to the *measurement* of linear stretching.

4   Processing

Our experiments for this paper involve shape matching based on bending and stretching models for graph surfaces which are meant to model a portion of the smoothly curved LV wall measured from $T_p(S)$, and bending models for complete 3D surface data obtained from DSR. To deal with data inconsistencies and measurement errors, we compute surface characteristics assuming locally quadric patches. In computing the surface characteristics for the graph surface case, we employ techniques given in [3].

For the case of actual 3D DSR contour data, although the approach is the same, the methodology is quite different as we will describe. For computing surface characteristics from 3D data, we first find $T_p(S)$ starting from an estimate of the local covariance matrix. Diagonalizing the covariance matrix will give us the variance of the data in each direction (eigenvalues) and the corresponding principal axes (eigenvectors). Points in the neighborhood in 3D space are then projected onto this plane. A linear least squares quadric fit is performed subsequently and local bending energies are computed from the coefficients of the fit.

Once the above quantities are found, we are in a position to find local displacement vectors at each point by finding the point on the deformed surface that minimizes bending and deviation from conformal stretching in the stated coordinate system. By varying $(\delta u, \delta v)$ for a fixed (u, v), $\epsilon_{be}(u, v, u + \delta u, v + \delta v)$ and $\epsilon_{st}(u, v, u + \delta u, v + \delta v)$ can be measured and compared. The point that minimizes these quantities is the found match. The basic assumption is that important shape features only move within the resolution of a search region. In addition, in the stretching case, the search region must accomodate for the largest possible stretching that can occur on the surface patch.

4.1   Experimental Results

Results of application of the method are given in figures 2 and 3. Experiments illustrate performance of the algorithm in computing stretching and bending of surface patches over three frames of the four-dimensional volume in figure 2 and bending effects with DSR data in figure 3. In figure 2, the three surface patches on the top show two simulated bumps extending upward from the surface at three points in time. The bumps simulate extreme cases of shape features on the LV surface. Note that the bumps shift slightly to the right and towards the rear as you look from the bottom to the top surface patch. The match vectors show the result of using only the bending energy measure described before to track features between pairs of patches. In the second part of the figure the original surface is stretched twice forming three surfaces in time. The stretching term

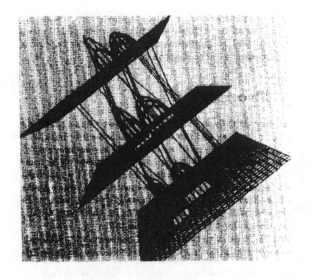

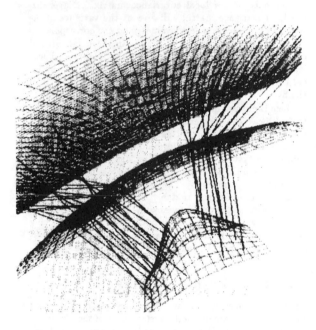

Figure 2: Motion computation using (graph) surface patches of 4D data. Top: the algorithm's performance in detecting motion of moving bumps by minimizing the bending energy. Bottom: Motion of points on the surface is computed by minimizing deviations from conformal stretching (see text).

is then used to predict where points on the first patch extend to on the second and top patches. Note that due to the smoothing effect over orientation discontinuities in the bending example, points close to bumps were also tracked. Surface matching based on bending requires an additional statement here. When there are no important landmarks that could be located, i.e., when there are ambiguities that might be present, the algorithm simply assumes minimal motion on the part of the ambiguous point, and hence finds the motion vector that has minimal length (this is the normal flow). The coordinate system partitions the surface patch into four equal quarters. Figure 3 shows application of the algorithm based on minimum bending energy to 3D DSR data. The example shows computed motion for two 3D frames locally adjacent in time using 5×5 quadric fits, and 17×9 search regions constructed around the closest point on $\hat{S}$ to the point of interest on S.

5 Conclusions

We have discussed three aspects of the problem of motion tracking of the LV endocardial wall: the image data, the motion models, and the computational algorithm. At the data level, MR and cine-CT are described as data types of choice for reasons outlined in section 2. Our algorithm currently characterizes surfaces with locally quadric approximations, although more accurate representations might be desirable in order to get better estimates of the various quantities.

In general, finding correct matches will not be sufficient for accurate estimation of the flow field due to noise in the flow estimation as well as the aperture problem (present in motion of 3D surfaces) for cases with bending. For this reason, once matches are found, in the spirit of [2], it may be necessary to associate confidences with the components of the flow and furthermore, propagate the flow estimates to adjacent regions of the surface. The confidences will be necessary in order to keep the components of the flow that are most likely to be correct, while smoothing over components that are not likely to be accurate. The fit error may provide us with a measure of confidence in the normal component of flow. Tangential components of flow also have confidences arising from principal curvatures of the surface. The match metric weighs the overall "data" term [2]. Currently, membrane smoothing has been implemented, without the confidences for the graph surface case.

Bending and stretching models are proposed for matching surface properties. This provides us with initial results of motion estimation from 3D data. Future formulations will assume more complete representations, and richer models. Gaining a better understanding of the left-ventricular motion in terms of modelling and analysis can be both diagnostically important and at the same time provide a suitable source of information for constructing techniques useful for analyzing motion of non-rigid objects in general.

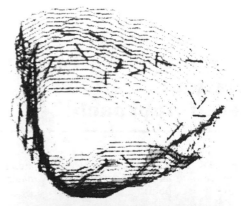

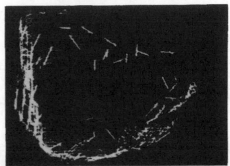

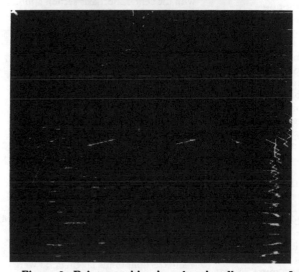

Figure 3: Point matching based on bending energy for DSR data. Note that different shades of grey are used to illustrate the different contour volumes of LV at the two successive time instants and the computed match vectors. The top two (same experiment) are vectors at the apical end of LV.

Acknowledgements

We would like to thank P. Anandan for many helpful discussions regarding motion analysis and confidences.

References

[1] J. K. Aggarwal. Motion and time-varying imagery – an overview. In *Proceedings of IEEE Workshop on Motion: Representation and Analysis*, 1986.

[2] P. Anandan. A computational framework and an algorithm for the measurement of visual motion. *International Journal of Computer Vision*, 2:283–310, 1989.

[3] P. Besl and R. Jain. Invariant surface characteristics for 3d object recognition. *Computer Vision, Graphics, and Image Processing*, 33:33–80, 1986.

[4] F. Bookstein. Principal warps: thin-plate splines and the decomposition of deformations. *IEEE Transactions on PAMI*, 1989.

[5] M. P. Do Carmo. *Differential Geometry of Curves and Surfaces*. Prentice-Hall, New Jersey, 1976.

[6] S. Collins and D. Skorton. *Cardiac Imaging and Image Processing*. McGraw Hill, New York, 1986.

[7] R. Courant and D. Hilbert. *Methods of Mathematical Physics*. Interscience, London, 1957.

[8] J. Duncan, R. Owen, L. Staib, and P. Anandan. Measurement of non-rigid motion using contour shape descriptors. In *Proceedings of Computer Vision and Pattern Recognition*, 1991.

[9] L. P. Eisenhart. *A treatize on Differential Geometry of Curves and Surfaces*. Ginn and Company, Boston.

[10] D. Goldgof, H. Lee, and T. Huang. Motion analysis of nonrigid surfaces. In *Proceedings of IEEE conference on Computer Vision and Pattern Recognition*, 1988.

[11] T. Huang. Modeling, analysis, and visualization of nonrigid object motion. In *International Conference on Pattern Recognition*, pages 361 – 364, Atlantic City, New Jersey, 1990.

[12] R. Millman and G. Parker. *Elements of Differential Geometry*. Prentice-Hall, Englewood Cliffs, New Jersey, 1977.

[13] S. Mishra, D. Goldgof, and T. Huang. Motion analysis and epicardial deformation estimation from angiography data. In *Computer Vision and Pattern Recognition*, pages 331–336, 1991.

[14] C. Slager, T. Hooghoudt, P. Serruys, j. Schuurbiers, J. Reiber, G. Meester, P. Verdouw, and R. Hugenholtz. Quantitative assessment of regional left ventricular motion using endocardial landmarks. *JACC*, 7(2):317 – 326, 1986.

[15] E. Zerhouni, D. Parish, W. Rogers, A. Yang, and P. Shapiro. Tagging of the human heart by multiplanar selective rf saturation for the analysis of myocardial contraction. In *Abstracts of the Annual Meeting of the Society of Magnetic Resonance in Imaging*, page 10, San Francisco, 1988.

Alistair A. Young, PhD • Leon Axel, PhD, MD

Three-dimensional Motion and Deformation of the Heart Wall: Estimation with Spatial Modulation of Magnetization—A Model-based Approach[1]

A method for in vivo estimation of the three-dimensional (3D) motion and deformation of the heart from tagged magnetic resonance images of the myocardium is presented. The method is based on a 3D deformable model fitted to the motion of tagged points in two views (short and long axes), which results in a comprehensive kinematic model of the dynamic geometry of the left ventricle. The method was applied to data obtained in four healthy volunteers, and data were pooled according to position within the model. Analytic modeling demonstrated that the calculated strain field was relatively invariant to the type of smoothing constraint applied; the greatest error was in the circumferential-radial shear strain. Displacement, torsion, and strain extracted from the model agreed with previous results of two-dimensional MR imaging analyses and 3D studies involving the implantation of radiopaque beads in canine myocardium. The model-driven approach provides an accurate and flexible technique for noninvasive estimation of 3D in vivo deformation of the human heart.

Index terms: Heart, function • Heart, MR, 52.1214 • Heart, ventricles • Magnetic resonance (MR), technology

Radiology 1992; 185:241–247

---

[1] From the Department of Radiology, Hospital of the University of Pennsylvania, 3400 Spruce St, Philadelphia, PA 19104. Received February 6, 1992; revision requested April 7; revision received May 21; accepted May 22. Supported by National Institutes of Health grant no. HL-43014 of the National Heart, Lung, and Blood Institute. Address reprint requests to L.A.
ⓒ RSNA, 1992

R ECENT developments in myocardial tagging with magnetic resonance (MR) imaging allow the creation and subsequent tracking of large numbers of material landmarks throughout the heart wall (1,2). With the spatial modulation of magnetization (SPAMM) technique (2,3), two orthogonal sets of parallel planes (sheets) of magnetic saturation, usually orthogonal to the imaging plane, are created in a short time by a sequence of nonselective radio-frequency pulses separated by magnetic field gradients. An imaging pulse sequence is then applied after a suitable delay, on the order of or less than the longitudinal T1. The motion of the tagging sheets is indicated by the displacement of dark bands in the image, corresponding to the intersection of the sheets with the imaging plane (Fig 1). Intersections of two sheets form tagging lines (Fig 2) that are initially orthogonal to the imaging plane. The intersections of these lines with the imaging plane can be tracked unambiguously in the image, yielding the two components of the motion parallel to the image plane (Fig 2).

To reconstruct the three-dimensional (3D) motion of material points, a number of two-dimensional tagged image sections must be obtained in at least two orientations, usually aligned parallel and perpendicular to the long axis of the LV. Some *a priori* knowledge of the deformation must be employed to interpolate information between points, sections, and views. Usually, this takes the form of a smoothness constraint, since the motion of each point reflects that of the underlying continuum. In this study, we applied a model-driven approach, whereby the LV is represented by a finite element model that is deformed to fit the displacements of the magnetic tags. This results in an accurate and efficient description of the 3D motion and geometry of the heart wall, which can be interrogated for kinematic variables at any material point.

MATERIALS AND METHODS

Imaging Protocol

Four healthy volunteers (aged 20–31 years; two male) underwent MR imaging with a 1.5-T MR imaging system (Signa; GE Medical Systems, Milwaukee). Images were obtained as two series of five parallel sections each, one oriented parallel to the long axis of the LV (long axis) and the other perpendicular to the long axis (short axis). Each section had thickness of 5 mm, and sections were spaced 10–15 mm apart, with the center short-axis section approximately at the middle portion of the LV and the center long-axis section approximately in the plane of the LV long axis, normal to the interventricular septum. Five images were acquired at each section location at equal temporal intervals from end diastole (time 1) to end systole (time 5), by using electrocardiographic (ECG) synchronization. The time 1 image was acquired 15 msec after generation of the tags (at detection of the ECG trigger). End systole was taken to be the time of least LV cavity area as seen in a short-axis cine scout study. Spin-echo images were obtained with an echo time of 27 msec and gradient moment nulling to compensate for motion effects. Each image was reconstructed as 256 × 256 pixels with a 24-cm field of view (0.92 mm/pixel). The SPAMM tagging planes were generated with a spacing of 7 mm and width of approximately 2 mm.

Intersections of the tagging grid were manually tracked through the five phases of each section with the aid of an image analysis package (3). The inner and outer contours of the LV were traced manually, to enclose the LV wall and septum (Fig 1). RV contours were also defined for time 1, as were the approximate locations of the LV apex and base (center of the LV at the

---

Abbreviations: ECG = electrocardiographic, LV = left ventricle, RV = right ventricle, SPAMM = spatial modulation of magnetization, 3D = three-dimensional.

---

base) on the central long-axis section at time 1. These were later used as fiducial markers to register the model to the anatomic features.

The Model

We adopted the standard piecewise polynomial representation used extensively in computer-aided design, computer graphics, and the finite element method (4,5). If each element (patch) contains N nodes, the geometric field $\mathbf{x} = (x, y, z)$ within the element is given by an interpolation of the values at the nodes (5):

$$\mathbf{x}(\xi) = \sum_{n=1}^{N} \psi_n(\xi)\mathbf{x}_n, \qquad (1)$$

where ξ are element coordinates, ψ_n are element basis functions, and $\mathbf{x}_n$ are nodal values. These models can efficiently describe the complex 3D geometry and fiber architecture of the heart (6) and are suitable for finite element analysis of stress and activation (5,7). The nodal parameters may be fitted to geometric data $\mathbf{x}_d$ by linear least squares (6,8,9). Given the material coordinates ξ_d corresponding to each data point $\mathbf{x}_d$, the following error function is minimized:

$$E(\mathbf{x}) = S(\mathbf{x}) + \sum_{d=1}^{D} \sum_{i=1}^{3} \gamma_{di}[x_i(\xi_d) - x_{di}]^2, \qquad (2)$$

where x_{di} is the ith component of the dth data point and γ_{di} is the associated weight. Equation (1) is minimized by setting the derivatives with respect to $\mathbf{x}_n$ to zero and solving the resulting set of "normal equations" for $\mathbf{x}_n$. $S(\mathbf{x})$ is a quadratic smoothing constraint included to regularize the problem, which is ill-posed due to the sparse distribution of the data (8,9). Since the element coordinates are also material coordinates (ie, they move with the muscle), detailed kinematic information is directly obtained from two states ($\mathbf{x}$ and $\mathbf{X}$), defining deformed and undeformed configurations (10,11).

The following sections describe the use of the model in reconstructing the geometry and motion of the LV. A flow diagram of the entire process is given in Figure 3. The geometry is defined by fitting surfaces to the inner and outer contours. Tag intersection points are then located within the geometry, which is deformed to match the tag displacements.

Geometric Fits

To register one heart to another, a fixed reference "cardiac" coordinate system is defined by using time 1 (end diastole) images in a manner independent of the number, location, and orientation of the image planes. The long axis of the LV is defined by the line passing through the centroids of the most basal and most apical short-axis endocardial contours. The apex and base landmarks (defined on the central long-axis section), as well as the

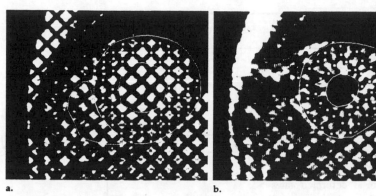

a.   **b.**

Figure 1. SPAMM short-axis images at the middle portion of the ventricle at **(a)** time 1 (end diastole) and **(b)** time 5 (end systole). Inner and outer contours of the left ventricle (LV) and initial inner contour of the right ventricle (RV) (in **a** only) are outlined in green. Small squares denote tracked intersections.

centroid of the RV contours, are projected onto this long axis (Fig 4). The origin of the cardiac coordinate system is placed one-third of the distance from base to apex projections. The x axis is oriented toward the apex projection, and the y axis is aligned parallel to the line joining the RV centroid and its projection (Fig 4).

The geometry of the LV is determined by fitting inner and outer surfaces to contours drawn on the short- and long-axis images. The procedure is similar to that previously described (5,6,8). In brief, the surfaces are defined in a polar (prolate spheroidal) coordinate system (λ, μ, θ), by using the same origin and long axis as the cardiac coordinate system, in which surfaces of constant radius are ellipsoids. Only the radial field $\lambda(\xi_1, \xi_2)$ is fitted, ξ_1 and ξ_2 being fixed linear functions of the circumferential and longitudinal coordinates, respectively. The placement of the origin of the cardiac coordinate system allows the polar system to be scaled so that the apex projection assumes a radial coordinate of $\lambda = 1$ and the aortic-mitral valve plane approximates a longitudinal coordinate of $\mu = 120°$ (6) The RV centroid has a circumferential coordinate of $\theta = 0°$. The element coordinates of the data points are given by projection along radial directions onto an initial constant-radius surface. A typical element topology has 16 elements for each surface, with nodes equally spaced in the angular and azimuthal directions. A particular material point referenced by element coordinates (ξ_1, ξ_2) thus refers to approximately the same anatomic location in each heart.

The λ field was fitted to the contour data by using Equation (2) with $S(\lambda)$ given by the weighted spline kernel:

$$S(\lambda) = \int \alpha\left[\left(\frac{\partial\lambda}{\partial\xi_1}\right)^2 + \left(\frac{\partial\lambda}{\partial\xi_2}\right)^2\right]$$
$$+ \beta\left[\left(\frac{\partial^2\lambda}{\partial\xi_1^2}\right)^2 + 2\left(\frac{\partial^2\lambda}{\partial\xi_1\partial\xi_2}\right)^2 + \left(\frac{\partial^2\lambda}{\partial\xi_2^2}\right)^2\right] d\xi_1 d\xi_2, \qquad (3)$$

with α and β controlling the surface tension and curvature, respectively (8,12).

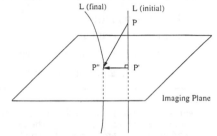

Figure 2. Relationship between imaged and material displacements. Point P on the tagging line L is initially imaged as P' and finally as P''. P and P'' are the same material point, two components of whose motion are given by the displacement of P' to P''. The motion of the material point initially at P' is generally not imaged due to through-plane motion.

The inner and outer surfaces are then joined by a linear interpolation in the radial direction, and the 3D geometry is converted back to the cardiac (rectangular Cartesian) reference frame. This results in a 3D model whose element coordinates are aligned along circumferential (ξ_1), longitudinal (ξ_2), and transmural (ξ_3) directions (Fig 5).

Reconstruction Fits

Whereas the geometry of the model is defined by the contours, motion is determined solely by the tag grid intersections, as follows. The subsequent motion of material points imaged at time 1 are not known, since the points generally move out of the imaging plane (Fig 2). Tagged points imaged at subsequent times ($t > 1$), however, provide displacement information because their projections at time 1 onto the imaging planes are known. We can therefore obtain the missing (through-plane) motion by a "reconstruction" fit of the displacement from a geometry defined at $t > 1$ back to time 1. The $t > 1$ geometry is obtained by fitting surfaces to the inner and outer contours as above. The

351

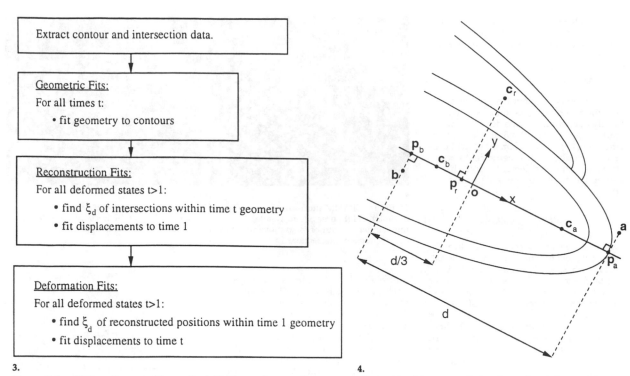

Extract contour and intersection data.

Geometric Fits:

For all times t:

- fit geometry to contours

Reconstruction Fits:

For all deformed states t>1:

- find ξ_d of intersections within time t geometry
- fit displacements to time 1

Deformation Fits:

For all deformed states t>1:

- find ξ_d of reconstructed positions within time 1 geometry
- fit displacements to time t

3.

4.

Figures 3, 4. **(3)** Flow diagram of the method. **(4)** The cardiac coordinate system. Centroids of the most apical and most basal short-axis inner contours are c_a and c_b, respectively. The centroid of the RV contours is c_r. The projections of these points into the long axis are p_a, p_b, and p_r. The origin is at **o**. User-defined apex and base markers are **a** and **b** , respectively. d = distance from base to apex projections along the long axis.

element coordinates of the intersection data points are determined in the 3D polar geometry by using the linear relationships $\theta(\xi_1)$, $\mu(\xi_2)$, and $\lambda(\xi_3)$. The conversion from polar to cardiac coordinates introduces small errors in the element data locations, which are corrected by means of Newton iteration.

For simplicity, the reconstruction fit is performed in a reference frame aligned to the imaging planes ("fitting coordinates"). This frame shares the same origin as the cardiac coordinate system but is rotated to make the xz coordinate plane parallel to the long-axis image planes and the yz plane parallel to the short-axis sections. The error function (Eq [2]) has data weights γ_{di} set to $(1, 0, 1)$ $(i = 1, 2, 3)$ for long-axis data and $(0, 1, 1)$ for short-axis data. Essentially, this fits the x displacement field to the x displacements of the long-axis data points, the y field to the short-axis y displacements, and the z field to data from both short- and long-axis images.

Deformation Fits

The above procedure applied to each time $t > 1$ results in a series of time 1 geometries, one for each subsequent time. This confuses the development of strain from end diastole to end systole and makes registration between hearts difficult. It is therefore desirable to deform a single reference geometry, defined by using time 1 contours, to fit displacements to each subsequent time. The 3D locations of

the intersection data at $t = 1$ are fully determined by the imaged displacements and the through-plane displacement estimated by the reconstruction fit. Because all the components of motion are given, all data weights then are $(1, 1, 1)$. This allows use of the same normal equations for each field, because only the right-hand side changes. The same equations for each time cannot be used, however, because the data sets are different.

Smoothing Constraints

There remains the question of which smoothing term $S(\mathbf{x})$ is appropriate for this problem. In this study, we considered three forms, which we termed spline, global, and body smoothing. Spline smoothing takes the form of Equation (3), used for the geometric fits. Contributions from each coordinate field are summed, and the integration is performed over the whole 3D object. Spline smoothing is computationally fast, produces normal equations which are separable into x, y, and z components (so each is fitted separately), and is quadratic in the nodal parameters (leading to linear least squares problems). It is also analogous to the small displacement deformation energy of a thin plate under bending and tension (12). This analogy, however, does not hold for finite deformations, and strains are introduced for large, rigid body rotations.

Global smoothing seeks to minimize the rate of change of the deformation gradient tensor F, defined with respect to the global

(fitting) coordinate system as

$$F_{ij} = \frac{\partial x_i}{\partial X_j} = \sum_k \frac{\partial x_i}{\partial \xi_k} \frac{\partial \xi_k}{\partial X_i}, \tag{4}$$

where $\mathbf{x}$ and $\mathbf{X}$ are position vectors of the same material point in the deformed and undeformed states, respectively (9,10,13). The form of $S(\mathbf{x})$ is (14):

$$S(\mathbf{x}) = W \int \sum_{k,i,j} \left(\frac{\partial F_{ij}}{\partial \xi_k}\right)^2 d\xi, \tag{5}$$

where w is a weight. The main advantage of this measure is that unlike Equation (3), it is invariant to arbitrary rigid body motion (14). Finite rigid body rotations do not affect the calculated strain field. It remains quadratic in the displacement parameters, and the resulting normal equations are still linear and separable. This results in a strain field that is as near to homogeneous as the data will allow; any variation of strain with respect to the coordinate directions is thus entirely due to the data and not the applied smoothing. The main disadvantage of global smoothing is that it will penalize deformations that are quite homogeneous in a material-oriented coordinate system (eg, aligned with the muscle fibers) but are nonhomogeneous in the global coordinate system. For example, torsion in cylindrical polar coordinates is homogeneous in the longitudinal and circumferential directions but nonhomogeneous in a rectangular Cartesian system. Thus, LV torsion, known to occur during systole (15,16), is penalized by this smoothing constraint.

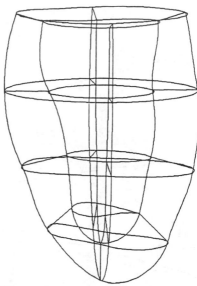

Figure 5. Wire frame plot shows element boundaries of the 3D model at time 1. Inner and outer LV surface models are joined by a linear transmural variation. Viewpoint is slightly elevated and in front of the septum.

Table 1

Error between True and Predicted Data for Reconstruction Fit, by Type of Smoothing Constraint

A: Spline

	α			
β	0.000	0.001	0.010	0.100
0.001	1.167	1.296	1.745	2.176
0.010	1.244	1.260	1.383	1.882
0.100	1.616	1.618	1.638	1.809

B: Global

w	Result
0.001	0.828
0.010	0.818
0.100	0.819
1.000	0.833

C: Body

w	Result
0.001	0.456
0.010	0.437
0.100	0.438
1.000	0.445

Note.—Data are averaged over all elements; w = weight.

Table 2

Error between True and Predicted Data for Reconstruction Fit, by Smoothing Constraint

A: Spline

	α			
β	0.000	0.001	0.010	0.100
0.001	0.351	0.353	0.363	0.413
0.010	0.357	0.358	0.363	0.422
0.100	0.570	0.571	0.579	0.667

B: Global

w	Result
0.001	0.349
0.010	0.349
0.100	0.353
1.000	0.354

C: Body

w	Result
0.001	0.347
0.010	0.347
0.100	0.342
1.000	0.348

Note.—Data are averaged over central eight elements; w = weight.

An alternative is to use Equation (5) but refer F to local "body" coordinates that are defined in some natural way, for example, aligned in circumferential, longitudinal, and radial directions, or with the muscle fibers (9). If y and Y are position vectors in the deformed and undeformed states in such a body coordinate system, then the deformation gradient tensor referred to body coordinates (as opposed to F) is

$$F^*_{ij} = \frac{\partial y_i}{\partial Y_j}. \qquad (6)$$

This, however, leads to a nonlinear least squares problem in the nodal parameters x_n. A linear approximation can be obtained by

$$F^*_{ij} = \sum_k \frac{\partial y_i}{\partial x_k} \frac{\partial x_k}{\partial Y_j} \qquad (7)$$

and approximation of $\partial y_i / \partial x_k$ with $\partial Y_i / \partial X_k$. Substitution of Equation (7) into Equation (5) leads to a smoothing constraint that yields a more correct solution in the case of pure torsion, but which is no longer invariant to large, rigid body rotations. It is quadratic but not separable, so all x, y, z fields need to be fitted simultaneously.

Analytic Test Case

We applied the 3D motion reconstruction procedure to a simulated test case involving known displacements and an analytically described strain field. As in McCulloch and Omens (10), we prescribed an axisymmetric deformation of a thick-walled incompressible cylinder such that a material point (R, Θ, Z) in the undeformed state displaces to (r, Θ, z) in the deformed state as follows:

$$r = r(R); \quad \theta = \phi R + \Theta + \gamma Z + \epsilon; \text{ and}$$
$$z = \omega R + \lambda Z + \delta. \qquad (8)$$

Due to incompressibility, the radial function r(R) is given by

$$r^2 = \frac{R^2 - R_1^2}{\lambda} - r_1^2. \qquad (9)$$

The cylinder was chosen to have an initial inner radius (R_1) of 15 mm, initial outer radius of 33 mm, and undeformed length of 100 mm; deformed inner radius (r_1) of 10 mm; and deformed length of 85 mm. The kinematic parameters were chosen to exaggerate the qualitative motion of the human heart: $\phi = -0.278°$/mm, $\gamma = 0.3°$/mm, $\epsilon = 9.167°$, $\omega = 0.278$, $\lambda = 0.8$, and $\delta = 4.167$ mm.

Imaging planes were defined at z = 20, 30, 40, 50, and 60 mm to simulate short-axis images, and y = −20, −10, 0, 10, and 20 mm for the long-axis images ($y = r \cdot \sin\theta$). Data points were simulated as if created by a 7-mm tagging grid: Short-axis data consisted of points whose initial X, Y, and final z are known (final x, y, and initial Z can be calculated from Equation [8]), and long-axis data were defined by known initial X, Z, and final y. The missing components (ie, the Z component of the short-axis data and the Y component of the long-axis data) were estimated by fitting a model defined in the deformed state to the known X, Y from the short-axis data and X, Z from the long-axis data. The model was defined in rectangular Cartesian coordinates so as to approximate the smallest cylinder encompassing the deformed data points. As pre-

viously, it comprised 16 3D elements with bicubic Hermite interpolation in the circumferential-longitudinal directions and linear variation in the radial direction. Finally, a model of the initial undeformed cylinder was fitted to the deformed data by using the reconstructed undeformed material points given by the reconstruction fit.

RESULTS

Analytic Test Case

The root mean squared distance between predicted (fitted) material points and their analytically calculated positions is given in Table 1 for various smoothing weights in each of the three smoothing terms applied to the reconstruction fit. A large contribution to the error is the poorly constrained Y coordinate in regions above and below the short-axis planes. The error averaged over elements containing both short- and long-axis data (Table 2) is relatively invariant over a wide range of smoothing weights in each case. This error is due mainly to the approximation of the nonlinear radial displacement field with a linear variation.

In the final deformation fit, the average distance between the true and predicted deformed data was approximately 0.3 mm over all the cases in Table 1. In Figure 6, transmural (radial) strain variation in the equatorial

353

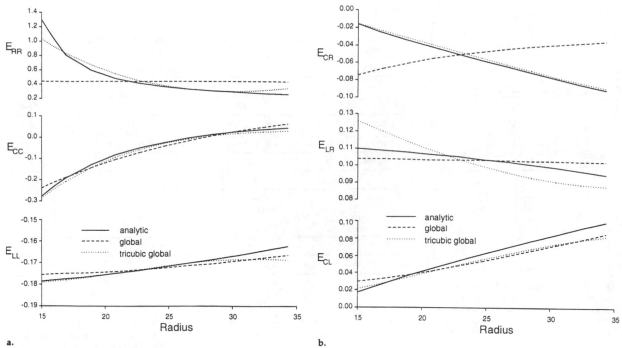

Figure 6. Comparison of analytic (true) and calculated strain variation (E) with respect to undeformed radius, for **(a)** normal strains and **(b)** shear strains. Strains are referred to body coordinates aligned in the circumferential (C), longitudinal (L), and radial (R) directions. *Global* refers to global smoothing constraint with linear transmural interpolation, and *tricubic global* refers to global smoothing constraint with cubic transmural interpolation.

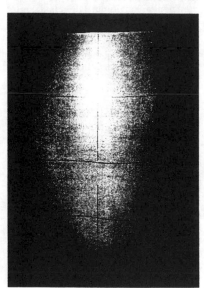

Figure 7. Shaded outer LV surface with element boundaries marked by red lines. Viewpoint is slightly elevated, with the septum on the right.

region of the model is compared with the analytical solution. Figure 6a shows the true and predicted normal components of the Lagrangian strain tensor $E = 0.5(F^T F - I)$ (9–11,13) referred to body coordinates, where F^T = transposition of F and I is the identity tensor. Figure 6b shows the comparison between shear strains. In this region (containing both short- and long-axis data), the estimated strain profiles are similar regardless of smoothing constraint, so only the global smoothing case is shown. All strains are modeled accurately, except for the radial normal strain and the circumferential-radial shear strain. The error in these strains is due to the enforcement of a linear transmural variation; they are reduced in the case of a model with a cubic radial variation (as well as circumferential and longitudinal), which also is shown in Figure 6.

Normal LV

Figure 5 shows a typical $t = 1$ configuration obtained from surface fits of the outer and inner LV contours. In general, there was greater difficulty in defining the inner contour, and short- and long-axis contours could be misregistered by up to 5 mm at points where they should have intersected. This is due to the lack of contrast between blood and muscle in some regions and the inability to resolve trabeculation of the LV endocardium. For this reason, the contours were not used to reconstruct motion or deformation but only to gain an approximate description of the geometry. The surface fits were performed by using spline smoothing with weights $\alpha = \beta = 0.01$ for the outer surface and $\alpha = \beta = 0.1$ for the inner surfaces, due to the greater uncertainty in the inner boundary location. Figure 7 shows a shaded surface display of an epicardial surface fit, with element boundaries marked in red.

Figure 8 shows typical forward fits from times 2–5. An average of 421 data points were fitted in the $t = 2$ state, dropping to 351 points at $t = 5$. The average root mean squared error between tracked and predicted data positions at $t = 5$ was 0.78 mm. Interobserver comparisons indicated a root mean squared error between users (0.85 mm) in the location of intersections. All of the general features of motion seen in the two-dimensional analysis (3,17) are also seen in the 3D model, including LV torsion and the relative immobility of the apex compared with the base. The displacement of points from the most basal short-axis section was 13.9 mm ± 2.4 (mean ± 1 standard deviation) between $t = 1$ and $t = 5$, while that of the most apical section was 5.5 mm ± 3.1. The rotation of points around the base about their centroid was $-1.7° \pm 3.9$, while that of points around the apex was $16.9° \pm 8.3$ (anticlockwise

354

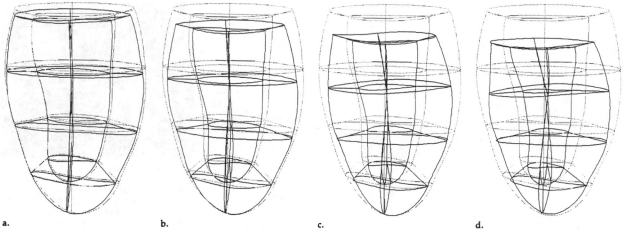

Figure 8. Deformation fits at **(a)** time 1 ($\cdots$) to time 2 (———), **(b)** time 1 ($\cdots$) to time 3 (———), **(c)** time 1 ($\cdots$) to time 4 (———), and **(d)** time 1 ($\cdots$) to time 5 (———). Viewpoint is slightly elevated and in front of the septum.

positive, looking from the apex).

The model provides a wealth of kinematic information in addition to motion. The six independent components of the Lagrangian strain tensor (9,13), averaged over the four hearts, are plotted against distance around the equatorial circumference at the middle of the wall of the LV (Fig 9). The greatest principal strain, associated with the largest final dimension of the "virtual ellipse" formed by deforming a small sphere centered at the material point, was always aligned in the approximate transmural direction and was thus associated with wall thickening. The least principal strain (greatest contraction or smallest final dimension of the ellipse) was oriented approximately 30° below the circumferential direction.

In interrogation of the model, it is important that the proximity of the data be indicated. One method is to define a data proximity field $p(\xi)$, which indicates the radius of the smallest sphere centered at $x(\xi)$, which encloses at least four noncoplanar short-axis data points and at least four noncoplanar long-axis data points. Thus, if $p(\xi)$ is small, we are guaranteed that all strain components are well constrained by the data. Figure 10 shows a Hammer projection plot (5) of the least principal strain contoured with the proximity function, which is coded in color.

DISCUSSION

The accuracy of the technique we used depends on the resolution and density of the data. Theoretically, the complexity of the model (number of elements and order of the basis func-

tions) can be adjusted so that the error between model and data is arbitrarily small. The interstripe spacing, however, is currently insufficient to track more than two points across most of the ventricular wall; hence, transmural variation was constrained to be linear. A 16-element model was chosen because it reproduced the deformed tag locations to within the interobserver error. The mean error of 0.78 mm is smaller than the pixel size (0.92 mm) and interobserver error (0.85 mm); further reduction of the error is unlikely to yield useful information. Experiments with a 12-element mesh yielded greater errors. The fits at time 5 are usually more poorly defined than at time 4, due to the relaxation of the stripes, blurring due to respiration, and errors in gating. Often, 50 data points are lost from time 4 to time 5. More accurate fits later into systole and perhaps diastole might be obtained with a cine SPAMM pulse sequence, in which the stripes are known to last longer (18), or with breath-hold imaging to reduce respiration artifacts.

The misregistration of the contours is most likely due to the difficulty in determining the true endocardial contour. Better contours could be obtained on images without tags, which confuse the contour. Also, signal intensity of blood could be differentiated from that of muscle through presaturation.

It is possible to also incorporate displacement information from points located along the stripes (between intersections) in the reconstruction fit as follows. An arbitrary number of data points may be defined along the stripe in the deformed ($t > 1$) state,

with their location completely specified, thus allowing ξ_d to be calculated. At $t = 1$, each data point must lie on the plane defined by the original tagging sheet. If n_d is the normal to the tagging plane on which x_d lies, then the error function is

$$E(\mathbf{x}) = S(\mathbf{x}) + \sum_{d=1}^{D} [\mathbf{n}_d \cdot (\mathbf{x}(\xi_d) - \mathbf{x}_d)]^2.$$

(10)

This effectively minimizes the distance between $\mathbf{x}(\xi_d)$ and the tagging plane. If the tagging planes are not aligned to the coordinate directions, the fit will be coupled. The data point $\mathbf{x}_d$ may lie anywhere on the plane; if a line-tracking algorithm is used, $\mathbf{x}_d$ would be expected to be close to the true position at $t = 1$.

The cylinder simulations show that while body smoothing most closely models the deformation in regions above and below the short-axis planes, the calculated strains are relatively independent of smoothing in regions containing both short- and long-axis data. As the resolution and density of the data sets improve, less reliance need be made on smoothing constraints. The choice of kinematic parameters gives the cylinder a more inhomogeneous deformation than occurs naturally in the human heart. Thus, the error in regions unconstrained by the data is larger than that expected in the normal heart, given perfect data. Another feature of the cylinder deformation is the very large endocardial normal radial strain (E_{RR} in Figure 6). This is due to incompressibility; the fact that these strains are not observed in the normal heart indicates that the blood content of

355

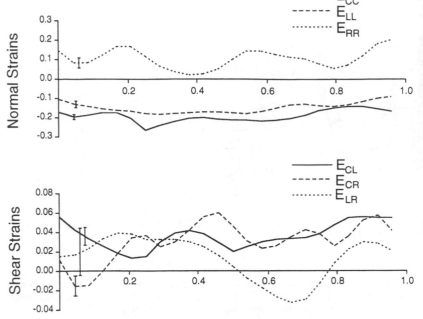

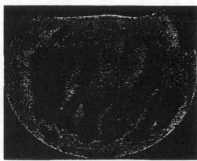

Figure 10. Hammer projection plot with contours showing the least principal strain at the middle portion of the wall. This projection cuts the wall surface longitudinally from base to apex at the center of the septum and lays the surface flat with an equal-area projection. The apex is a point at the bottom and the base traverses the top. From left to right are septal, anterior, lateral, posterior, and septal regions. The colored field indicates proximity to the data: red is < 10 mm, light blue is < 20 mm, and dark blue is > 20 mm.

Circumferential Distance

Figure 9. Strain variation (E) with respect to distance around the equatorial circumference of the middle portion of the heart wall. Mean values of four hearts $\pm$ 1 standard error of the mean are indicated by bars. Strains are referred to body coordinates aligned in the circumferential (C), longitudinal (L), and radial (R) directions. Distance is normalized so that 0 and 1 refer to the central septum, 0.25 is anterior, 0.5 is lateral, and 0.75 is posterior.

endocardial regions decreases during systole.

The mean rotation of the apex relative to the base was 18.6°, which is consistent with results of previous studies in which MR tagging and bead implantation methods were used. Buchalter et al (16) measured the two-dimensional rotation of magnetic tags in MR imaging and found a relative rotation of 19.1° at the epicardium and 11.2° at the endocardium. Hansen et al (15) tracked radiopaque markers implanted at the middle portion of the wall in the LV and found a rotation of 15° near the apex, compared with 17° in this study. The least principal strain (greatest contraction) was oriented consistently below the circumferential direction at about −30° (anticlockwise relative to the circumferential); this agrees with bead studies performed in the canine LV. Waldman et al (19) measured the homogeneous strains within tetrahedra formed by implanted beads in the anterior canine LV and found the principal angle of maximum shortening to vary from −45° at the epicardium to 0° at the endocardium. To resolve the transmural variation with

magnetic tags, the interstripe width must at least be halved.

In conclusion, the model-based approach to 3D analysis of myocardial deformation can yield a comprehensive kinematic data base on heart wall motion, which until this point has not been available without invasive means. ■

Acknowledgment: We thank David Rahdert, MS, for many interesting discussions on smoothing and data constraints.

References

1. Zerhouni E, Parish DM, Rogers WF, Yang A, Shapiro EP. Human heart: tagging with MR imaging—a method for noninvasive assessment of myocardial motion. Radiology 1988; 169:59–63.
2. Axel L, Dougherty L. Heart wall motion: improved method of spatial modulation of magnetization for MR imaging. Radiology 1989; 172:349–350.
3. Axel L, Gonçalves R, Bloomgarden D. Regional heart wall motion: two-dimensional analysis and functional imaging with MR imaging. Radiology 1992; 183:745–750.
4. Zienkiewicz OC, Morgan K. Finite elements and approximation. New York: Wiley, 1982.
5. Hunter PJ, Smaill BH. The analysis of cardiac function: a continuum approach. Prog Biophys Mol Biol 1988; 52:101–164.
6. Nielsen PMF, Le Grice IJ, Smaill BH, Hunter PJ. Mathematical model of geometry and fibrous structure of the heart. Am J Physiol 1991; 260:H1365–H1378.
7. McCulloch AD, Guccione JM, Rogers JM, Hunter PJ. Three-dimensional finite element analysis of stress and activation in the heart

(abstr). Proceedings of an Engineering Mechanics Specialty Conference. American Society of Civil Engineers, Columbus, Ohio, May 19–22,1991.
8. Young AA, Hunter PJ, Smaill BH. Epicardial surface estimation from coronary cineangiograms. Comput Vision Graph Image Proc 1989; 47:111–127.
9. Hashima AR, Waldman LK, Young AA, McCulloch AD. Nonhomogeneous analysis of epicardial strain distributions during acute myocardial ischemia in the dog. J Biomech 1992 (in press).
10. McCulloch AD, Omens JH. Nonhomogeneous analysis of three-dimensional transmural finite deformation in canine left ventricle. J Biomech 1991; 24:539–548.
11. Young AA, Hunter PJ, Smaill BH. Estimation of epicardial strain using the motions of coronary bifurcations in biplane cineangiography. IEEE Trans Biomed Eng 1992; 39:526–531.
12. Terzopoulos D. The computation of visible-surface representations. IEEE Trans Pattern Anal Machine Intell 1988; 10:417–438.
13. Spencer AJM. Continuum mechanics. White Plains, NY: Longman, 1980.
14. Young AA, Axel L. Non-rigid heart wall motion using MR tagging (abstr). Proceedings of the IEEE Computer Society Conference on Computer Vision and Pattern Recognition, Champaign, Ill, June 15–18, 1992.
15. Hanson DE, Daughters GT, Alderman EL, Ingels NB, Stinson EB, Miller DC. Effect of volume loading, pressure loading and inotropic stimulation on left ventricular torsion in humans. Circulation 1991; 83:1315–1326.
16. Buchalter MB, Weiss JL, Rogers WJ, et al. Noninvasive quantification of left ventricular rotational deformation in normal humans using magnetic resonance imaging myocardial tagging. Circulation 1990; 81:1236–1244.
17. Axel L, Bloomgarden D, Cheng C-N, Gonçalves R, Kraitchman D, Reichek N. MRI of normal regional heart wall motion. In: Book of abstracts: Society of Magnetic Resonance in Medicine 1991. Berkeley, Calif: Society of Magnetic Resonance in Medicine, 1991; 13.
18. Dougherty L, Axel L. Cine spatial modulation of magnetization imaging of heart wall motion (abstr). Radiology 1989; 173(P):276.
19. Waldman LK, Nossan D, Villareal F, Covell JW. The relationship between transmural deformation and local myofiber direction in the canine left ventricle. Circ Res 1988; 63:550–562.

Modeling, Analysis, and Visualization of Left Ventricle Shape and Motion by Hierarchical Decomposition

Chang Wen Chen, *Member, IEEE*, Thomas S. Huang, *Fellow, IEEE*, and Matthew Arrott

Abstract—This paper presents an approach to the modeling, analysis, and visualization of left ventricle motion and deformation. Our modeling of left ventricle shape and motion as a hierarchical representation enables us to develop a promising noninvasive technique for monitoring heart dynamics where both image analysis and image synthesis are involved. The proposed hierarchical motion model of left ventricle is constructed by combining several existing simple models and is able to capture major motion and deformation components of the left ventricle. The hierarchical decomposition characterizes the left ventricle motion and deformation in a coarse-to-fine fashion and leads to computationally efficient estimation algorithms. We estimate the global rigid motion of the left ventricle by establishing a time-varying object-centered coordinate system. The global deformations of the left ventricle are obtained by fitting the given data to superquadric modeling primitives. The local deformations are estimated by a tensor-description approach that is based on the locally deformable surface obtained by constructing spherical harmonic local surface from the residues of global shape estimation. We also describe in this paper methods of image synthesis and dynamic animation for visualizing the estimated results of the time-varying left ventricle shape, motion, and deformations. These animation results are consistent with the apparent motion pattern of the left ventricle and therefore show the success of our hierarchical decomposition based approach.

I. INTRODUCTION

LEFT ventricle motion and deformation analysis from image sequences provides an invaluable noninvasive technique for monitoring the dynamic behavior of human heart. To develop a clinically useful system that is able to analyze the given image sequence as well as display the estimated results, we need to apply the rigid and nonrigid object motion analysis algorithms evolved in the field of computer vision as well as the display and animation techniques investigated in the fields of computer graphics and scientific visualization. It is natural that development of such a system requires the integration of image analysis and image synthesis techniques. However, motion estimation of a beating heart from the image sequence is

Manuscript received December 7, 1992; revised January 20, 1993. This work was supported by the NSF under Grant IRI-89-08255. The computation and animation are carried out at NCSA, University of Illinois at Urbana-Champaign. Recommended for acceptance by Editor-in-Chief A. K. Jain.

C. W. Chen is with the Department of Electrical Engineering, University of Rochester, Rochester, NY 14627-0231.

T. S. Huang is with the Beckman Institute and Coordinated Science Laboratory, University of Illinois at Urbana-Champaign, Urbana, IL 61801. He is now with the Autodesk, Inc., Sausalido, CA 94965.

M. Arrott was with the National Center for Supercomputing Applications, University of Illinois at Urbana-Champaign, Champaign, IL 61820.

IEEE Log Number 9215853.

difficult since the heart undergoes a complex dynamic process throughout the cardiac cycle. How to display the estimation results is also a challenging problem because of the time-varying three-dimensional and tensor-based representations of the motion and deformation parameters.

There are four major methods of acquiring image data for extracting 3-D time-varying information of the heart. They are: echocardiography [1], cineangiography [2], [3], computed tomography [4], and nuclear magnetic resonance imaging [5]. Among these attempts of using imaging techniques for monitoring the dynamic behavior of the human heart, it appears that biplane cineangiography is at present the best in terms of both computational requirement and image quality. Several researchers have already been working on angiographic data-based approaches, and the results are rather promising. Kim et al. [6] used biplane coronary artery bifurcation points as natural markers for the kinematic analysis of heart motion. Coppini et al. [7] extended that approach and developed a method for a 3-D kinematic description of the local deformation of the heart surface by the end-diastole and end-systole configurations. Goldgof, Lee, and Huang [8] applied 3-D Gaussian curvature to analyze the heart surface by recovering the stretching factor from the angiographic data. However, all these researchers confined their approaches to the local region of the heart in order to implicitly eliminate the global movement effects, and global motion estimation was never addressed. Recently, Chen and Huang [9] started to apply algorithms developed in computer vision research and presented a new algorithm for heart motion analysis. They suggested that both global motion and local deformation of the beating heart should be considered and proposed a scheme to decouple the global motion from the local deformations.

This paper presents a scheme for left ventricle shape and motion modeling, analysis, and visualization using angiographic data. We are given the 3-D coordinates of the bifurcation points obtained through biplane cineangiography. The correspondences of these bifurcation points are obtained by tracking the coronary artery over a cardiac cycle. The detail of how these points are tracked can be found in recent papers [2], [10]. We propose in this paper a hierarchical motion model that is able to combine various cardiac motion and deformation models into a unified one. We also develop coarse-to-fine estimation algorithms based on the hierarchical decompositions. The hierarchical modeling has been motivated by the intentions to utilize *a priori* knowledge of the cardiac

Reprinted from *IEEE Trans. Pattern Analysis and Machine Intelligence*, Vol. 16, No. 4, Apr. 1994, pp. 342–356.

motion and reorganize such knowledge into a hierarchy of representations. The modeling of heart motion and deformation plays a central role in this estimation procedure. However, it is the hierarchical decomposition that allows us to convert a complex motion estimation problem into several stages of well-defined and simpler estimation procedures. Furthermore, the idea of hierarchical decomposition of shape and motion can also be applied to a wide variety of nonrigid objects with the necessary modification of motion and deformation classifications to suit the particular objects under consideration.

Model-based estimation of heart motion and shape has been investigated by many researchers. In the earlier study of left ventricle dynamics, simple shape primitives such as spheres and cylinders were assumed and motion descriptions were limited to volume changes of the left ventricle over a cardiac cycle [7], [11]. These simple models have been modified later, and more complex models have been investigated [12]. However, the estimation results based on these models represent only fragmentary characteristics of complex heart motion and deformations since they are based on either crude shape information or local motion information. In this paper, we intend to combine different shape and motion models into a hierarchical representation in an attempt to systematically characterize the complex nature of the heart motion. We have arranged the hierarchy in such a way that the decomposition of motion estimation leads to a series of well-defined estimation procedures.

In Section II, we introduce the motion and shape modeling primitives for our model-based approach. We propose a hierarchical motion model and two types of shape modeling primitives; each characterizes the global deformable surface and the local deformable surface, respectively. In Section III, we present the hierarchical decomposition approach, which converts the original complex estimation problem into a series of well-defined and relatively simple parameter estimation problems. The successful decomposition of the hierarchical representation of the motion and deformations enables us to develop computationally efficient estimation algorithms. The implementation details of this model-based motion and deformation analysis are described in Section IV. This section includes a recursive algorithm developed to produce a good estimate of global motion and deformation even when the given data points are distributed with bias, and an algorithm for the estimation of local deformations that global shape modeling primitives are unable to characterize. Section V shows the estimation results obtained by the algorithms developed in Sections III and IV. Visualization techniques for analyzing the estimated left ventricle motion and deformations are presented in Section VI. We describe how we can synthesize the 3-D dynamics of the left ventricle by means of enhancing the spatial dimensionality and color coding the local deformations. Section VII concludes this paper with some discussions on future research directions.

II. Left Ventricle Motion and Shape Modeling

The advantage of modeling in image sequence-based cardiac research is twofold. First, *a priori* knowledge of the heart motion and shape can be easily incorporated into the modeling primitives. Second, the modeling primitives are generally parameterized so that we are able to devise well-defined parameter estimation algorithms. In the following, we first present a hierarchical motion model that combines various simple motion models. Then we introduce the left ventricle shape modeling primitives that correspond to different levels of shape representations. We also identify the relationship between the level of shape representation and the hierarchy of motion description in order to show the correlation between the shape modeling and the motion modeling.

A. Left Ventricle Motion Modeling

The importance of motion modeling has long been recognized by the cardiac researchers. Based on various motion models, the noninvasive evaluation of cardiac dynamics using image sequences such as cineangiograms has been investigated. Most motion and deformation models are simple in the sense that they are based on crude approximation or localized information. Many simple motion models provide fairly good qualitative intuition but not quantitative characterization of heart dynamics. The complexity of the motion model has grown over the years of research. However, no unified model that combines localized models into a generalized one has been proposed. We present here a hierarchical motion model, a superposition of several simple models, in an attempt to characterize the overall dynamics of the heart. In the following, we first review existing motion models that are based on only partial information of heart dynamics. Then we discuss how the hierarchical motion model can be derived from these simple motion models. The advantages of hierarchical motion modeling are also explored so that the philosophy of hierarchical modeling can be applied to the implementation of estimation algorithms.

Existing Motion Models: Existing models of left ventricle motion and deformation can be roughly divided into two major categories: global motion and deformation models, and local deformation models. The global motion and deformation models generally describe the overall changes in the ventricular shape, size, and orientation [13]. Although global rigid motion of the heart is part of the heart dynamics, cardiac researchers have been focusing mainly on the global deformations, such as volume change, shape dilation and twisting. For a crude estimate of global cardiac dynamics, simple models of motion and deformation have been considered good enough. One typical example of such models is the pressure-volume model [14], which indicates the global dynamic changes of the left ventricular wall. Another example is the linear transformation model, which computes the global deformation (ventricular ejection fractions) based on eigenvolumes calculated from implanted markers [13].

The local deformation models concentrate on the local fibrous structure and stress distribution of the left ventricle wall [6], [15]. To isolate local deformations from chamber global translation and rotation, these models are usually based on a reconstructed local cardiac coordinate system. Two popular methods have been employed in the analysis of the left ventricle local deformation. Tensor analysis of the local deformation is applied when the correspondences of the markers on the surface of left ventricle are available or can be established [7], [16], [17]. Otherwise, finite element method is a good alternative since it is capable of interpolating the data points into nodes of nearby elements and estimating the deformation based on these nodal values of displacement [11], [15].

These models, global or local, reflect only partially the complex dynamic behavior of the left ventricle. It is necessary to combine many aspects of these simple models into a generalized model in order to more completely characterize the left ventricle dynamics.

The Hierarchical Motion Model: Our hierarchical motion model decomposes a general motion into two major parts: global movement and local movement. The global movement is further decomposed into global rigid motion and global nonrigid motion, while the local movement is decomposed into local rigid motion and local deformations. Such a generalized motion model is built via the rearrangement of individual global and local motion models into a hierarchy of motion and deformations. This motion hierarchy can be applied to other nonrigid object motion analysis problems as well. However, in the case of left ventricle motion analysis, this motion model includes several well-recognized cardiac motion patterns, especially the patterns of global and local deformations. These patterns have been used separately in existing motion models, and each has been confirmed by medical observations or biomedical engineering experiments.

We now identify the components of the hierarchical motion model for the left ventricle. Global rigid motion of the left ventricle is parameterized by the overall chamber translation and rotation. Global nonrigid motion consists of dilation (scaling) deformation in three orthogonal directions and twisting deformation about the long axis of the left ventricle. Local rigid motion and nonrigid deformation can be described together using the well-known Helmholz theorem of kinematics [18], which represents the local deformation by stretching tensors in a localized volume element. Naturally, we will employ the tensor description-based method in our local deformation estimation algorithms.

B. Left Ventricle Shape Modeling

The left ventricle as a whole is a nonrigid object, and it is well known that its shape changes periodically over each cardiac cycle. The shape change of the left ventricle is due to the global and local deformations during the pumping of the heart. Naturally, deformation modeling of the left ventricle, global or local, can be realized by shape modeling of the left ventricle, if one is able to incorporate these deformation parameters into the shape modeling primitives. Therefore, many cardiac researchers have implemented the left ventricle deformation analysis algorithms through modeling the left ventricle surface by simple shape primitives, such as sphere and cylinder [19], [20]. However, the success of existing shape-modeling-based approaches are limited due to the oversimplified surface primitives that are in sharp contrast to the complex nature of the left ventricle dynamics.

We present here two types of shape modeling primitives; each describes a different level of shape representation, or deformation description. For global deformation analysis, global shape is modeled by the superquadric modeling primitives. Superquadric shape modeling primitives presented in this paper are considered better than the existing simple shape models, such as spheres or cylinders, since their parameters are capable of describing the global deformations that simple shape models are unable to characterize. However, due to the intrinsic axial symmetric property of the superquadrics, they are still not flexible enough to characterize local deformations, which are different from one surface patch to another. For local deformation analysis, we propose a local surface estimation scheme based on spherical harmonic fitting of the residual distances computed from the given data and the fitted superquadric surface. These residual distances are the measures of the deviation of the global superquadric surface from the given data. A finite expansion of spherical harmonic basis functions is chosen in such a way that the fitted surface is a good interpolation of these residual distances in terms of both surface smoothness and variation. In other words, the spherical harmonic shape modeling is used to characterize the details of the left ventricle shape that superquadric modeling primitives are unable to characterize. The combination of these two shape modeling primitives forms the left ventricle shape that captures the global as well as local surface properties.

Superquadric Shape Modeling: We propose here a parameterized family of shapes, known as superquadrics, as the global shape modeling primitives. In contrast to existing models, they are flexible enough to capture the globally deformable nature of the left ventricle. They have been used for shape representation in computer graphics [21],[22] as well as computer vision [23], [24], [25], [26]. A superquadric surface is the spherical product of two superquadric curves and can be defined in vector form as follows:

$$S(\theta, \phi) = \begin{bmatrix} x \\ y \\ z \end{bmatrix} = \begin{bmatrix} a_x \cos^{\epsilon_1}(\theta) \cos^{\epsilon_2}(\phi) \\ a_y \cos^{\epsilon_1}(\theta) \sin^{\epsilon_2}(\phi) \\ a_z \sin^{\epsilon_1}(\theta) \end{bmatrix}, \quad (1)$$

where $-\frac{\pi}{2} \leq \theta \leq \frac{\pi}{2}$ and $-\pi \leq \phi \leq \pi$. Parameters θ and ϕ correspond to latitude and longitude angles, respectively, expressed in the object-centered spherical coordinate system. Angle ϕ lies in the $x - y$ plane, while θ corresponds to the angle between the vector $S(\theta, \phi)$ and the $x - y$ plane. Scale parameters a_x, a_y, a_z define the size of the superquadrics in the x, y, and z directions, respectively, ϵ_1 is the squareness parameter along the z-axis, and ϵ_2 is the squareness parameter in the $x - y$ plane. By varying these parameters, superquadrics can model a large set of standard building blocks such as spheres, cylinders, and parallelopipeds as well as shapes in between. An implicit equation of the superquadrics can be obtained by manipulating the components of the vector in (1),

$$\left(\left(\frac{x}{a_x} \right)^{\frac{2}{\epsilon_2}} + \left(\frac{y}{a_y} \right)^{\frac{2}{\epsilon_2}} \right)^{\frac{\epsilon_2}{\epsilon_1}} + \left(\frac{z}{a_z} \right)^{\frac{2}{\epsilon_1}} = 1. \quad (2)$$

The modeling power of superquadrics is augmented by the application of various deformation operations to the basic models [27]. In particular, certain classes of deformed superquadrics are able to model nonrigid objects that are nonsymmetric. A typical example of deformation operation that can be applied to the basic superquadrics is the tapering deformation. If a point (x, y, z) is transformed to (X, Y, Z), the tapering deformation can be written as

$$X = f_x(z)x$$
$$Y = f_y(z)y$$
$$Z = z, \qquad (3)$$

where $f_x(z)$ and $f_y(z)$, the tapering functions, are usually piecewise linear functions of z. An object's cross section increases its size when the derivative of the tapering function is positive and decreases its size when the derivative is negative.

Twisting and bending deformations can also be applied to the basic superquadrics to model the complex nature of the left ventricle shape. The basic superquadrics of (1) along with possible deformation transformations define the parametric model that we use for left ventricle motion analysis. The parameters we need to recover in this model include three rotation parameters and three translation parameters for global motion, three scale parameters and two squareness parameters for basic superquadrics, and additional shape deformation parameters for deformed superquadrics.

As previously indicated, the choice of modeling primitive depends heavily on our *a priori* knowledge of the object. The modeling primitive plays an important role in recovering global motion, especially when the 3-D feature points are distributed with bias. In the case of the left ventricle, *a priori* shape knowledge leads us to choose an ellipsoid with tapering and twist deformations to model the left ventricle shape. Although the modeling of the left ventricle as a tapered and twisted ellipsoid will not model all localized deformations, it is a good approximation of the global shape. The tapering deformation allows us to model the varying cross sectional areas perpendicular to the long axis of the left ventricle. For simplicity's sake, we make the tapering functions the same for two global axes:

$$f_x(z) = f_y(z) = kz + 1, \qquad (4)$$

where k is a tapering constant and $-\frac{1}{a_z} < k < \frac{1}{a_z}$. The axial twist deformation models the shape change caused by torsion of the left ventricle during the ejection phase. Its functional form is usually linear with respect to the axis z. The introduction of twist deformation to model the shape of left ventricle is justified in [28] and [29].

Spherical Harmonic Shape Modeling: The superquadric modeling primitives presented earlier capture only the global deformations of the left ventricle. The residual distances computed from the fitted global shape and the given data are the measures of local deformations that the superquadric modeling primitives are unable to capture. To analyze the local deformation of the left ventricle shape in the neighborhood of the data points, these discretely distributed residual distances should be interpolated over their neighborhood surface patches. We introduce here the spherical harmonic shape modeling primitives in order to construct a smooth surface from the residual distances.

According to Ballard and Brown [30], spherical harmonic surfaces are closed surfaces that are functions on the sphere and can be decomposed into a set of orthogonal functions. Spherical harmonics may be parameterized by two numbers, m and n; thus they are a doubly infinite set of functions that are continuous, orthogonal, single valued, and complete on the sphere. The basis functions $U_{mn}(\phi, \theta)$ and $V_{mn}(\phi, \theta)$ are defined in a spherical coordinate system as

$$U_{nm}(\phi, \theta) = \cos m\phi P_{n,m}(\cos \theta) \qquad (5)$$
$$V_{nm}(\phi, \theta) = \sin m\phi P_{n,m}(\cos \theta), \qquad (6)$$

where $P_{n,m}(\cdot)$ is the general Legendre function and given by

$$P_{n,m}(x) = (1 - x^2)^{\frac{m}{2}} \frac{d^m}{dx^m} P_n(x) \qquad (7)$$

and $P_n(\cdot)$ is the Legendre polynomial of degree n.

In combination, the spherical harmonics are able to produce various well-behaved functions. To represent an arbitrary shape, the radius $r(\phi, \theta)$ in spherical coordinate system can be written as a linear sum of spherical harmonic base functions:

$$r(\phi, \theta) \approx \sum_{n=1}^{N} \sum_{m=0}^{n} [A_{nm} U_{nm}(\phi, \theta) + B_{nm} V_{nm}(\phi, \theta)]. \qquad (8)$$

In other words, any continuous surface on the sphere may be represented by a set of real coefficients A_{nm} and B_{nm}.

We propose spherical harmonics as shape modeling primitives for left ventricle deformation analysis mainly because they can produce a closed surface with well-defined functional properties. One distinct nature of the spherical harmonic modeling primitives different from the superquadric modeling primitives is their ability to capture the details of local surface patch without enforcing any kind of symmetric constraints. Moreover, the size of the coefficient set can be chosen so that the spherical harmonic modeling primitives characterize enough details in a localized region. Therefore, the reconstruction of the surface details that superquadric modeling primitives fail to capture enables us to analyze local deformation of the left ventricle based on spherical harmonic modeling.

To estimate the local deformations from a spherical harmonic fitted surface, we propose to establish the displacement fields of left ventricle surface over the cardiac cycle. The details of how we estimate the displacement fields will be presented in Section IV. The spherical harmonic surfaces will be combined with the displacement field to produce correspondences of surface points so that tensor-description-based analysis can be applied to local surface patches.

III. MODEL-BASED MOTION AND DEFORMATION ANALYSIS

In the previous section, we presented motion and shape modeling primitives for the left ventricle. Our objective of introducing these modeling primitives is to devise a model-based approach for estimating left ventricle motion and deformations. Through modeling, we are able to incorporate into the model *a priori* knowledge of left ventricle motion and shape. Furthermore, the modeling primitives are generally parameterized so that the model-based approach can be easily implemented.

In this section, we first present the hierarchical decomposition of the proposed motion model. The philosophy of the simple motion-model-based approaches is isolating different components of motion and deformations by adopting a simple model that describes only the component of motion or deformation of particular interest. In contrast, our hierarchical decomposition of motion does not isolate the motion and deformation components. The well-defined hierarchy of the motion model provides the interconnections between each of these components. This model based analysis of left ventricle motion and deformation is expected to produce better estimation results because of the hierarchical structure of the motion model.

A. Motion Analysis by Hierarchical Decomposition

Various generalized motion models have been proposed in the analysis of nonrigid motion in the field of computer vision. One popular approach to nonrigid motion analysis based on a generalized model analysis is the overall motion parameterization without identifying and utilizing the interrelations of each of the components of motion or deformations in the whole parameter set. It is obvious that such an overall parameterization approach is difficult to implement since it usually involves a nonlinear optimization with a large number of parameters. In the following, we first discuss the need for motion decomposition when a generalized motion model is used for nonrigid motion analysis. We argue that the overall parameterization approach is suitable only for motion analysis of nonrigid objects whose pattern of motion is not clear. To perform the model-based motion analysis of the left ventricle, we present the hierarchical decomposition of the our motion model described in Section II. Through decomposition, our estimation scheme reflects the interrelation of each motion and deformation component in our hierarchical motion model and leads to the implementation of coarse-to-fine estimation algorithms.

The Needs for Motion Decomposition: Terzopoulos *et al.* [31], [32] are among the first computer vision and graphics researchers [23], [31], [32], [33] to start working on nonrigid object motion analysis based on motion and surface modeling. They developed algorithms [31], [34] that are able to recover the geometric shape of the object at different time instants using intrinsic and extrinsic constraints. Recently, they have extended their previous approach and proposed a family of modeling primitives called deformable superquadrics [35], [36]. This is a unified motion and shape model with the parameters of global motion, global deformation, and local deformations. These classified motion and deformations are combined into an overall set of parameters that is estimated simultaneously through manipulation of dynamic equations derived for the purpose of implementation only. Chen and Huang [37] have independently proposed a unified motion model similar to that of Terzopoulos [35] when developing estimation algorithms for left ventricle motion analysis based on computer vision techniques. However, they have imple-

mented their estimation algorithms by decomposing the global motion from the local deformations. Such a decomposition is based on the interrelations between motion and deformation components of the left ventricle and leads to computationally efficient estimation algorithms.

The deformable superquadrics proposed by Terzopoulos *et al.* [35], [36] is an elegant formulation of dynamic 3-D surface modeling. However, the motion and deformation parameters so recovered do not reflect the interrelations of each component of nonrigid motion and deformations. The model can be applied to many practical problems that involve shape fitting as well as motion analysis. However, this approach is not practical for general nonrigid motion analysis, mainly due to the complex overall optimization implementation of dynamic equations used in their energy minimizing schemes. For many nonrigid objects, it is possible to implement a decomposition of optimization algorithm if the knowledge of the motion pattern of the object is available. It is also not practical to apply their approach directly to model-based heart motion analysis for following reasons. First of all, since the pattern of left ventricle motion is approximately known, the recovery of such motion patterns instead of overall motion and deformations becomes necessary. Second, the global deformations, including expansion/contraction and twisting, are all in terms of a localized coordinate system with its origin on the center of contraction. This kind of global deformation directly reflects the functioning of a beating heart but is generally different from the deformation parameters recovered from the deformable superquadrics unless the origin of the superquadrics, in fact, coincides with the center of contraction. In our work, we also make use of the modeling primitive superquadrics, but only after we have established the object-centered coordinate system. That means we will separate the global rigid motion estimation from the global nonrigid motion estimation process. Finally, we will show later that, by hierarchical decomposition, the implementation of the estimation scheme can be converted into a series of simple or linear estimation algorithms. The implementation of these simpler algorithms is easier than the approach based on deformable superquadrics that combines all of the parameters into one single set. Therefore, instead of directly applying the hierarchical motion model, we devise a hierarchical decomposition of motion model based on *a priori* knowledge of the motion patterns of the left ventricle.

Hierarchical Decomposition Approach: Our hierarchical motion model includes four parts: global rigid motion, global deformation, local rigid motion, and local deformation. The goal of hierarchical decomposition is to devise algorithms that can estimate each part individually. We described earlier the necessity and advantages of such decomposition in the case of left ventricle motion analysis based on the hierarchical model. Here we will discuss the interrelation of these four components of left ventricle motion and how the interrelation can be used in our concrete implementation of the proposed hierarchical decomposition.

We first examine carefully the overall motion and deformation patterns of the left ventricle known to cardiac researchers. Although many models of left ventricle motion and deformation have been proposed, until recently there was no attempt being made to recognize the interrelations among different motion and deformation components of heart dynamics. Potel *et al.* [38] are among the first few researchers who looked into the overall dynamics of the left ventricle and identified the relationship among different motion and deformation components. According to their findings, a moving coordinate system seems to describe the left ventricle motion better than a fixed coordinate system. This suggests that the left ventricle does have a global rigid motion in addition to the well-known global deformation, such as expansion/contraction, and local deformations. They also found that, at each time instant, about 90% of the entire left ventricle wall motion is directed toward the center of contraction, the origin of the moving spherical coordinate system. This tells us that the expansion and contraction in terms of the center of contraction are far more significant than the circumferential rotation or twisting motion that have also been observed in their research. All of these findings prompted our idea of hierarchical motion decomposition, which allows us to devise a series of efficient estimation algorithms. We shall show later that some of the hierarchical decomposition scheme can be derived analytically based on the Potel's findings.

Three basic assumptions have been adopted in our hierarchical decomposition of overall motion and deformations. These assumptions are summarized as follows.

1) Among the various global and local deformation—such as expansion or contraction, twisting, bending, and local stretching, and so on—the deformation due to expansion or contraction accounts for a commanding high percentage of the total deformation.

2) The global shape of the left ventricle can be approximated as an ellipsoid with tapering and twisting deformations. The local deformations can be defined as the minimum deviation from the global shape.

3) The local deformations are spatially smooth, or, in other words, the neighboring areas have similar local stretching deformation in terms of both direction and magnitude.

These three assumptions have all been confirmed by medical observations. The first assumption is the crucial one and has been supported by Potel's findings. The second assumption is based on many medical observations and experiments that the global shape of the left ventricle can be roughly approximated as ellipsoid [13]. However, our modeling primitives are not as restrictive as these ellipsoid models, since we allow the tapering and twisting deformations to be performed on the ellipsoid models to capture the varying sizes of cross section and transverse or shear stresses during contraction. The third assumption has also been widely used in cardiac research and shown to match medical observations [7].

Here is an outline of our hierarchical motion decomposition, which divides the model-based estimation of left ventricle motion into three stages. First, the global rigid motion of the left ventricle is computed by constructing an object-centered moving coordinate system. The origin of the coordinate system is defined as the center of contraction and the orientation of the coordinate system as the principal axes. We will show in Section III–B that the origin and the orientation of the coordinate system calculated directly from the 3-D data are approximately invariant to the global deformations, assuming that the twisting deformations are small compared with the rigid motion and expansion or contraction during a cardiac cycle. Upon compensation of global rigid motion, the left ventricle undergoes global as well as local deformations. Then, the global deformations are estimated by performing superquadric surface fitting on the time-varying object-centered coordinate system. The superquadric surface fittings will capture the global deformation characteristics of the left ventricle shape, including expansion/contraction and twisting. Finally, the spherical harmonic fitting of residual distances is performed to characterize the local deformations of the left ventricle that global surface modeling primitives are unable to capture. In this stage, we will combine the global superquadric surface with the spherical harmonic interpolated residual surface to form an overall surface on which the tensor-based deformation analysis is carried out.

B. Global Rigid Motion Analysis

In the first stage of hierarchical decomposition, we propose to estimate the global rigid motion of the left ventricle by extracting the global rigid motion from the overall motion. In the following, we present the estimation of the left ventricle centroid and principal axes, which serve as the origin and orientation of the object-centered moving coordinate system. We show that the global rigid motion of the left ventricle between two consecutive time instants can be easily calculated from the estimated moving coordinate system for each time instant.

Estimation of Left Ventricle Centroid: According to our first assumption, the contribution of local deformation and global twisting to the overall motion is small compared with the global rigid motion and global expansion or contraction. This means that the motion of the centroid of these data points is mainly due to global rigid motion and global expansion or contraction. It can be shown further that pure expansion or contraction of the left ventricle contributes null to the motion of the centroid. Therefore, the centroid computed from the data points can be a good approximation for the origin of the moving coordinate system.

Suppose there are n points of interests on the surface of the left ventricle with coordinates $(x_i, y_i, z_i), i = 1, \cdots n$; then, the centroid of these points will be

$$
\begin{aligned}
x_m &= \tfrac{1}{n} \sum_1^n x_i \\
y_m &= \tfrac{1}{n} \sum_1^n y_i \\
z_m &= \tfrac{1}{n} \sum_1^n z_i.
\end{aligned}
\tag{9}
$$

The centroid computed from data points using (9) is used to represent the center of contraction of the left ventricle. The displacement of the centroid over two time instants represents the translation vector of the global rigid motion. Based on the estimated centroid, the principal axes can be estimated and the object-centered coordinate system can therefore be constructed.

Estimation of Left Ventricle Principal Axes: As discussed above, the translation vector of the global motion over consecutive time instants can be determined by the centroids of the data sets. However, to determine the rotation matrix of global motion, we need more information than the location of the centroids. It is well known in the motion analysis of rigid objects that the correspondences between two noncolinear vectors over two time instants is sufficient to determine the rotation matrix. Thus, for the purpose of determining the rotation matrix of global motion, we need to find the principal axes that are invariant to the expansion or contraction of the left ventricle, so that the relative orientation of these axes over the consecutive time instants represents the global rotation of left ventricle.

For a given set of 3-D points on the surface of an object, a principal axis can be defined as an axis that goes through the centroid of these points with its orientation in such direction that the sum of the squared distances between the axis and the individual points is minimum. Assume that the directional cosines of the axis are α, β, γ. Then the parameters are the solutions of the following constrained optimization problem:

$$Minimize : \sum_{i=1}^{n} \| D \times (P_i - P_m) \|^2$$
$$subject\ to : \| D \| = 1, \tag{10}$$

where $D = (\alpha, \beta, \gamma)$, P_i's are position vectors representing the *i*th 3-D points, P_m is the position vector of the centroid, and $\times$ is the vector cross product. In fact, $\| D \times (P_i - P_m) \|$ is the distance between point P_i and the axis that goes through the centroid P_m with directional vector D. After some algebraic manipulation, the above optimization problem is converted into the problem of minimizing a quadratic objective function, as follows:

$$Min : a_{11}\alpha^2 + a_{22}\beta^2 + a_{33}\gamma^2 + (a_{12} + a_{21})\alpha\beta$$
$$(a_{13} + a_{31})\alpha\gamma + (a_{23} + a_{32})\beta\gamma$$
$$subject\ to : \alpha^2 + \beta^2 + \gamma^2 = 1 \tag{11}$$

where

$$a_{11} = \sum_{i=1}^{n} \left[(y_i - y_m)^2 + (z_i - z_m)^2 \right] \tag{12}$$

$$a_{12} = a_{21} = -\sum_{i=1}^{n} (x_i - x_m)(y_i - y_m) \tag{13}$$

$$a_{13} = a_{31} = -\sum_{i=1}^{n} (x_i - x_m)(z_i - z_m) \tag{14}$$

$$a_{22} = \sum_{i=1}^{n} \left[(x_i - x_m)^2 + (z_i - z_m)^2 \right] \tag{15}$$

$$a_{23} = a_{32} = -\sum_{i=1}^{n} (y_i - y_m)(z_i - z_m) \tag{16}$$

$$a_{33} = \sum_{i=1}^{n} \left[(x_i - x_m)^2 + (y_i - y_m)^2 \right], \tag{17}$$

or in matrix form,

$$minimize : D^T A D \tag{18}$$
$$subject\ to : \| D \| = 1.$$

Equivalently, the problem now is to find the smallest eigenvalue of A, a 3×3 symmetric and positive definite matrix. The solution to the optimization problem will be the eigenvector that corresponds to the smallest eigenvalue of the matrix. The 3×3 symmetric matrix is of the following form:

$$A = \begin{bmatrix} a_{11} & a_{12} & a_{13} \\ a_{21} & a_{22} & a_{23} \\ a_{31} & a_{32} & a_{33} \end{bmatrix}. \tag{19}$$

Suppose that the expansion or contraction factor between two consecutive time instants is k. Then, according to (6) through (14), the relationship between the two matrixes A and A' will be $A' = k^2 A$, where A and A' are matrixes used to find the principal axes that correspond to two consecutive time instants. Therefore, the eigenvectors of A and A' are clearly the same. This shows that the rotation of the estimated principal axis represents global rigid rotation of the left ventricle if the contributions due to global twisting and local deformations can be neglected since the expansion or contraction does not contribute to the rotation of the axis.

We indicated earlier that two noncolinear vectors associated with the surface are needed to determine the rotation matrix of global motion. We have already discussed how to locate an axis that is approximately invariant to certain global and local deformation. Note that the objective function we used in the above optimization problem is the sum of the squared distances from the points of interests to an axis we intended to determine. For the same reason, we can determine an axis such that the objective function is actually maximized. The solution of this optimization problem is the eigenvector of the constructed matrix corresponding to the largest eigenvalue. Furthermore, since A is a symmetric, positive definite matrix, the two axes are orthogonal because they are the eigenvectors corresponding to smallest and largest eigenvalues. Therefore, the noncolinearity requirement of the vectors is satisfied and global rotation can be determined using these two estimated principal axes.

Global Rigid Motion Computation: Assume that we have already found the centroids and principal axes that are associated with the bifurcation points over the successive time instants. Then, the translation vector and the rotation matrix of the equivalent global motion of the left ventricle surface between successive time instants can easily be identified from the position and the orientation change of these axes.

The translation vector of the global motion is simply the difference between the two centroids. For the rotation matrix, it is the change in orientation of the principal axes between two consecutive time instants. Since these two principal axes estimated from the given set of points are orthogonal, we can construct a mutually orthogonal 3-D coordinates fixed to the left ventricle surface by using the two principal axes and their cross product as the third axis. Now, the rotation matrix of the global motion becomes the transformation matrix of the coordinate system from one time instant to the next. In matrix form, the global motion parameters can be written as

$$
T = \begin{bmatrix} x'_m \\ y'_m \\ z'_m \end{bmatrix} - \begin{bmatrix} x_m \\ y_m \\ z_m \end{bmatrix} \tag{20}
$$

$$
R = [e'_1 \quad e'_2 \quad (e'_1 \times e'_2)][e_1 e_2 (e_1 \times e_2)]^T, \tag{21}
$$

where (x_m, y_m, z_m) and (x'_m, y'_m, z'_m) are the centroids, e_1, e_2, and e'_1, e'_2 are principal axes of the left ventricle at two consecutive time instants. The main assumption for estimating the global rigid motion has been that, in addition to global rigid motion, the component of global expansion or contraction is much larger in magnitude than the rest of the possible deformations.

C. Global Deformation Analysis

Suppose that we have successfully found the translation vectors and rotation matrixes of the global rigid motion over successive time instants. Then, the position and orientation of the left ventricle are all known at these time instants. Upon transformation of original data to the object-centered coordinate system using the rigid motion parameters, we are ready to perform the global deformation analysis through fitting the transformed data to the superquadric modeling primitives. Generally, the parameters to be estimated in the superquadric surface fitting would include six parameters for position and orientation since the given data are usually with respect to a fixed coordinate system due to the fixed spatial position of the imaging devices. It is therefore a great advantage in the shape recovery process based on superquadrics that we know the position and orientation of the object. In recent research on recovering superquadric model from 3-D information [24], [25], [26], [27], various error of fit measures have been investigated, all leading to nonlinear optimization algorithms. By reducing the number of parameters involved, we reduce the dimension of search space, reduce the computational complexity, and increase the probability of convergence to the right solution.

Among various optimization schemes in recovering superquadrics investigated by many researchers, the most common one is based on the *inside–outside* function defined as:

$$
f(x, y, z) = \left(\left(\frac{x}{a_x} \right)^{\frac{2}{\epsilon_2}} + \left(\frac{y}{a_y} \right)^{\frac{2}{\epsilon_2}} \right)^{\frac{\epsilon_2}{\epsilon_1}} + \left(\frac{z}{a_z} \right)^{\frac{2}{\epsilon_1}}, \tag{22}
$$

where if $f(x_0, y_0, z_0) = 1$, then (x_0, y_0, z_0) is on the surface; if $f(x_0, y_0, z_0) < 1$, then (x_0, y_0, z_0) lies inside the surface; if $f(x_0, y_0, z_0) > 1$, then (x_0, y_0, z_0) lies outside the surface. The objective function for the optimization is defined as:

$$
Minimize : \sum_{i=1}^{n} |f(x, y. z) - 1|^2, \tag{23}
$$

where the summation is over all known 3-D points.

D. Local Motion and Deformation Analysis

The well-known Helmholz decomposition states that [18], locally, the motion of a sufficiently small volumetric element of a deformable body can be decomposed into the sum of a translation, a rotation, and an expansion (contraction) in three orthogonal directions. Notice that the translation and rotation here are that of the small element and therefore are different from the global rigid motion of the whole deformable body, assuming that the deformable object undergoes both local deformations and global movement. For a given reference coordinate system, the mathematical expression of the local deformation based on tensor transformation can be written as

$$
P_{i+1} = T_i(P_i) + R_i(P_i)P_i + E_i(P_i)P_i, \tag{24}
$$

where P_i and P_{i+1} are point vectors within the small volumetric element at time instant i and $i + 1$, respectively. T_i is a translation vector, R_i a rotation tensor, and E_i an expansion tensor, all varying with space and time. However, within a local small volumetric element, T_i, R_i, and E_i can be considered approximately the same for all points. Furthermore, the rotation tensor R_i is orthonormal and the expansion tensor symmetric. It has been shown in [17] that local deformation of the cardiac wall can be approximated as homogeneous changes and described by the tensor model of deformable object, as illustrated above.

There are 12 unknowns in (24). For each 3-D point correspondence, three equations can be established to specify the relationship of motion and deformation between two successive time instants using (24). Hence, in order to determine all twelve unknowns, four point correspondences within the local element are needed. Assuming that the deformable surface is specified by the sample points on the surface and the correspondences of these points over consecutive time instants are given, then the tensor analysis parameters can be estimated over each local surface patch containing at least four points. Equation (24) is nonlinear with respect to the three rotation parameters, and no closed form solution is known. However, as Chen and Huang [9] pointed out, if small angle rotation is assumed, the original nonlinear problem can be transformed into a linear one. The rotation matrix can be approximately expressed as

$$
R = R_z R_y R_x \approx \begin{bmatrix} 1 & -\gamma & \beta \\ \gamma & 1 & -\alpha \\ -\beta & \alpha & 1 \end{bmatrix}, \tag{25}
$$

where α, β, γ are rotation angles around $x-, y-, z-$axis, respectively. Then, (24) reduces to a set of linear equations. Singular value decomposition method may be introduced to overcome the possible ill condition of the system. According to [18], the eigenvectors of the expansion tensor E_i give the directions of extreme deformation, and the corresponding eigenvalues specify the amounts of deformation.

IV. IMPLEMENTATION OF ESTIMATION ALGORITHMS

We have discussed our methodology for motion and deformation analysis of left ventricle from angiographic data using hierarchical decomposition. The idea of decomposing a complex and nonlinear problem into several simple or linear stages has been applied throughout the development of these estimation algorithms. We describe here the implementation of some of these algorithms and discuss their simplicity and robustness. One special feature of this approach is its ability to provide a good estimate of left ventricle global motion and shape even when the given bifurcation points derived from angiographic data are distributed with bias.

A. A Recursive Algorithm for Global Motion and Deformation Analysis

The global rigid motion analysis algorithm presented in Section III–B is based on 3-D coordinates of the data points at successive time instants. We have implicitly assumed that these data points are uniformly distributed on the surface of the left ventricle. In reality, however, the data points used are bifurcation points extracted from the biplane angiogram sequences. The estimate of the centroid of the left ventricle using the proposed scheme based on only bifurcation points is inaccurate since these bifurcation points do not cover the whole surface of left ventricle. The inaccurate estimate of the centroid then causes faulty computation of the object orientation and global deformations. Therefore, the estimation of the object centroid is critical. In this section, we present a recursive algorithm that can adjust the centroid estimate based on the knowledge that has been incorporated in the global shape modeling primitives of the left ventricle.

Combat the Bias via Modeling Primitives: In the bifurcation point-based heart motion analysis, we notice that complete and unbiased 3-D data points are not available due to the structural configuration of left ventricle coronary arteries. Fortunately, along with the biased data, *a priori* shape information of the left ventricle can also be used in the development of estimation algorithms. In Section II the *a priori* shape knowledge of the left ventricle has been incorporated into global shape modeling primitives, which are used to estimate the global deformation of the left ventricle. Although the global deformation estimation is based on the results of global rigid motion estimation, the shape modeling primitives can also be used to develop a recursive algorithm for improved estimation of global rigid motion and global deformations. Our recursive algorithm intends to use the shape information of the left ventricle incorporated in the global shape modeling primitives to guide the adjustment of the estimated centroid until the fitted surface has the smallest error of fit, which implies that the fitted surface is considered consistent with *a priori* knowledge of the left ventricle shape.

Let us examine carefully the given 3-D data, which consist of coronary artery bifurcation points of the left ventricle. It is known that the coronary arteries of the left ventricle encircle only about three-quarters of the left ventricle surface. Hence, the 3-D bifurcation points are distributed with bias on the surface of left ventricle. The algorithm for estimating global rigid motion presented in Section III–B provides unacceptable results if we use only the bifurcation points that are distributed with bias. Here, a recursive algorithm is proposed that utilizes *a priori* knowledge of the left ventricle shape in the esti-

mation process and produces potentially unbiased estimation results.

The recursive algorithm is implemented by incrementally adjusting the estimated centroid. The adjustment of estimated centroid is accomplished through the application of *a priori* knowledge of left ventricle shape and the data acquisition limitations. After analyzing the geometric position of the coronary arteries, we know that the actual centroid of the left ventricle is different from the geometric center of the given bifurcation points. Compared with the estimated centroid directly using (9), the actual centroid is located further away from the side of the left ventricle surface encircled by the coronary arteries. This side of the surface is identified as the side in which the size parameter of the surface primitives, estimated from fitting the given data, is the smallest. Our argument is based on the observation that a left ventricle modeled by the surface primitives may be elongated along only the long axis of the left ventricle. This *a priori* knowledge is utilized to guide the adjustment of the estimated centroid towards the direction in which we believe the actual centroid should be located. This adjusted centroid, together with the newly estimated principal axes, is used to fine tune the left ventricle shape again through surface fitting. The updated error-of-fit measure, computed using (23), is used to control the adjustment to prevent over adjusting. If the updated error of fit is greater or equal than the previous one, then the centroid may have been over adjusted. One cycle of such adjustment is considered as one step in a recursive algorithm to be described in the following. We show in Section V that the results obtained by this recursive algorithm are much better in terms of their compatibility with the apparent shape knowledge of the left ventricle.

A Recursive Algorithm: In the above, we presented a scheme to adjust the biased centroid estimate according to the available left ventricle shape information. Since the optimal adjustment often cannot be accomplished in just one step, we propose a recursive algorithm that adjusts the estimated parameters incrementally until they are in accordance with *a priori* knowledge of the left ventricle. A single step of the adjustment includes centroid adjustment, principal axes modification, and error-of-fit computation. Based on the current error of fit, we decide whether the adjustment is in the correct direction and the amount of adjustment is right. The adjustment will continue until the error-of-fit measure stops decreasing. Intuitively, this recursive algorithm for estimating global motion and object shape will converge to the right solution. A solid theoretical study of the convergence properties of the recursive algorithm is yet to be made, but the estimation results presented in Section V show the desired convergence in our application of this recursive algorithm to left ventricle motion analysis.

This recursive algorithm consists of the following steps:

Step 1: Estimate the centroid and the principal axes using the algorithms proposed for the ideal case, in which only the given 3-D coordinates of bifurcation points are used.

Step 2: Recover the global shape of the left ventricle using the position (centroid) and orientation (principal axes) parameters via the superquadric-modeling-based approach and calculate the error of fit.

Step 3: Adjust the position parameters according to the *a priori* knowledge of the distribution of bifurcation points and estimate the new orientation parameters.

Step 4: Recover the global shape parameters using the adjusted position and orientation parameters and calculate the error of fit again.

Step 5: Stop the recursive algorithm if the current error of fit is greater than or equal to the previous one; otherwise go to Step 3 and continue the recursive algorithm.

The recursive estimation algorithm provides us the adjusted centroid, adjusted principal axes, and adjusted parameters for superquadric modeling primitives. For a given pair of centroid and principal axes set, the global rigid motion of the left ventricle can be obtained using (20) and (21). The global deformation parameters can be obtained by comparing the parameters of the superquadric surfaces at two consecutive time instants.

B. Spherical Harmonic Interpolation of Deformable Surface

The recursive algorithm presented in the previous subsection produces the global rigid motion parameters and the global deformation parameters for the left ventricle. However, the left ventricle shape obtained from the recursive algorithm represents only the global shape at a given time instant. The local deformations, which are different from one localized surface patch to another, have been smoothed out in this globally oriented modeling approach because of the axial symmetry property of the modeling primitives. A fine tuning of the surface estimation is thus needed in order to accurately describe the local deformable left ventricle surface. In particular, the local deformable surfaces are very much needed for the tensor analysis based on the correspondences of local feature points.

We notice that the given bifurcation points are not necessarily on the fitted surface of the left ventricle represented by the shape modeling primitives. The distances between these points and the estimated surface provide information on the estimation residues for the localized region around these points. To obtain a better representation of the left ventricle surface, the distances between these points and the estimated surface are interpolated over the spherical coordinate system as a function of spherical coordinates (ϕ, θ) to produce a residual surface for each time instant. These residual surfaces are added to their corresponding global shapes estimated in previous subsections to compose a more accurate description of the left ventricle surface.

Several things must be taken care of when we produce the residual surface from the estimated global shape and the given data points. First of all, the distances between the estimated superquadric surface and the given points are calculated along the radial direction since we intend to interpolate these dis-

tances over the spherical coordinates (ϕ, θ). Second, these bifurcation points are distributed over only three-quarters of the left ventricle surface. This means that we have to pad some zero residues for that side of the residual surface where there are no bifurcation points. Finally, these points can be inside or outside the estimated surface and thus a base value has to be set for these distances in order to produce a surface that has a one-to-one mapping onto the unit sphere.

Suppose the 3-D coordinates of the given points are (x_i, y_i, z_i), $i = 1, \cdots, n$, the estimated global shape is specified by the parameters (a_x, a_y, a_z, k), and the base value is set as b_0; then the following is a mathematical procedure of producing sample points that are used to interpolate the residual surface. The spherical coordinates of these bifurcation points are calculated as

$$
\begin{bmatrix} \phi_i \\ \theta_i \\ r_d(\phi_i, \theta_i) \end{bmatrix} = \begin{bmatrix} \arctan(\frac{y_i}{x_i}) \\ \arctan(\frac{\sqrt{x_i^2+y_i^2}}{z}) \\ \sqrt{x_i^2 + y_i^2 + z_i^2} \end{bmatrix}. \tag{26}
$$

The radial component of their corresponding points on the estimated superquadric surface with the same longitudinal and latitudinal coordinates as the given bifurcation points can be calculated as shown in (27) at the bottom of this page, where $f_x(\theta_i) = f_y(\theta_i) = (ka_z \sin(\theta_i) + 1)$ is the tapering function.

On that side of the estimated surface where there are no bifurcation points, we have no information indicating the difference between the estimated global surface and local deformed surface. To get a closed residual surface that represents the estimation residue distribution over the whole surface of the estimated global shape, we need to zero-pad some residual distances. Thus, the residual sample points are defined as follows:

$$
\begin{cases} r_i = r_d(\phi_i, \theta_i) - r_s(\phi_i, \theta_i), & i = 1, \cdots, n; \\ r_i = 0, & i = n+1, \cdots, p. \end{cases} \tag{28}
$$

As we have already pointed out, the given bifurcation points may be inside or outside the estimated surface, and therefore the above defined r_i's may not necessarily be positive. Since the interpolation of residual surface is over the whole spherical coordinate system, a one-to-one mapping between the residual surface and the unit sphere is generally required. Under this assumption, the interpolation algorithm will require that the sample points be all positive. To meet this condition, we need to set a base value for all the sample points such that the radial coordinate of all sample points become positive by adding such a base value. A natural choice of the base value is the average of estimated global shape size parameters since it represents the approximate size of left ventricle. Therefore, the radial coordinate of these sample points is represented as

$$
d_i = r_i + b_0 > 0 \quad i = 1, \cdots, p, \tag{29}
$$

where b_0 can be set as $\frac{1}{3}(a_x + a_y + a_z)$.

$$
r_s(\phi_i, \theta_i) = \sqrt{f_x^2(\theta_i)a_x^2 \cos^2 \theta_i \cos^2 \phi_i + f_y^2(\theta_i)a_y^2 \cos^2 \theta_i \sin^2 \phi_i + a_z^2 \sin^2 \theta_i} \tag{27}
$$

Now we are ready to interpolate these sample points to form the residual surface. Among these p points, n of them are calculated as the distances between the given bifurcation points and estimated superquadric surface, and $p - n$ of them are exactly on the surface of a sphere with radius b_0.

In Section II–B, we indicated that the radius $r(\phi, \theta)$ of an arbitrary surface in spherical coordinate system can be written as a linear sum of spherical harmonic base functions:

$$r_a(\phi, \theta) \approx \sum_{n=1}^{N} \sum_{m=0}^{n} [A_{nm} U_{nm}(\phi, \theta) + B_{nm} V_{nm}(\phi, \theta)]. \quad (30)$$

If we denote the coefficients of the above approximation by α_i and the basis functions as $B_i(\phi, \theta)$, then the approximation will be:

$$r_a(\phi, \theta) \approx \sum_{i=1}^{M} \alpha_i B_i(\phi, \theta). \quad (31)$$

The number of coefficients M may be large depending upon the order of approximation N. In the case of left ventricle, according to Coppini et al [7], we can take the order of approximation $N = 3$ ($M = 16$) to get a satisfactory interpolation over the given sample points. The objective function for the interpolation is therefore of the following form:

$$\epsilon = \sum_{j=1}^{p} \left[r_a(\phi_j, \theta_j) - \sum_{i=1}^{16} \alpha_i B_i(\phi_j, \theta_j) \right]^2. \quad (32)$$

Least squares methods are applied to get the coefficients of the interpolation. In this case, the sample points are set as $r_a(\phi_i, \theta_i) = d_i, i = 1, \cdots, p$ by the definition given in (29). This algorithm is easy to implement since the coefficients to be estimated can be obtained by solving a system of linear equations.

The surface obtained using (32) is a superposition of a sphere with radius b_0 and the interpolated error distances. For any given longitudinal and latitudinal coordinates, the corresponding residual distances can be calculated from the interpolated surface. For example, if the given longitudinal and latitudinal coordinates are (ϕ_i, θ_i), then the residual distances will be:

$$r_e(\phi_i, \theta_i) = r_a(\phi_i, \theta_i) - b_0. \quad (33)$$

If we represent the estimated global shape by its radial coordinate as a function of longitudinal and latitudinal coordinates, we can get a deformable surface by combining (27) and (33). The deformable surface can be written as follows:

$$r_l(\phi, \theta) = r_s(\phi, \theta) + r_e(\phi, \theta), \quad (34)$$

where $-\pi < \phi \leq \pi$ and $0 \leq \theta \leq \pi$.

C. Displacement Field Estimation and Tensor Analysis

We indicated in Section III–D that four-point correspondences within a localized surface are needed to perform the tensor-based deformation analysis. In the case of estimating left ventricle motion and deformation from coronary artery bifurcation points, we are given the correspondences of these bifurcation points over consecutive time instants within a cardiac cycle. As we have already pointed out, these bifurcation points are sparsely and biasedly distributed over the surface of left ventricle. To analyze the local deformation using the tensor-based approach, these correspondences are again interpolated over their neighborhood to obtain a displacement field that specifies how each point on the estimated left ventricle surface moves from one time instant to another.

The algorithm developed in Section IV–B produces surfaces that are represented by their radial components and are functions of longitudinal and latitudinal coordinates (ϕ, θ). It is natural that the displacement fields to be established for each consecutive time instant are also expressed as the longitudinal and latitudinal coordinates variations for each point. These variations are in turn functions of the spatial position, or functions of longitudinal and latitudinal coordinates since the radial coordinate of given point is fixed by the constraint that the point is on the estimated surface. Without loss of generality, we can write:

$$\begin{cases} \phi_{t+1} = \phi_t + \Delta\phi(\phi_t, \theta_t) \\ \theta_{t+1} = \theta_t + \Delta\theta(\phi_t, \theta_t), \end{cases} \quad (35)$$

where t and $t + 1$ denote two consecutive time instants associated with the displacement field. The functions $\Delta\phi(\phi_t, \theta_t)$ and $\Delta\phi(\phi_t, \theta_t)$ can also be approximated by spherical harmonics as we did for the interpolation of local deformations. The sample points we use for the interpolation are the displacements of the given bifurcation points. This algorithm again is implemented by solving a system of linear equations.

Once we have established the displacement field, we can calculate its corresponding point in the next time instant for any given point using (35). A tensor-based approach for local deformation estimation can be performed based on the left ventricle surface estimated in Section IV–B and the displacement field specified above. Given four point correspondences on a localized surface, (24) and (25) are combined to derive a system of 12 linear equations. The local translation, local rotation, and local expansion tensor can be obtained simultaneously by solving this system of linear equations. The magnitudes and directions of extreme deformation within the localized surface patch can be represented by the eigenvalues and corresponding eigenvectors of the expansion tensor.

V. ESTIMATION RESULTS

We present here the estimation results of the angiographic data-based left ventricle motion and deformation analysis. The estimated trajectory of the left ventricle centroid is shown in Fig. 1. A complete cardiac cycle consists of 16 consecutive image frames, but we have obtained only 10 of these 16 image frames. The estimated trajectory shows that the left ventricle centroid has a tendency to move back to its starting position at the eighth time instant and therefore corresponds well to the supposed periodic motion of the heart. Figs. 2 and 3 show the 3-D view and top view of the estimated left ventricle global shape without and with the recursive algorithm. The results indicate that the estimated global shape using the recursive

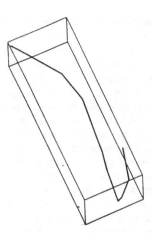

Fig. 1. 3-D view (left) and 2-D projection (right) of the estimated centroid trajectory.

algorithm is much closer to the intuitive shape of a left ventricle.

The numerical results of estimated local deformation is difficult to present since the left ventricle surface is composed of many pieces of small quadrilateral patches and each would be quantified by a vector system of extreme deformations. One way of analyzing and understanding such estimated results is to animate the moving surface and its quadrilateral meshes using scientific visualization techniques. The details of the animation are discussed in Section VI. We have produced a videotape based on the animation that shows the motion and deformation of left ventricle estimated by the proposed algorithms developed in this paper.

VI. VISUALIZATION OF DYNAMIC LEFT VENTRICLE GEOMETRY

Scientific visualization is a very effective tool both for interpreting image data and for generating images from complex multidimensional data sets. It embraces both image understanding and image synthesis. The visual representation of the data often reveals more insight than the numerical data itself. However, visualization of data poses not only a question of how we should represent numerical data but also, more importantly, what we should represent, since the visual domain is limited in how much can be shown at any moment in time. Once we have decided what we want to look at, the "how to" is a matter of communication and technology. Communication deals with data representation and the format of the visual presentation. Technology deals with the mechanics that we have at our disposal to carry the communication forward.

In this research, once we have obtained the estimation results for the left ventricle shape, motion and deformation, we need to present the 3-D geometry in such a way that evolution of spatially varying left ventricle surface or volume is clearly reflected by the estimated results. Since the motion and deformation of a beating heart is a time-varying 3-D process, these estimation results are difficult to present numerically. It is appropriate to inspect and analyze the numerical results visually by generating an animation of a beating heart using the

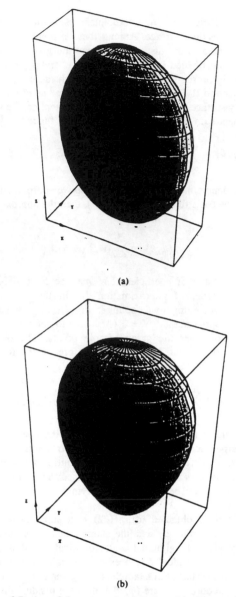

(a)

(b)

Fig. 2. 3-D view of the estimated global shape (a) without and (b) with recursive algorithm.

estimated left ventricle model driven by the estimated motion and deformation parameters. With the help of visualization tools, we can observe the estimation results at various stages of the analysis; this allows the computation to be interactive. Also, the display of the estimated left ventricle surface reveals the performance of the estimation algorithm, which is not apparent from numerical representation. Furthermore, the visualization of spatial-varying left ventricle surface or volume with encoded deformation quantities provides the physicians convenient means of clinical evaluation and understanding.

In the following, we first discuss the representation of a beating left ventricle as 3-D geometry. Several techniques are applied in the generation of such 3-D geometry so that the visual effects of the dimensionality is enhanced. We then present schemes we use to code the local deformations

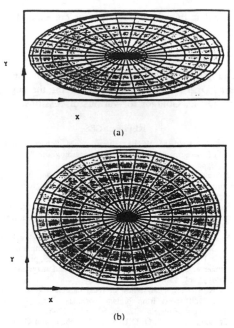

(a)

(b)

Fig. 3. Top view of the estimated global shape (a) without and (b) with recursive algorithm.

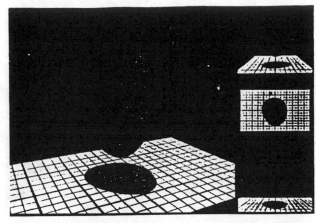

Fig. 4. A typical frame of the animation sequence of left ventricle global rigid motion and global deformation.

represented by tensor quantities. One easy way of coding these tensor quantities is to extract scalar quantities from the tensor and represent them by visually sensitive quantities, such as color.

A. Beating Left Ventricle as a 3-D Geometry

When visualizing 3-D forms, it is useful to give each form a three dimensional context, as opposed to the use of black background. The context, or *stage*, reinforces the dimensionality of the form against the inherit ambiguity and loss of information caused by the projection of the 3-D geometric shape onto the 2-D image plane. In our approach to the left ventricle motion analysis, the 3-D surface or volume of the left ventricle at each time instant is estimated. We inspect these 3-D geometric forms using visualization techniques to improve the depth and fidelity of the constructed image.

In the visualization of left ventricle geometry, we surrounded the estimated form of the heart with three orthogonal planes. This was done in the same fashion and for the same reasons that a 2-D graph is surrounded by its axes. However, for a 3-D geometric form that is time varying, the context or stage will not be enough to reflect the dimensionality of the geometric motion and deformation. To reinforce the dimensionality of time-varying property, we then cast orthogonal projections of the form onto each of the planes as shadow objects. These shadow objects serve two purposes. The first is to visually establish the relationship of the form with the surrounding planes. The second purpose is that the shadows and the planes are themselves 2-D plots of the position or extent of deformation of the form on the given projection planes. The projection planes are gridded so as to give a reference for motion and deformation of the geometric form. A typical frame of this animation sequence is shown in Fig. 4.

B. Visualization of Tensor-Represented Deformation

When we analyze the heart motion and deformation based on the angiographic data, the estimated heart form is visualized as a shaded polygonal mesh on the surface in order to identify each localized surface area. The polygons are outlined to denote the extent of the underlining quadrilateral mesh. The outlines also serve to give depth to the geometric form. The estimated local deformations associated with each quadrilateral patch are represented by stretching tensors. Although a stretching tensor can be depicted as a vector system at the center of the quadrilateral, such a representation would be unclear or too minute on a global scale. These tensor quantities must be converted into some scalar quantity and linked to visually sensitive quantities, such as color or intensity.

Following are the details of how we have investigated the visualization of local deformations. First we applied color to the polygon mesh as a function of area change of the quadrilaterals. The color ranged from blue for negative area change to yellow for positive area change. The color swing was through red, which represented no area change. The color map was based on the LAB color space, where red and green are the extents of one axis, yellow and blue are the extents of the perpendicular axis, and luminance is the vertical axis. We used this visualization of area change to guide us into regions of interest to look at the quadrilateral mesh in close up. This was to analyze the stretch tensors in these regions of interest, in which we could show the directions and magnitudes of extreme deformations using a vector system at the center of that quadrilateral patch. A typical frame of this animation is shown in Fig. 5.

The visualization part of research is performed at the National Center for Supercomputing, NCSA, the University of Illinois Urbana-Champaign. The data representation software is an internal product of the Visualization Group at NCSA. The choreography and render software used is part of the Wavefront Technology "Advanced Visualizer" software package. The image sequences were assembled on an Abekas A64 digital video disk system, and the video was mastered on a Bocsh D1 digital video record deck. Post production of

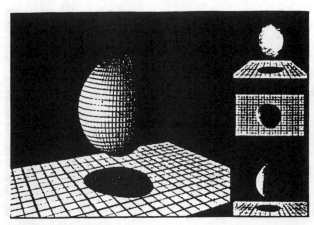

Fig. 5. A typical frame of the animation sequence of left ventricle local deformations coded by color.

the video was done in conjunction with the Media Services Group at NCSA.

VII. CONCLUSION

We have presented a hierarchical-decomposition-based approach to the modeling, analysis, and visualization of left ventricle motion and deformation using angiographic data. In modeling left ventricle motion and shape, we have combined several existing simple motion models into a hierarchy of motion and deformations. Such a hierarchical approach can also be applied to motion analysis of other nonrigid objects. Our left ventricle motion model characterizes all major motion and deformation components that are confirmed by medical observations and thus is more realistic than any of the existing simple models. More importantly, the hierarchical decomposition enables us to convert the seemingly complex estimation procedure of the coupled parameterization into coarse-to-fine estimation subprocedures. Each of these subprocedures is well defined and relatively simple so that computationally efficient algorithms can be implemented. We have also developed an animation procedure for left ventricle dynamic geometry by means of scientific visualization techniques to inspect and analyze the estimation results of such time-varying 3-D processes. Our animation of left ventricle dynamic shape is generated through enhancing the spatial dimensionality and color coding the vector-represented local deformations.

In summary, we have shown that the bifurcation points obtained from biplane cineangiography can be used for left ventricle motion and deformation analysis, even though they are sparse and distributed with bias. However, denser and more uniformly distributed data are still desired. Currently, we are investigating the analysis of left ventricle motion and deformation using dynamic computed tomographic data. The volumetric nature of the computed tomographic data provides us accurate 3-D shape description of the left ventricle. Furthermore, the hierarchical decomposition of the left ventricle motion and deformation can be easily adapted to the computed tomographic data case. However, the difficulty lies in the estimation of 3-D displacement field from the time-varying volumetric data in order to establish the correspondences over consecutive image frames.

ACKNOWLEDGMENT

The authors wish to thank the referees for their helpful comments, Dr. L. D. R. Smith for providing the angiographic data, and Dr. D. Goldgof for various discussions.

REFERENCES

[1] J. Liu, K. Affeld, M. W. Engelhorn and M. Schartl, "Animated 3-D model of the human heart based on echocardiograms," in *Proc. Aachen Conf. Signal Processing*, pp. 155–158, 1987.

[2] D. J. Stevenson, L. D. R. Smith, and G. Robinson, "Working towards the automatic detection of blood vessels *x*-ray angiograms," *Pattern Recogn. Lett.*, vol. 6, pp. 107–112, 1987.

[3] T. Saito, M. Misaki, K. Shirato, and T. Takishima, "Three-dimensional quantitative coronary angiography," *IEEE Trans. Biomed. Eng.*, vol. 37, pp. 768–777, Aug. 1990.

[4] R. S. Acharya, P. B. Heffeman, R. A. Robb, and H. Wechsler, "High-speed 3-D imaging of the beating heart using temporal estimation," *Comput. Vision, Graphics Image Processing*, vol. 39, pp. 279–290, 1987.

[5] P. Lanzer et al., "Cardiac imaging using gated magnetic resonance," *Radiology*, vol. 150, pp. 121–127, 1984.

[6] H. C. Kim et al., "Estimation of local cardiac wall deformation and regional wall stress from biplane coronary cineangiograms," *IEEE Trans. Biomed. Eng.*, vol. 32, pp. 503–512, 1985.

[7] G. Coppini, M. Demi, G. D'Urso, A. L'Abbate, and G. Valli, "Tensor description of 3-D time varying surfaces using scattered landmarks: An application to heart motion," in *Time-Varying Image Processing and Moving Object Recognition*, V. Cappellini, Ed. New York: Elsevier, 1987.

[8] D. Goldgof, H. Lee, and T. S. Huang, "Motion analysis of nonrigid surfaces," in *Proc. IEEE Conf. Computer Vision and Pattern Recognition*, Ann Arbor, MI, pp. 375–380, June 1988.

[9] C. W. Chen and T. S. Huang, "Epicardial motion and deformation estimation from coronary artery bifurcation points," in *Proc. 3rd Int. Conf. Computer Vision*, Osaka, Japan, pp. 456–459, Dec. 1990.

[10] A. A. Young, P. J. Hunter, and B. H. Smaill, "Epicardial surface estimation from coronary angiograms," *Comput. Vision, Graphics, Image Processing*, vol. 47, pp. 111–127, 1989.

[11] F. C. P. Yin, "Applications of finite-element method to ventricular mechanics," *CRC Crit. Rev. Biomed. Eng.*, vol. 12, pp. 311–342, 1985.

[12] S. K. Mishra, D. B. Goldgof, and T. S. Huang, "Nonrigid motion analysis and epicardial deformation estimation from angiographic data," in *Proc. IEEE Conf. Computer Vision and Pattern Recognition*, pp. 331–336, 1991.

[13] J. M. Wattenbarger et al., "Ventricular ejection fractions of linear transformation and ellipsoid models," *Amer. J. Physiol.*, vol. 255, pp. 197–201, 1988.

[14] T. F. Moriarty, "The law of Laplace, its limitations as a relation for diastolic pressure, volume, or wall stress of the left ventricle," *Circ. Res.*, vol. 46, pp. 321–331, 1980.

[15] I. J. Legrice, B. H. Smaill, and P. J. Hunter, "Mathematical model of geometry and fibrous structure of the heart," *Amer. J. Physiol.*, vol. 260, pp. 1365–1378, 1991.

[16] K. G. F. Bookstein and A. Buda, "Mean tensor analysis of left ventricular wall motion," *Comput. in Cardiol.*, pp. 513–516, 1984.

[17] G. Meier, M. Ziskin, W. Santamore, and A. Bove, "Kinematics of the beating heart," *IEEE Trans. Biomed. Eng.*, vol. 27, pp. 319–329, 1980.

[18] A. Sommerfeld, *Mechanics of Deformable Bodies*. New York: Academic, 1950.

[19] S. S. Cassidy and M. Ramanathan, "Dimensional analysis of the left ventricle during peep: Relative septal and lateral wall displacements," *Amer. J. Physiol.*, vol. 246, pp. 792–805, 1984.

[20] T. Arts and R. S. Reneman, "Dynamics of left entricular wall and mitral valve mechanics—a model study," *J. Biomech. (U.S.)*, vol. 22, pp. 261–271, 1989.

[21] A. H. Barr, "Superquadrics and angle-preserving transformation," *IEEE Comput. Graph. Appl.*, vol. 1, pp. 11–23, Jan. 1981.

[22] A. H. Barr, "Global and local deformations of solid primitives," *Comput. Graph.*, vol. 18, pp. 21–30, July 1984.

[23] A. Pentland, "Perceptual organization and the representation of natural form," *Artificial Intell.*, pp. 293–331, 1986.

[24] F. Solina and R. Bajcsy, "Shape and function," *Intelligent Robots and Computer Vision: Fifth in a Series (1986)*, vol. 726, pp. 284–91, 1986.

[25] R. Bajcsy and F. Solina, "Three dimensional object representation revisited," in *Proc. First ICCV*, London, pp. 231–240, June 1987.

[26] A. D. Gross and T. E. Boult, "Error of fit measures for recovering parameteric solids," in *Proc. 2nd ICCV*, Tampa, FL, pp. 690–94, Dec. 1988.

[27] A. Gupta, L. Bogoni, and R. Bajcsy, "Quantitative and qualitative measures for the evaluation of the superquadric models," in *Proc. Workshop on Interpretation of 3-D Scenes*, Austin, TX, pp. 162–69, Nov. 1989.

[28] T. Arts, S. Meerbaum, R. S. Reneman, and E. Corday, "Torsion of the left ventricle during the ejection phase in the intact dog," *Cardiovasc. Research*, vol. 18, pp. 183–193, 1984.

[29] M. B. Buchalter *et al.*, "Noninvasive quantification of left-ventricular rotational deformation in normal humans using magnetic-resonance-imaging myocardial tagging," *Circulation*, vol. 81, pp. 1236–1244, 1990.

[30] D. Ballard and C. Brown, *Comput. Vision*. Englewood Cliffs, New Jersey: Prentice, 1982.

[31] D. Terzopoulos, A. Witkin, and M. Kass, "Constraints deformable models: recovering 3-D shape and nonrigid motion," *Artificial Intell.*, vol. 36, pp. 91–123, 1988.

[32] D. Terzopoulos, A. Witkin, and M. Kass, "Symmetry-seeking models and 3-D object recognition," *Int. J. Comput. Vision*, vol. 1, pp. 211–221, 1987.

[33] S. Chen and M. Penna, "Shape and motion of nonrigid bodies," *Comput. Vision, Graphics, Image Processing*, vol. 36, pp. 175–207, 1986.

[34] D. Terzopoulos and A. Witkin, "Physically based models with rigid and deformable components," *IEEE Comput. Graphics Appl.*, pp. 41–51, 1988.

[35] D. Terzopoulos and M. Metaxas, "Dynamic 3D models with local and global deformations: deformable superquadrics," in *Proc. 3rd Int. Conf. Computer Vision*, Osaka, Japan, pp. 606–615, Dec. 1990.

[36] D. Metaxas and D. Terzopoulos, "Constrained deformable superquadrics and nonrigid motion tracking," in *IEEE Conf. Computer Vision and Pattern Recognition*, Maui, HI, pp. 337–343, June 1991.

[37] C. W. Chen and T. S. Huang, "Nonrigid object motion and deformation estimation from three-dimensional data," *Int. J. Imaging Syst. Technol.*, vol. 2, pp. 385–394, 1990.

[38] M. J. Potel, S. A. MacKay, J. M. Rubin, A. M. Aisen, and R. E. Sayre, "Three-dimensional left ventricular wall motion in man coordinate systems for representing wall movement direction," *Investigative Radiol.*, vol. 19, pp. 499–509, 1984.

Chang Wen Chen (S'86–M'92) received the BS degree from the University of Science and Technology of China in 1983, the MSEE degree from the University of Southern California, Los Angeles, in 1986, and the PhD degree from the University of Illinois, Urbana-Champaign, in 1992, all in electrical engineering.

He was a Research Assistant in the Signal and Image Processing Institute, University of Southern California, in 1986. From January 1987 to July 1992, he was a Research Assistant at the Coordinated Science Laboratory and the Beckman Institute, University of Illinois. In the summers of 1989 and 1990, he was employed at the National Center for Supercomputing Applications, Champaign, IL, working with the Visualization Service and Development Group. In August 1992 he joined the faculty of the Department of Electrical Engineering, University of Rochester, Rochester, NY. His current research interests include biomedical image understanding, image sequence processing and analysis, image and video coding, digital signal processing, medical imaging, computer vision, computer graphics, scientific visualization, and artificial intelligence.

Dr. Chen is a member of SPIE and Tau Beta Pi.

Thomas S. Huang (S'61–M'63–SM'76–F'79) received the BS degree from National Taiwan University, Taipei, Taiwan, and the MS and ScD degrees from the Massachusetts Institute of Technology (MIT), Cambridge, MA, all in electrical engineering.

He was on the Faculty of the Department of Electrical Engineering at MIT from 1963 to 1973, and on the Faculty of the School of electrical engineering and Director of its laboratory for Information and Signal Processing at Purdue University, West Lafayette, IN, from 1973 to 1980. In 1980 he joined the University of Illinois, Urbana-Champaign, where he is now Professor of Electrical and Computer Engineering and Research Professor at the Coordinated Science Laboratory, and at the Beckman Institute. During his sabbatical leaves, he has worked at the MIT Lincoln Laboratory, the IBM T. J. Watson Research Center, and the Rheinishes Landes Museum, Bonn, Germany; he has also held Visiting Professor positions at the Swiss Institutes of Technology in Zürich and Lausanne, University of Hannover, Hannover, Germany, and INRS-Telecommunications, University of Quebec, Montreal, Canada. He has served as a consultant to numerous industrial firms and government agencies, both in the United States and abroad. His professional interests lie in the broad area of information technology, especially the transmission and processing of multidimensional signals.

Dr. Huang has published 11 books and over 300 papers in network theory, digital filtering, image processing, and computer vision. He is a Fellow of the Optical Society of America and has received a Guggenheim Fellowship (1971–72), an A. V. Humboldt Foundation Senior U. S. Scientist Award (1976–77), and a Fellowship from the Japan Association for the Promotion of Science (1986). He also received the IEEE Signal Processing Society's Technical Achievment Award in 1987 and the Society Award in 1991. He was a founding editor and is currently an area editor of the *International Journal of Computer Vision, Graphics, and Image Processing*, and editor of the Springer Series in Information Sciences, published by Springer-Verlag.

Matthew Arrott received the BA degree in 1983 from Harvard University, Cambridge, MA.

He currently is with Autodesk Inc. as a development manager responsible for the graphics subsystem. Prior to his current position, he worked as a Senior Graphics Programmer and Project Leader for the Visualization Group at the National Center for Supercomputing Applications, Champaign, IL. He has also worked as a Graphics Programmer at Wavefront Technologies Inc., and as an animator at Digital Productions.

Mr. Arrott is a member of ACM.

Frequency-Based Nonrigid Motion Analysis: Application to Four Dimensional Medical Images

Chahab Nastar and Nicholas Ayache

Abstract—We present a method for nonrigid motion analysis in time sequences of volume images (4D data). In this method, nonrigid motion of the deforming object contour is dynamically approximated by a physically-based deformable surface. In order to reduce the number of parameters describing the deformation, we make use of a modal analysis which provides a spatial smoothing of the surface. The deformation spectrum, which outlines the main excited modes, can be efficiently used for deformation comparison. Fourier analysis on time signals of the main deformation spectrum components provides a temporal smoothing of the data. Thus a complex nonrigid deformation is described by only a few parameters: the main excited modes and the main Fourier harmonics. Therefore, 4D data can be analyzed in a very concise manner. The power and robustness of the approach is illustrated by various results on medical data. We believe that our method has important applications in automatic diagnosis of heart diseases and in motion compression.

Index Terms—Medical image analysis, nonrigid motion, deformable models, modal analysis, Fourier analysis, compression, dynamic data, four-dimensional images, cardiac imagery, automatic diagnosis.

---◆---

1 INTRODUCTION

1.1 Motivation and Organization

IN this article, we propose a unified approach for non-rigid motion estimation from time sequences of three-dimensional images [5], i.e., 4D data, by taking into account both spatial and temporal frequencies of a deformable geometric model.

Our method has important applications in automatic diagnosis of heart diseases and in 4D data compression, as we shall see in the experimental section. Our method involves three steps:

1) Recover the deformation field between each pair of successive 3D images,
2) Express the modal coefficients (or amplitudes) of the deformation at each time t,
3) Express Fourier coefficients of the time-varying modal amplitudes.

The information contained in the data can then be compressed, by discarding spatial modes and/or temporal Fourier harmonics.

The basic justification of the approach relies on the following observations: most smoothly deforming structures mainly have low-frequency excited modes; this justifies Step 2. Furthermore, for periodic motions like heart motion, modal amplitudes as a function of time are periodic and sine-like;[1] this justifies Step 3.

For Steps 1 and 2, it is possible to constrain the modes beforehand, by letting a deformable model evolve along low-order modes. The advantage is, of course, a reduced numerical complexity and a low-order smoothing of the deformation allowing its robust recovery. Note that Step 1 can be performed not only by our deformable model, but also by optical flow or any other technique providing the motion field [10].

The following example can serve as a motivation to our work. Let us consider (Fig. 1) the canine 4D heart data provided by the dynamic spatial reconstructor (DSR, a high speed X-ray CT scanner). We used this data as an input to our method. It consists of 18 volume (or 3D) images during a single cardiac cycle. Each volume image has a spatial resolution of $98 \times 100 \times 110$. Dye was injected into the left ventricle, which shows up as a light gray color. Note the difficulty of interpretation of such complex and huge data by physicians. The challenge was to analyze such a tremendous amount of information (19,404,000 bytes, with each voxel being coded on one byte) and supply physicians with a few quantitative parameters describing the motion. We shall see in the experimental section of this paper how we tried to meet these objectives.

The article is organized as follows:

In Section 2, we introduce our deformable model for nonrigid motion estimation, develop its governing equations and outline its properties.

In Section 3, we present the modal analysis of the model, allowing a closed-form recovery of the motion by a few parameters: the modal amplitudes. We show how these amplitudes may be used to characterize deformations. Section 3.2, which describes the *analytic modes*, may be required only for in depth reading.

- *The authors are with INRIA, B.P. 105, 78153 Le Chesnay Cédex, France. E-mail: {chahab.nastar; nicholas.ayache}@inria.fr.*

Manuscript received Mar. 14, 1995; revised July 25, 1995.
Recommended for acceptance by A. Singh.
For information on obtaining reprints of this article, please send e-mail to: transpami@computer.org, and reference IEEECS Log Number P96085.

1. Note that our method is not restricted to periodic motions. For nonperiodic motions there is generally no need in performing the Fourier analysis (step 3).

Reprinted from *IEEE Trans. Pattern Analysis and Machine Intelligence*, Vol. 18, No. 11, Nov. 1996, pp. 1067–1079.

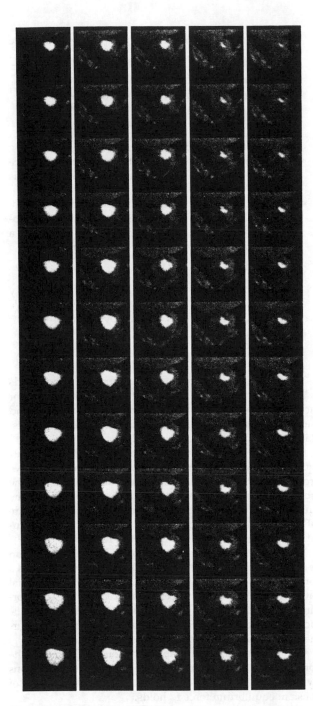

Fig. 1. 4D data displaying a 3D dog ventricle in motion. Each 2D image is an axial slice in the *x y* plane. The *z* coordinate is along the vertical axis, while the *t* coordinate is along the horizontal axis.

In Section 4, we propose a Fourier analysis for the time-varying main modal amplitudes; this is particularly well suited for cyclic motions (e.g., heart motion). An example involving 4D medical data is presented.

We conclude and propose future work in Section 5.

1.2 Related Work

A lot of research work is related to our work. First of all, we want to mention the pioneering work of Terzopoulos et al. on snakes and deformable physics-based models [24], [26], [42], [45]. This work was mainly dedicated to tracking and animation problems rather than analysis.

A second category of research work is related to the analysis of deformations. Our work was initially inspired by the pioneering work of Pentland et al. on the use of modal deformations to describe deformations [36], [37]. The main differences with our approach is that our modes have a simpler physical meaning (they can be interpreted as the harmonics of the free vibrations basis of the deformable object) while Pentland's modes are more dedicated to animation [38]. Also, we have derived a method to compute our modes beforehand, as a function of the topology of the deformable object only, allowing a much faster computation (Pentland's modes require the knowledge of the exact shape of the original object and, therefore, have to be computed online).

Our work can be seen as providing a coherent unifying framework between these first two categories of publications, allowing to both track and analyze a deformable 3D motion.

In addition to these references, we have to mention the work of Cootes et al. [15], [16], [17], done independently of, and concurrently with, ours which provides an interesting alternative to the solution of both the tracking and the analysis of the deformation. We also have to mention the work of Bardinet [7] and Metaxas [27], [35], among others, who use deformable parametric models like superquadrics to track and analyze deformable objects. Their work is limited to the class of objects which can be easily represented by such parametric models, which include the left cardiac ventricle. A number of methods to track 3D data were proposed in the past few years. Duncan et al. [2], [39], [40], and Benayoun et al. [9], [10], used differential constraints; Goldgof [23] and Chen [13] used a coarse-to-fine approach; Bookstein [12] and Szeliski and Lavallee [41] proposed energy based methods; Creswell [18] and Amini [1] suggested data-dedicated methods. All these approaches can be seen as complementary to ours, in the sense that the tracking result they provide could be completed by our proposed analysis. It would however be interesting to compare all these approaches on a specific and common database. This could be the topic of a future work.

2 A DEFORMABLE MODEL FOR MOTION ESTIMATION

In this section, we introduce our physically based deformable model which we use for tracking nonrigid motion of dynamic structures in time sequences of 2D or 3D medical images.

We consider both the surface and volume properties of the objects at hand. We restrict ourselves to elastic deformations, i.e., we assume that the object recovers its reference configuration as soon as all applied forces causing deformation are removed. In general, we seek a trade off between precise modeling and computational efficiency. Therefore, simplifying assumptions will be introduced in the modeling.

2.1 Mass-Spring Meshes

Modeling an elastic boundary can be achieved by a mesh of N virtual masses on the contour. Each mass is attached to its neighbors by perfect identical springs of stiffness K and natural length l_0 [23], [46].

These springs achieve a *polygonal approximation* and model the *surface* properties of the object.

Generalizing the model to 3D contours (surfaces) is straightforward: We can either model "quadrilateral" or "diagonal" meshes[2] (see Fig. 2).

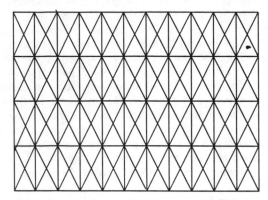

Fig. 2. "Diagonal" mesh.

If necessary, we can improve the modeling by attaching extra springs between non-neighbor nodes in order to model *volume* properties inside the object. These springs constrain the general shape of the object within its deformation, making a template shape out of it [11], [48].

The boundary modeled as above will also be called a *structure*. Such a structure can be easily deformed to match the contour of an object of interest, thus performing a *segmentation* step. If we take a series of images displaying the deformation of the object through time, the structure can achieve simultaneously both *segmentation* and *tracking* of the object surface through time.

2.2 Governing Equations

The system under study is made of the N virtual masses located at time t at points $(M_1(t), M_2(t), ..., M_N(t))$.

The fundamental equation of dynamics states that the vector addition of all applied forces on M_i is equal to its mass m_i multiplied by its acceleration. Let A be the origin of the reference system. Then:

$$\sum_j \mathbf{f}_j(M_i, t) = m_i \frac{d^2}{dt^2} \overrightarrow{AM_i} = m_i \ddot{\mathbf{M}}_i \qquad (1)$$

Let us now describe the applied forces on each node M_i:

- Elastic force between M_i and its connected nodes.

$$\mathbf{f}_e(M_i, t) = -K \left\{ \sum_{j \in C_i} U_{ij}(t) - l_0 \sum_{j \in C_i} \frac{U_{ij}(t)}{\| U_{ij}(t) \|} \right\} \qquad (2)$$

where K is the stiffness constant, $U_{ij}(t) = \overrightarrow{M_j M_i}(t)$ is the vector separation of nodes M_j and M_i at time t, and C_i is the set of nodes connected to node M_i.

- Fluid damping force, proportional to node velocity:

$$\mathbf{f}_d(M_i, t) = -c_i \frac{d}{dt} \overrightarrow{AM_i} = -c_i \dot{\mathbf{M}}_i \qquad (3)$$

where c_i is the damping constant.

- Image force $\mathbf{f}_{im}(M_i, t)$. This is the main external force that has the system attracted by image features. This force is defined in Section 2.3.

- Suppose the natural length l_0 of the springs is fixed. Since we wish to give the system an initial equilibrium configuration, we need to apply on each node a force balancing the action of the elastic force:

$$\mathbf{f}_{eq}(M_i) = -\mathbf{f}_e(M_i, t_0) \qquad (4)$$

This force is similar to the force that our fingers apply to an elastic rubber to keep it in a specific shape. We assume that this force is constant over time.

Finally, (1) yields the governing equation:

$$\mathbf{f}_e(M_i, t) + \mathbf{f}_d(M_i, t) + \mathbf{f}_{im}(M_i, t) + \mathbf{f}_{eq}(M_i) = m_i \ddot{\mathbf{M}}_i \qquad (5)$$

The governing equation, expressed for all N nodes, leads to a *nonlinear* system of *coupled* differential equations (for each node, the x, y, and z displacements are coupled, and the displacement of a node depends on its neighbors displacement, as it appears clearly in (2)).

One possible approach is the resolution of these complex equations by an iterative procedure [43]. In this paper, we propose to set $l_0 = 0$. This assumption does not restrict the arbitrary initial configuration of the structure because of the equilibrium force $\mathbf{f}_{eq}$. Indeed, this force keeps the structure inflated so that it does not shrink to a point. Thus, the natural state of the system is its initial configuration.

The advantage of this assumption is that our model can be considered within the framework of *linear elasticity*. As a consequence, we end up with a set of *linear* differential equations with node displacements *decoupled* in each coordinate, regardless of the magnitude of the displacements. Moreover, these linear equations are a prerequisite to further quantitative analysis of the motion (see Section 3).

On the other hand, our approximation is valid only if the spring orientations undergo small angular variations (typically less than 15 degrees), so that our assumption of constant equilibrium force $\mathbf{f}_{eq}$ holds.[3]

Finally, in 3D, the deformation of the system is governed by the $3N$-dimensional differential matrix equation:

$$\mathbf{M\ddot{U}} + \mathbf{C\dot{U}} + \mathbf{KU} = \mathbf{F}(t) \qquad (6)$$

where $\mathbf{U}$ is a vector storing nodal displacements $\mathbf{M}$, $\mathbf{C}$, and $\mathbf{K}$ are, respectively, the mass, damping, and stiffness matrices of the system, and $\mathbf{F}$ is the image force which has the object attracted by image edges. Equation (6) is the finite element formulation of the deformation process. Note that the equilibrium forces do not explicitly appear in the governing equation.

---

2. The shear-resisting cross springs may be useful to avoid self-intersection problems during the deformation of the surface.

3. Similar limitations can be found in the model described in [36], [37].

2.3 Image Force

In the original formulation of the "snake," the authors propose a convolution of the image with a smoothing filter that causes artificial blurring, so that the active contour can be attracted by the edges from a distance [24].

Unlike these methods, we introduce a force at each node M_i that points to *the closest boundary point P_i in the image* [14], [20], [22], [25]. Several Euclidean distance algorithms can help us extract this force in each voxel of the image [19], [47]. At node M, this force is set to:

$$f_{im}(M, t) = \alpha \overrightarrow{M(t)P(t)} \tag{7}$$

where α is a constant scalar. This force can be seen as a virtual spring of natural length zero and of stiffness α joining M to P. Hence, both internal and external forces are elastic, making the modeling coherent.

The advantage is that we speed up the convergence of the model toward image edges; one can consider edge extraction and distance computation as a data-to-force transformation which is performed as a preprocessing.

2.4 Integration Scheme

In 3D, the $3N$-order matrix equations decouple into three directional matrix equations of order N:

$$\begin{cases} M\ddot{U}_x + C\dot{U}_x + KU_x = F_x(t) \\ M\ddot{U}_y + C\dot{U}_y + KU_y = F_y(t) \\ M\ddot{U}_z + C\dot{U}_z + KU_z = F_z(t) \end{cases} \tag{8}$$

where M, C, and K are from now on N-order matrices, and U_μ and F_μ ($\mu = x, y, z$) are, respectively, the N-order displacement field and image force in the μ direction. From now on, we will omit the indexes, and all matrix equations will be of order N. It is assumed that three equations corresponding the three space directions have to be solved.

We integrate the governing equations with an explicit Euler scheme:

$$\begin{cases} \ddot{U}(t) = M^{-1}(F(t) - C\dot{U}(t) - KU(t)) \\ \dot{U}(t + \Delta t) = \dot{U}(t) + \Delta t\ddot{U}(t) \\ U(t + \Delta t) = U(t) + \Delta t\dot{U}(t + \Delta t) \end{cases} \tag{9}$$

where Δt is the time step of the simulation. The initial values of displacement and velocity are generally set to zero. Note that the mass matrix is diagonal and therefore its inversion is trivial and only has to be processed once. The damping constant is chosen so that the system is slightly overdamped [44]. Convergence is achieved once the image force balances the internal elastic forces.

In any numerical integration scheme, numerical stability requires the time step Δt to be inferior to a critical value Δt_{cr} which is defined by the mass and stiffness properties of the system:

$$\Delta t \leq \Delta t_{cr} = \frac{T_N}{\gamma} \tag{10}$$

where $T_N = \frac{2\pi}{\omega_N}$ is the smallest period of the finite element mesh, and γ is a constant depending on the scheme. The Euler method is conditionally stable, i.e., needs small time steps ($\gamma \geq 2$). In order to make a more accurate computation, we decrease the time step and set $\gamma \geq 10$. Note that a larger time step can be used when high-frequency components of the deformable model are discarded (see Section 3).

2.5 Results on Medical Data

We have tested our method on a set of ultrasound images of the left ventricle of a human heart. The tracking of the mitral valve is indeed a problem of major interest in medical imaging since heart-attacks can generally be predicted from abnormal motion of the valve. Each image has a resolution of 256×256 pixels. First, a polar edge extraction is performed on the images [6]. Then, for each image, the distance field is computed on every pixel. Thus we can segment the initial valve. We then add volume springs for making our model a template; this will make the tracking more robust. Finally we track the valve through time and display the estimated displacement field on the valve surface (Fig. 3). The program runs in *real-time* on 2D data.

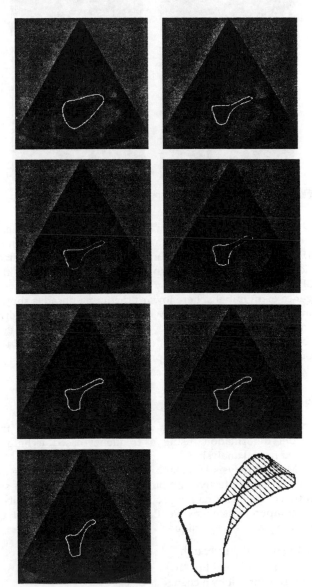

Fig. 3. Initial segmentation and tracking of the mitral valve.

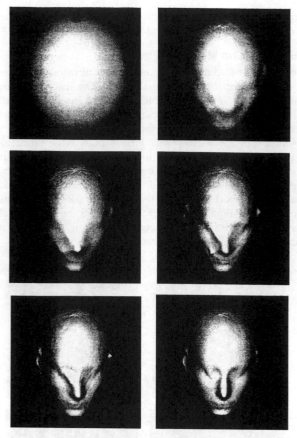

Fig. 4. Convergence of an initial sphere toward the human head.

The method has similarly been tested on a 3D Magnetic Resonance image of the human head, with a resolution of $158 \times 158 \times 158$ voxels. We make use of the 3D generalization of Canny's edge detector [28], [29], then compute the 3D distance maps and finally run the program. The convergence of an initial sphere toward the human head is shown in Fig. 4. It runs at *interactive rates* on a DEC-ALPHA workstation; convergence is achieved in eight seconds. Note that this segmentation example does not really make use of the power of our dynamic approach; it is provided here to demonstrate model properties.

3 MODAL ANALYSIS AND APPLICATIONS

In this section we focus on a quantitative analysis of the model deformation, using a frequency-based technique called modal analysis.

Modal analysis is a standard engineering technique allowing more effective computations and a closed-form solution of the deformation process [8]. It was first introduced in computer vision by Pentland's team [36], [37]. Let us now explain this technique.

3.1 General Approach

Instead of solving directly the equilibrium equation (6), one can transform it by a change of basis:

$$\mathbf{U} = \mathbf{P}\tilde{\mathbf{U}} \qquad (11)$$

where $\mathbf{P}$ is the square nonsingular transformation matrix of order N to be determined, and $\tilde{\mathbf{U}}$ is referred to as the *generalized displacements* vector. One effective way of choosing $\mathbf{P}$ is setting it to $\boldsymbol{\Phi}$, a matrix whose entries are the eigenvectors of the generalized eigenproblem:

$$\mathbf{K}\phi = \omega^2 \mathbf{M}\phi \qquad (12)$$

$$\mathbf{U}(t) = \boldsymbol{\Phi}\tilde{\mathbf{U}} = \sum_{i=1}^{N} \tilde{u}_i(t)\phi_i \qquad (13)$$

Equation (13) is referred to as the modal superposition equation. ϕ_i is the ith mode, $\tilde{u}_i$ its *amplitude*, and ω_i its frequency. Fig. 5 displays a sample of six frequency-increasing modes of a cylinder, all of them having the same amplitude.

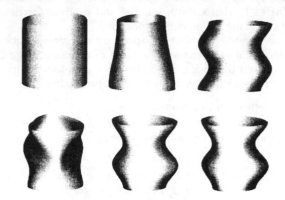

Fig. 5. A sample of frequency-increasing modes of a cylinder (constant amplitude).

Note that the modes of a generalized eigenproblem involving real symmetric matrices can be chosen to be orthonormal vectors [8]. The new modal basis simultaneously diagonalizes $\mathbf{M}$ and $\mathbf{K}$, and provided that matrix $\tilde{\mathbf{C}} = \boldsymbol{\Phi}^T \mathbf{C} \boldsymbol{\Phi}$ is diagonal as well,[4] the governing matrix-form equations decouple into N scalar equations:

$$\ddot{\tilde{u}}_i(t) + \tilde{c}_i \dot{\tilde{u}}_i(t) + \omega_i^2 \tilde{u}_i(t) = \tilde{f}_i(t) \qquad (14)$$

The amplitudes $\left(\tilde{u}_i(t)\right)_{i=1,\ldots,N}$, are obtained by solving these equations at time t, and the displacement of the structure nodes is obtained by the modal superposition equation.

In practice, we wish to approximate nodal displacements $\mathbf{U}(t)$ by $\hat{\mathbf{U}}(t)$, the truncated addition of the p low-frequency modes, where $p \ll N$.

$$\hat{\mathbf{U}}(t) \approx \sum_{i=1}^{p} \tilde{u}_i(t)\phi_i \qquad (15)$$

Vectors $(\phi_i)_{i=1,\ldots,p}$ form the *reduced modal basis* of the system. This is the major advantage of modal analysis: It allows a closed-form solution by selecting a few number of low-frequency modes [8], [31], [32]. Therefore a compact description of the motion is provided by *spatial smoothing*. Fig. 6 illustrates modal superposition on the real example of the mitral valve.

---

4. This condition, called the Rayleigh condition, is satisfied as soon as the damping matrix $\mathbf{C}$ is a linear combination of the mass and stiffness matrices. Rayleigh damping is generally assumed for any standard engineering problem [8].

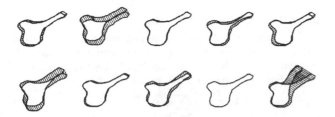

Fig. 6. Nine low-order amplitude-moderated eigenmodes describing the motion of the valve; their superposition (bottom-right) is a good approximation of valve motion.

Note that superimposing p low-frequency equations of the type (14) allows the time step to be larger; we choose:

$$\Delta t \leq \Delta t_{cr} = \frac{T_p}{\gamma} \tag{16}$$

where $T_p = \frac{2\pi}{\omega_p} \gg T_N$. As a consequence, the convergence of the model is numerically much faster with modal analysis than with direct integration of the governing equations.

Due to orthonormality of the modes, the approximation error is:

$$\left(\mathbf{U} - \hat{\mathbf{U}}\right)^2 = \sum_{i=p+1}^{N} \tilde{u}_i^2 \tag{17}$$

This means that the approximation error is a rapidly decreasing function of the truncation frequency p.

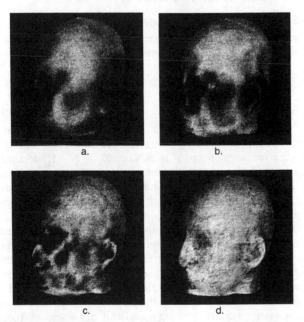

a.   b.

c.   d.

Fig. 7. Approximation error distribution for the low-order deformation of a sphere into the human head. Darker regions indicate more important errors, while lighter regions represent best-recovered ones. a. Computation using 60 modes. b. 243 modes. c. 468 modes. d. 2790 modes. (Exact computation needs 37,683 modes).

The distribution of the approximation error along the surface for increasing values of p is shown in Fig. 7. Darker colors outline regions with bigger error. The model being

initially a sphere, one can observe that the error is more important in the regions that need a locally important deformation of the sphere (nose, eyes, ears), while more spherical regions (top of the head) are better approximated, as expected. Note however that the level of accuracy can be easily controlled, at the expense of additional modes.

3.2 Analytic Modal Analysis

Even as a precalculation, solving the generalized eigenproblem is very costly as soon as we consider 3D boundaries (surfaces). For instance, if we consider a mesh of 100×100 nodes, *a generalized eigenproblem where the size of the matrices is $10,000 \times 10,000$ has to be solved*. It is clear that *the analytic expression of the modes* would noticeably reduce the computations [30]. This leads us to consider the theory of solid state physics, where similar problems are encountered at a microscopic level (ionic vibrations of a crystal lattice). If we parameterize our deformable curves by arc length, and similarly our deformable surfaces by natural coordinates, we get periodic boundary conditions which depend on the surface topology. This allows the analogy between our deformable model and a crystal lattice.

3.2.1 Free Vibrations of a Chain

The classical theory of vibration of a crystal lattice is based on the *harmonic approximation*, a theory which assumes that the first non-vanishing correction to the equilibrium potential energy is quadratic [3]:

$$V^{harm} = \frac{1}{2} \sum_{\substack{\bar{R}, \bar{R}' \\ \mu, \nu}} u_\mu(\bar{R}) D_{\mu\nu}(\bar{R} - \bar{R}') u_\nu(\bar{R}') \tag{18}$$

where $u_\mu(\bar{R})$ is the displacement in the μ direction of the ion whose mean position is $\bar{R}$, and $\mathbf{D}$ is the Hessian matrix of the interaction energy.

Consider now a set of ions distributed along a *closed* chain at points separated by a distance a, so that the lattice vectors are $R = na$ for $n \in \{1, \ldots, N\}$. If only neighboring ions interact, we may take the harmonic potential energy to have the form:

$$V^{harm} = \frac{1}{2} K \sum_{n=1}^{N} \left[u(na) - u((n+1)a) \right]^2 \tag{19}$$

where $K = v''(a)$ is the stiffness constant of the system, $v(x)$ being the interaction energy of two ions at distance x along the chain. The free vibrations of the lattice are governed by:

$$M\ddot{u}(na) = -\frac{\partial V^{harm}}{\partial u(na)} = K\left(u((n+1)a) + u((n-1)a) - 2u(na)\right) \tag{20}$$

These are precisely the equations that would be satisfied if each ion were connected to its neighbors by perfect massless springs of stiffness K (and equilibrium length a, although the equations are in fact independent of the equilibrium length of the spring).

We seek solutions to (20) of the form $Ae^{i(kna - \omega t)}$. This yields the dispersion equation which gives the relationship between spatial (k) and temporal (ω) frequencies:

$$\omega^2(p) = \frac{4K}{M} \sin^2\left(\frac{k(p)a}{2}\right) \tag{21}$$

The periodicity of the closed chain is expressed by $u[(n + N)a] = u(na)$. We now obtain the set of independent solutions:

$$k(p)a = \frac{2p\pi}{N} \qquad p \in \mathcal{B}(N) \qquad (22)$$

where $\mathcal{B}(N)$ is the first Brillouin zone.

$\mathcal{B}(N)$ is equal to $\left\{-\frac{N}{2} + 1, ..., \frac{N}{2}\right\}$ for N even, and $\left\{-\frac{N-1}{2}, ..., \frac{N-1}{2}\right\}$ for N odd.

The general solution of the free vibrations of the closed chain is the linear combination of the former solutions:

$$u(na, t) = \sum_{p \in \mathcal{B}(N)} A(p)e^{i(k(p)na - \omega(p)t)} \qquad (23)$$

$$= \sum_{p \in \mathcal{B}(N)} A(p)e^{-i\omega(p)t} e^{ik(p)na} \qquad (24)$$

The case of the open chain is very similar. We sum up the expression of the free vibrations for both types of chains in Table 1.

TABLE 1
DISPLACEMENT OF THE NODES OF A FREE VIBRATING CHAIN

	$k(p)a$	$p \in$	$u(na, t)$
closed	$\dfrac{2p\pi}{N}$	$\mathcal{B}(N)$	$\sum_p A(p)e^{-i\omega(p)t}e^{ik(p)na}$
open	$\dfrac{p\pi}{N}$	$\{0, ..., N-1\}$	$\sum_p A(p)e^{-i\omega(p)t}e^{-\frac{k(p)a}{2}}\cos\left(k(p)na - \frac{k(p)a}{2}\right)$

3.2.2 Nonlinear Waves in Discrete Media

When k is small compared with π/a (i.e., when the wavelength is large compared to the interparticle spacing), ω is linear in k (from (21)):

$$\omega = a\sqrt{\frac{K}{M}}|k| \qquad (25)$$

This is the type of behavior we are accustomed to in the case of light waves and ordinary sound waves. If ω is linear in k, then the group velocity is the same as the phase velocity (equal to $c = a\sqrt{\frac{K}{M}}$), and both are independent of frequency. Note that if we approximate finite differences by derivatives:

$u((n + 1)a) - u(na) \simeq a\partial u/\partial x(na)$
$u((n - 1)a) - u(na) \simeq a\partial u/\partial x((n - 1)a)$
$u((n + 1)a) - u(na) + u((n - 1)a) - u(na) \simeq a^2\partial^2 u/\partial x^2 \qquad (26)$

in (20), we end up with a wave equation of velocity c:

$$\frac{\partial^2 u}{\partial x^2} = \frac{1}{c^2}\frac{\partial^2 u}{\partial t^2} \qquad \text{with} \quad c = a\sqrt{\frac{K}{M}} \qquad (27)$$

One of the characteristic features of waves in discrete media, however, is that the nonlinearity ceases to hold at wavelengths short enough to be comparable with the interparticle spacing. In the present case ω falls below ck as k increases, and the group velocity drops to zero when $|k|$ reaches π/a.

3.2.3 Analytic Modes for Curves

In the more general case of damped and forced vibrations (which is the case of our governing equations), time dependency is not harmonic, and has to be computed separately. For a closed chain, (23) becomes:

$$u(na, t) = \sum_{p \in \mathcal{B}(N)} \tilde{u}_p(t)e^{ik(p)na} \qquad (28)$$

Comparing (28) with the modal superposition (13) yields the analytic expression of the modes for a closed chain. Note that since time and space dependency are separate in (28), modal analysis is the decomposition of the displacement in a basis of *standing waves* which are the vibration modes of the system.

TABLE 2
ANALYTIC EIGENVALUES AND EIGENVECTORS FOR CLOSED AND OPEN CURVES

	$\omega^2 \times M/4K$	$\phi(p)$
closed	$\sin^2\left(\dfrac{p\pi}{N}\right)$	$\left[..., \cos\dfrac{2p\pi n}{N}, ...\right]^T$
open	$\sin^2\left(\dfrac{p\pi}{2N}\right)$	$\left[..., \cos\dfrac{p\pi(2n-1)}{2N}, ...\right]^T$

Table 2 sums up the frequencies (eigenvalues) and modes (eigenvectors) for closed and open curves.

3.2.4 Analytic Modes for Surfaces

The generalization to surface meshes is done by mixing all possible pairs of boundary conditions; it yields three different surface topologies:

open and open	$\rightarrow$	torus topology,
closed and closed	$\rightarrow$	plane topology,
closed and open	$\rightarrow$	cylinder topology

The analytic expressions for these topologies are summed up in Table 3, where the set of variation of the mode parameters p and p' is $\mathcal{B}(N)$ or $\{0, ..., N - 1\}$, depending on the boundary conditions.

Note that we implicitly develop the surface expressions for quadrilateral meshes, and that the modes have to be normalized to unity.

Finally, analytic modal analysis has both theoretical and practical implications. Theoretically, it shows that modal analysis is a specific form of Fourier decomposition of the deformation in a basis of standing waves (28). From a more practical point of view, analytic expressions of the modes are an efficient tool for *real time* eigenvector extraction as soon as the surface topology and the mass and stiffness properties of the model are defined.

3.2.5 Analytic Modes for Volumes

Suppose we wish to model a deformable volume. This may be typically the case for nonrigid motion recovery in a whole 3D image [10]. Therefore we model a volume mesh of size $N \times N' \times N''$. The volume has "open" boundary conditions in all three directions.

Thus, it is easy to generalize the results for the deformable plane, defining this time the modes with three pa-

	$\omega^2 \times M/4K$	$\phi(p)$
plane	$\sin^2 \dfrac{p\pi}{2N} + \sin^2 \dfrac{p'\pi}{2N'}$	$\left[\ldots, \cos \dfrac{p\pi(2n-1)}{2N} \cos \dfrac{p'\pi(2n'-1)}{2N'}, \ldots \right]^T$
torus	$\sin^2 \dfrac{p\pi}{N} + \sin^2 \dfrac{p'\pi}{N'}$	$\left[\ldots, \cos\left(\dfrac{2p\pi n}{N} + \dfrac{2p'\pi n'}{N'} \right), \ldots \right]^T$
cylinder	$\sin^2 \dfrac{p\pi}{2N} + \sin^2 \dfrac{p'\pi}{N'}$	$\left[\ldots, \cos \dfrac{p\pi(2n-1)}{2N} \cos \dfrac{2p'\pi n'}{N'}, \ldots \right]^T$

rameters p, p', and p'' varying, respectively, in $\{0 \ldots N-1\}$, $\{0 \ldots N'-1\}$, and $\{0 \ldots N''-1\}$.

The eigenvalues are:

$$\omega^2(p, p', p'') = \frac{4K}{M} \left(\sin^2 \frac{p\pi}{2N} + \sin^2 \frac{p'\pi}{2N'} + \sin^2 \frac{p''\pi}{2N''} \right) \quad (29)$$

while the eigenvectors have the following expression:

$$\phi(p, p', p'') =$$
$$\left[\ldots, \cos \frac{p\pi(2n-1)}{2N} \cos \frac{p'\pi(2n'-1)}{2N'} \cos \frac{p''\pi(2n''-1)}{2N''}, \ldots \right]^T \quad (30)$$

with $n \in \{1, \ldots, N\}$, $n' \in \{1, \ldots, N'\}$, and $n'' \in \{1, \ldots, N''\}$.

3.3 The Deformation Spectrum and Its Applications

DEFINITION. *The deformation spectrum of a motion is the graph representing the value of the modal amplitudes as a function of mode rank: $\tilde{u}_i(t) = f(i)$ [33]. The deformation spectrum is initially drawn for a deformation occurring between two image frames: It describes which modes are excited, and how, in order to deform one object into another. It also gives an indication of the strain energy, as we have:*

$$E_{strain} = \frac{1}{2} \mathbf{U}^T \mathbf{K} \mathbf{U} = \frac{1}{2} \sum_{i=1}^{N} \omega_i^2 \tilde{u}_i^2 \quad (31)$$

Note that rigid motion has zero strain energy. Let us now define the term *similar deformations*. Two deformations are similar when the corresponding displacement fields $\mathbf{U}_1$ and $\mathbf{U}_2$ are similar within a rigid transform, i.e., if we can find a rotation matrix $\mathbf{R}$ and a translation vector $\mathbf{T}$ such that:

$$\| \mathbf{U}_1 - (\mathbf{R}\mathbf{U}_2 + \mathbf{T}) \| < \epsilon \quad (32)$$

for a small value of ϵ.

TABLE 3
Analytic Therefore, it is natural to state that, provided that the dimensionality p of the reduced modal basis is suitably chosen, *two similar deformations have similar deformation spectra*. However, we cannot compare the deformations of two objects placed in arbitrary configurations in the same global reference frame. Thus the modal computations have to be developed in the object reference frame, defined by its *center and axes of inertia*.

In the following, we get rid of the rigid modes in order to study exclusively the deformations. Thus we will refer to the deformation spectrum as the set of total amplitudes of the first p deformable and low-frequency modes. Once the spectra are computed, we can define a distance measure between the spectra. We choose the Euclidean distance d, such that lower amplitudes are given less importance than higher ones:

$$d(D_1, D_2) = \frac{1}{p} \sqrt{\sum_{i=1}^{p} \left(\tilde{u}_i(D_1) - \tilde{u}_i(D_2) \right)^2} \quad (33)$$

where D_1 and D_2 are the labels of the deformations. Distance d gives a *relative* value of how different the two deformations are.

3.3.1 Similarity

Fig. 8 shows two similar deformations and their spectrum; in this example, $\mathbf{R}$ is a 90-degree rotation matrix and $\mathbf{T}$ is arbitrary.

These are the deformations of the initial deformable model for segmenting the mitral valve contour in Fig. 3.

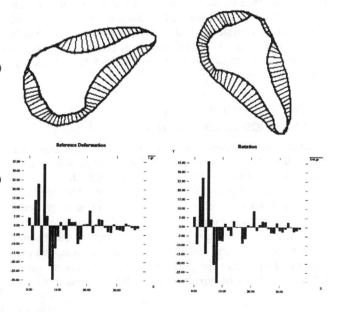

Fig. 8. Similar deformations D_1 and D_2 and their spectrum.

3.3.2 Robustness

In order to test the robustness of the spectra in the presence of noise, we add a Gaussian noise of standard deviation σ to the initial 3D diastole, then deform the diastole into the systole, draw the spectrum and compare it to the spectrum of the true deformation.

The results are very promising (Fig. 9): For $\sigma = 0.1$ the difference between the original spectrum and the corrupted one is almost invisible ($d = 0.01$); for $\sigma = 1$ very slight differences appear ($d = 0.10$); for $\sigma = 5$ the main excited modes are still the same ($d = 0.44$).

Note the very chaotic visual representations of the corrupted shapes, while the modal spectra still succeed in extracting the significant deformation information.

3.3.3 Classification

In order to test the matching of a specific deformation to a group of predefined deformations, we can consider several *admissible* deformations[5] X_i of a reference shape like the valve (Fig. 10). Under the assumption of Gaussian distribution, we can then classify a test deformation Y as belonging or not to the set $\mathcal{D} = \{..., X_i, ...\}$ by using the *Mahalanobis distance* [4], [21]:

$$d_M^2(Y, \mathcal{D}) = (Y - \overline{X})^T W^{-1}(Y - \overline{X}) \qquad (34)$$

where W is the covariance matrix of the admissible deformations $\mathcal{D}$, and $\overline{X}$ the mean admissible deformation.

By comparing with a χ^2 table of q degrees of freedom, where q is the rank of the covariance matrix,[6] we can determine a confidence measure for acceptation ($d_M^2(Y, \mathcal{D}) < \epsilon$) or rejection of the test deformation as being part of the predefined admissible deformations. Fig. 11 shows the classification of four deformations. The *confidence* that we have in our classification (derived from the χ^2 table) is also indicated. Note that visually, we would classify the four deformations the way the system has done it (that is, reject the first three deformations, and accept the fourth). Note finally that though this set of deformations has been artificially generated, the application of the method to a clinically-significant case is straightforward.

4 TIME EVOLUTION OF THE MAIN MODAL AMPLITUDES

A single deformation spectrum gives a *static* information about the spatial frequencies of the motion, whereas the time parameter t is not really taken into account.

However, temporal evolution is really what we are interested in. A *dynamic* deformation process can be much better described and interpreted if we have a time sequence of images. Therefore, we can draw T consecutive deformation spectra for $T + 1$ frames of images showing the temporal evolution of the deformation process. For a chosen mode i, we are interested in the time signals: $\tilde{u}_i(t)$ for different values of i.

---

5. By deformation we mean the vector of total modal amplitudes, in other terms the deformation spectrum.
6. If $q < p$ then $W - 1$ is the pseudo-inverse of W.

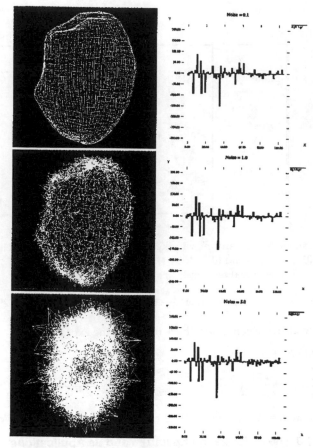

Fig. 9. Corrupted initial diastole deformed to the systole (not shown here), and its spectrum, for different values of noise σ ($\sigma = 0.1$, $\sigma = 1$, $\sigma = 5$).

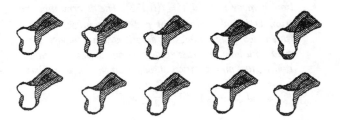

Fig. 10. Ten admissible deformations of the valve.

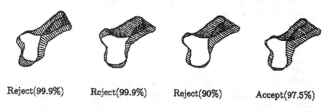

Reject(99.9%)　　Reject(99.9%)　　Reject(90%)　　Accept(97.5%)

Fig. 11. Classification of four deformations, with the confidence values.

Let us track the moving ventricle (cf. Fig. 1) through all image frames. We wish to find a minimum number of parameters describing this sequence. Can we compress the 4D data information for its further analysis, storage, or transmission?

Let us denote by $(P_0, ..., P_T)$ the positions of this surface during the $T + 1$ frames of the cardiac cycle. Therefore, $3N \times (T + 1)$ parameters describe the 4D data (i.e., 345,600 parameters with $N = 6,400$ and $T = 17$).

Let us now track the ventricle in the reduced modal space. We obtain T truncated spectra that store the low-frequency modal amplitudes through the cycle. 4D data is now stored in $3N + T \times p$ parameters (i.e., 20,985 parameters with $p = 105$). The numerical value of p is chosen so that each truncated spectrum has 90% of the energy of the corresponding non-truncated spectrum.

We wish to discard as many modes as possible. Therefore we define a criterion for keeping only the most excited modes among the p low-frequency modes. We compute the energy of an amplitude through the cycle:

$$L^2(i) = \int_0^T \tilde{u}_i(t)^2 \, dt \tag{35}$$

The larger L^2, the more important the contribution of the corresponding amplitude. In our experiment with this data, the first nine values of L^2 were much larger than the other ones. $q = 9$ was then an obvious threshold for us to choose.

Let us draw the temporal evolution of the q selected modal amplitudes. They are represented by groups of three in Fig. 12.

These curves have, globally, a single period sine shape, which is an expectable result for low-frequency modes during a cardiac cycle. Their shape is quite like the ventricle volume curve as a function of time during a cardiac cycle. The shape of these curves encourage us to perform a fast Fourier Transform: Most probably only a few Fourier harmonics will describe the time evolution of the curves.

In order to illustrate this point, let us choose one among these $q = 9$ spectral components (or modal amplitudes). Fig. 12 (bottom right) shows the time evolution of this particular amplitude. Fig. 13 displays the real (top left) and imaginary (top right) parts of the corresponding Fourier Transform; we observe that indeed only low-frequency Fourier harmonics are excited. Therefore we keep the harmonics of rank 0, 1, and 2 of the Fourier spectra (thus, with symmetry considerations, a total of $H = 5$ harmonics, see Fig. 13 bottom left and bottom right); we then reconstruct the time signal in Fig. 14.

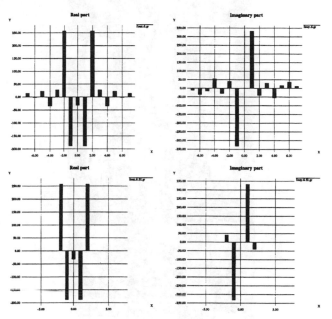

Fig. 13. Fourier (top) and Truncated Fourier (bottom) spectra of the modal amplitude displayed in Fig. 12, bottom-right.

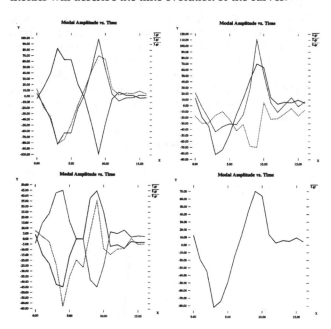

Fig. 12. Top-left, top-right and bottom-left: Each figure displays the time evolution of three main modal amplitudes through a cardiac cycle. In total, the nine main amplitudes are displayed. Bottom right: time evolution of a particular modal amplitude.

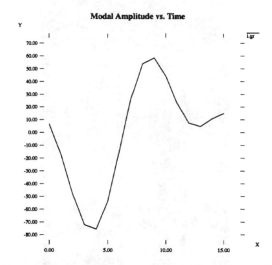

Fig. 14. Reconstruction of the time evolution of the modal amplitude in Fig. 12 bottom-right from truncated Fourier spectra.

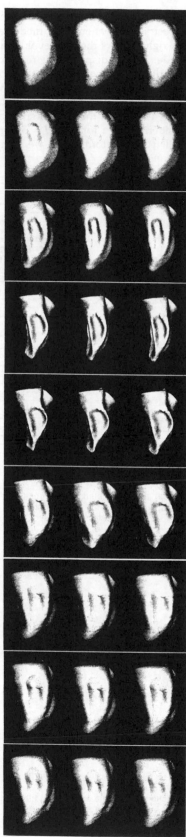

As for motion compression, instead of keeping a whole 3D image at every frame (that makes $t_x\, t_y\, t_z = 1,078,000$ parameters per frame) we now keep only $H \times q/(T + 1) = 2.5$ parameters per frame. This compression of 4D data is impressive: It means that, provided that we keep the first shape, we are able to synthesize the motion with 2.5 parameters per frame. This 4D data is then described by $3N + H \times q = 19,245$ parameters instead of $(T + 1) \times t_x\, t_y\, t_z = 19,404,000$, which makes a compression of more than 10^3, for a cardiac cycle whose duration is approximately one second. If the analysis was extended over a much longer period (e.g., 10 minutes), the compression rate would continuously increase toward the asymptotic value of $1,078,000/2.5$, i.e., approximately 4.10^5 *per frame*. If we compare the total compression with the transmission of all the 3D images over the 10 minutes, we would get an asymptotic compression factor superior to 10^9.

On the top of the compression ability, the synthetic information that our spatiotemporal processing provides allows comparison of nonrigid motion by comparing very few parameters. The method is indeed useful not only for compression, but also for analysis of dynamic motion for diagnosis purposes.

The evolution of the left ventricle model over a cardiac cycle is displayed in Fig. 15. In each row, we observe: Left, the evolution of the model in the real space (6); center, the approximation with $q = 9$ modes (spatial smoothing); right, spatiotemporal processing with nine modes and five Fourier harmonics.

Finally, Fig. 16 displays the mean Euclidean error between the real-space mesh (complete computation) and respectively spatial smoothing (modal recovery) and spatiotemporal smoothing (modal and Fourier recovery). Note that this error (in voxels) is extremely small. The position of the two peaks indicate that the error is maximum in the middle of diastolic and systolic shapes: This is because the change in the overall shape is maximum in those frames. An interesting topic would be the study of the error range, and its relationship with the number of modes and Fourier harmonics.

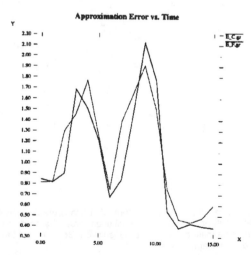

Fig. 15. Space-time evolution of the left ventricle model. In each row: Left: Finite element formulation. Center: Modal recovery. Right: Modal plus Fourier recovery.

Fig. 16. Evolution of the approximation error (in voxels) during a cardiac cycle, for modal recovery (solid line) and modal plus Fourier recovery (dotted line).

5 CONCLUSION

In this article, we presented a frequency-based analysis of nonrigid motion by coupling modal analysis (outlining the main spatial frequencies of the motion), and Fourier analysis (outlining the main temporal frequencies, mainly for cyclic motions).

Nonrigid motion is first estimated by a physically based deformable model.

The modal decomposition of the deformation, made real-time and precise by using the analytic expressions of the modes, leads to the definition of the deformation spectrum, which is a compact description of the deformation allowing its straightforward comparison and classification (identifying pathologic and normal deformations).

We then introduced a temporal analysis of nonrigid motion from 4D data by recovering the temporal evolution of the main modal amplitudes by a Fourier analysis.

The method provides a very nice description of 4D data by very few parameters (a few modal amplitudes and a few Fourier harmonics). It has important applications in medical analyis of nonrigid motion (mainly for automatic diagnosis purposes), and also provides a tremendous compression of multidimensional nonrigid motion, mainly for storage or transmission purposes.

Our future work will focus on the clinical use and validation of this framework, and its transfer toward concrete medical applications, in particular in the cardiology field.

ACKNOWLEDGMENTS

We wish to thank Dr. Richard Robb at Biomedical Imaging Resource, Mayo Foundation/Clinic, for providing the DSR data. This work was supported in part by a grant from Digital Equipment Corporation.

REFERENCES

[1] A.A. Amini, R. Curwen, R.T. Constable, and J.C. Gore, "MR Physics-Based Snake Tracking and Dense Deformations from Tagged Cardiac Images," *AAAI 1994 Spring Symp. Series. Application of Computer Vision in Medical Image Processing*, Stanford Univ., March 1994.

[2] A.A. Amini and J.S. Duncan, "Bending and Stretching Models for LV Wall Motion Analysis Form Curves and Surfaces," *Image and Vision Computing*, vol. 10, no. 6, pp. 418–430, 1992.

[3] N.W. Ashcroft and M.D. Mermin, *Solid State Physics*. Saunders College Publishing Int'l Ed., 1976.

[4] N. Ayache, *Artificial Vision for Mobile Robots—Stereo-Vision and Multisensory Perception*. MIT Press, 1991.

[5] N. Ayache, "Medical Computer Vision, Virtual Reality and Robotics—Promising Research," *Image and Vision Computing*, vol. 13, no. 4, pp. 295–313, May 1995.

[6] N. Ayache, I. Cohen, and I. Herlin, "Medical Image Tracking," *Active Vision*, chapter 17. MIT Press, Dec. 1992.

[7] E. Bardinet, L.D. Cohen, and N. Ayache, "Superquadrics and Free-Form Deformations: A Global Model to Fit and Track 3D Medical Data," *First Conf. Computer Vision, Virtual Reality and Robotics in Medicine (CVRMed '95)*, N. Ayache, ed., vol. 905, Nice, France, Apr. 1995. Springer Verlag.

[8] K.J. Bathe, *Finite Element Procedures in Engineering Analysis*. Prentice-Hall, 1982.

[9] S. Benayoun, N. Ayache, and I. Cohen, "Adaptive Meshes and Nonrigid Motion Computation," *Int'l Conf. Pattern Recognition*, Jerusalem, Israel, March 1994.

[10] S. Benayoun, C. Nastar, and N. Ayache, "Dense Non-Rigid Motion Estimation in Sequences of 3D Images Using Differential Constraints," *First Conf. Computer Vision, Virtual Reality and Robotics in Medicine (CVRMed '95)*, N. Ayache, ed., vol. 905, Nice, France, Apr. 1995. Springer Verlag.

[11] A. Blake, R. Curwen, and A. Zisserman, "Affine-Invariant Contour Tracking with Automatic Control of Spatiotemporal Scale," *IEEE Proc. Fourth Int'l Conf. Computer Vision*, pp. 66–75, Berlin, Germany, May 1993.

[12] L. Bookstein, "Principal Warps: Thin-Plate Splines and the Decomposition of Deformations," *IEEE Trans. Pattern Analysis and Machine Intelligence*, vol. 11, no. 6, pp. 567–585, June 1989.

[13] C.W. Chen, T.S. Huang, and M. Arrott, "Modeling, Analysis, and Visualization of LV Shape and Motion by Hierarchical Decomposition," *IEEE Trans Pattern Analysis and Machine Intelligence*, vol. 16, no. 7, Apr. 1994.

[14] I. Cohen, L.D. Cohen, and N. Ayache., "Using Deformable Surfaces to Segment 3D Images and Infer Differential Structures," *Computer Vision, Graphics, and Image Processing*, vol. 26, no. 2, pp. 242–263, 1992.

[15] T.F. Cootes, C.J. Taylor, D.H. Cooper, and J. Graham, "Active Shape Models—Their Training and Application," *Computer Vision and Image Understanding*, vol. 61, no. 1, pp. 38–59, Jan. 1995.

[16] T.F Cootes, A. Hill, C.J Taylor, and J. Haslam, "The Use of Active Shape Models for Locating Structures in Medical Images," *Proc. 13th Int'l Conf. Information Processing in Medical Imaging*, Flagstaff, Ariz., June 1993.

[17] T.F. Cootes and C.J. Taylor, "Combining Point Distribution Models with Shape Models Based on Finite Element Analysis," *Image and Vision Computing*, vol. 13, no. 5, 1995.

[18] L.L. Creswell, S.G. Wyers, J.S. Pirolo, W.H. Perman, M.W. Vannier, and M.K. Pasque, "Mathematical Modeling of the Heart Using Magnetic Resonance Imaging," *IEEE Trans. Medical Imaging*, vol. 11, no. 4, pp. 581–589, 1992.

[19] P.E. Danielsson, "Euclidean Distance Mapping," *Computer Vision, Graphics, and Image Processing*, vol. 14, pp. 227–248, 1980.

[20] H. Delingette, M. Hebert, and K. Ikeuchi, "Shape Representation and Image Segmentation Using Deformable Surfaces," *IEEE Proc. Computer Vision and Pattern Recognition*, pp. 467–472, Lahaina, Maui, Hawaii, June 1991.

[21] R.O. Duda and P.E. Hart, *Pattern Classification and Scene Analysis*. John Wiley and Sons, 1973.

[22] A. Guéziec, "Large Deformable Splines Crest Lines and Matching," *Proc. Fourth Int'l Conf. Computer Vision*, Berlin, May 1993.

[23] W.-C. Huang and D.B. Goldgof, "Adaptive-Size Physically Based Models for Nonrigid Motion Analysis," *Proc. Computer Vision and Pattern Recognition. IEEE Computer Society Conf.*, pp. 833–835, Champaign, Ill., June 1992.

[24] M. Kass, A. Witkin, and D. Terzopoulos, "Snakes: Active Contour Models," *Int'l J. Computer Vision*, vol. 1, pp. 321–331, 1987.

[25] F. Leitner, I. Marque, S. Lavallée, and P. Cinquin, "Dynamic Segmentation: Finding the Edge with Snake-Splines," *Proc. Int'l Conf. Curves and Surfaces*, pp. 1–4, Chamonix, France, June 1990. Academic Press.

[26] T. McInerney and D. Terzopoulos, "A Dynamic Finite Element Surface Model for Segmentation and Tracking in Multidimensional Images with Application to Cardiac 4D Image Analysis," *J. Computerized Medical Imaging and Graphics*, vol. 19, no. 1, pp. 69–83, 1995.

[27] D. Metaxas and D. Terzopoulos, "Shape and Non-Rigid Motion Estimation Through Physics-Based Synthesis," *IEEE Trans. Pattern Analysis and Machine Intelligence*, vol. 15, no. 6, pp. 580–591, 1993.

[28] O. Monga and R. Deriche, "3D Edge Detection Using Recursive Filtering," *Proc. Computer Vision and Pattern Recognition*, San Diego, June 1989.

[29] O. Monga, R. Deriche, G. Malandain, and J-P. Cocquerez, "Recursive Filtering and Edge Closing: Two Primary Tools for 3D Edge Detection," *Proc. First European Conf. Computer Vision (ECCV)*, Antibes, France, Apr. 1990.

[30] C. Nastar, "Vibration Modes for Nonrigid Motion Analysis in 3D Images," *Proc. Third European Conf. Computer Vision (ECCV '94)*, Stockholm, May 1994.

[31] C. Nastar and N. Ayache, "Fast Segmentation, Tracking, and Analysis of Deformable Objects," *Proc. Fourth Int'l Conf. Computer Vision (ICCV '93)*, Berlin, May 1993.

[32] C. Nastar and N. Ayache, "Non-Rigid Motion Analysis in Medical Images: A Physically Based Approach," *Proc. 13th Int'l Conf. Information Processing in Medical Imaging (IPMI '93)*, Flagstaff, Ariz., June 1993.

[33] C. Nastar and N. Ayache, "Classification of Nonrigid Motion in 3D Images Using Physics-Based Vibration Analysis," *Proc. IEEE Workshop Biomedical Image Analysis*, Seattle, June 1994.

[34] C. Nastar and N. Ayache, "Time Representation of Deformations: Combining Vibration Modes and Fourier Analysis," *Lecture Notes in Computer Science 994: Object Representation in Computer Vision.* Springer-Verlag, 1995.

[35] J. Park, D. Metaxas, and L. Axel, "Volumetric Deformable Models with Parametric Functions: A New Approach to the 3D Motion Analysis of the LV from MRI-SPAMM," *Proc. Fifth Int'l Conf. Computer Vision* (ICCV '95), Boston, June 1995.

[36] A. Pentland and B. Horowitz, "Recovery of Non-Rigid Motion and Structure," *IEEE Trans. Pattern Analysis and Machine Intelligence*, vol. 13, no. 7, pp. 730–742, July 1991.

[37] A. Pentland and S. Sclaroff, "Closed-Form Solutions for Physically-Based Shape Modeling and Recognition," *IEEE Trans. Pattern Analysis and Machine Intelligence*, vol. 13, no. 7, pp. 715–729, July 1991.

[38] A. Pentland and J. Williams, "Good Vibrations: Modal Dynamics for Graphics and Animation," *Computer Graphics*, 1989.

[39] P. Shi, G. Robinson, A. Chakraborty, L. Staib, R. Constable, A. Sinuasa, and J. Duncan, "A Unified Framework to Assess Myocardial Function from 4D Images," *Proc. First Conf Computer Vision, Virtual Reality, and Robotics in Medicine* (CVRMed '95), N. Ayache, ed., vol. 905, Nice, France, Apr. 1995. Springer Verlag.

[40] P. Shi, A. Amini, G. Robinson, A. Sinusas, C.T. Constable, and J. Duncan, "Shape-Based 4D Left Ventricular Myocardial Function Analysis, *Proc IEEE Workshop on Biomedical Image Analysis*, Seattle, Wash., June 1994.

[41] R. Szeliski and S. Lavallée, "Matching 3D Anatomical Surfaces with Non-Rigid Volumetric Deformations," *Proc. AAAI 1994 Spring Symp. Series. Application of Computer Vision in Medical Image Processing*, Stanford Univ., March 1994.

[42] D. Terzopoulos and K. Fleischer, "Deformable Models," The Visual Computer, vol. 4, pp. 306–331, 1988.

[43] D. Terzopoulos and K. Waters, Physically Based Facial Modeling, Analysis, and Animation," *J. Visualization and Computer Animation*, vol 1, pp. 73-80, 1990.

[44] D. Terzopoulos and K. Waters, "Analysis and Synthesis of Facial Image Sequences Using Physical and Anatomical Models," *IEEE Trans. Pattern Analysis and Machine Intelligence*, vol. 15, no. 6, pp. 569–579, 1993.

[45] D. Terzopoulos, A. Witkin, and M. Kass, "Constraints on Deformable Models: Recovering 3D Shape and Nonrigid Motion," *AI J.*, vol. 36, pp. 91–123, 1988.

[46] M. Vasilescu and D. Terzopoulos, "Adaptive Meshes and Shells," Proc. Computer Vision and Pattern Recognition, *Proc. IEEE Computer Society Conf.*, June 1992, pp. 829–832, Champaign, Ill.

[47] Q.Z. Ye, "The Signed Euclidean Distance Transform and Its Applications," *Int'l Conf. Pattern Recognition*, pp. 495–499, 1988.

[48] A.L. Yuille, D.S. Cohen, and P.W. Hallinan, "Feature Extraction from Faces Using Deformable Templates," *Proc. Computer Vision and Pattern Recognition*, San Diego, June 1989.

Chahab Nastar is a senior research scientist at Institut National de Recherche en Informatique et Automatique (INRIA), Rocquencourt, France.

He received the *Diplôme d'Ingénieur* from *l'Ecole Nationale des Ponts et Chaussées* in Paris in 1991 and the PhD degree in mathematics and computer science in 1994. His research, conducted at INRIA, focused on medical image analysis.

In 1994–95, Dr. Nastar joined the MIT Media Laboratory as a postdoctural fellow, developing new techniques for image matching and recognition. Dr. Nastar returned to INRIA in 1996, where his current research interests include computer vision, eigentechniques, object recognition, face recognition, content-based image retrieval, and augmented reality.

Nicholas Ayache is a research director at INRIA, Sophia-Antipolis, France, where he has lead the EPIDAURE research group on medical image analysis and robotics since 1989. He is also teaching graduate courses on computer vision at the University of Paris XI, *Ecole Centrale*, *Ecole des Ponts*, *Ensta*, and *Ecole des Mines*. He is also consulting for a number of private companies, including *Matra-Cap-Systemes* and Focus-Medical.

Dr. Ayache received his PhD in 1983, and his *Thèse d'Etat* in 1988, both in computer science from the University of Paris XI, on topics related to model-based object recognition, passive stereovision, and multisensor fusion. His current research interests are medical image processing and analysis, shape and motion representation, rigid and nonrigid registration, tracking and analysis of deformable objects, and image guided and simulated therapy.

Dr. Ayache is currently coeditor-in-chief of the *Journal of Medical Image Analysis* (Oxford University Press), a member of the editorial board of the *International Journal of Computer Vision* (Kluwer), associate editor of *Medical Imaging* (IEEE), and area editor of the *Journal of Computer Vision and Image Understanding* (Academic Press). He also served on the editorial board of the *IEEE Transactions on Robotics and Automation* (1990–93).

Dr. Ayache is the author of the books *Artificial Vision for Mobile Robots* (MIT Press) and *Vision stéréioscopique et perception multisensorielle* (Inter-Editions). He chaired the first International Conference on Computer Vision, Virtual Reality and Robotics in Medicine (CVRMed), held in Nice, France, in April 1995 and serves on the editorial board of a number of conferences on medical imaging, computer vision, visualization, and robotics, including ECCV, ICCV, VBC, MRCAS, and MMVR.

The Hybrid Volumetric Ventriculoid: A Model for MR-SPAMM 3-D Analysis

Thomas O'Donnell[†], Alok Gupta[*], Terry Boult[‡]

† Columbia University, NY, NY, USA

* Siemens Corp. Research, Princeton, NJ, USA   ‡ Lehigh University Bethlehem, PA, USA

Abstract

In this paper we introduce the Hybrid Volumetric Ventriculoid (HVV), a model for quantatatively analyzing 3-D Left Ventricular (LV) geometry and motion from tagged MR (SPAMM) images. It is the only model which is both hybrid and volumetric. It is hybrid in that it is comprised of a global (parametric) component and a local (explicit) component which form a composite model capable of resembling an LV with arbitrary precision. Among other advantages, this formulation allows the model to provide a concise description of the LV's gross shape for comparison with a "normal" population while at the same time being detailed enough to recover local material measures (i.e., strain). Since the HVV is volumetric it may be deformed directly from myocardial MR tag intersection displacements without prior processing. Deformation is cast as an energy minimization in which lower energies imply a better fit. Our paradigm extends the state of the art myocardial motion recovery to directly include myocardial contour information. This improves the overall model fit by helping to overcome the inherent sparsity of MR-tag data. We apply an HVV to volunteer multi-slice, multi-phase SPAMM data sets taken from orthogonal views and report LV strain as well as motion parameters quantifying myocardial thickening.

1 Introduction and Related Work

Myocardial geometry and motion are considered extremely useful in the diagnosis of cardiac disease. These attributes have been exploited successfully in a variety of clinical settings for the detection of congenital anomalies such as septal defects, chamber enlargement, and the diagnosis of ischemia as well as arhythmia and infarctions.

In standard MR, the deforming heart tissue appears homogeneous. This absence of landmarks prevents the recovery of motion within the myocardium. Advances in magnetic resonance imaging have resulted in a form of non-invasive tagging (e.g. SPAMM - SPatial Modulation of Magnetization) which allows the creation of transient material markers (or tags) in heart tissue (see Figure 1). The tags form a grid

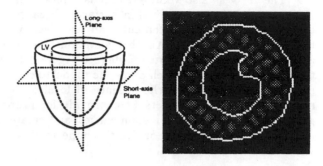

Figure 1: Right: In this short axis view of the left ventricle (left) taken approximately halfway between end-diastole (ED) and end-systole (ES), tagged tissues appear as a black grid. An initially rectangular grid was laid down at ED. The movement of the underlying myocardial tissue causes the grid to deform over the cardiac cycle. We use the displacement of the grid intersection over time to recover the myocardial motion. (Also shown is the contour of the left ventricle, highlighted by hand in white)

in the MR imaging plane. By tracking the SPAMM grid intersection points over time we can extract a 2-D projection of the true 3-D motion. While most MR machines are capable of providing a tagging protocol, the analysis of the motion of tags is commonly left to the physician's eye.

To estimate 3-D cardiac motion researchers have exploited acquisitions of the same heart taken from different views registered in time [3]. Each view is multi-slice, covering the LV spatially, and multi-phase over the cardiac cycle from ED to ES. Differing views (usually orthogonal, short axis and long axis) are needed to garner all three components of motion. The reconstruction of this motion requires a 3-D model based approach.

In this paper, we introduce the Hybrid Volumetric Ventriculoid (HVV), a new formulation for modeling LV motion and geometry. It is the only model that is both hybrid and volumetric. The HVV is hybrid in that it is comprised of a global (parametric) component and a local (explicit) component which form a composite model capable of resembling an LV with arbitrary precision. The global component is able to provide concise descriptions of overall shape and movement. These descriptions can be used to compare an LV under study with a "normal" population to detect and classify abnormalities. The model also shares the other advantages of the hybrid formulation: a local component to describe fine detail, and the ability to fit more rapidly and with increased topological stability compared with purely local models.

The HVV is also volumetric; it is "thick-walled" and not an infinitesimally thin surface. Because of this, the SPAMM displacements can act directly on the model to deform it. Another distinguishing characteristic of the HVV are its offsets (see Figure?) from the global component which allow the model to closely resemble the LV even in the absence of local component activity. These offsets help provide for proper geometric model-data correspondencies and create a more appropriate default or "rest" shape in the absence of constraining data.

The HVV recovery paradigm also extends the state of the art to directly include myocardial contour information. SPAMM displacement information alone is adequate to deform the body of the model but is insufficient at the endo and epi cardia where the tag intersections do not clearly delineate the myocardial border. We overcome the sparseness of tag information by fitting the model to myocardial contour data as well as the tag intersection displacements once the displacements alone have deformed the model. We claim that the fit using the SPAMM 3-D displacements facilitates appropriate contour-model correspondences, thus improving the overall model fit.

Axel and Young pioneered this analysis [5] by deforming a volumetric Finite Element (FEM) model of the LV with the projected 2-D tag-intersection displacements taken from two orthogonal SPAMM acquisitions. MR tags are quite sparse, however, and the recovery of myocardial borders in their model may have been hindered by the paucity of data. In addition, due to their purely local Finite Element Method (FEM) formulation they could not directly provide a concise description of the overall LV movement.

Park, Metaxas, and Young [2] applied a hybrid model to Axel's processed results to recover such an overall description. Their's was a surface model, however, and could only report on an infinitesimally thin layer in the myocardium. And, it could only be fit to pre-processed dense data since the raw 3-D displacement information is spread through the heart wall, not concentrated in a single layer.

In the next section we describe the HVV model

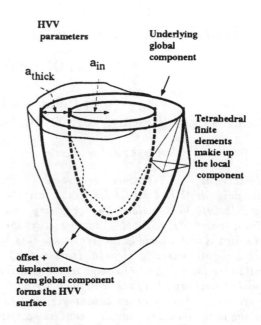

Figure 2: The thick HVV model for the LV.

and follow this with a discussion of its associated recovery paradigm. In section 4 results of two experiments on multi-view SPAMM acquisitions are presented and we conclude with a discussion of our work in section 5.

2 The Hybrid Volumetric Ventriculoid

The HVV is composed of an implicit parametric global component and and a set of volumetric finite elements which express both offsets and local deformations away this underlying shape (see Figure 2).

2.1 The Global Component

Our development of the global component of the HVV was inspired by superellipsoid *surface* models [1]. We expand upon these models by including an additional implicit parameter, $\alpha : 0 \rightarrow 1$, which turns the infinitesimally thin surface of a superellipsoid into a solid, thick wall. A point $S(x, y, z)$ on the global component of the HVV is described by

$$
\begin{aligned}
x(u, v, \alpha) &= a_1(u, \alpha) \cos^{\varepsilon_1}(u) \cos^{\varepsilon_2}(v) \\
y(u, v, \alpha) &= a_2(u, \alpha) \cos^{\varepsilon_1}(u) \sin^{\varepsilon_2}(v) \\
z(u, v, \alpha) &= a_3(\alpha) \sin^{\varepsilon_1}(u) \\
&\qquad 0 \le u \le \pi/2 \quad -\pi \le v \le \pi, \quad (1)
\end{aligned}
$$

where the parameters, a_1, a_2, a_3, are defined as functions of the dimensions of the inner wall, the wall thickness and its variation along u.

$$a_1(u, \alpha) = a_{1_{\text{in}}} + \alpha \left(a_{1_{\text{thick}}} + a_{1_{\text{coeff}}} \sin(u + \frac{\pi}{2}) \right)$$

$$a_2(u, \alpha) = a_{2_{\text{in}}} + \alpha \left(a_{2_{\text{thick}}} + a_{2_{\text{coeff}}} \sin(u + \frac{\pi}{2}) \right)$$

$$a_3(u, \alpha) = a_{3_{\text{in}}} + \alpha \, a_{3_{\text{thick}}} \qquad (2)$$

At $\alpha = 0$ and 1 the model describes the inner walls and outer walls respectively.

Our global component is further augmented with the deformations tapering, bending and twist using the variations of these formulations found in [4].

Thus the global component of the HVV is a *fully volumetric* and capable of describing functionally any point in space between its inner and outer walls. By specifying a particular value of α iso-surfaces inside the intermural volume may be described. Defining the global component in this way allows wall thickness becomes a model parameter. And, inner and outer wall twist may be combined to report differential twist.

2.2 The Local Component

The local component of the HVV is made up of both *offsets* and *local deformations* which differ from one another. We introduce *offsets* (from the global component) to the standard hybrid model formulation in order to create a default or "rest" shape which resembles the object undergoing recovery. Our inclusion results in a significantly more accurate default shape than could be modeled with the implicit parametric global component alone (even with its global deformations). *Local deformations*, on the other hand, serve to tailor the model to the detail of an individual LV instance. Unlike offsets, local deformations and are assigned a material smoothing penalty.

This penalty encourages smooth deformations from the "rest" shape by attempting to maintain initial internodal distances. Both the offsets and local deformations of the HVV are described using 3-D tetrahedral finite elements which are stationed *in* the intermural volume.

3 The Recovery Process

Our approach to recovering the 3-D motion of the tagged tissue builds on the work by Young and Axel

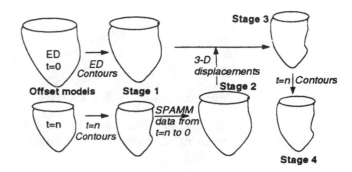

Figure 3: A diagram of the fitting process. See text for details.

[5]. We make use of hand-segmented contour data describing the endo and epicardial borders of the LV and the 2-D projected displacements of LV tissues garnered from two (or three) mutually orthogonal multi-slice, multi-phase SPAMM acquisitions.

The technique is comprised of four stages (see Figure 3). First, individual HVVs are deformed to fit contour data from the different phases in the cardiac cycle (Note that these HVVs have local offsets which make their default shape closely resemble an LV). In Stage 2 the fitted HVVs from phases (*phase* > 1) are each deformed to resemble the initial phase (*phase* = 1) according to the 2-D displacement information from multiple orthogonal SPAMM acquisitions. By fitting a single model representing a single phase to multiple orthogonal sets of 2-D displacements we are able to infer *3-D* displacements for that phase. (Note that a set of 2-D displacements are constrained from affecting the model out of their plane). In Stage 3 the 3-D displacements are reversed. This is because in the previous stage we fit *phase* > 1 HVVs backwards in time to *phase* = 1. We now reverse the displacement directions and deform the model forward in time. Finally, in Stage 4 the HVVs are fit to both the contour data and forward-in-time 3-D displacements associated with that phase to improve the overall fit.

Model deformation at all stages follows the approach developed by Metaxas and Terzopoulos [4]. Model deformations are set to mimic physical deformations through the simulation of Lagrangian dynamics.

4 Results

We applied the HVV to a volunteer SPAMM acquisition to extract concise descriptions of the LV's gross movement as well as its local strain.

All images were acquired on a Siemens MAGNE-

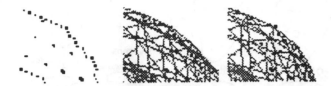
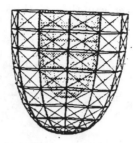
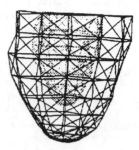

Figure 4: Left: Data. Middle: Closeup of the model prior to the final stage fit to contour data. Right: Same shot after the final fit.

TOM Vision 1.5 T MRI system with a standard 25 mT/m gradient system. An ECG triggered 2-D gradient echo cine pulse sequence with velocity compensation was utilized. In-plane resolution was 1.74*1.17 mm and slice thickness 10 mm. The tag grid was applied within 20 msec immediately following the R-wave trigger. The tags were 2 mm wide, and spaced 9 mm apart. 6 cardiac phases were acquired, covering from ED to ES with 60 msec temporal resolution. Identical imaging parameters were used for the long-axis and short-axis acquisitions.

The results of fitting the HVV models to the data are shown for all the six phases with overlaid data in Figure 6. Salient model characteristics describing the inner ventricular diameter, and wall thickness both in the short axis ($a1_{in}$ and $a1_{thick}$, respectively) and long axis ($a3_{in}$ and $a3_{thick}$, respectively) over the phase are reported below. This indicates a greater extension in the long axis direction as compared to the short axis.

Parameter	t=0	t=2	t=5
$a1_{in}$	2.64	2.57	2.22
$a1_{thick}$	4.08	4.06	4.01
$a3_{in}$	8.044	8.02	7.83
$a3_{thick}$	6.66	6.65	6.58

We found strain to be higher in the base of the LV (typical tensor norm of 4.39) as compared to the apex (2.68). We are currently developing a graphical routine to display these results.

As shown in Figure 4 the additional use of contour data in the Stage 4 of our fitting paradigm improves the overall model fit. In this way the inherent sparseness of the SPAMM data may be overcome.

5   Conclusions

We have demonstrated the feasibility of the HVV in recovering the 3-D motion of a human LV. The model has the advantages of being *both* hybrid and volumetric and is capable reporting an overall description of heart movement as well as local strain.

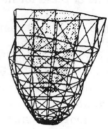
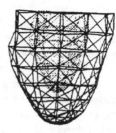

Figure 5: The fit to ED contour data in Stage 1 of the paradigm.

Figure 6: Stage4 (final) fits to volunteer data on ED and ES phases.

6   Acknowledgements

We wish to thank Dr. Lon Simonetti for acquiring the SPAMM data sets and Dr. Gareth Funka-Lea for his help in the tracking of the SPAMM grid intersections.

References

[1] A. H. Barr. Superquadrics and angle-preserving transformations. *IEEE Computer Graphics and Applications*, 1(1):11–23, 1981.

[2] J. Park, D. Metaxas, and A. Young. Deformable models with parameter functions: Application to heart-wall modeling. In *Proceedings of the IEEE CVPR, Seattle, Washington*, pages 437–442, 1994.

[3] J. Pipe J. Boes and T. Chenevert. Method for measuring three-dimensional motion with tagged mr imaging. *Radiology*, 181:591–595, 1991.

[4] D. Terzopoulos and D. Metaxas. Dynamic 3D models with local and global deformations: Deformable superquadrics. *IEEE Transactions on Pattern Analysis and Machine Intelligence*, 13(7):703–714, 1991.

[5] A.A. Young and L. Axel. Three-dimensional motion and deformation of the heart wall: Estimation with spatial modulation of magnetization - a model-based approach. *Radiology*, 185(1):241–247, 1992.

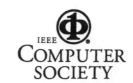

IEEE
COMPUTER
SOCIETY

Press Activities Board

IEEE Computer Society Publications

The world-renowned IEEE Computer Society publishes, promotes, and distributes a wide variety of authoritative computer science and engineering texts. These books are available from most retail outlets. The IEEE Computer Society is seeking new practitioner-oriented and leading-edge research titles in computer science and computer engineering. Visit the Online Catalog, http://computer.org, for a list of products and new author information.

Submission of proposals: For guidelines and information on the IEEE Computer Society books, send e-mail to cs.books@computer.org or write to the Project Editor, IEEE Computer Society, P.O. Box 3014, 10662 Los Vaqueros Circle, Los Alamitos, CA 90720-1314. Telephone +1 714-821-8380. FAX +1 714-761-1784.

IEEE Computer Society Proceedings

The IEEE Computer Society also produces and actively promotes the proceedings of more than 130 acclaimed international conferences each year in multimedia formats that include hard and softcover books, CD-ROMs, videos, and on-line publications.

For information on the IEEE Computer Society proceedings, send e-mail to cs.books@computer.org or write to Proceedings, IEEE Computer Society, P.O. Box 3014, 10662 Los Vaqueros Circle, Los Alamitos, CA 90720-1314. Telephone +1 714-821-8380. FAX +1 714-761-1784.

Additional information regarding the Computer Society, conferences and proceedings, CD-ROMs, videos, and books can also be accessed from our web site at http://computer.org/cspress

8/24/98